Stedman's
ONCOLOGY
WORDS

FIFTH EDITION

INCLUDES
HEMATOLOGY,
HIV, & AIDS

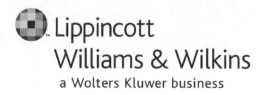

Lippincott
Williams & Wilkins
a Wolters Kluwer business

Publisher: Julie K. Stegman
Senior Product Manager: Eric Branger
Associate Managing Editor: Cecilia González
Typesetter: Josephine Bergin
Printer & Binder: RR Donnelley

Copyright © 2006 Lippincott Williams & Wilkins
351 West Camden Street
Baltimore, Maryland 21201-2436

Printed in China

Fifth Edition, 2007

Library of Congress Cataloging-in-Publication Data
Stedman's oncology words : includes hematology, HIV, and AIDS—5th ed.
    p. ; cm. — (Stedman's word books)
    Includes bibliographical references.
    ISBN 13: 978-0-7817-7382-9
    ISBN 10: 0-7817-7382-2
    1. Oncology—Terminology. 2. Hematology—Terminology. 3. AIDS (Disease)—Termi-
nology. I. Stedman, Thomas Lathrop, 1853–1938. II. Title: Oncology words. III. Series.
    [DNLM: 1. Medical Oncology—Terminology—English. 2. Acquired Immunodeficiency
Syndrome—Terminology—English.   3. HIV Infections—Terminology—English.   4.
Hematology—Terminology—English. QZ 15 S81215 2006]
    RC254.5.S84 2006
    616.99'40014—dc22

                                                                                    2006000978

                                                                            10 11 12
                                                                    4 5 6 7 8 9 10

Stedman's
ONCOLOGY
WORDS

FIFTH EDITION

INCLUDES
HEMATOLOGY,
HIV, & AIDS

Contents

Contents

Acknowledgements

An important part of our editorial process is the involvement of medical transcriptionists — as advisors, reviewers, and/or editors.

We extend special thanks to Nicole G. Peck, CMT, and Jeanne Bock, CMT, for editing the manuscript, helping resolve many difficult questions, and contributing material for the appendix sections. We are grateful to our MT Editorial Advisory Board members, who were instrumental in the development of this reference: Barbara Batchelder; Kathy Duggins, MT; and Cynthia Mann, MT. They recommended sources and shared their valuable judgment, insight, and perspective.

Our appreciation goes to the following reviewers who helped to enhance the A-to-Z content for this edition: Marty Cantu, CMT; Jeanne Bock; Nicola C. Y. Ho; Robin Koza; and Bev Oberline.

We also extend thanks to Jeanne Bock for working on the appendix. Additional thanks to Helen Littrell for performing the final prepublication review. Lisa Fahnestock played an integral role in the process by reviewing the content files for format, updating the content, and providing a final quality check.

As with all our *Stedman's* word references, this resource incorporates the suggestions and expertise of our many contacts in the medical transcriptionist community. Thanks to all of our advisory board participants, reviewers, and editors; AAMT meeting attendees; and others who have written us with requests and comments — keep talking, and we'll keep listening.

Editors' Preface

Cancer — such an ominous word that strikes a powerful chord of fear and sadness in our hearts. Every day we hear of someone who has passed away after suffering from cancer, whether it's a celebrity we don't personally know or a neighbor or loved one whom we knew and cared for deeply. Though cancer still ravages the lives of so many, we can all be thankful that research and technology in this field of medicine have advanced and continue to advance exponentially.

AIDS — another dreaded disease that makes our hearts heavy and often causes us to feel hopeless and helpless. This disease still affects the lives of too many people, but research and medical advances have resulted in an increased number of antivirals and other treatments, thereby dramatically extending the life expectancy and improving the quality of life of those individuals diagnosed with HIV and AIDS.

In this new edition of *Oncology Words* we worked to include many of the new treatments, medicines, and other terminology related to these two diseases, as well as those used in the specialties of oncology and hematology. We hope you will find these additions an enhancement to the previous edition. We believe the sample reports and the comprehensive appendix sections found in this edition will be a tremendous help to you in the transcription of accurate, quality medical records. For an expanded source of more terms, please refer to the expanded line of Stedman's Word Books.

We would like to express our sincere thanks to Tiffany Piper, Cecilia González, and Lisa Fahnestock for all their help in keeping this edition on track and in working through the kinks we encountered along the way. Our thanks would not be complete without including the Editorial Advisory Board, the research contributors, and all the medical transcriptionists who use this book and have provided us with suggestions of items for inclusion in this edition.

Nicole Peck, CMT
Jeanne Bock, CSR, MT

Publisher's Preface

Stedman's Oncology Words, Fifth Edition, offers an authoritative assurance of quality and exactness to the wordsmiths of the healthcare professions — medical transcriptionists, medical editors and copyeditors, health information management personnel, court reporters, and the many other users and producers of medical documentation.

In *Stedman's Oncology Words, Fifth Edition*, we feature and expand the topics of oncology, hematology, HIV, and AIDS. Users will find thousands of words encompassing the terminology specific to chemotherapies, drugs, eponyms, devices, instrumentation, new techniques, operations, lab tests, clinical trials, and abbreviations. The appendix sections, substantially enhanced over the previous edition, provide anatomical illustrations with useful captions and labels; equipment; lab values; chemotherapy drug treatments; clinical trials; cancer classification/grading/staging systems; drug abbreviations and names; NCI Comprehensive Care Centers; sample reports; common terms by procedure; and drugs by indication.

This compilation of more than 55,000 terms, fully cross-indexed for quick access, includes over 1,800 more terms than the previous edition. The extensive A-to-Z list was developed from manufacturers' literature, scientific reports, books, journals, CDs, and Web sites (please see list of References on page xvii).

We at Lippincott Williams & Wilkins strive to provide you with the most up-to-date and accurate word references available. Your use of this word book will prompt new editions, which we will publish as often as updates and revisions justify. We welcome your suggestions for improvements, changes, corrections, and additions — whatever will make this Stedman's product more useful to you. Please complete the postage-paid card in this book for future suggestions and recommendations, or visit us online at www.stedmans.com.

Explanatory Notes

Medical transcription is an art as well as a science. Both approaches are needed to correctly interpret the dictation of a physician, whose language is a product of education, training, and experience. This variety in medical language means that there are several acceptable ways to express certain terms, including jargon. *Stedman's Oncology Words, Fifth Edition*, provides variant spellings and phrasings for many terms. These elements, in addition to complete cross-indexing, make this edition a valuable resource for determining the validity of terms as they are encountered.

Alphabetical Organization
Alphabetization of main entries is letter by letter as spelled, ignoring punctuation, spaces, prefixed numbers, or other special characters. For example:

chloroacetate esterase-butyrate esterase stain
8-chloro-cAMP
2-chlorodeoxyadenosine (2CDA)
chloroethyl nitrosourea (CNU)

Terms beginning or ending with Greek letters show the Greek letters spelled out and listed alphabetically. For example:

alpha, α
    a. particle
    a. radiation

In subentry alphabetization, the abbreviated singular form or the spelled-out plural form of the noun main entry word is ignored.

Format and Style
All main entries are in **boldface** to expedite locating a sought-after term, to enhance distinction between main entries and subentries, and to relieve the textual density of the pages.

Irregular plurals and variant spellings are shown on the same line as the singular or preferred form of the word. For example:

esophagus, pl. esophagi
dissociation, disassociation

Hyphenation

As a rule of style, multiple eponyms (e.g., Schüller-Christian disease) are hyphenated. Also, hyphens have been added between a manufacturer and one or more eponyms (e.g., Vital-Metzenbaum dissecting scissors). Please note that in many cases hyphenation is a question of style, not of accuracy, and thus is a matter of choice.

Possessives

Possessive forms have been dropped in this reference for the sake of consistency and conformance with the guidelines of the American Association for Medical Transcription (AAMT) and other groups. Please note, however, that in many cases retaining the possessive, like hyphenating, is a question of style, not of accuracy, and thus is a matter of choice. To form the possessive of a word in the singular, add an apostrophe and an "s" to the end of the word, and to form the possessive of a word in the plural, and only an apostrophe.

Cross-indexing

The word list is in an index-like main entry–subentry format that contains two combined alphabetical listings:

(1) A noun main entry–subentry organization, which is typical of the A–Z section of medical dictionaries like Stedman's:

germ	**mass**
g. cell neoplasm	atomic m.
g. cell testicular tumor	benign m.
g. cell tumor (GCT)	bleeder in tumor m.

(2) An adjective main entry–subentry organization, which lists words and phrases as you hear them. The main entries are the adjectives or modifiers in a multiword term. The subentries are the nouns around which the terms are constructed and to which the adjectives or modifiers pertain:

genomic
  g. assay
  g. disease management
  g. DNA

cerebellar
  c. atrophy
  c. degeneration
  c. ectopia

This format provides the user with more than one way to locate and identify a multiword term. For example:

transfusion
  erythrocyte

erythrocyte
  e. transfusion

prophylactic
  p. chemotherapy

chemotherapy
  prophylactic c.

It also allows the user to see together all terms that contain a particular descriptor, as well as all types, kinds, or variations of a noun entity. For example:

field
  coplanar f.
  f. disease
  f. drift

joint
  diarthrodial j.
  j. effusion
  elbow j.

Wherever possible, abbreviations are separately defined and cross-referenced. For example:

FBA
  fluorescent bacteriophage assay

fluorescent
  f. bacteriophage assay (FBA)

assay
  fluorescent bacteriophage a. (FBA)

Note on Gene Terms

Conventionally, all letters in human gene names are capitalized and the entire term is italicized (*TSC1, TSC2*). It is also acceptable to write gene names as "TSC1 gene" or "TSC2 gene." Roman (non-italicized) text indicates a protein, but the addition of the word "gene" indicates that one is referring to the gene encoding that protein. So, it is appropriate to write *"TSC1"* or "TSC1 gene" but *not "TSC1* gene." In this word book, we have listed gene names without the italics and followed by the word "gene" so that these terms could be cross-referenced.

References

In addition to the lists of our MT Editorial Advisory Board members (from their daily transcription work), we used the following sources for new terms in *Stedman's Oncology Words, Fifth Edition*.

Books

Abraham, Jame, James L. Gulley, and Carmen J. Allegra. Bethesda Handbook of Clinical Oncology. Baltimore: Lippincott Williams & Wilkins, 2005.

Armitage, James O. Atlas of Clinical Hematology. Baltimore: Lippincott Williams & Wilkins, 2003.

Bartlett, John G. The Johns Hopkins Hospital 2004 Guide to Medical Care of Patients with HIV Infection, 11th Edition. Baltimore: Lippincott Williams & Wilkins, 2003.

Berek, Jonathan S., Neville F. Hacker, and Timothy C. Hengst. Practical Gynecologic Oncology, 4th Edition. Baltimore: Lippincott Williams & Wilkins, 2004.

Casciato, Dennis Albert. Manual of Clinical Oncology, 5th Edition. Baltimore: Lippincott Williams & Wilkins, 2004.

Chabner, B. A. and Dan L. Longo. Cancer Chemotherapy and Biotherapy, 3rd Edition. Baltimore: Lippincott Williams & Wilkins, 2001.

Khatri, Vijay P. Clinical Scenarios in Surgical Oncology. Baltimore: Lippincott Williams & Wilkins, 2005.

Lister, Sara and Lisa Dougherty. The Royal Marsden Hospital Manual of Clinical Nursing Procedures, 6th Edition. Boston: Blackwell Publishing, 2004.

O'Connell, Casey and Vanessa Lynn Dickey. Blueprints Hematology and Oncology. Bethesda Handbook of Clinical Oncology. Baltimore: Lippincott Williams & Wilkins, 2005.

Perez, Carlos A., Robert C. Young, Richard R. Barakat, Maurie Markman, Marcus E. Randall, and William J. Hoskins. Principles and Practice of Gynecologic Oncology, 4th Edition. Baltimore: Lippincott Williams & Wilkins, 2004.

Pizzo, Philip A. and David G Poplack. Principles and Practice of Pediatric Oncology, 5th Edition. Baltimore: Lippincott Williams & Wilkins, 2005.

Rodgers, Griffin P. and Neal S. Young. Bethesda Handbook of Clinical Hematology. Baltimore: Lippincott Williams & Wilkins, 2004.

Shelton, Brenda K., Constance R. Ziegfeld, and Mikaela M. Olsen. Manual of Cancer Nursing: The Sidney Kimmel Comprehensive Cancer Center at Johns Hopkins, 2nd Edition. Baltimore: Lippincott Williams & Wilkins, 2004.

Stine, Gerald J. AIDS Update 2003: An Annual Overview of Acquired Immune Deficiency Syndrome. San Francisco: Benjamin-Cummings Publishing Company, 2002.

Turgeon, Mary Louise. Clinical Hematology: Theory and Procedures, 3rd Edition. Baltimore: Lippincott Williams & Wilkins, 1999.

Vogel, Wendy H., Margery A. Wilson, and Michelle S. Melvin. Advanced Practice Oncology and Palliative Care Guidelines. Baltimore: Lippincott Williams & Wilkins, 2003.

Yang, Katherine Y., Larissa Graff, and Aaron B. Caughey. Blueprints Notes & Cases--Pathophysiology: Renal, Hematology and Oncology. Baltimore: Lippincott Williams & Wilkins, 2003.

Images

Agur, A. M. and M. J. Lee. Grant's Atlas of Anatomy, 10th Edition. Baltimore: Lippincott Williams & Wilkins, 1999.

Born, K., J. Fuller, and J. Schaller-Ayers. A Nursing Approach, 2nd Edition. Philadelphia: J. B. Lippincott Company, 1994.

Brant, W. E. and C. A. Helms. Fundamentals of Diagnostic Radiology, 2nd Edition. Baltimore: Williams & Wilkins, 1998.

Caldwell, Susan. In Stedman's Medical Dictionary, 27th Edition. Baltimore: Lippincott Williams & Wilkins, 2000.

Daffner, R. H. Clinical Radiology: The Essentials, 2nd Edition. Baltimore: Williams & Wilkins, 1998.

Hardy, Neil O. In Stedman's Medical Dictionary, 27th edition. Baltimore: Lippincott Williams & Wilkins, 2000.

LifeART Super Anatomy Collection 3, CD-ROM. Baltimore: Lippincott Williams & Wilkins.

LifeART Super Anatomy Collection 4, CD-ROM. Baltimore: Lippincott Williams & Wilkins.

LifeART Super Anatomy Collection 5, CD-ROM. Baltimore: Lippincott Williams & Wilkins.

LifeART Super Anatomy Collection 7, CD-ROM. Baltimore: Lippincott Williams & Wilkins.

McKenzie, S. B. Textbook of Hematology, 2nd Edition. Baltimore: Williams & Wilkins, 1996.

MediClip Clinical Cardiopulmonary, CD-ROM. Baltimore: Lippincott Williams & Wilkins.

MediClip Clinical OBGYN, CD-ROM. Baltimore: Lippincott Williams & Wilkins.

Roche Lexikon Medizin, 2nd Edition. Munich, Germany: Urban & Schwarzenburg, 1993.

Rosdahl, D. B. Textbook of Basic Nursing, 7th Edition. Philadelphia: Lippincott Williams & Wilkins, 1999.

Schenk, Jackson M. In Stedman's Medical Dictionary, 27th Edition. Baltimore: Lippincott Williams & Wilkins, 2000.

Journals

American Journal of Clinical Oncology, Lippincott Williams & Wilkins, 2003–2005.

American Journal of Clinical Oncology Cancer Clinical Trials, Lippincott Williams & Wilkins, 2004.

CA: A Cancer Journal for Clinicians, American Cancer Society, 2002–2003.

Cancer, John Wiley & Sons, Inc., 2002–2005.

Clinical Dysmorphology, Lippincott Williams & Wilkins, 2002.

Journal of the American Association of Medical Transcriptionists, Lippincott Williams & Wilkins, 2005.

The Latest Word, WB Saunders Co., 2005.

Let's Talk Terms, Journal of the American Association of Medical Transcriptionists, Lippincott Williams & Wilkins, 2004.

Web Sites

www.bms.com

www.hpisum.com/perspectives

www.cancer.gov

www.drugs.com

www.gehealthcare.com

www.hpisum.com

www.mtdesk.com

www.cancer.gov/cancercenters/centerslist.html#L1

www.usoncology.com/OurServices/search.asp

www.cancer.gov/search/ViewClinicalTrials.aspx?cdrid=67279&version=patient&protocolsearchid=1962898

www.clinicaltrials.gov

www.cancer.gov/templates/drugdictionary.aspx?expand=A

www.dictionary.rare-cancer.org/chemotherapy-acronyms.php?letter=a

www.cancerpage.com/centers/Drug/combination.asp

www.hci.utah.edu/patientdocs/hci/drugs/Chemoregimen/combocancer.html

Newsletters

Medquist

α (*var. of* alpha)

A
    chromogranin A (CgA)
    coenzyme A (CoA)
    concanavalin A
    cyclin A
    cyclosporin A (CsA, CSA)
    erb A
    immunoglobulin A (IgA)

A10
    antineoplaston A10

17-1A
    chimeric 17-1A (C17-1A)
    17-1A monoclonal antibody

A₁
    hemoglobin A_1

A₂
    hemoglobin A_2

A-80
    glycoprotein A-80

AA
  anaplastic astrocytoma
  ara-C and Adriamycin
  atypical angiomyolipoma

AAA
  acquired aplastic anemia

AACR
  American Association for Cancer
    Research

AAF
  2-acetylaminofluorene

AAG
  17-(allylamino)-17-
    demethoxygeldanamycin

AAI
  ankle-arm index

AAML
  atypical angiomyolipoma

AAV
  adenoassociated virus

Ab
  antibody

Ab1 antibody
Ab2 antibody
abacavir
    central nervous system-
      penetrating a.

abarelix
abarelix-depot-M
Abbokinase catheter
Abbot assay
ABC
  adenosine triphosphate-binding cassette
  Adriamycin, BCNU, cyclophosphamide

ABC drug transporter family
ABC transporter

ABCD
  Adriamycin, bleomycin, CCNU,
    dacarbazine
  amphotericin B colloidal dispersion

abciximab
ABCM
  Adriamycin, bleomycin,
    cyclophosphamide, mitomycin C

ABCT
  ATP-binding cassette transporter
    ABCT efflux pump

ABCVEP-I
  Adriamycin, bleomycin,
    cyclophosphamide, vincristine,
    etoposide, prednisolone I

ABCVEP-II
  Adriamycin, bleomycin,
    cyclophosphamide, vincristine,
    etoposide, prednisolone II

ABDIC
  Adriamycin, bleomycin, dacarbazine,
    CCNU, prednisone
  Adriamycin, bleomycin, DTIC, CCNU,
    prednisone

abdomen
  acute a.

abdominal
  a. abscess
  a. abscess drainage catheter
  a. adenopathy
  a. adhesion
  a. air collection
  a. angina
  a. aorta
  a. aortic aneurysm
  a. aortography
  a. cavity
  a. diffuse calcification
  a. distention
  a. fibromatosis
  a. great vessel
  a. hemorrhage
  a. hysterectomy
  a. irradiation
  a. lymph node biopsy
  a. mass
  a. pain
  a. plain film
  a. roentgenography
  a. sonography
  a. space
  a. strip radiotherapy
  a. trauma

abdominal *(continued)*
   a. vascular calcification
   a. viscus
   a. wall
   a. wall calcification
   a. wall defect
   a. wall desmoid tumor
   a. wall hernia
abdominis
abdominopelvic
   a. cavity
   a. mass
abdominoperineal resection (APR)
abdominosacral resection
abduction-external rotation fracture
abductor muscle
ABDV
   Adriamycin, bleomycin, DTIC, vinblastine
Abelcet (ABLC)
Abelson murine leukemia virus
Abenol
Abernethy sarcoma
aberrant
   a. cell
   a. crypt focus
   a. crypt focus lesion
   a. intrahepatic bile duct
   a. right subclavian artery
aberration
   metabolic a.
abetalipoproteinemia
ABH
   Ativan, Benadryl, Haldol
   ABH blood group carbohydrate antigen
ABH/Lewis-related antigen
ABH(O) cell surface antigen
ABI
   ankle-brachial index
   ABI fluorescence dye
   ABI PRISM 3700 DNA analyzer
ability
   syncytium-inducing a.
   tumor-targeting a.
ab initio
Abitrate
Abitrexate
ABL
   acute basophilic leukemia
abl
   abl oncogene
   abl protooncogene/oncogene
ablastin
ablation
   adrenal a.
   androgen a.
   cryosurgical a.
   laser a.

   marrow a.
   ovarian a. (OA)
   parathyroid tumor a.
   percutaneous ethanol a.
   percutaneous tumor a.
   radioactive iodine a.
   radiofrequency a. (RFA)
   radiofrequency interstitial tissue a. (RITA)
   saline-enhanced radiofrequency a.
   a. therapy
   thermal a.
   thyroid nodule a.
   total androgen a.
   total hormonal a.
   transurethral needle a. (TUNA)
   tumor a.
ablative
   a. neurosurgery
   a. therapy
ABLC
   Abelcet
   amphotericin B lipid complex
ABMR
   autologous bone marrow rescue
ABMS
   autologous bone marrow support
ABMT
   allogeneic bone marrow transplant
   allogeneic bone marrow transplantation
   autologous bone marrow transplant
   autologous bone marrow transplantation
ABMTR
   Autologous Blood and Marrow Transplant Registry
abnormal
   a. bright signal
   a. fetal urogenital tract
   a. localization of immature precursors (ALIP)
   a. staining
abnormality
   acquired a.
   arterial blood gas a.
   bladder congenital a.
   bone a.
   breast a.
   caliceal a.
   cardiopulmonary a.
   cellular a.
   clonal cytogenetic a.
   complex cytogenetic a.
   cytogenetic a.
   diverticulation a.
   endocrine a.
   extremity a.
   high-signal a.
   histopathologic a.
   hormonal a.

immune function a.
migrational a.
neurologic a.
nuclear membrane a.
ophthalmologic a.
protein-binding a.
taste a.
abnormally
a. contracting region
a. thin skull
ABO
ABO blood group
ABO incompatibility
abortive
a. calyx
a. neurofibromatosis
abortus
Brucella a.
ABOS
Adriamycin, bleomycin sulfate,
vincristine, streptozocin
ABP
Adriamycin, bleomycin, prednisone
ABPP
bropirimine
Abrams biopsy needle
abrasion
cortical a.
tooth a.
Abraxane
Abrikosov, Abrikossoff
A. tumor
abrogated immune response
ABS
Affect Balance Scale
ABS2000 blood typing system
abscess, pl. **abscesses**
abdominal a.
amebic a.
anchovy paste a.
anular a.
aortic anulus a.
appendiceal a.
brain a.
breast a.
Brodie a.
chocolate sauce a.
chronic breast a.
diverticular a.
a. drainage
epidural a.
granulomatous a.
liver a.

Pautrier a.
renal a.
scrotal a.
abscissa
abscission needle
abscopal effect
absent
a. kidney
a. radius thrombocytopenia inhibitor
absolute
a. alcohol
a. blood flow
a. cell count
a. curative resection
a. dose intensity (ADI)
a. ethanol
a. granulocyte count (ACG)
a. linearity
a. lymphocyte value
a. neutrophil count (ANC)
a. noncurative resection
a. polycythemia
a. reticulocyte count
absorbable gelatin
absorbed
a. dose
a. plasma
absorbent
antibody a.
absorber
exudate a.
Hollister wound exudate a.
absorptiometry
dual-energy x-ray a. (DEXA,
DXA)
absorption
a. coefficient
Compton a.
a., distribution, metabolism,
excretion (ADME)
drug a.
electromagnetic a.
fluorescent treponemal antibody a.
(FTA-ABS)
ABTA
American Brain Tumor Association
abuse
intravenous drug a. (IVDA)
abutment connection surgery
ABV
actinomycin D, bleomycin, vincristine
Adriamycin, bleomycin, vinblastine

NOTES

ABVD
Adriamycin, bleomycin, vinblastine, dacarbazine
Adriamycin, bleomycin, vincristine, dacarbazine
ABVD-MP
Adriamycin, bleomycin, vinblastine, dacarbazine, methylprednisolone
ABVE
Adriamycin, bleomycin, vincristine, etoposide
ABVP
Adriamycin, bleomycin sulfate, vinblastine, prednisone
Adriamycin, bleomycin sulfate, vincristine, prednisone
ABX-CBL monoclonal antibody
ABX-EGF monoclonal antibody
AC
acromioclavicular
Adriamycin and carmustine
Adriamycin and CCNU
Adriamycin and cisplatin
alcoholic cirrhosis
anterior commissure
anticoagulant
AC joint
AC vaccine
A/C
assist/control
A/C recombinant
ACA
anticardiolipin antibody
acanthocyte
acanthocytosis
hereditary a.
acantholytic dermatosis
acanthoma
basosquamous cell a.
acanthosis
glycogen a.
a. nigricans
acanthotic lesion
Acapodene
acardia
ACAT
automated computerized axial tomography
ACC
adenoid cystic carcinoma
adrenocortical carcinoma
alveolar cell carcinoma
ACC/AHA
American College of Cardiology/American Heart Association
accelerated
a. approval
a. fractionated radiation therapy
a. fractionated radiotherapy

a. fractionation
a. hyperfractionated radiation
a. hyperfractionated radiation therapy
a. hyperfractionated radiotherapy
a. hyperfractionated thoracic radiotherapy (AHFTRT)
a. hyperfractionation (AHF)
a. partial breast irradiation (APBI)
a. phase
a. phase gain
a. radiation therapy
a. radiotherapy with carbogen and nicotinamide (ARCON)
a. superfractionated radiotherapy
acceleration
liver acquisitions with volume a. (LAVA)
accelerator
a. factor
linear a. (LINAC)
low-energy linear a.
Mobetron mobile, self-shielded electron a.
proserum prothrombin conversion a.
prothrombin a.
serum prothrombin conversion a.
stereotactic linear a.
Varian a.
Accellon sampler
accentuation
access
central venous a.
translumbar a.
accessory
a. adhesion molecule
a. fissure
a. hemidiaphragm
a. hepatic vein
a. lobe
a. lymph node
a. middle cerebral artery
a. muscle
a. nerve
a. ossicle
a. ossification center
a. spleen
accident
Chernobyl nuclear a.
accrual
bone mineral a.
a. method for survival analysis
trial a.
Accucore II biopsy needle
accumulation
cytoplasmic a.
tracer a.
accumulative phase
AccuProbe system

accurate beam modeling
Accuray robotic device
Accutane/Rezulin cocktail
Ac-D-Ac
    Adriamycin, daunorubicin, Adriamycin
ACE
    Adriamycin, cyclophosphamide,
     etoposide
    angiotensin-converting enzyme
       ACE chemotherapy protocol
       ACE inhibitor
acemannan
    lyophilized a.
Acephen
acervuloma
Aceta
acetabula (pl. of acetabulum)
acetabular
    a. cavity
    a. column
    a. fossa
    a. posterior wall fracture
    a. protrusion
    a. residual dysplasia
    a. rim fracture
    a. roof
acetabuli
    protrusio a.
acetabulum, pl. acetabula
acetaminophen
    a., aspirin, caffeine
    a. and codeine
    a. and diphenhydramine
    hydrocodone and a.
    oxycodone and a.
    a. and phenyltoloxamine
    propoxyphene and a.
acetanilide
acetate
    aminophenylmercuric a.
    buserelin a.
    calcium a.
    cellulose a. (CA)
    cortisone a.
    cyproterone a. (CPA)
    depomedroxyprogesterone a.
     (DMPA)
    desmopressin a.
    goserelin a.
    leuprolide a. (LA)
    leuprorelin a.
    medroxyprogesterone a. (MPA)
    megestrol a. (MA)

    melengestrol a.
    melphalan, 5-fluorouracil,
     medroxyprogesterone a. (MFP)
    methylprednisolone a.
    octreotide a.
    paramethasone a.
    potassium a.
    sodium a.
    tetradecanoyl phorbol a.
acetomorphine
acetone
acetrizoate
acetrizoic acid
2-acetylaminofluorene (AAF)
acetylation
    histone a.
acetylator
acetylcholine
acetylcysteine
acetylsalicylic acid (ASA)
acetyltransferase
    chloramphenicol a.
ACFM
    automated cardiac flow measurement
A/C/F recombinant
AcFuCy
    actinomycin D, 5-fluorouracil,
     cyclophosphamide
ACG
    absolute granulocyte count
achalasia
    esophageal a.
Aches-N-Pain
achievable
    as low as reasonably a. (ALARA)
Achilles tendon
achlorhydria
    watery diarrhea, hypokalemia, a.
     (WDHA)
achlorhydric anemia
achondroplasia
    heterozygous a.
    homozygous a.
    hyperplastic a.
achoresis
achrestic anemia
achromic erythrocyte
achylic anemia
ACID
    Adriamycin, cyclophosphamide,
     imidazole, dactinomycin
acid
    acetrizoic a.

NOTES

acid (*continued*)
    acetylsalicylic a. (ASA)
    all-*trans*-retinoic a. (ATRA)
    alpha-lipoic a. (ALA)
    aminocaproic a.
    5-aminolevulinic a. (ALA)
    arachidonic a.
    arsanilic a.
    ascorbic a.
    aspartic a.
    azelaic a. (AZA)
    benzoic a.
    betulinic a.
    bile a.
    caffeic a.
    cis-retinoic a. (CRA)
    9-*cis*-retinoic a.
    13-*cis*-retinoic a. (13-CRA)
    dehydroascorbic a.
    dehydrocholic a.
    deoxyribonucleic a. (DNA)
    diatrizoic a.
    diethylenetriamine pentaacetic a.
      (DTPA)
    double-stranded proviral
      deoxyribonucleic a.
    eicosanoid fatty a.
    eicosapentaenoic a.
    ellagic a.
    a. elution
    ethacrynic a. (EA)
    ethylene diamine tetraacetic a.
      (EDTA)
    ethylene diamine tetramethylene
      phosphonic a. (EDTMP)
    fatty a.
    ferrous salt and ascorbic a.
    ferrous sulfate, ascorbic acid,
      vitamin B complex, folic a.
    flavone acetic a. (FAA)
    flufenamic a.
    folic a.
    folinic a. (FA)
    fusidic a.
    glutamic a.
    glutaric a.
    glycyrrhetinic a.
    hepatic 2,6-dimethyl
      iminodiacetic a.
    hippuric a.
    homocholic a.
    homovanillic a. (HVA)
    human immunodeficiency virus
      ribonucleic a.
    hyaluronic a.
    4-hydroperoxycyclophosphamide a.
    hydroperoxyeicosatetraenoic a.
      (HPETE)
    5-hydroxyindoleacetic a. (5-HIAA)

    6-hydroxyindoleacetic a. (6-HIAA)
    a. labile DNA
    lipid-associated sialic a.
    mefenamic a.
    messenger ribonucleic a.
    myristic a.
    nalidixic a.
    nonhuman bile a.
    nucleic a.
    oleic a.
    omega-3 polyunsaturated fatty a.
    oxidation of fatty a.'s
    p-aminobenzoic a.
    paraaminobenzoic a. (PABA)
    phenoxyacetic a.
    plasma human immunodeficiency
      virus ribonucleic a.
    plasma uric a.
    pleural fluid hyaluronic a.
    podophyllin and salicylic a.
    prostanoic a.
    pteroylglutamic a.
    pyrogallic a.
    retinoic a. (RA)
    ribonucleic a. (RNA)
    salicylic a.
    serum methylmalonic a.
    short-chain fatty a. (SCFA)
    sialic a.
    sparfosic a.
    Tc-diethylenetriamine pentaacetic a.
    technetium-99m diethylenetriamine
      pentaacetic a. (^{99m}Tc-DTPA)
    a. test
    tetraazacyclododecanetetraacetic a.
      (DOTA)
    thromboanoic a.
    tranexamic a.
    trans-retinoic a. (TRA)
    trichloroacetic a.
    tumor necrosis factor-alpha
      messenger ribonucleic a.
    uric a.
    ursodeoxycholic a. (UDCA)
    valproic a.
    vanillylmandelic a. (VMA)
    zoledronic a.

acid-base disorder

acidemia
    asymptomatic lactic a.
    isovaleric a.
    lactic a.

acid-fast
    a.-f. bacillus (AFB)
    a.-f. stain

acidic fibroblast growth factor (aFGF)
acidified serum lysis test
acidophil

acidophilic
- a. adenoma
- a. cytoplasm
- a. leukocyte
- a. structure

acidosis
- lactic a.
- metabolic a.

ACIDS
- acquired cellular immune deficiency syndrome

acid-Schiff
- periodic a.-S. (PAS)
- a.-S. stain

aciduria
- glutaric a. type I

Acilac

acinar
- a. cell
- a. cell adenocarcinoma
- a. cell carcinoma
- a. cell tumor
- a. sarcoidosis

acinarization

Acinetobacter lwoffii

acinus, pl. **acini**
- neoplastic acini

ACIP
- Asymptomatic Cardiac Ischemia Pilot
- ACIP protocol

ACIS
- automated cellular imaging system

ACIT
- allogeneic cellular immune therapy
- ACIT system

acitretin

acivicin

Ackermann needle

aclarubicin (ACR)
- a. HCl

aclasis
- diaphysial a.

ACM
- Adriamycin, cyclophosphamide, methotrexate

ACNU
- nimustine

ACOAP
- Adriamycin, cyclophosphamide, Oncovin, cytosine arabinoside, prednisone

ACOP
- Adriamycin, cyclophosphamide, Oncovin, prednisone
- Adriamycin, Cytoxan, Oncovin, prednisone

ACOPP
- Adriamycin, cyclophosphamide, Oncovin, prednisone, procarbazine
- Adriamycin, cyclophosphamide, Oncovin, procarbazine, prednisone

acoustic
- a. canal
- a. enhancement
- a. gel
- a. imaging
- a. impedance
- a. lens
- a. meatus
- a. nerve
- a. nerve sheath tumor
- a. neurinoma
- a. neuroma
- a. noise
- a. pressure
- a. pressure amplitude
- a. response technology
- a. schwannoma
- a. shadow
- a. velocity
- a. voice analysis
- a. wave

acoustical shadowing

ACPA
- anticytoplasmic autoantibody
- ACPA blood test

AcQsim CT simulator

acquired
- a. abnormality
- a. agammaglobulinemia
- a. aplastic anemia (AAA)
- a. cellular immune deficiency syndrome (ACIDS)
- a. drug resistance
- a. factor deficiency
- a. hemolytic anemia (AHA)
- a. hemophilia
- a. hepatocerebral degeneration
- a. hypercoagulable state
- a. hypogammaglobulinemia
- a. ichthyosis
- a. immune deficiency
- a. immunity

NOTES

acquired *(continued)*
  a. immunodeficiency syndrome (AIDS)
  a. immunodeficiency syndrome health assessment questionnaire (AIDS-HAQ)
  a. methemoglobinemia
  a. neutropenia
  a. prothrombotic disorder
  a. renal cystic disease
  a. spinal stenosis
  a. thrombophilic state
  a. von Willebrand disease (AvWD)
acquisita
  hypertrichosis lanuginosa a.
acquisition
  data a.
  dynamic a.
  a. matrix
  multiple gated a. (MUGA)
  polarity-altered spectral selective a. (PASTA)
  single-point a.
  spiral CT a.
  static image a.
  a. time
  a. window
ACR
  aclarubicin
  American College of Radiology
acral
  a. erythema
  a. lentiginous melanoma
  a. palmoplantar keratosis
acral-lentiginous melanoma
acridine orange
acrocephalosyndactyly, acrocephalosyndactylia
  Pfeiffer a.
  Saethre-Chotzen a.
acrochordon
acrodermatitis enteropathica
acrokeratosis
  paraneoplastic a.
  a. paraneoplastica
acrolein
acromegaly
acromesomelic
acrometastasis
acromioclavicular (AC)
  a. joint
  a. joint separation
  a. space
acromiocoracoid
acromion process
acroosteolysis
acropachy
acrospiroma
acrylamide gel

acrylic
  a. microsphere
  a. nucleotide reverse transcriptase inhibitor
ACS
  American Cancer Society
ACS:180 BR breast cancer screening test
ACSB
  AIDS and Cancer Specimen Bank
ACSR
  AIDS and Cancer Specimen Resource
ACT
  actinomycin
  activated clotting time
  activated coagulation time
  adoptive cellular therapy
act
  Compassionate Use A.
Actalyke activated clotting time test
ACTC, ACT-C
  actinomycin C
ACTD, ACT-D
  actinomycin D
ACTG
  AIDS Clinical Treatment Group
    ACTG 076 protocol
ACTG 214
  AIDS Clinical Treatment Group 214
ACTG 325
  AIDS Clinical Treatment Group 325
ACTG 334
  AIDS Clinical Treatment Group 334
ACTG 349
  AIDS Clinical Treatment Group 349
ACTH
  adrenocorticotropic hormone
Acthar
ACTH-producing adenoma
Acticoat
  A. composite dressing
  A. foam dressing
Actimmune
actin
  antismooth muscle a.
  muscle a.
  muscle-specific a. (MSA)
  a. protein
  smooth muscle a. (SMA)
actinic
  a. granuloma
  a. keratosis
  a. reticuloid
actinomycin (ACT)
  a. C (ACTC, ACT-C)
  a. D (ACTD, ACT-D)
  a. D, bleomycin, vincristine (ABV)
  a. D, 5-fluorouracil, cyclophosphamide (AcFuCy)

DTIC and a. (DTIC-ACTD)
a. D, vincristine, Platinol (AVP)
ifosfamide, vincristine, a. (IVA)
vincristine and a. D (VA)
actinomycosis
actinophage
actin-positive spindle cell neoplasm
action
  drug a.
  phase-specific a.
Actiprofen
Actiq Oral Transmucosal
Activase
  Cathflo A.
activated
  a. clotting time (ACT)
  a. clotting time test
  a. coagulation time (ACT)
  a. endothelial cell
  a. partial thromboplastin time (APTT)
  a. protein C resistance assay
  a. T-cell transfer
activating protein-1 (AP-1)
activation
  cell a.
  a. factor
  functional a.
  immune a.
  intracellular a.
  lyl-1-oncogene a.
  lyt-10 oncogene a.
  a. mapping
  oncogene a.
  polyclonal a.
  task a.
  transcriptional a.
  viral-mediated cellular a.
activation-associated antigen
activation-induced cell death (AICD)
activator
  BCI-Immune a.
  class II transcriptional a. (CIITA)
  lymphocyte a.
  polyclonal a.
  tissue plasminogen a. (TPA)
  transcriptional a.
  urokinase-type plasminogen a. (uPA)
active
  a. anal intercourse
  a. immunity
  a. immunization

a. nonspecific immunotherapy
a. specific immunotherapy (ASI)
a. transcription factor
activity, pl. **activities**
  antiestrogenic a.
  antiproliferative a.
  antitumor a.
  antiviral a.
  a. assay sphingomyelinase
  bacteriostatic a.
  binding a.
  bone morphogenetic a.
  cancer cell-derived blood coagulating a. 1 (CCA-1)
  ceramide synthase a.
  cytolytic a.
  activities of daily living (ADL)
  endogenous biotin a.
  endogenous peroxidase a.
  estrogenic a.
  Fas-ligand-mediated cytotoxic a.
  immunoradiometric assay of antigen a.
  intrinsic tyrosine kinase a.
  in vitro antiviral a.
  lymphoproliferative a.
  lymphotoxin antitumor a.
  macrophage phagocytic a.
  macrophage tumoricidal a.
  melanoma-inhibitory a. (MIA)
  MHC class I-restricted cytolytic a.
  natural killer a.
  NK a.
  perforin-mediated cytotoxic a.
  platelet procoagulant a.
  proliferative a.
  sequence-specific anti-HIV a.
  sexual a.
  telomerase a.
  tumoricidal a.
  veto a.
Actonel
actuarial survival
ACTUR
  Automated Central Tumor Registry
acuity
acuminatum, pl. **acuminata**
  Camptotheca acuminata
  condyloma a.
acupuncture
Acuson linear array transducer
acute
  a. abdomen

NOTES

9

acute *(continued)*
- a. allergic extrinsic alveolitis
- a. anaphylaxis
- a. basophilic leukemia (ABL)
- a. biphenotypic leukemia
- a. bronchopulmonary asthma
- a. cellular xenograft rejection
- a. chest syndrome
- a. cholecystitis
- a. diffuse bacterial nephritis
- a. disseminated encephalomyelitis
- a. diverticulitis
- a. encephalopathy
- a. eosinophilic leukemia
- a. erythroblastic leukemia
- a. focal bacterial nephritis
- a. fracture
- a. granulocytic leukemia (AGL)
- a. hemolytic transfusion reaction
- a. hepatitis
- a. HIV exanthem
- a. hypocellular leukemia
- a. hypogranular promyelocytic leukemia
- a. inflammatory disease
- a. interstitial nephritis (AIN)
- a. intravascular hemolysis
- a. lethal carditis
- a. lymphoblastic leukemia (ALL)
- a. lymphoblastic lymphoma
- a. lymphoblastic myelogenous leukemia
- a. lymphocytic leukemia (ALL)
- a. lymphoid leukemia
- a. megakaryoblastic leukemia (AMegL)
- a. megakaryocytic leukemia
- a. mixed lineage leukemia
- a. monoblastic leukemia (AML, AMOL)
- a. monocytic leukemia (AML, AMOL)
- a. myeloblastic leukemia (AMBL)
- a. myeloblastic myelogenous leukemia
- a. myelocytic leukemia (AML)
- a. myelofibrosis
- a. myelogenous leukemia (AML)
- a. myeloid leukemia (AML)
- a. myelomonoblastic leukemia (AMMOL)
- a. myelomonocytic leukemia
- a. myocardial infarction
- a. neuropathy
- a. nonlymphoblastic leukemia (ANLL)
- a. nonlymphocytic leukemia (ANLL)
- a. nonlymphoid leukemia
- a. nonsuppurative ascending cholangitis
- a. normovolemic hemodilution
- a. pain
- a. pancreatitis
- a. panmyelosis
- a. phase reactant
- a. progranulocytic leukemia
- a. promyelocytic leukemia (APL, APML)
- a. radiation bone marrow syndrome
- a. respiratory distress syndrome (ARDS)
- a. retroviral syndrome
- a. seroconversion syndrome
- a. splenic tumor
- a. suppurative ascending cholangitis
- a. suppurative sialadenitis
- a. suppurative thyroiditis
- a. testicular torsion
- a. traumatic aortic injury
- a. tubular necrosis
- a. tumor lysis (ATL)
- a. tumor lysis syndrome
- a. undifferentiated leukemia (AUL)

ACV
    amifostine, cisplatin, vinblastine

ACVBP
    Adriamycin, cyclophosphamide, vindesine, bleomycin, prednisone

acyanotic heart disease

acyclic
- a. metal chelate complex
- a. nucleoside phosphonate

acyclovir sodium

acylfulvene

AD
    Alzheimer disease
    autosomal dominant

ADA
    adenosine deaminase

Adagen

Adalat CC

adamantinoma

adamantinomatous craniopharyngioma

Adamkiewicz
    arteries of A.
    A. artery

adaptation

adapted standard mammography unit

adapter
    Rutner nephroscopy a.
    Y a.

adaptive
- a. correction
- a. remodeling

adaptogen

ADBC
    Adriamycin, DTIC, bleomycin, CCNU

ADC
AIDS-dementia complex
analog-to-digital converter
antibody-directed catalysis
ADCC
antibody-dependent cell cytotoxicity
antibody-dependent cell-mediated
cytotoxicity
antibody-dependent cellular cytotoxicity
addiction disorder
addictive
a. androgen
a. behavior
Addis count
Addison
A. disease
A. syndrome
Addison-Biermer anemia
additive
Hemo-Dial dialysate a.
a. solution (AS)
a. solution red cell
additivity
mode I, II a.
add-on treatment
addressed
regional lymph nodes cannot be a.
(NX)
adduct
Schiff base a.
adduction
adductor
a. brevis
a. canal
a. hallucis
a. longus
a. magnus
a. pollicis
a. tubercle
ADE
ara-C, daunorubicin, etoposide
Adeflor
adefovir
adenectomy
adenine
a. arabinoside (ara-A)
9-2-phosphonylmethoxyethyl a.
(PMEA)
a. phosphoribosyl transferase
9-R-2-phosphonylmethoxypropyl a.
(PMPA)
adenitis

adeno
a. p53 therapy
a. p53 therapy of recurrent
glioblastoma
adenoacanthoma
endometrial a.
adenoassociated
a. virus (AAV)
a. virus vector
adenocarcinoma
acinar cell a.
aggressive digital papillary a.
ampullary a.
apocrine a.
Barrett esophagus-associated a.
(BEAC)
basal cell a.
bronchiolar a.
cervical a.
ciliated cell a.
Clara cell a.
clear cell a.
colorectal a.
cystic a.
distal rectal a. (DRA)
duct cell a.
endometrial secretory a.
endometrioid a.
a. of esophagus
fetal a.
follicular a.
gastrointestinal tract a.
goblet cell-type a.
hepatoid a.
intraluminal a.
invasive a.
kidney a.
Klatskin biliary a.
Lucké a.
mesonephric a.
metastatic a.
minimal deviation a.
moderately differentiated a.
a. of Moll
mucinous a.
mucoid a.
nonmucinous a.
oncocytic a.
pancreatic a.
pancreatic ductal a. (PDAC)
papillary a.
polymorphous low-grade a. (PLGA)
renal a.

NOTES

adenocarcinoma *(continued)*
>scirrhous a.
>secretory a.
>serous a.
>sialo-type pancreatic a.
>sinonasal a. (SNA)
>a. in situ (AIS)
>stomach a.
>synchronous colonic a.
>tubular a.
>a. of uterus
>villoglandular a.
>vulvar adenocystic a.
>a. with squamous differentiation

adenocystic carcinoma
adenoepithelioma
adenofibroma
adenofibromyoma
adenoid
>a. cystic carcinoma (ACC)
>a. squamous cell carcinoma
>a. tumor

adenoidal lesion
adenoidal-pharyngeal-conjunctival (A-P-C)
adeno-interferon gamma
adenoleiomyofibroma
adenolipoma
adenoma
>acidophilic a.
>ACTH-producing a.
>adnexal a.
>adrenal cortex a.
>adrenocortical a.
>aldosterone-producing a. (APA)
>apocrine a.
>autonomous a.
>basal cell a.
>basophilic a.
>black a.
>a. of breast
>bronchial a.
>bronchoalveolar cell a.
>carcinoma ex pleomorphic a.
>carotid sheath a.
>chromophilic a.
>chromophobe a.
>colloid a.
>colorectal a.
>Cushing a.
>cystic pituitary a.
>ductal a.
>duodenal Brunner gland a.
>ectopic parathyroid a.
>embryonal a.
>endoscopic removal of duodenal Brunner gland a.
>eosinophilic a.
>a. fibrosum

>growth hormone-producing a.
>high-grade dysplastic a.
>islet cell a.
>lactating a.
>Leydig cell a.
>macrofollicular a.
>a. malignum
>metachronous a.
>microcystic a.
>microfollicular a.
>monomorphic a.
>nephrogenic a.
>a. of nipple
>ovarian tubular a.
>oxyphilic a.
>papillary cystic a.
>parathyroid a.
>Pick tubular a.
>pituitary a. (PA)
>pleomorphic a.
>plurihormonal a.
>polypoid a.
>prolactin-producing a.
>prostatic a.
>salivary gland pleomorphic a.
>sebaceous a.
>a. sebaceum
>somatotrophic a.
>sweat duct a.
>synchronous a.
>testicular tubular a.
>thyroid a.
>thyrotropin-producing a.
>tubular a.
>tubulopapillary a.
>tubulovillous a.
>undifferentiated cell a.
>unicryptal a.
>villotubular a.
>villous a.

adenomatoid
>a. hyperplasia
>a. nodule
>a. odontogenic tumor

adenomatous
>a. colonic polyp
>a. goiter
>a. hyperplasia
>a. polyp (AP)
>a. polyposis coli
>a. polyposis coli gene mutation assay
>a. polyposis of colon (APC)
>a. polyposis syndrome

adenomyoma
adenomyomatosis
adenomyosarcoma
adenomyosis in uterine enlargement

adenopathy
  abdominal a.
  axillary a.
  cervical a.
  hilar a.
  paratracheal a.
  secondary axillary a.
adenopolyposis coli gene
adenosarcoma
  müllerian a.
adenosine
  a. analog
  a. arabinoside
  a. deaminase (ADA)
  a. deaminase deficiency
  a. 5'-diphosphate (ADP)
  a. diphosphoribosyl transferase
    (ADPRT)
  a. monophosphate (AMP)
  a. 5'-triphosphate (ATP)
  a. triphosphate-binding cassette
    (ABC)
adenosis
adenosquamous carcinoma
adenovector
adenoviral
adenovirus
  a. colitis
  a. infection
  a. pneumonia
  a. vector
  a. vector expressing the RSV-1
    thymidine kinase gene AdV.RSV-
    TK
adenylosuccinate synthetase/lyase
ADEPT
  antibody-directed enzyme prodrug
  therapy
ADH
  antidiuretic hormone
  atypical ductal hyperplasia
AdHCC
  advanced hepatocellular carcinoma
adherence
  immune a.
  leukocyte a.
adhesin
adhesion
  abdominal a.
  cellular a.
  a. molecule
adhesive
  a. arachnoiditis

  a. atelectasis
  a. capsulitis
  a. platelet
  polymerizing tissue a.
  tissue a.
adhesive/sealant
  BioGlue a./s.
ADI
  absolute dose intensity
adiabatic fast passage (AFP)
ADIC, A-DIC
  Adriamycin and dacarbazine
  Adriamycin and DTIC
Ad-IFN gamma
adipocyte damage
adipose
  a. sarcoma
  a. tissue
  a. tumor
adiposis inhibitor factor
aditus ad antrum
adjusted survival rate
adjuvant
  a. analgesic
  a. analgesic drug
  a. chemoradiation
  a. chemotherapy
  a. chronotherapy
  complete Freund a. (CFA)
  Detox a.
  Freund complete a. (FCA)
  a. immunotherapy
  incomplete Freund a. (IFA)
  a. irradiation
  multiple a.
  a. polychemotherapy
  a. postradiation therapy
  a. treatment
  a. treatment option
adjuvanticity
AdjuVax-100a
ADL
  activities of daily living
  adrenoleukodystrophy
ADL-AMN
  adrenoleukodystrophy-
  adrenomyeloneuropathy
Adlone Injection
ADME
  absorption, distribution, metabolism,
  excretion
administration
  bolus a.

NOTES

13

administration *(continued)*
>drug a.
>Food and Drug A. (FDA)
>Health Care Financing A. (HCFA)
>intradermal a.
>intralesional a.
>intralymphatic radioactivity a.
>intraperitoneal drug a.
>intraspinal a.
>passive a.

admix

admixture lesion

adnexa
>lymphoma of ocular a.
>ocular a.

adnexal
>a. adenoma
>a. carcinoma
>a. cyst
>a. embryo
>a. lesion
>a. lymphoid proliferation
>a. mass
>a. metastasis
>a. tumor

adnexectomy

ADOAP, AD-OAP, AdOAP
>Adriamycin, Oncovin,
>   arabinosylcytosine, prednisone

ADOC
>Adriamycin, docetaxel, Oncovin,
>   cyclophosphamide

AdoHcy
>S-adenosylhomocysteine

AdoHcyase
>S-adenosylhomocysteine hydrolase

adolescent
>a. breast
>a. cancer
>a. nulliparous patient
>A. and Pediatric Pain Tool Scale
>a. surveillance case definition

ADOP, AdOP
>Adriamycin, Oncovin, prednisone

adopter molecule Shc

adoptive
>a. cell transfer
>a. cell transfer therapy
>a. cellular therapy (ACT)
>a. immunity
>a. immunotherapy

adozelesin

ADP
>adenosine 5′-diphosphate

ADPRT
>adenosine diphosphoribosyl transferase

ADR
>Adriamycin

adverse drug reaction
>ara-C + ADR

adrenal
>a. ablation
>a. artery
>a. calcification
>a. cortex
>a. cortex adenoma
>a. cortical carcinoma
>a. cyst
>a. cystic mass
>a. failure
>a. feminizing syndrome
>a. gland
>a. gland biopsy
>a. gland cancer
>a. hemorrhage
>a. hyperplasia
>a. incidentaloma
>a. insufficiency
>a. medullary disease
>a. metastasectomy
>a. metastasis
>a. myelolipoma
>a. neoplasm
>a. pheochromocytoma
>a. rest
>a. scintigraphy
>a. tumor
>a. vein
>a. virilizing syndrome

adrenalectomy
>contralateral synchronous a.
>ipsilateral synchronous a.
>laparoscopic a.

adrenergic
>a. blocker
>a. receptor

adrenoceptor

adrenocortical
>a. adenoma
>a. carcinoma (ACC)
>a. disease
>a. hyperplasia
>a. macrocyst
>a. neoplasm
>a. rest cell tumor
>a. secretion

adrenocorticoid

adrenocorticotropic hormone (ACTH)

adrenocorticotropin microadenoma

adrenogenital syndrome

adrenoleukodystrophy (ADL)

adrenoleukodystrophy-
>**adrenomyeloneuropathy (ADL-AMN)**

adrenomyeloneuropathy (AMN)

Adriamycin (ADR)
>Adriamycin, daunorubicin, A. (Ac-
>   D-Ac)

ara-C and A. (AA)

L-asparaginase, prednisone, Oncovin, cytarabine, A. (LAPOCA)

A., BCNU, cyclophosphamide (ABC)

A., bleomycin, CCNU, dacarbazine (ABCD)

A., bleomycin, cyclophosphamide, mitomycin C (ABCM)

A., bleomycin, cyclophosphamide, vincristine, etoposide, prednisolone I (ABCVEP-I)

A., bleomycin, dacarbazine, CCNU, prednisone (ABDIC)

A., bleomycin, DTIC, CCNU, prednisone (ABDIC)

bleomycin, DTIC, Oncovin, prednisone, A. (B-DOPA)

A., bleomycin, DTIC, vinblastine (ABDV)

A., bleomycin, prednisone (ABP)

A., bleomycin sulfate, vinblastine, prednisone (ABVP)

A., bleomycin sulfate, vincristine, prednisone (ABVP)

A., bleomycin sulfate, vincristine, streptozocin (ABOS)

A., bleomycin, vinblastine (ABV)

A., bleomycin, vinblastine, dacarbazine (ABVD)

A., bleomycin, vinblastine, dacarbazine, methylprednisolone (ABVD-MP)

A., bleomycin, vincristine, dacarbazine (ABVD)

A., bleomycin, vincristine, etoposide (ABVE)

A. and carmustine (AC)

A. and CCNU (AC)

CCNU, cyclophosphamide, methotrexate, A. (CCMA)

CCNU, ifosfamide, A. (CIA)

chlorambucil, vinblastine, procarbazine, prednisone, etoposide, vincristine, A. (ChlVPP/EVA)

A. and cisplatin (AC)

cisplatin, cyclophosphamide, A. (CisCA)

cisplatin, etoposide, cyclophosphamide, A. (CECA)

cisplatin, etoposide, Cytoxan, A. (CECA)

cyclophosphamide and A. (CA)

A., cyclophosphamide, etoposide (ACE)

A., cyclophosphamide, imidazole, dactinomycin (ACID)

A., cyclophosphamide, methotrexate (ACM)

cyclophosphamide, methotrexate, 5-fluorouracil, prednisone, vincristine, A. (CMFP-VA)

A., cyclophosphamide, Oncovin, cytosine arabinoside, prednisone (ACOAP)

A., cyclophosphamide, Oncovin, prednisone (ACOP)

cyclophosphamide, Oncovin, prednisone, A. (COPA)

A., cyclophosphamide, Oncovin, prednisone, procarbazine (ACOPP)

A., cyclophosphamide, Oncovin, procarbazine, prednisone (ACOPP)

cyclophosphamide, Oncovin, procarbazine, prednisone, A. (COPPA)

A., cyclophosphamide, vindesine, bleomycin, prednisone (ACVBP)

cytarabine plus A.

Cytoxan, hydroxyurea, actinomycin D, methotrexate, Oncovin, calcium folinate, A. (CHAMOCA)

A., Cytoxan, Oncovin, prednisone (ACOP)

A. and dacarbazine (ADIC, A-DIC)

A., daunorubicin, Adriamycin (Ac-D-Ac)

A., docetaxel, Oncovin, cyclophosphamide (ADOC)

A. and DTIC (ADIC, A-DIC)

A., DTIC, bleomycin, CCNU (ADBC)

epinephrine and A. (epi-ADR)

etoposide, vinblastine, A. (EVA)

A., 5-fluorouracil, methotrexate (AFM)

A., 5-fluorouracil, methotrexate with leucovorin rescue

A., ifosfamide, dacarbazine, mesna

ifosfamide, Platinol, A. (IPA)

A., Leukeran, Oncovin, methotrexate, actinomycin D, dacarbazine (ALOMAD)

MeCCNU and A. (MAD)

NOTES

Adriamycin *(continued)*
  methotrexate, Oncovin,
    cyclophosphamide, A. (MOCA)
  methyl-CCNU, 5-fluorouracil, A.
    (MeFA)
  mitomycin, 5-fluorouracil, A.
    (MIFA)
  A., Oncovin, arabinosylcytosine,
    prednisone (ADOAP, AD-OAP,
    AdOAP)
  A., Oncovin, prednisone (ADOP,
    AdOP)
  A., Oncovin, prednisone, etoposide
    (AOPE)
  Oncovin, procarbazine,
    prednisone, A. (OPPA)
  Oncovin, (vincristine), citrovorum
    factor, A.
  A. and Platinol (AP)
  A., Platinol, etoposide (APE)
  Platinol, ifosfamide, A. (PIA)
  A. plus BCNU
  A. plus L-PAM
  A. plus L-phenylalanine mustard
    (Adria + L-PAM, Adria + L-PAM)
  A., prednisone, Oncovin (APO)
  prednisone, Oncovin, cytarabine, A.
    (POCA)
  A. RDF
  sequential high-dose methotrexate
    followed by 5-FU in combination
    with A. (FAMTX)
  A., Solu-Medrol, ara-C, Platinol
    (ASAP)
  A., Solu-Medrol, high-dose ara-C,
    Platinol (ASHAP, A-SHAP)
  vinblastine, etoposide,
    prednisone, A. (VEPA)
  A., vinblastine, methotrexate
    (AVM)
  A. and vincristine (AV)
  vincristine, actinomycin A,
    cyclophosphamide, A. (VACA)
  vincristine, actinomycin D,
    cyclophosphamide, A. (VACA)
  vincristine, actinomycin D,
    ifosfamide, A. (VAIA)
  vincristine, BCNU, A. (VBA)
  A., vincristine, cyclophosphamide,
    5-fluorouracil (AVCF)
  A., vincristine, cytarabine,
    dexamethasone (AVAD)
  A., vincristine, mitomycin C
    (AVM)
  A., vincristine, procarbazine (AVP)
  VP-16, Oncovin,
    cyclophosphamide, A. (VOCA)
Adria + L-PAM
  Adriamycin plus L-phenylalanine mustard

Adrucil Injection
adsorption
  aluminum hydroxide a.
ADT
  androgen deprivation therapy
adult
  a. breast
  A. Hematopoietic Stem Cell
    Transplant Program
  a. polycystic kidney disease
  a. respiratory distress syndrome
    (ARDS)
  a. T-cell leukemia (ATL)
  a. T-cell leukemia/lymphoma
    (ATLL)
  a. T-cell lymphoma (ATL)
advanced
  a. epithelial ovarian cancer
  a. hepatocellular carcinoma
    (AdHCC)
  A. Interventional Systems (AIS)
  a. multiple-beam equalization
    radiography
advance directive
advancement flap
Advanta bed
Advantage4D PET/CT applicator
Advantage Fusion application
AdvantageSim 6.0 simulation software
Advantx LC/LP cardiac biplane system
adventitia
  tunica a.
adventitial
  a. cell
  a. fibroplasia
adverse drug reaction (ADR)
Advexin
advice
  against medical a. (AMA)
advocate
  patient a.
AdV.RSV-TK
  adenovirus vector expressing the
    RSV-1 thymidine kinase gene
    AdV.RSV-TK
  AdV.RSV-TK and ganciclovir
    combination
adynamic ileus
aegyptius
  Haemophilus a.
aeration
aerobe
aerobic Gram-negative rod
aerodigestive
  a. cancer
  a. tract
  upper a. (UAD)
aerogenes
  Enterobacter a.

Aeroseb-Dex
aerosol
> Virazole A.

aerosolized pentamidine
Aerospray hematology slide
> **stainer/cytocentrifuge**

aeruginosa
> *Burkholderia a.*
> *Pseudomonas a.*

AF
> aggressive fibromatosis

AFAP
> attenuated familial adenomatous
> polyposis

AFB
> acid-fast bacillus
> aortofemoral bypass
> aspirated foreign body

AFE
> 5-aminolevulinic acid-induced
> fluorescence endoscopy

Affect Balance Scale (ABS)
afferent
> a. loop syndrome
> a. lymphatic drainage

affinity
> drug-binding a.

affinity-based method
aFGF
> acidic fibroblast growth factor

afibrinogenemia
AFIP
> Armed Forces Institute of Pathology

aflatoxin
AFM
> Adriamycin, 5-fluorouracil, methotrexate
> AFM with leucovorin rescue

A-form RNA-DNA hybrid
AFP
> adiabatic fast passage
> alpha fetoprotein
> AFP tumor marker

African
> A. Burkitt lymphoma
> A. iron overload
> A. Kaposi sarcoma
> A. swine fever
> A. traditional medicine
> A. trypanosomiasis

AFRT
> altered fractionation radiotherapy

Aftate Antifungal
afterglow

afterload
afterloader
> Fletcher a.
> Henschke a.
> microSelectron-HDR a.

afterloading
> a. catheter
> computer-assisted controlled a.
> a. probe
> a. radiation
> a. tandem and ovoid
> a. technique

aftosa
AFX
> atypical fibroxanthoma

AG3340
> AG3340 in combination with
> mitoxantrone and prednisone
> AG3340 in combination with
> Novantrone and prednisone

Ag
> antigen
> silver

against medical advice (AMA)
agammaglobulinemia
> acquired a.
> Bruton sex-linked a.
> common variable a.
> congenital a.
> Swiss-type a.
> X-linked a.

aganglionic
> a. megacolon
> a. segment

aganglionosis
agar
> a. gel electrophoresis
> Geliperm a.
> MacConkey a.
> Middlebrook a.
> Mycosel a.
> Schaedler blood a.

AGCUS, AGUS
> atypical glandular cell of unknown
> significance

age
> bone a.
> a., distant metastases, extent, size
> (AMES)

age-dependent rise
aged serum
Agenerase

NOTES

agenesis
  tibial a.
agenetic fracture
agent
  alkylating a.
  antiangiogenesis a.
  antiangiogenic a.
  antibacterial a.
  anticholinergic a.
  anticlotting a.
  antidiarrheal a.
  antiemetic a.
  antifungal a.
  antiherpetic a.
  antiinflammatory a.
  antimalarial a.
  antimicrotubule a.
  antineoplastic a.
  antiparasitic a.
  antiplatelet a.
  antiproliferative a.
  antiretroviral a.
  antitelomerase a.
  antitoxoplasmosis a.
  antiviral a.
  bifunctional alkylating a.
  bioreductive a.
  Bittner a.
  cardioprotective a.
  chelating a.
  chemopreventive a.
  chemotherapeutic a.
  cobalt-bleomycin imaging a.
  Combidex MRI contrast a.
  Cremophor EL emulsifying a.
  cycle-nonspecific a.
  cycle-specific a.
  cytotoxic chemotherapeutic a.
  delta a.
  Eaton a.
  ectoapyrases class of
    anticlotting a.'s
  foamy a.
  gastrointestinal a.
  glutathione-depleting a.
  high-dose alkylating a.
  hormonal a.
  HumaSPECT cancer imaging a.
  hydroxyephedrine imaging a.
  hypomethylating a.
  hypoxic cell cytotoxic a.
  imidazotetrazine a.
  immune-stimulating a.
  immunosuppressant a.
  intravascular a.
  LDH a.
  low molecular weight oxidizing a.
  lympholytic a.
  mitotic spindle a.

  mobilizing a.
  NeoSpect diagnostic imaging a.
  NeoTect imaging a.
  neuroleptic a.
  nonalkylating a.
  nonmyelosuppressive a.
  Norwalk a.
  OctreoScan 111 radioactive
    imaging a.
  oncogenic a.
  ONYX-015 anticancer a.
  oxazaphosphorine alkylating a.
  platinating a.
  platinum-containing a.
  potent differentiating a.
  progestational a.
  psychotropic a.
  retinoic acid metabolism
    blocking a. (RAMBA)
  targeting a.
  Thorotrast contrast a.
  Tru-Scint AD imaging a.
  vascular-disrupting a. (VDA)
  vasopermeation enhancement a.
    (VEA)
  Verluma diagnostic imaging a.
ageusia
agger nasi air cell
agglomerans
  Enterobacter a.
agglutinate
agglutination
  a. assay
  chick-cell a.
  latex a.
  lectin a.
  platelet a.
agglutinative
agglutinin
  cold a.
  helix pomatia a. (HPA)
  immune a.
  peanut a.
  Rh a.
  soybean a. (SBA)
  wheat germ a.
agglutinogen
aggregate
  ferritin a.
  fibrinoplatelet a.
aggregation
  a. antibody-antigen complex
  erythrocyte a.
  familial a.
  platelet a.
aggregometer
aggressin
aggressive
  a. blastic natural killer leukemia

A

a. blastic NK leukemia
a. digital papillary adenocarcinoma
a. fibromatosis (AF)
a. good-prognosis non-Hodgkin lymphoma (AGPNHL)
a. histology lymphoma (AHL)
a. infantile fibromatosis

aggressiveness
tumor cell a.

agitation
severe a.

AGL
acute granulocytic leukemia

agnogenic myeloid metaplasia (AMM)

AgNOR
argyrophilic stain for nucleolar organizer region
AgNOR stain

agonist
dopamine a.
gonadotropin-releasing hormone a.
LHRF a.
LHRH a.
luteinizing hormone-releasing factor a.
luteinizing hormone-releasing hormone a.
opioid a.
SC-68420 dual receptor a.

agonist-antagonist
mixed opioid a.-a.

agoraphobia

AGPNHL
aggressive good-prognosis non-Hodgkin lymphoma

agranular leukocyte

agranulocytosis
toxic a.

agretope

Agrylin

AGT
aminoglutethimide

AGUS (*var. of* AGCUS)

AHA
acquired hemolytic anemia
autoimmune hemolytic anemia

ahaustral

AHD
autoimmune hemolytic disease

AHF
accelerated hyperfraction

AHFTRT
accelerated hyperfractionated thoracic radiotherapy

AHG
antihemophilic globulin

AHL
aggressive histology lymphoma

AHPCT
autologous hematopoietic progenitor cell transplantation

AHSCT
autologous hematopoietic stem cell transplantation

A-HydroCort Injection

AI
apoptotic index
aromatase inhibitor

Aicardi syndrome

AICD
activation-induced cell death

AICP
androgen-independent prostate carcinoma

AICR
American Institute for Cancer Research

aid
Foille Medicated First A.
pharmacologic a.
Sensability breast self-examination a.

aide
Calm Formula Sleep A.
Calm Forte Sleep A.
Insomnia Formula Sleep A.

AIDS
acquired immunodeficiency syndrome
AIDS and Cancer Specimen Bank (ACSB)
AIDS and Cancer Specimen Resource (ACSR)
AIDS Clinical Treatment Group (ACTG)
AIDS Clinical Treatment Group 214 (ACTG 214)
AIDS Clinical Treatment Group 325 (ACTG 325)
AIDS Clinical Treatment Group 334 (ACTG 334)
AIDS Clinical Treatment Group 349 (ACTG 349)
AIDS Clinical Treatment Group 076 protocol
AIDS enteropathy
feline AIDS

NOTES

AIDS *(continued)*
    AIDS group home
    hemophilia-associated AIDS
    Joint United Nations Programme
      on HIV/AIDS (UNAIDS)
    AIDS patient care
    AIDS PCNSL
    person with AIDS (PWA)
    AIDS prodrome
    AIDS risk-reduction model
    AIDS service organization (ASO)
    transfusion-related AIDS (TRAIDS)
    AIDS Vaccine Evaluation Group
      (AVEG)
    AIDS Vaccine Evaluation Unit
      (AVEU)
AIDS-associated KS
AIDS-dementia complex (ADC)
AIDS-HAQ
    acquired immunodeficiency syndrome
    health assessment questionnaire
AIDS/HIV Treatment Directory
AIDS-KS
    AIDS-related Kaposi sarcoma
AIDSphobia
AIDS-related
    AIDS-r. complex (ARC)
    AIDS-r. Kaposi sarcoma (AIDS-KS)
    AIDS-r. lymphomatous meningitis
    AIDS-r. primary central nervous
      system lymphoma
    AIDS-r. virus (ARV)
AIDSVAX B/B vaccine
AIHA
    autoimmune hemolytic anemia
AIL
    angiocentric immunoproliferative lesion
    angioimmunoblastic lymphadenopathy
AILD
    angioimmunoblastic lymphadenopathy
      with dysproteinemia
AIM
    L-asparaginase, ifosfamide, methotrexate
AIN
    acute interstitial nephritis
    anal intraepithelial neoplasia
AIPC
    androgen-independent prostate cancer
    androgen-independent prostate carcinoma
AI-PCa
    androgen-independent prostate carcinoma
air
    a. bronchogram
    a. collection
    a. contrast
    a. contrast barium enema
    a. contrast view
    a. embolism
    a. encephalography

    a. esophagram
    a. exchange
    a. filtration system
    a. gap
    a. space disease
    a. space enlargement
    a. trapping
air-bone-tissue boundary
airborne transmission
air-crescent sign
air-filled lung
air-fluid
    a.-f. level
    a.-f. line
air-gap
    a.-g. radiography
    a.-g. technique
air-kerma
    integrated reference a.-k. (IRAK)
    a.-k. rate constant
    a.-k. strength
    total reference a.-k. (TRAK)
airspace-filling pattern
airway
    3-dimensional display of a.'s
    a. obstruction
    a. pattern
    a. stenting
AIS
    adenocarcinoma in situ
    Advanced Interventional Systems
    Applied Immune Sciences
      AIS CELLector CD8 Cell Culture
      Device
AITP
    autoimmune thrombocytopenic purpura
AJCC
    American Joint Committee on Cancer
AJCC/UICC classification
akathisia
akinesis
Akineton
AK-Mycin
ALA
    alpha-lipoic acid
    American Lung Association
    5-aminolevulinic acid
ala, pl. **alae**
alanine aminotransferase (ALT)
ALA-PDT
    5-aminolevulinic acid photodynamic
      therapy
ALARA
    as low as reasonably achievable
albendazole
albicans
    azole-resistant *Candida a.*
    Candida a.

albuginea
tunica a.
albumin
Bence Jones a.
a. human 5%, 25%
human serum a.
macroaggregated a. (MAA)
radioactive iodinated serum a.
(RISA)
^{99m}Tc macroaggregated a.
technetium-99m macroaggregated
albumin (^{99m}Tc-MAA)
Albuminar
albuminemia
albuminuria
Bamberger hematogenic a.
Albumotope ^{131}I
Albunex
albus
Staphylococcus a.
ALCASE
Alliance for Lung Cancer Advocacy,
Support, and Education
ALCL
anaplastic large cell lymphoma
alcohol
absolute a.
aliphatic a.
a. injection
isopropyl a.
perillyl a.
polyvinyl a.
a. subarachnoid block
alcoholic
a. cardiomyopathy
a. cirrhosis (AC)
a. gastritis
Aldactazide
Aldactone
Aldara
Alder-Reilly inclusion
aldesleukin
aldocyclophosphamide
aldosterone-producing adenoma (APA)
aldosterone secretion rate (ASR)
aldosteronoma
Aldrich syndrome
alemtuzumab
alendronate
high-dose ketoconazole plus a.
a. sodium
alert bracelet

alethine
beta a.
aleukemic
a. leukemia
a. myelosis
a. presentation
aleukocythemic leukemia
aleukocytosis
Alexa
A. 1000 breast diagnostic system
A. 1000 breast lesion diagnostic
device
Alexagram breast lesion diagnostic test
Alexander technique
alexin
alfa
darbepoetin a.
drotrecogin a.
epoetin a.
a. interferon
interferon a.
a. interferon-n1
a. interferon-n3
recombinant interferon a. (IFLFA,
rIFN-A)
thyrotropin a.
alfa-2a
interferon a.-2a (IFNa)
alfa-2b
cisplatin, 5-fluorouracil, leucovorin,
interferon a.-2b (PFL-IFN)
interferon a.-2b
recombinant interferon a.-2b
alfacalcidol
alfalfa
alfa-n1
interferon a.-n1
alfa-n3
interferon a.-n3
Alfenta
alfentanil
Alferon
A. LDO
A. N
algorithm
artificial neural network a.
blocked beam a.
bone a.
Clarkson scatter-summation a.
EPL a.
genetic a.
geometric optimization a.

NOTES

algorithm *(continued)*
    high spatial resolution a.
    UroScore staging a.
Alibert-Bazin
    A.-B. form
    A.-B. form of mycosis fungoides
alignment
    bony a.
alimentary
    a. tract
    a. tract calcification
alimentation
    intravenous a.
Alimta
ALIP
   abnormal localization of immature
    precursors
aliphatic alcohol
aliquot
alitretinoin
Alius-Grignaschi anomaly
alive
    withdrawn a.
Alkaban-AQ
alkali denaturation assay
alkaline
    a. denaturation
    a. electrophoresis
    a. phosphatase (AP)
    a. phosphatase-antialkaline
     phosphatase (APAAP)
    a. phosphatase isoenzyme tumor
     marker
alkaloid
    ergot a.
    opium a.
    periwinkle a.
    plant a.
    pyrrolizidine a.
    Vinca a.
alkalosis
    metabolic a.
    watery diarrhea with
     hypokalemic a. (WDHA)
Alka-Mints
alkane sulfonate
Alkeran
alkylate DNA
alkylating agent
alkylation
    busulfan a.
alkylator therapy
alkylphosphocholine
ALL
    acute lymphoblastic leukemia
    acute lymphocytic leukemia

    p190 and p210 BCR/abl variants
     of Philadelphia chromosome-
     positive ALL
allantoin vaginal cream
all-donor chimerism
allele
    class I, II a.
    DQB1 a.
    DRB1 a.
    HA-1^A a.
    HA-1^H a.
    minisatellite a.
    wild-type a.
allele-specific
    a.-s. oligonucleotide (ASO)
    a.-s. oligonucleotide assay
allelic heterogeneity
allergen
allergic
    a. bronchopulmonary aspergillosis
    a. contact dermatitis
    a. disease
    a. granulomatosis
    a. granulomatous angiitis
    a. lung disorder
    a. reaction
allergization
allergosis
alliance
    Colon Cancer A.
    International Cancer A.
    A. for Lung Cancer Advocacy,
     Support, and Education
     (ALCASE)
alloantibody
alloantigen L^d
allocation
    fresh tissue a.
    a. of treatment
allodonor lymphocyte infusion
allogeneic, allogenic
    a. antigen
    a. antigen candidate
    a. blood transfusion
    a. bone marrow cell
    a. bone marrow transplant (ABMT)
    a. bone marrow transplantation
     (ABMT)
    a. cellular immune therapy (ACIT)
    a. disease
    a. donor
    a. engraftment
    a. peripheral cell transplant
    a. stem cell
    a. stem cell transplantation
    a. tumor cell immunization
    a. tumor cell vaccine

allograft
bone-chip a.
pancreatic a.
a. rejection
renal a.
tumor a.
allogroup
alloimmune
a. disease
a. hemolytic anemia
alloimmunization
PNH prep a.
AlloMune system
allopathic medicine
alloplast
allopurinol sodium
alloreaction
alloreactivity
allosensitization
allosteric inhibitor
allotope
allotransplantation
allotransplant recipient
allotype
allotypic marker
Allovectin-7
all-*trans*-retinoic
a.-*t.*-r. acid (ATRA)
a.-*t.*-r. acid in combination with interferon
a.-*t.*-r. acid, daunomycin, arsenic trioxide sequential therapy
a.-*t.*-r. acid/interferon-alfa 2a combination
17-(allylamino)-17-demethoxygeldanamycin (AAG)
ALN
axillary lymph node
ALND
axillary lymph node dissection
Aloe Vesta moisturizing skin care product
AL(OH)$_3$+deoxycholate
Aloka 650 ultrasound scanner
ALOMAD
Adriamycin, Leukeran, Oncovin, methotrexate, actinomycin D, dacarbazine
alopecia
drug-induced a.
a. mucinosa
a. mucinosa/follicular mucinosis (AM/FM)

Aloprim
Alora Transdermal
Aloxi
alpha, α
A. Chymar
a. cradle
a. fetoprotein (AFP)
a. fetoprotein tumor marker
a. granule
a. islet cell neoplasm
macrophage inflammatory protein-1 a. (MIP-1a, MIP-1 alpha)
a. methyltyrosine
a. naphthyl
a. particle
a. radiation
recombinant human MIP-1 a.
a. tocopherol
transforming growth factor a. (TGF-alpha)
alpha-1
a.-1 antitrypsin
a.-1 antitrypsin deficiency
alpha-1-antichymotrypsin-prostate-specific antigen
alpha-2 antiplasmin
alpha-actinin protein
alpha-adrenergic blocker
alpha-anilinophenyl-acetamide
Alpha-Beta
alpha-tocopherol beta-carotene
alpha-catenin
alpha-chymotrypsin
alpha-emitting radionucleotide
alpha-etiocholanolone
alpha-heavy-chain disease
alpha-lipoic acid (ALA)
alpha-M2
radiolabeled peptide a.-M2
alpha$_2$-macroglobulin
alpha-methyldopa
alpha-methyltyrosine
alpha-n
Wellferon lymphoblastoid interferon IFN a.-n
alpha-naphthyl
a.-n. acetate esterase
a.-n. butyrate esterase
AlphaNine SD
5-alpha-reductase inhibitor
Alpha-Tamoxifen
alpha-thalassemia

NOTES

alpha-tocopherol
    a.-t. antioxidant
    a.-t. beta-carotene (Alpha-Beta, ATBC)
    A.-t. Beta-Carotene Cancer Prevention Study
Alphavirus
alprazolam
ALPS
    autologous leukapheresis, processing, storage
    ALPS container
ALS
    antilymphocyte serum
ALT
    alanine aminotransferase
alteplase
alteration
    gustatory a.
    platelet aggregation a.
altered
    a. fractionation radiotherapy (AFRT)
    a. immunophenotype
    a. mental state
ALternaGel
Alternaria
alternariosis
    cutaneous a.
alternating triple therapy (ATT)
alternative
    a. donor
    a. medicine
    a. treatment activist manifesto
alternator
ALT-RCC
    autolymphocyte-based treatment for renal cell carcinoma
altretamine
Alu-Cap
aluminum
    a. carbonate
    a. hydroxide
    a. hydroxide adsorption
    a. phosphate
Alu-Tab
alvei
    Hafnia a.
alveolar
    a. canal
    a. cell carcinoma (ACC)
    a. disease
    a. duct
    a. echinococcosis
    a. epithelial hyperplasia
    a. foramen
    a. hemorrhage
    a. hypersensitivity
    a. infiltrate

    a. macrophage
    a. microlithiasis
    a. mucosal carcinoma
    a. nerve
    a. pattern
    a. pneumonia
    a. process
    a. proteinosis
    a. pulmonary edema
    a. rhabdomyosarcoma
    a. ridge
    a. sac
    a. sarcoidosis
    a. soft part sarcoma (ASPS)
alveolaris
    Echinococcus a.
alveolarization
alveoli (*pl. of* alveolus)
alveolitis
    acute allergic extrinsic a.
    chronic diffuse sclerosing a.
    chronic fibrosing a.
    desquamative fibrosing a.
    diffuse sclerosing a.
    extrinsic allergic a.
alveologram
alveolus, pl. **alveoli**
alvircept sudotox
alymphocytosis
alymphoplasia
    Nezelof type of thymic a.
    thymic a.
ALZ-50
    marker ALZ-50
Alzheimer disease (AD)
^{241}Am
    americium
AMA
    against medical advice
    antimitochondrial antibody
    autoregressive moving average
amantadine
amastia
amaurosis fugax
amazia
Ambicor inflatable prosthesis
Ambien
ambient
    a. wing
    a. wing of quadrigeminal cistern
ambiguus
    situs a.
AmBisome
AMBL
    acute myeloblastic leukemia
amboceptor
ambulatory infusion pump
Amcill
Amcort Injection

amdoxovir
Amdray
ameba, pl. **amebae**
amebiasis
amebic
    a. abscess
    a. dysentery
    a. granuloma
    a. infection
ameboma
amegakaryocytic thrombocytopenia
AMegL
    acute megakaryoblastic leukemia
amelanotic
    a. melanoma
    a. tumor
amelioration
ameloblastic
    a. adenomatoid tumor
    a. epithelium
    a. fibroma
    a. fibrosarcoma
    a. sarcoma
ameloblastoma
    extragnathic a.
ameloblastomatous differentiation
amenorrhea
    chemotherapy-related a. (CRA)
    hypothalamic a.
    primary a.
amenorrhea-galactorrhea
America
    Leukemia Society of A.
    Lymphoma Research Foundation of A.
    Radiological Society of North A. (RSNA)
Americaine
American
    A. Association for Cancer Research (AACR)
    A. Brain Tumor Association (ABTA)
    A. Cancer Society (ACS)
    A. College of Cardiology/American Heart Association (ACC/AHA)
    A. College of Radiology (ACR)
    A. Foundation for AIDS Research (AMFAR)
    A. Institute for Cancer Research (AICR)
    A. Joint Committee for Cancer Staging and End Results Reporting
    A. Joint Committee on Cancer (AJCC)
    A. Lung Association (ALA)
    A. Musculoskeletal Tumor Society (MSTS)
    A. Society of Clinical Oncology (ASCO)
    A. Society of Hematology (ASH)
    A. Society of Neuroradiology (ASN)
    A. Society of Preventive Oncology (ASPO)
    A. Society for Therapeutic Radiology and Oncology (ASTRO)
    A. Stop Smoking Intervention Study for Cancer Prevention (ASSIST)
    A. Thoracic Society (ATS)
    A. Urological Association (AUA)
    A. Urological Association classification
americium (^{241}Am)
Amersham
    A. CDCS A-type needle
    A. J tube
AMES
    age, distant metastases, extent, size
    AMES scoring
Ames test
A-methaPred Injection
amethopterin
AMFAR
    American Foundation for AIDS Research
AM/FM
    alopecia mucinosa/follicular mucinosis
Amicar
amicrobic
Amicus blood collection separator
amide
    angiotensin a.
    desacetyl vinblastine a. (DAVA)
amifostine
    a., cisplatin, vinblastine (ACV)
    a. pretreatment
amikacin
Amikin
amiloride
amine
    aryl aromatic a.

NOTES

amine *(continued)*
    heterocyclic aromatic a. (HAA)
    a. precursor uptake
    a. precursor uptake and
      decarboxylation (APUD)
    sympathomimetic a.
amino
    a. acid sequence
    a. acid therapy
    a. acid triplet
    a. terminus
aminoacridine
9-aminocamptothecin
aminocaproate esterase
aminocaproic acid
aminoglutethimide (AGT)
aminoglycoside
aminohydroxypropylidene diphosphate (APD)
aminolevulinic
5-aminolevulinic
    5-a. acid (ALA)
    5-a. acid-induced fluorescence
      endoscopy (AFE)
    5-a. acid photodynamic therapy
      (ALA-PDT)
aminooxypentane (AOP)
    a. regulated-on-activation normal T-
      expressed and secreted (AOP-
      RANTES)
aminopeptidase (AP)
    leucine a. (LAP)
aminophenylmercuric acetate
aminopterin syndrome
aminopyrine
aminothiadiazole
aminotransferase
    alanine a. (ALT)
    aspartate a. (AST)
amiodarone
Amitone
amitriptyline
    a. and chlordiazepoxide
    a. and perphenazine
AML
    acute monoblastic leukemia
    acute monocytic leukemia
    acute myelocytic leukemia
    acute myelogenous leukemia
    acute myeloid leukemia
AML-2-23 monoclonal antibody
amlexanox
amlodipine
AMM
    agnogenic myeloid metaplasia
AMMOL
    acute myelomonoblastic leukemia
ammonium chloride

AMN
    adrenomyeloneuropathy
AMN107 aminopyrimidine inhibitor
amniography
amniotic fluid embolism
amobarbital
AMOL
    acute monoblastic leukemia
    acute monocytic leukemia
amonafide
amoxapine
amoxicillin and clavulanate potassium
Amoxil
AMP
    adenosine monophosphate
amp
    Jaa A.
amphicrine cell carcinoma
Amphojel
Amphotec
amphotericin
    a. B
    a. B cholesteryl sulfate complex
    a. B colloidal dispersion (ABCD)
    a. B lipid complex (ABLC)
    a. B toxicity
ampicillin and sulbactam
Ampicin
Amplatz
    A. angiography needle
    A. dilator set
    A. double-J stent
    A. dual-stiffness Malecot catheter
    A. long tapered Teflon dilator
    A. mechanical thrombolysis catheter
    A. radiolucent handle
    A. renal dilator
    A. stiffening wire
    A. tapered pyeloureteral stent
    A. tapered-tip coaxial dilator
    A. through-and-through basket
    A. TLA needle
Amplatz-Lund retrievable filter
amplicon template
amplification
    c-erbB2 a.
    gene a.
    HER-2 protein a.
    tyramide signal a. (TSA)
amplified oncogene
amplifier T lymphocyte
Ampligen
Amplimexon
amplitude
    acoustic pressure a.
    a. mode
    a. modulation
amprenavir
ampulla, pl. ampullae

a. of Vater
a. of Vater cyst
ampullar
ampullary
a. adenocarcinoma
a. carcinoma
a. stenosis
AMSA
amsacrine
AMSA, prednisone, chlorambucil
(APC)
amsacrine (AMSA, mAMSA, m-AMSA)
Amsidyl
Amsterdam Criteria
amylase level
amyl nitrite
amyloid
a. arthropathy
a. deposit
a. deposition
a. light chain
a. oral cavity disease
a. tumor
amyloidoma
intracerebral a.
amyloidosis
familial a.
a. of multiple myeloma
myeloma-induced a.
primary systemic a.
renal a.
secondary a.
systemic a.
Amytal
AN-238 cytotoxic somatostatin analog
ANA
antinuclear antibody
ANA test
anabolic
a. phosphorylation
a. steroid
Anacin
Anadrol
anaerobe
anaerobic infection
anagen effluvium
anagrelide hydrochloride
anakinra
anakmesis
anal
a. canal
a. condyloma
a. endosonography

a. gland carcinoma
a. herpes
a. intercourse
a. intraepithelial neoplasia (AIN)
a. margin
a. pterygoid
a. region cancer
a. rimming
a. sex
a. sphincter
a. squamous cell carcinoma
a. squamous intraepithelial lesion
a. triangle
a. verge
a. wart
anal-digital intercourse
analgesia
epidural a.
patient-controlled a. (PCA)
patient-controlled epidural a.
(PCEA)
analgesic
adjuvant a.
a. nephropathy
nonopioid a.
opioid a.
a. syndrome
anallergic
anal-manual intercourse
analog, analogue
adenosine a.
AN-238 cytotoxic somatostatin a.
anti-human S5 a.
camptothecin a.
CCI-79 rapamycin a.
cisplatin a.
a. combination
coumarin a.
cyclosporine a.
deoxypyrimidine nucleoside a.
dideoxypurine a.
diffusible somatostatin a.
dipyridodiazepinone a.
epothilone B a.
GnRH a.
heteroatom-substituted a.
hydrazide a.
LHRH a.
monophosphated acyclic adenine
nucleoside a.
nucleoside a.
platinum a.
purine a.

NOTES

analog *(continued)*
    pyrimidine a.
    RMP-7 bradykinin a.
    somatostatin a.
    synthetic a.
    thalidomide a.
    thymidine a.
    triphosphate a.
    vitamin D a.
analog-to-digital converter (ADC)
analysis, pl. **analyses**
    accrual method for survival a.
    acoustic voice a.
    aneusomy a.
    automated hematology a.
    bootstrap a.
    cell block a.
    cell cycle kinetic a.
    chromosome a.
    Classification and Regression Tree a.
    Cox regression a.
    cytofluorimetric a.
    cytogenetic a.
    decision a.
    2-dimensional structure a.
    DNA content a.
    dose intensity a.
    dot blot a.
    fetal blood a.
    fluorescence-based single strand conformation a.
    fluorescent multiplexed polymerase chain reaction a.
    genotypic a.
    heteroduplex a.
    high-throughput tissue microarray a.
    histologic a.
    histopathologic a.
    immunoblot a.
    immunocytochemical a.
    immunofluorescence a.
    immunogenotypic a.
    immunohistochemical a.
    immunophenotypic a.
    isobologram a.
    karyometric a.
    karyotypic a.
    Khan scatter a.
    K-ras a.
    linear regression a.
    linkage a.
    ModFit DNA a.
    molecular genetic a.
    morphologic a.
    multicolor data a.
    multidimensional a.
    multivariate logistic regression a.
    nonlinear least squares regression a.
    Northern blot a.
    nucleotide sequence a.
    p53 a.
    phylogenetic a.
    piecewise regression a.
    proportional hazard model a.
    quantitative cell dispersion a.
    recursive partitioning a.
    regression a.
    restriction fragment length polymorphism a.
    SELDI-TOF a.
    sibpair linkage a.
    single-strand conformation polymorphism a.
    Southern blot a.
    S-phase a.
    surface-enhanced laser desorption and ionization time-of-flight a.
    TaqMan a.
    trend line a.
analyte
analytic
    a. reconstruction
    subjective, objective, management, a. (SOMA)
analyzer
    ABI PRISM 3700 DNA a.
    coagulation a.
    Cobas Mira a.
    Coulter S-plus a.
    KC1 Delta coagulation a.
    Synchron LX20 pro chemical a.
anamnestic response
Anandron
ANAP
    anionic neutrophil-activating peptide
anaphase
anaphylactic blood transfusion reaction
anaphylactoid
    a. crisis
    a. reaction
anaphylaxis
    acute a.
anaplasia
anaplastic
    a. astrocytoma (AA)
    cerebellar a.
    a. ependymoma
    a. large cell Ki-1-positive lymphoma
    a. large cell lymphoma (ALCL)
    a. mixed glioma
    a. oligoastrocytoma
    a. oligodendroglioma
    a. plasmacytoma

a. sarcoma
a. thyroid carcinoma
Anapolon
Anaprox
anastomosis, pl. **anastomoses**
    arterial a.
    arteriovenous a.
    biliary-enteric a.
    colorectal a.
    direct coloanal a.
    end-to-end a.
    end-to-side a.
    microvascular a.
    percutaneous portocaval a.
    portopulmonary venous a.
    portosystemic a.
    ureteroureteral a.
anastomotic
    a. aneurysm
    a. arterial circle
    a. leak
    a. stenosis
    a. stricture
anastrozole
anatomic
    a. barrier
    a. fracture
    a. snuffbox
anatomical variant
anatomy
    immune system a.
    zonal a.
Anbesol
    Maximum Strength A.
ANC
    absolute neutrophil count
ANCA
    antineutrophilic cytoplasmic antibody
Ancef
anchovy paste abscess
Ancobon
anconeus muscle
Ancotil
ancrod
androblastoma
Androcur Depot
Andro-Cyp
Androderm Transdermal System
androgen
    a. ablation
    a. ablation therapy
    addictive a.
    a. blockade

a. deprivation
a. deprivation therapy (ADT)
a. insensitivity syndrome
intraprostatic a.
a. receptor
a. suppression
a. suppression therapy (AST)
androgen-dependent prostate cancer
androgen-independent
    a.-i. prostate cancer (AIPC)
    a.-i. prostate carcinoma (AICP, AIPC, AI-PCa)
Android-10
Android-25
Android-F
Andro-L.A. Injection
Andronate
Andropository-200
Andropository Injection
androstane
androstanediol glucuronide
androstenedione
Andryl
anechoic thrombus
anejaculatory
anemia
    achlorhydric a.
    achrestic a.
    achylic a.
    acquired aplastic a. (AAA)
    acquired hemolytic a. (AHA)
    Addison-Biermer a.
    alloimmune hemolytic a.
    aplastic a.
    aregenerative a.
    autoimmune hemolytic a. (AHA, AIHA)
    Baghdad Spring a.
    Banti splenic a.
    Bartonella a.
    Biermer a.
    Blackfan-Diamond a.
    cameloid a.
    cancer-associated a.
    chlorotic a.
    a. of chronic disease
    chronic hemolytic a. (CHA)
    Chvostek a.
    cold-type autoimmune hemolytic a.
    congenital aplastic a.
    congenital dyserythropoietic a.
    congenital hypoplastic a. (CHA)
    constitutional aplastic a.

NOTES

anemia *(continued)*
    Cooley a.
    Coombs-negative hemolytic a.
    crescent cell a.
    cytogenic a.
    Czerny a.
    Diamond-Blackfan a.
    dimorphic a.
    drepanocytic a.
    Dresbach a.
    drug-induced immune hemolytic a.
    dyserythropoietic a.
    Edelmann a.
    elliptocytotic a.
    erythronormoblastic a.
    Estren-Dameshek a.
    extravascular hemolytic a.
    extrinsic hemolytic a.
    Faber a.
    Fanconi a.
    globe cell a.
    ground itch a.
    Heinz body hemolytic a.
    hemolytic a.
    Herrick a.
    hookworm a.
    hyperproliferative a.
    hypersplenic a.
    hypochromic a.
    hypoplastic a.
    hypoproliferative a.
    iatrogenic a.
    idiopathic hypochromic a.
    immune hemolytic a.
    immune-mediated a.
    inherited hemolytic a.
    intrinsic hemolytic a.
    iron-deficiency a.
    Jaksch a.
    Josephs-Diamond-Blackfan a.
    Lederer a.
    leukoerythroblastic a.
    macrocytic a.
    march a.
    megaloblastic a.
    microangiopathic hemolytic a.
    miner's a.
    mountain a.
    myelopathic a.
    myelophthisic a.
    neonatal a.
    a. neonatorum
    normochromic a.
    normocytic a.
    normocytic, normochromic a.
    nosocomial a.
    paraneoplastic a.
    pernicious a. (PA)
    phenylhydrazine a.

    phlebotomy-related a.
    polar a.
    pyridoxine-responsive a.
    radiation a.
    refractory a.
    Rundles-Falls a.
    Runeberg a.
    scorbutic a.
    severe aplastic a. (SAA)
    sickle cell a. (SCA)
    sideroblastic a.
    simple achlorhydric a.
    spur cell a.
    thrombopenic a.
    tropical macrocytic a.
    von Jaksch a.
    warm-and-cold-type autoimmune
      hemolytic a.
    warm-antibody acquired autoimmune
      hemolytic a.
    warm-type autoimmune hemolytic a.
    Witts a.
anemic hypoxia
anergic
anergy
    T-cell a.
    a. test
anesthesia
    epidural a.
    general a.
    halothane a.
    local a.
    1-lung a.
    regional a.
    saddle block a.
anesthetic
    epidural a.
    eutectic mixture of local a.'s
      (EMLA)
    general a.
    local a.
    Orajel Brace-Aid oral a.
    regional a.
    topical a.
aneuploid
    a. colorectal carcinoma
    a. NBX tumor
aneuploidy
    DNA a.
    tumor a.
aneurysm
    abdominal aortic a.
    anastomotic a.
    aortic a.
    arterial a.
    arteriovenous a.
    bacterial a.
    berry a.
    bifurcation a.

A

brain a.
cerebral a.
intracranial a. (ICA)
aneurysmal
a. bone cyst
a. clip
a. dilatation
a. proportion
aneurysmectomy
aneurysmogram
aneurysmograph
aneusomy analysis
Anexsia
ANF
antinuclear factor
Anger gamma camera system
angiitis, angitis
allergic granulomatous a.
frosted branch a.
granulomatous a.
lymphocytic a.
angiitis-granulomatosis disorder
angina
abdominal a.
a. pectoris (AP)
angioblastic lymphadenopathy
angioblastoma
angiocardiography
exercise radionuclide a.
angiocentric
a. immunoproliferative disorder
a. immunoproliferative lesion (AIL)
a. lymphoproliferative lesion
a. NK-cell lymphoma
a. T-cell lymphoma
Angiocol
angiodynography
angiodysgenetic
angiodysplasia
angioedema
angioendotheliomatosis
malignant a.
neoplastic proliferating a.
angioendotheliosis
angiofibroma
giant cell a.
juvenile nasopharyngeal a. (JNPA)
angiofollicular
a. lymph node hyperplasia
a. lymphoid hyperplasia
a. and plasmacytic polyadenopathy
angiogenesis
endogenous inhibitor of a.

a. inhibitor
neoplastic a.
tumor a.
angiogenic
a. cell
a. factor
a. stimulus
angiogenin
angiograph
angiographic
a. guidewire
a. occlusion
a. success
a. Teflon dilator
a. 2-wire snare
angiography
aortic arch a.
axial a.
balloon occlusion pulmonary a.
basilar a.
biplane a.
bronchial a.
a. catheter
cerebral a.
computed tomographic a.
digital subtraction a.
spiral CT a.
angioimmunoblastic
a. lymphadenopathy (AIL)
a. lymphadenopathy-like T-cell lymphoma
a. lymphadenopathy with dysproteinemia (AILD)
a. lymphadenopathy with dysproteinemia-like T-cell lymphoma
a. T-cell lymphoma (ATCL)
angioinfarction
angioleiomyoma
angiolipofibroma
angiolipoma
epidural a.
spinal epidural a.
angiolithic sarcoma
angiolymphoid hyperplasia
angioma, pl. angiomata
arterial a.
capillary a.
cherry a.
encephalic a.
extracerebral cavernous a.
a. lymphaticum
a. serpiginosum

NOTES

31

angioma *(continued)*
    spider a.
    superficial a.
    telangiectatic a.
    a. venosum racemosum
    venous a.
angiomatoid
    a. malignant fibrous histiocytoma
    a. tumor
angiomatosis
    bacillary a.
    bacillary epithelioid a. (BEA)
    cystic a.
    encephalotrigeminal a.
    epithelioid a.
    retinal a.
angiomatous
    a. disease
    a. lymphoid hamartoma
Angiomax
angiomyofibroblastoma
angiomyofibroma
angiomyofibrosarcoma
angiomyoid
    a. lesion
    a. proliferation
angiomyolipoma
    atypical a. (AA, AAML)
    renal a.
angiomyoma
angiomyosarcoma
angiomyxoma
angioneuromyoma
angioosteohypertrophy syndrome
angiopathy
    cerebral amyloid a.
angioplasty
    aortoiliac a.
    balloon dilation a.
    percutaneous excimer laser
      coronary a. (PELCA)
    percutaneous low-stress a.
    renal a.
AngioRad ^{192}Ir wire source
angioreticuloma
angiosarcoma
    a. bone tumor
    hepatic a.
    uterine a.
angioscopic guidance
angioscopy
angiostatin with radiation therapy
angiotensin
    a. amide
    a. III (AT-III)
angiotensin-converting enzyme (ACE)
angiotropic large cell lymphoma
angitis *(var. of* angiitis)

angle
    basal a.
    beam a.
    cardiophrenic a.
    carinal a.
    cerebellopontine a.
angularis
ani (*pl. of* anus)
anicteric bile duct
anidulafungin
aniline
    a. fuchsin
    a. gentian violet
    a. red
anionic neutrophil-activating peptide (ANAP)
aniridia
anisakiasis
anisochromia
anisocytosis
anisoleukocytosis
anisopoikilocytosis
anisotropic tissue
anisotropy factor
ankle
    a. joint
    a. mortise fracture
ankle-arm index (AAI)
ankle-brachial
    a.-b. index (ABI)
    a.-b. pressure measurement
ankylosing
    a. hyperostosis
    a. spondylitis
ankylosis
    bony a.
ankyrin deficiency
ANLL
    acute nonlymphoblastic leukemia
    acute nonlymphocytic leukemia
ANN
    artificial neural network
Ann
    A. Arbor classification
    A. Arbor classification of Hodgkin
      disease staging
    A. Arbor/Cotswold staging
      classification
    A. Arbor staging system I-IV
annamycin
    liposomal a.
anneal
annealing
    simulated a.
annihilation
    a. photon
    a. radiation
annular *(var. of* anular)
annulus *(var. of* anulus), pl. **annuli**

Anodynos-DHC
anogenital
- a. cancer
- a. squamous intraepithelial neoplasia
- a. wart

anoikis
anomala
Hansenula a.
anomalous
- a. antigen expression
- a. branching
- a. innominate artery compression syndrome
- a. junction
- a. left coronary artery
- a. origin
- a. pulmonary venous return
- a. serum chemistry

anomaly, pl. **anomalies**
- Alius-Grignaschi a.
- anorectal a.
- atrioventricular junction a.
- congenital a.
- Fox-Fordyce a.
- Huët-Pelger nuclear a.
- May-Hegglin a.
- microgastria-limb reduction a.
- Pelger a.
- Pelger-Huët a.
- Steinbrinck a.

anorchia
anorectal
- a. anomaly
- a. atresia
- a. fistula
- a. herpes
- a. lymphoma
- a. malformation
- a. melanoma
- a. tuberculosis

anorectum
cloacogenic carcinoma of a.
anorexia
- a. nervosa
- paraneoplastic a.

anoxia
- cellular a.
- cerebral a.

anoxic encephalopathy
Ansaid Oral
anserinus
pes a.

antagonist
- endothelin-receptor a.
- estrogen a.
- folate a.
- folic acid a.
- 5-HT$_3$ receptor a.
- 5-hydroxytryptamine type 3 receptor a.
- IL-1 receptor a.
- insulin a.
- integrin a.
- LHRH a.
- neurokinin-1 receptor a.
- opioid a.
- progesterone receptor a.
- RG 12915 serotonin a.
- serotonin a.

antagonistic pattern
antalgic gait
Antazone
antecedent
plasma thromboplastin a.
antecolic
antecubital
- a. approach
- a. fossa
- a. vein

antedate
anteflexed uterus
antegrade
- a. catheterization
- a. ejaculation
- a. flow
- a. puncture
- a. pyelogram
- a. venography

anterior
- a. cerebral artery
- a. choroidal artery
- a. clear space
- a. column fracture
- a. commissure (AC)
- a. commissure ligament
- a. communicating artery
- a. condylar canal
- a. condyloid foramen
- a. cruciate ligament
- a. exenteration
- a. horn cell disease
- a. iliac crest
- a. junction line
- a. labroligamentous periosteal sleeve

NOTES

anterior (*continued*)
   a. labroligamentous periosteal sleeve avulsion
   a. mediastinal mass
   a. osteophyte
   a. palatine foramen
   a. sacral foramen
   a. sagittal diameter
   a. scalloping
   a. scalloping of vertebrae
   a. spinal artery
   a. spinal artery syndrome
   a. spinal ligament
   a. spinal ligament calcification
   a. tibial bowing
   a. tibial tendon
   a. tracking
anterior-posterior repair
anterolateral
   a. abdominal wall
   a. compression fracture
   a. system
anteroposterior (AP)
   a. projection
anteroposterior/posteroanterior (AP/PA)
anterovertebral
antetracheal node
anteverted uterus
antherpetic (*var. of* antiherpetic)
anthracenedione
anthracosilicosis
   conglomerate a.
anthracosis
anthracotic material
anthracycline
   a. cardiomyopathy
   liposomal a.
   morpholino a.
   semisynthetic a.
anthracycline-based
   a.-b. induction chemotherapy
   a.-b. therapy
anthracycline-nave metastatic breast cancer
anthracycline-refractory metastatic breast carcinoma
anthramycin
anthrapyrazole
   DuP 937 a.
   DuP 996 a.
anthraquinone
anthrax
Anthron heparinized catheter
anthropometric
   a. measure
   a. test
anti-ABO antibody
antiacetylcholine receptor antibody

antiandrogen
   nonsteroidal a. (NSAA)
   steroidal a.
   a. withdrawal
antianemia
   a. factor
   a. principle
antiangiogenesis
   a. agent
   a. factor
   a. gene therapy
antiangiogenic
   a. agent
   a. molecule
   a. therapy
antiantibody formation
antiantitoxin
antiapoptotic
   a. effect
   a. property
   a. signaling pathway
antiarrhythmic
anti-B19 antibody test
anti-B4-blocked ricin
antibacterial agent
antibasement membrane antibody
anti-B-cell antibody
antibiosis
antibiotic
   antitumor a.
   broad-spectrum a.
   duocarmycin a.
   a. prophylaxis
   semisynthetic duocarmycin a.
   a. therapy
antibiotic-resistant bacteria
antibioticus
   Streptomyces a.
antiblastic perfusion
antibody, pl. **antibodies (Ab)**
   Ab1 a.
   Ab2 a.
   ABX-CBL monoclonal a.
   ABX-EGF monoclonal a.
   AML-2-23 monoclonal a.
   17-1A monoclonal a.
   anti-ABO a.
   antiacetylcholine receptor a.
   antibasement membrane a.
   anti-B-cell a.
   anti-CALLA, hybridoma a.
   anticardiolipin a. (ACA)
   anti-CD52 a.
   anti-CD18 humanized a.
   anti-CD22 a.
   anti-CD31 monoclonal a.
   anticentromere a.
   anti-CNA a.
   anticytoplasmic a.

anti-D a.
anti-DNA a.
anti-EBV a.
anti-E-cadherin monoclonal a.
anti-EGFr a.
antiepidermal growth factor receptor
  monoclonal a.
antifibrin a.
antifibronectin a.
antigranulocyte a.
anti-HER-2 monoclonal a.
anti-HIV a.
anti-HLA a.
anti-HTLV-I a.
antiidiotype a.
antiimmunocytokeratin a.
anti-IRF-1 a.
anti-IRF-2 a.
antimitochondrial a. (AMA)
antineuronal a.
antineutrophilic cytoplasmic a.
  (ANCA)
antinuclear a. (ANA)
anti-PD-ECGF monoclonal a.
antiphenyloxazolone a.
antiphospholipid a. (APA)
antispermicidal monoclonal a.
anti-T12 a.
anti-Tac a.
antithymidylate synthase
  polyclonal a.
antithyroglobulin a.
antityrosinase a.
antivascular endothelial growth
  factor monoclonal a.
anti-Yo serum a.
autologous a.
automated enzyme immunoassay for
  antinuclear a.
Bexxar radiolabeled monoclonal a.
bifunctional a.
bispecific a.
blocking a.
BR64 a.
BR96 a.
BrE-1 a.
BrE-2 a.
BrE-3 a.
Campath humanized monoclonal a.
2C3 anti-VEGF a.
caspase-9 a.
CC49 monoclonal a.
CD3 monoclonal a.

CD5+ monoclonal a.
CD45Ro a.
cell-bound a.
cell-fixed a.
cell-mediated a.
chelated a.
chimeric anti-GD3 a.
chimeric L6 monoclonal a.
cold a.
combining-site a.
complement-fixing a. (CFA)
cryptosporidiosis a.
CSLEX1 monoclonal a.
cyclophosphamide, total body
  irradiation, monoclonal antibodies
cytophilic a.
CytoTAb polyclonal a.
cytotoxic a.
DAB389 a.
a. deficiency syndrome
a. deposition
Di-dgA-RFB4 monoclonal a.
direct fluorescent a. (DFA)
Donath-Landsteiner a.
Duffy a.
EGF-receptor specific monoclonal a.
envelope a.
antibodies to Epstein-Barr virus
  transactivator protein (ZEBRA)
erythrocyte a.
F_2 a.
fluorescein isothiocyanate-conjugated
  secondary a.
fluorescent antinuclear a. (FANA)
fluorophore-linked a.
a. formation
Forssman a.
gastric tumor marker a.
GBM a.
G25 monoclonal a.
HBME-1 a.
hemagglutinating a.
heterogenetic a.
heterophil a.
high-affinity a.
HIK1083 a.
HIV a.
HMB45 a.
human antimouse a. (HAMA)
human immunodeficiency virus a.
humanized anticancer bispecific a.
humanized antihuman IL-2
  receptor a. (anti-Tac)

NOTES

antibody *(continued)*
humoral a.
hybridoma a.
^{131}I antitenascin monoclonal a.
I-B1 radiolabeled a.
idiotype a.
IFN-alfa-2b a.
IgA a.
IgY a.
^{131}I-labeled anti-CD20 a.
^{131}I-labeled anti-CD45 a.
^{131}I-labeled B-cell-specific anti-CD20 monoclonal a.
immune a.
immunofluorescence a. (IFA)
isophil a.
Kell a.
Kidd a.
kidney-fixing a.
Ki-67 monoclonal a.
a. labeling
Leu monoclonal a.
Lewis a.
a. linkage method
LKM1 a.
Lutheran a.
Lym-1 monoclonal a.
lymphotoxic a.
M344 a.
Mc1 a.
Mc5 a.
mitochondrial a.
MoAb 425 a.
monoclonal a. (MAb, MoAb)
monoclonal a. B43.13
monoclonal a. B72.3
murine L6 monoclonal a.
natural a.
neutralizing a.
nonmitogenic humanized anti-CD3 a.
NR-LU-10 a.
OKB7 monoclonal a.
OKT3 anti-CD3 monoclonal a.
Oncolym radiolabeled monoclonal a.
opsonizing a.
Orthoclone OKT3 monoclonal a.
Ortho-mune a.
osteosarcoma antigen-associated monoclonal a.
a. panel
PGM 37 a.
PM-81 monoclonal a.
polyclonal CD3 a.
pretargeted a.
radiolabeled monoclonal a.
a. radionucleotide
a. radionucleotide conjugate

a. reaction site
recombinant anti-p185HER2 monoclonal a. (rhuMAb HER-2)
a. response
Rh a.
ricin-blocked a.
RSV-specific monoclonal a.
SM3 a.
SMART M195 a.
targeted radiotherapy using ^{131}I anti-CD20 a.
thrombomodulin a.
a. titer
Toxoplasma IgG a.
TSH-displacing a.
virus-neutralizing a.
warm-reactive a.
antibody-antigen complex
antibody-based detection system
antibody-dependent
a.-d. cell cytotoxicity (ADCC)
a.-d. cell-mediated cytotoxicity (ADCC)
a.-d. cellular cytotoxicity (ADCC)
a.-d. enhancement
antibody-directed
a.-d. catalysis (ADC)
a.-d. enzyme prodrug therapy (ADEPT)
antibody-positive
HTLV-I a.-p.
a.-p. woman
anticachectic effect
anti-CALLA, hybridoma antibody
anticancer
a. drug
a. vaccine
anticarcinogen
anticardiolipin antibody (ACA)
anti-cathepsin D autoantibody assay
anti-CD18 humanized antibody
anti-CD22 antibody
anti-CD31 monoclonal antibody
anti-CD33
bismuth-213-HuM195 a.-CD33
M195 monoclonal antibody a.-CD33
recombinant engineered human a.-CD33
anti-CD52 antibody
anti-CD3 stimulated peripheral blood lymphocyte
anti-CEA
a.-CEA antibody immunoscintigraphy
^{99m}Tc a.-CEA
anticentromere antibody
anticholinergic
a. agent
a. drug

anticipatory vomiting
anticlotting agent
anti-CNA antibody
anticoagulant (AC)
    lupus-like a.
    a. protein
anticoagulation
anticonvulsant
anticrotalus serum
anticryptosporidium
    bovine a.
anti-cytochrome P4502D6 assay
anticytokeratin
    monoclonal a. (MAK-6)
anticytoplasmic
    a. antibody
    a. antibody test
    a. autoantibody (ACPA)
anti-D antibody
antidepressant
    selective serotonin reuptake
      inhibitor a.
    SSRI a.
    tricyclic a. (TCA)
antidiarrheal agent
antidiuretic hormone (ADH)
anti-DNA antibody
antidotally beneficial
antidote
    Hall a.
anti-EBV antibody
anti-E-cadherin monoclonal antibody
anti-EGFr antibody
anti-ELAM-1
    monoclonal mouse anti-ELAM-1
antiembolism stockings
antiemetic agent
antiepidermal
    a. growth factor receptor
    a. growth factor receptor
      monoclonal antibody
antiepileptic
antiestrogen
    nonsteroidal a.
    pure a.
    a. therapy
antiestrogenic
    a. activity
    a. property
antiferritin
    a. antibody linked to [131]I
    yttrium-90-labeled a.
antiferromagnetism

antifibrin antibody
antifibrinolysin
antifibronectin antibody
antifolate
    multitargeted a. (MTA)
antifungal
    Aftate A.
    a. agent
    Breezee Mist A.
    echinocandin a.
    a. prophylaxis
    a. therapy
antigen (Ag)
    ABH blood group carbohydrate a.
    ABH/Lewis-related a.
    ABH(O) cell surface a.
    activation-associated a.
    allogeneic a.
    alpha-1-antichymotrypsin-prostate-
      specific a.
    autologous tumor rejection a.
    B-cell lineage a.
    B7-DC a.
    beef heart a.
    blood cell a.
    blood group a.
    B-ly-7 a.
    breast cancer a.
    cancer a. (CA)
    cancer a. 125 (CA125, CA-125)
    cancer-associated serum a. (CASA)
    a. capture assay
    carbohydrate a. 19-9
    carcinoembryonic a. (CEA)
    carcinoid embryonic a.
    CD a.
    CD18 a.
    CD21 a.
    CD33 a.
    CD34 a.
    CD52 a.
    CD5 surface a.
    cell-bound a.
    class II histocompatibility a.
    common acute leukemia a.
    common acute lymphoblastic
      leukemia a. (CALLA)
    common leukocyte a.
    complexed prostate-specific a.
      (cPSA)
    conjugated a.
    cutaneous lymphocyte a.
    cytokeratin membrane a.

NOTES

antigen *(continued)*
  cytoplasmic CD3 a.
  cytoskeletal a.
  a. deficiency
  delta a.
  a. determinant
  DF3 a.
  differentiation a.
  diphtheria a.
  Duffy a.
  E a.
  early a.
  early prostate cancer a. (EPCA)
  endogenous a.
  endothelial localization of a.
  env a.
  epithelial membrane a. (EMA)
  Epstein-Barr nuclear a. (EBNA)
  exogenous a.
  a. expression
  extractable nuclear a.
  factor VII a. (VII:Ag)
  factor IX a. (IX:Ag)
  factor X a. (X:Ag)
  factor VIII-related a.
  fecal carcinoembryonic a.
  Forssman a.
  Frei a.
  Fy a.
  GD2 cancer-associated a.
  Gm a.
  gp100 melanoma a.
  Gross cell surface a.
  H a.
  H-2 a.
  Hangar-Rose skin test a.
  Helmes 3 a.
  hematopoietic cell surface a.
  hepatitis-associated a. (HAA)
  hepatitis B surface a. (HBsAg)
  heterogeneic a.
  heterologous a.
  heterophil a.
  histocompatibility a.
  HIV viral a.
  HLA-L a.
  homologous a.
  human hematopoietic progenitor
    cell a.
  human immunodeficiency virus a.
  human leukemia-associated a.
  human leukocyte a. (HLA)
  human leukocyte a. B27 (HLA-
    B27)
  human leukocyte a. B57 (HLA-
    B57)
  human leukocyte Cw5 a.
  HUTCH-1 a.
  H-Y a.

  Ia a.
  idiotypic a.
  IIIB-based gp120 a.
  International Workshop and
    Conference on Human Leukocyte
    Differentiation A.'s
  intracellular a.
  isogeneic a.
  isophil a.
  K a.
  Ki-1 a.
  Ki-67 nuclear a.
  Km a.
  Kveim a.
  L26 a.
  large granular lymphocyte a.
  late a.
  LD a.
  Le blood group a.
  Leu-8 a.
  leukocyte common a.
  Lewis A, Y a.
  Lewis blood group a.
  lineage-associated a.
  Ly a.
  Lyb a.
  lymphocyte function a.
  lymphocyte function-associated a.
    (LFA)
  lymphocyte function-associated a. 1
    (LFA-1)
  lymphocyte function-associated a. 2
    (LFA-2)
  lymphocyte function-associated a. 3
    (LFA-3)
  lymphogranuloma venereum a.
  Lyt a.
  lytic-associated nuclear a. (LANA)
  M a.
  M344 a.
  Mac-1 a.
  macrophage lineage a.
  major histocompatibility complex a.
  mammary serum a. (MSA)
  matrix a.
  melanoma-associated a.
  melanoma-specific a.
  MHC class II a.
  minor histocompatibility a.
  Mitsuda a.
  MO1 a.
  monoclonal antibody-defined a.
  monocyte lineage a.
  MUC1 a.
  mumps skin test a.
  myeloid-associated a.
  myeloid lineage a.
  myelomonocytic a.
  natural killer cell a.

NR a.
nuclear proliferation a.
O a.
oncofetal a.
organ-specific a.
osteosarcoma a.
Oz a.
pancreatic oncofetal a.
panhematopoietic cell a.
parenteral a.
perinuclear CD15 a.
phytohemagglutinin a.
preferential B-cell
  panhematopoietic a.
preferential T-cell
  panhematopoietic a.
a. presentation
proliferating cell nuclear a.
  (PCNA)
prostate-specific a. (PSA)
prostate-specific membrane a.
  (PSMA)
a. receptor
a. receptor gene
recombinant fowlpox virus encoding
  the gp100 melanoma a.
red blood cell a.
a. restriction
Rh factor a.
serum hepatitis a.
serum tissue polypeptide a. (S-
  TPA)
sialyl Lewis a.
sialyl-Tn a. (STn)
soluble a.
squamous cell carcinoma a. (SCC-
  Ag)
stem cell donor a.
surface-marker a.
TB a.
tetanus a.
Thomsen-Friedenreich T a.
thymic lymphocyte a.
tissue polypeptide a. (TPA)
a. titer
a. tolerance
transplantation a.
tuberculosis a.
tumor a.
tumor-associated a. (TAA)
tumor-associated glycoprotein-72 a.
tumor-associated transplantation a.
  (TATA)

tumor-derived a.
tumor-specific a. (TSA)
tumor-specific transplantation a.
  (TSTA)
tyrosinase melanoma a.
a. unmasking
antigen-antibody complex
antigenemia
  HIV a.
  immune complex-dissociated p24 a.
  p24 a.
antigenetic
antigenic
  a. competition
  a. determinant
  a. drift
  a. modulation
  a. paralysis
  a. shift
  a. stimulation
  a. target
antigenicity
  lowered tumor a.
  tumor a.
antigen-presenting cell (APC)
antigen-processing gene Ii
antigen-pulsed autologous dendritic cell
antigen-sensitive cell
antigen-specific T cell
antigliadin
  a. IgA ELISA autoimmune test
  a. IgG ELISA autoimmune test
antigonadotropin
antigranulocyte antibody
anti-HAV
  a.-HAV IgG
  a.-HAV IgM
anti-HBc IgM
anti-HDV Ig
antihemagglutinin
antihemolytic
antihemophilic
  a. factor
  a. factor A
  a. factor human
  a. factor method M
  a. factor VIII FS
  a. globulin (AHG)
antihemorrhagic factor
antihepatitis
  a. A virus immunoglobulin G, M
  a. B core immunoglobulin G
  a. C virus-positive cirrhosis

NOTES

39

antihepatitis *(continued)*
   a. delta virus immunoglobulin
   a. E virus immunoglobulin
anti-HER-2 monoclonal antibody
antiherpetic, antherpetic
   a. agent
anti-HEV Ig
anti-HHV8 antibody titer
antihistamine
anti-HIV
   a.-HIV antibody
   a.-HIV immune serum globulin
   a.-HIV protease inhibitor
anti-HLA antibody
antihormone
anti-HTLV-I antibody
anti-Hu antineuronal autoantibody
anti-human
   a.-h. globulin
   a.-h. herpesvirus 8 antibody titer
   a.-h. immunodeficiency virus
      protease inhibitor
   a.-h. S5 analog
antihyperlipidemic
anti-ICAM-1
   monoclonal mouse a.-ICAM-1
antiidiotype
   a. antibody
   a. immune response
antiidiotypic
   a. affinity chromatography
   a. immunoglobulin response
antiimmunocytokeratin antibody
antiimmunoglobulin
antiinfective
antiinflammatory agent
antiinhibitor
   a. coagulant complex
   a. coagulant complex, vapor heated
anti-IRF-1 antibody
anti-IRF-2 antibody
anti-Kaposi sarcoma
anti-Lewisite
   British a.-L. (BAL)
antilymphocyte serum (ALS)
antimacrophage
antimalarial
   a. agent
   primaquine phosphate a.
antimetabolite
   a. induction
   purine a.
   pyrimidine nucleoside a.
antimicrotubule agent
antimitochondrial antibody (AMA)
antimitogenic signal
antimitotic drug
antimoniotungstate
anti-MY9-blocked ricin

antimycobacterial prophylaxis
antineoplastic
   a. agent
   a. combined chemotherapy protocol
   a. drug
   a. therapy
antineoplaston
   a. A10
   a. A10 and As2-1 therapy
   a. A10/low-dose methotrexate
      combination
   a. As2-1
antineuronal antibody
antineutrophilic cytoplasmic antibody
   (ANCA)
antinociceptive procedure
antinuclear
   a. antibody (ANA)
   a. factor (ANF)
antioncogene
antioxidant
   alpha-tocopherol a.
   extracellular a.
antiparasitic agent
anti-PD-ECGF monoclonal antibody
antiphenyloxazolone antibody
antiphosphatidylserine-prothrombin
   complex antibody testing
antiphospholipid antibody (APA)
antiphosphotyrosine
antiplasmin
   Stachrom a.
antiplatelet
   a. agent
   a. antibody assay
   a. therapy
antipleiotrophin therapy
antipneumocystis
antipolycythemic
antiprogestin
antiproliferative
   a. activity
   a. agent
   a. effect
   a. property
antiprotrusio cage
antipruritic
antireceptor
antiretroviral
   a. agent
   a. drug
   a. therapy (ART)
anti-rev construct
anti-RhD
anti-Ri syndrome
anti-Schiff stain
antisense
   bcl-2 a.
   a. drug

a. oligonucleotide
a. oligos
antisepsis
hand a.
antiserum, pl. **antisera**
human a.
antismooth muscle actin
antispermicidal monoclonal antibody
antistreptolysin
a. O (ASO)
a. O titer
anti-T12 antibody
anti-Tac
humanized antihuman IL-2 receptor
antibody
anti-Tac antibody
humanized anti-Tac
anti-Tac(Fv)-PE38 LMB-2
anti-TAP-72 immunotoxin
anti-T-cell therapy
antitelomerase
a. agent
a. antisense oligonucleotide
antithrombin (AT)
human a. III
a. III
antithymidylate synthase polyclonal antibody
antithymocyte globulin (ATG)
antithyroglobulin antibody
antitoxin response
antitoxoplasma therapy
antitoxoplasmosis agent
anti-toxo therapy
antitrypsin
alpha-1 a.
antitrypsin deficiency
antitumor
a. activity
a. antibiotic
a. cytotoxic lymphocyte
a. drug
a. effect
a. vaccine
antityrosinase antibody
antivascular endothelial growth factor monoclonal antibody
anti-VCAM-1
monoclonal mouse a.-VCAM-1
2C3 anti-VEGF antibody
antiviral
a. activity
a. agent

a. immunity
a. therapy
Antivirogram test procedure
anti-Yo serum antibody
Antoni neurilemoma
antra (*pl. of* antrum)
antral
a. beaking
a. exclusion
a. exclusion procedure
a. lavage
a. mucosa
a. mucosal diaphragm
a. mucosal thickening
a. padding
a. polyp
a. stricture
a. ulcer
a. web
Antril
antrochoanal polyp
antroduodenal motility
antropyloric canal
antrostomy
antrum, pl. **antra**
aditus ad a.
Anturane
anuclear cell
anular, annular
a. abscess
a. array
a. calcification
a. constricting lesion
a. disc
a. disc bulge
a. fiber
a. fibrosis
a. pancreas
a. phased-array hyperthermia
anulare
granuloma a.
anulus, pl. **anuli**
bulging a.
a. fibrosus tear
anuria
anus, pl. **ani**
ectopic a.
Anusol-HC Suppository
Anusol Ointment
anxiolysis
anxiolytic
nonbenzodiazepine a.
Anzemet

NOTES

AOP
aminooxypentane
AOPA
ara-C, Oncovin, prednisone, L-asparaginase
AOPE
Adriamycin, Oncovin, prednisone, etoposide
AOPE chemotherapy protocol
AOP-RANTES
aminooxypentane regulated-on-activation normal T-expressed and secreted
aorta, pl. **aortae**
abdominal a.
ascending a.
aortic
a. aneurysm
a. anulus abscess
a. aperture
a. arch
a. arch angiography
a. arch atresia
a. balloon pump
a. bifurcation
a. bifurcation prosthesis
a. body tumor
a. coarctation
a. dissection
a. flow volume
a. foramen
a. graft
a. injury
a. insufficiency
a. isthmus
a. kinking
a. knob
a. lymph node
a. motion artifact
a. nipple
a. node metastasis
a. opening
a. regurgitation
a. root
a. rupture
a. stenosis
a. thrombosis
a. transection
a. valve
a. valve atresia
a. valve echocardiography
a. valve lesion
a. valvular disease
a. wall necrosis
a. window
aorticopulmonary, aortopulmonary
a. window
a. window shunt
aorticorenal graft
aorticosympathetic paraganglion

aortic-pulmonic window
aortitis
bacterial a.
giant cell a.
syphilitic a.
aortobifemoral bypass
aortoenteric fistula
aortofemoral
a. bypass (AFB)
a. bypass graft
aortography
abdominal a.
ascending a.
aortoiliac
a. angioplasty
a. bypass graft
a. disease
a. inflow system
aortoplasty
aortopulmonary (*var. of* aorticopulmonary)
aortovisceral bypass
AP
adenomatous polyp
Adriamycin and Platinol
alkaline phosphatase
aminopeptidase
angina pectoris
anteroposterior
AP portal
AP projection
AP repair
AP-1
activating protein-1
AP-2 gamma protein
APA
aldosterone-producing adenoma
antiphospholipid antibody
Asserachrom APA
APAAP
alkaline phosphatase-antialkaline phosphatase
Apacet
APAF
apoptosis activating factor
apallic syndrome
Apatate
apathy
apatite deposition disease
APBI
accelerated partial breast irradiation
APBSCT
autologous peripheral blood stem cell transplantation
A-P-C
adenoidal-pharyngeal-conjunctival
A-P-C virus
APC
adenomatous polyposis of colon

AMSA, prednisone, chlorambucil
antigen-presenting cell
  APC gene
  APC gene mutation assay
  APC stool test
APD
  aminohydroxypropylidene diphosphate
APE
  Adriamycin, Platinol, etoposide
  ara-C, Platinol, etoposide
Apert syndrome
aperture
  aortic a.
  beam a.
  collimation a.
  a. diaphragm
apex, pl. **apices**
  a. of heart
aphasia
  Wernicke a.
apheresis
  single-donor a.
  subclavian a.
aphidicolin
Aphrodyne
aphrophilus
  Haemophilus a.
APHSCS
  autologous peripheral hematopoietic stem
  cell support
aphtha, pl. **aphthae**
  major aphthae
aphthous
  a. stomatitis
  a. ulcer
  a. ulceration
apical
  a. cap sign
  a. cardiac nodal enlargement
  a. granuloma
  a. lordotic projection
  a. lordotic view
  a. notch
  a. petrositis
  a. pleural thickening
  a. vagina
apices (*pl. of* apex)
apiospermum
  Scedosporium a.
APL
  acute promyelocytic leukemia
  APL 400-047 HIV-1 core structural
  protein

aplasia
  blood cell a.
  bone marrow a.
  a. cutis
  germinal a.
  idiopathic megakaryocytic a.
  pure red cell a.
  red cell a. (RCA)
  tibia a.
  uterine a.
aplastic
  a. anemia
  a. crisis
  a. lymph
Aplidin
APML
  acute promyelocytic leukemia
apnea
  sleep a.
apnea/bradycardia ratio
APO
  Adriamycin, prednisone, Oncovin
  APO chemotherapy protocol
Apo-Acetazolamide
Apo-Allopurinol
Apo-Alpraz
Apo-Amitriptyline
Apo-Amoxi
Apo-Ampi
Apo-ASA
Apo-Bisacodyl
APOC2 region
Apo-Cal
Apo-Carbamazepine
Apo-Cephalex
Apo-Chlorpromazine
Apo-Chlorthalidone
Apo-Cimetidine
Apo-Clorazepate
Apo-Cloxi
apocrine
  a. adenocarcinoma
  a. adenoma
  a. carcinoma
  a. cyst
  a. cystadenoma
  a. hidrocystoma
  a. sweat gland
Apo-Diclo
Apo-Diflunisal
Apo-Dipyridamole FC
Apo-Doxepin
Apo-Doxy Tabs

NOTES

Apo-Famotidine
Apo-Ferrous
    A.-F. Gluconate
    A.-F. Sulfate
Apo-Flurbiprofen
Apo-Folic
Apo-Furosemide
Apogee 800 ultrasound system
Apo-Gemfibrozil
Apo-Hydro
Apo-Ibuprofen
Apo-Imipramine
Apo-Indomethacin
Apo-ISDN
Apo-Keto-E
apolipoprotein
Apo-Minocycline
Apo-Naproxen
aponeurotic fibroma
Apo-Nifed
Apo-Nitrofurantoin
Apo-Oxazepam
apophylaxis
apophysial, apophyseal
    a. fracture
    a. injury
apophysis, pl. **apophyses**
Apo-Piroxicam
apoplexy
    pituitary a.
Apo-Prednisone
Apo-Primidone
Apo-Propranolol
apoptosis
    a. activating factor (APAF)
    a. assay
    Fas-mediated a.
    HIV-induced a.
    homing-induced a.
    staurosporine-induced a.
apoptotic
    a. cell
    a. cell death
    a. index (AI)
    a. response
Apo-Ranitidine
Apo-Sulfamethoxazole
Apo-Sulfatrim
Apo-Sulfinpyrazone
Apo-Sulin
Apo-Tamox
Apo-Tetra
Apo-Triazide
Apo-Trihex
Apo-Trimip
Apo-Zidovudine

AP/PA
    anteroposterior/posteroanterior
    AP/PA portal
apparatus, pl. **apparatus**
    Bio-Rad Sequi-Gen a.
    contractile a.
    Golgi a.
    Skatron a.
    Warburg a.
apparent
    a. diffusion coefficient
    a. paramagnetism
appearance
    apple core a.
    apple peel a.
    applesauce a.
    ball-in-hand a.
    beaded a.
    beaked a.
    bone-within-bone a.
    candle drippings a.
    cystic a.
    echopenic a.
    harlequin a.
    moccasin a.
    owl's eye a.
    scalloped a.
    shaggy a.
    strandlike a.
appendage
    atrial a.
    skin a.
appendectomy
appendiceal
    a. abscess
    a. cancer
appendices (*pl. of* appendix)
appendicitis
appendicolith
appendicular
    a. sign
    a. skeleton
appendix, pl. **appendices**
    a. mucocele
apple
    a. core appearance
    a. core carcinoma
    a. peel appearance
applesauce appearance
application
    Advantage Fusion a.
    Hawkeye SPECT a.
    surface-dose a.
applicator
    Advantage4D PET/CT a.
    Bloedorn a.
    brachytherapy balloon a.
    colpostat a.
    Delrin a.

double-balloon a.
Henschke seed a.
intracavitary balloon a.
Mallinckrodt Institute of Radiology
  Afterloading Vaginal A.
  (MIRALVA)
Mick seed a.
Syed-Puthawala-Hedger
  esophageal a.
tandem a.
Wang a.
Applied Immune Sciences (AIS)
apposition
approach
antecubital a.
Bentley-Milan a.
brachial artery a.
cytokine-based a.
genetic a.
integrated trimodality a.
molecular a.
neurosurgical a.
nonpharmacological a.
psychological a.
ray tracing a.
therapeutic a.
Trager a.
transcubital a.
transgluteal a.
transvaginal a.
appropriate resection
approval
accelerated a.
APR
abdominoperineal resection
aprepitant
neurokinin-1 antagonist a.
NK$_1$ antagonist a.
aprinocarsen
aprotinin
aPS antibody testing
Aptosyn
APTT
activated partial thromboplastin time
APUD
amine precursor uptake and
  decarboxylation
apudoma
APV
average peak velocity
AquaMEPHYTON Injection
Aquaplast cast
Aquasol A, E

Aquatensen
aqueduct
cerebral a.
a. of Sylvius
aqueductal
a. obstruction
a. stenosis
aqueous
estrone a.
penicillin G, parenteral, a.
a. solution
Testosterone A.
Theelin A.
ara-A
adenine arabinoside
ara-AC
azacytosine arabinoside
arabinofuranosylcytosine
arabinoside
adenine a. (ara-A)
adenosine a.
azacytosine a. (ara-AC)
cytosine a. (ara-C, CA)
high-dose a. C (HiDAC)
high-dose cytosine a. (HI-DAC,
  HiDAC)
iodoazomycin a.
arabinoside-liposome
cytosine a.-l.
arabinosylcytosine (ara-C)
cyclophosphamide, Oncovin,
  methotrexate, leucovorin, a.
  (COMLA)
arabinosyl guanosine (ara-G)
ara-C
arabinosylcytosine
cytarabine
cytosine arabinoside
ara-C + ADR
ara-C and Adriamycin (AA)
cyclophosphamide, Oncovin,
  methotrexate, Adriamycin, ara-C
  (COMA-A)
cyclophosphamide, Oncovin,
  methotrexate, leucovorin, ara-C
  (COMLA)
cyclophosphamide, Oncovin,
  methotrexate, leucovorin,
  etoposide, ara-C (COMET-A)
daunorubicin and ara-C (DA)
ara-C, daunorubicin, etoposide
  (ADE)

NOTES

45

ara-C *(continued)*
ara-C, daunorubicin, prednisolone, mercaptopurine
ara-C + DNR + PRED + MP
high-dose ara-C (HDARA-C)
ara-C + HU
ara-C, hydrocortisone, mesna, prednisone, VP-16, leucovorin
ara-C, Oncovin, prednisone, L-asparaginase (AOPA)
ara-C and Platinol
ara-C, Platinol, etoposide (APE)
ara-C plus hydroxyurea (ara-C/HU)
ara-C plus 6-thioguanine
time-release ara-C
ara-C 5′-triphosphate
vincristine, Adriamycin, prednisone, ara-C (VAPA)
vincristine, prednisone, cyclophosphamide, ara-C (VPCA)

arachidonic acid

arachnoid
a. cyst
a. granulation calcification
a. retrocerebellar pouch
a. space
a. villi
a. villi obstruction

arachnoiditis
adhesive a.
chemical a.
cystic a.
neoplastic a.

ara-C/HU
ara-C plus hydroxyurea

ara-cytidine

ara-G
arabinosyl guanosine

Aralen Phosphate With Primaquine Phosphate

Aranesp
A. I.V.
A. subcutaneous injection

arbovirus

aRb protein expression

ARC
AIDS-related complex

arc
coplanar a.
rotation a.
a. therapy
a. therapy technique
xenon a.

arc-beam pattern

arch
aortic a.
branchial a.
ductus a.

a. fracture
gill a.

architect
A. CA125 II tumor marker assay
A. CA 15-3 tumor marker assay
a. ci8200 immunoassay system
A. i2000 immunoassay system

architectural disorder

architecture
histologic a.
zonal a.

archive
genetic a.

arcitumomab

ARCON
accelerated radiotherapy with carbogen and nicotinamide

arcuate
a. artery
a. ligament

arcuatus
uterus a.

ARDS
acute respiratory distress syndrome
adult respiratory distress syndrome

area, pl. **areae, areas**
Broca a.
cells per unit a.
areae gastricae
hematopoietic cobblestone a.
a. hepatica fibrosa
multifocal a.
perianal a.
proliferation a.
skip a.
speech a.
total body surface a. (TBSA)
a. under the curve (AUC)
Wernicke a.

areal density

areca nut

Aredia

5a-reductase

aregenerative anemia

Arenavirus

areola, pl. **areolae**
Chaussier a.

argatroban injection

argentaffin
a. carcinoid tumor
a. staining

Argentinian hemorrhagic fever

Argesic-SA

argininosuccinate synthetase (ASS)

argon
a. destruction
a. laser

argon-pumped dye laser

Argyle
 A. feeding tube
 A. Ingram trocar catheter
argyrophilic stain for nucleolar organizer region (AgNOR)
Arimidex
 A., Tamoxifen, Alone or in Combination (ATAC)
 A., Tamoxifen, Alone or in Combination trial
Aristocort
 A. Forte Injection
 A. Intralesional Injection
 A. Oral
Aristolochia
Aristospan
 A. Intraarticular Injection
 A. Intralesional Injection
aritox
 zolimomab a.
Arixtra
Arizona Cancer Center multiple myeloma staging system
arm
 a. edema
 PinPoint stereotactic a.
armamentarium
Armand-Frappier strain
armed
 A. Forces Institute of Pathology (AFIP)
 A. Forces Institute of Pathology classification of testicular tumors
 a. macrophage
Arneth count
Arnoff external fixation device
Arnold body
Aromasin
aromatase inhibitor (AI)
aromatization
 total body a.
arotinoid
arousal
 sexual a.
arrangement
 palisade-like a.
Arranon injection
array
 anular a.
 DNA a.
 microchip DNA a.
 parallel a.'s

arrest
 cardiac a.
 cell-cycle a.
 maturation a.
 mps1-induced a.
arresten angiogenesis inhibitor
arrhenoblastoma
Arrhythmia Research Technology (ART)
arsanilic acid
arsenic
 a. poisoning
 a. trioxide (AsO$_3$, ATO)
ars moriendi
ART
 antiretroviral therapy
 Arrhythmia Research Technology
artefact (*var. of* artifact)
arterial
 a. anastomosis
 a. aneurysm
 a. angioma
 a. blood
 a. blood gas abnormality
 a. bypass graft
 a. calcification
 a. disease
 a. hypertension
 a. hypotension
 a. linear density
 a. NIVA
 a. noninvasive vascular assessment
 a. occlusion
 a. oxygen saturation (SaO$_2$)
 a. perfusion
 a. phase
 a. pulsatility
 a. sheath
 a. spasm
 a. stenosis
 a. supply
 a. wall
 a. wall dissection
 a. waveform
arterial-arterial fistula
arteries (*pl. of* artery)
arteriobiliary fistula
arteriogenic impotence
arteriogram
arteriography
 bilateral carotid a.
 bronchial a.
arteriolar narrowing
arteriole

NOTES

arteriomyomatosis
arteriopathy
arterioportal
    a. fistula
    a. venous shunting
arterioportobiliary fistula
arteriosclerosis
arteriosclerotic
    a. occlusive disease
    a. renal disease
arteriosinusoidal penile fistula
arteriosus
    ductus a.
arteriovascular calcification
arteriovenous (A-V)
    a. anastomosis
    a. aneurysm
    a. fistula (AVF)
    a. glomus complex
    a. hemangioma
    a. malformation
    a. shunt
arteritis, pl. **arteritides**
    giant cell a.
    granulomatous a.
artery, pl. **arteries**
    aberrant right subclavian a.
    accessory middle cerebral a.
    Adamkiewicz a.
    arteries of Adamkiewicz
    adrenal a.
    anomalous left coronary a.
    anterior cerebral a.
    anterior choroidal a.
    anterior communicating a.
    anterior spinal a.
    arcuate a.
    ascending pharyngeal a.
    atrial circumflex a.
    auricular a.
    axillary a.
    azygos anterior cerebral a.
    basal cerebral a.
    basilar a.
    brachial a.
    brachiocephalic a.
    branch pulmonary a.
    bronchial a.
    bulbourethral a.
    celiac a.
    cerebellar a.
    cerebellolabyrinthine a.
    cerebral a.
    cervical a.
    choroidal a.
    cortical a.
    cystic a.
    deendothelialized a.
    a. of Drummond

    duodenal a.
    ectatic carotid a.
    ethmoidal a.
    external carotid a.
    external iliac a.
    facial a.
    hemorrhoidal a.
    internal carotid a. (ICA)
    labial a.
    lingual a.
    main pulmonary a. (MPA)
    malposition of branch pulmonary a.
    nutrient a.
    pulmonary a. (PA)
    superior mesenteric a. (SMA)
arthritis, pl. **arthritides**
    coccidioidomycosis a.
    degenerative a.
    leukemic a.
    psoriatic a.
    rheumatoid a.
    septic a.
arthrography
    magnetic resonance a.
    MR a.
Arthropan
arthropathy
    amyloid a.
    hemophiliac a.
    Jaccoud a.
arthroplasty
arthropneumoradiography
arthroscopic
arthroscopy
arthrosis
arthrotomography
Arthus reaction
articular
    a. cartilage
    a. disorder
    a. facet
    a. mass
    a. mass separation fracture
    a. pillar fracture
    a. process
    a. surface
articulation
artifact, artefact
    aortic motion a.
    barium a.
    beam-hardening a.
    bone-hardening a.
    bowel gas a.
    calibration failure a.
    clothing a.
    computer-generated a.
    nuclear bubbling a.
    skin lesion a.
    ZEBRA a.

artificial
    a. neural network (ANN)
    a. neural network algorithm
ARV
    AIDS-related virus
aryepiglottic
    a. cyst
    a. fold
    a. fold neurofibroma
aryl aromatic amine
arylsulfatase A deficiency
arytenoid cartilage
arzoxifene
AS
    additive solution
    autologous stem
        AS red cell
As2-1
    antineoplaston As2-1
ASA
    acetylsalicylic acid
    Lortab ASA
    MSD Enteric-Coated ASA
ASAP
    Adriamycin, Solu-Medrol, ara-C, Platinol
asbestos fiber
asbestosis
    pulmonary a.
asbestos-related
    a.-r. mesothelioma
    a.-r. pleural disease
ascariasis
    binary a.
Ascaris
ascending
    a. aorta
    a. aortography
    a. colon
    a. medullary vein thrombosis
    a. pharyngeal artery
    a. ramus
Aschoff
    A. body
    A. cell
ascites
    chylous a.
    gelatinous a.
    pelvic a.
ascitic fluid
ASCO
    American Society of Clinical Oncology
Ascomycetes
ascorbic acid

ASCR
    autologous stem cell rescue
Ascriptin
ASCS
    autologous stem cell support
ASCUS
    atypical squamous cells of undetermined
        significance
asepsis
aseptic
    a. meningitis
    a. necrosis
ASH
    American Society of Hematology
ASHAP, A-SHAP
    Adriamycin, Solu-Medrol, high-dose ara-
        C, Platinol
Ashhurst-Bromer
    A.-B. classification
    A.-B. classification of ankle
        fractures
Ashkenazi Jew
ash leaf patch
ASI
    active specific immunotherapy
asialoglycoprotein receptor
Askin
    A. sarcoma
    A. tumor
ASLN
    axillary sentinel lymph node
as low as reasonably achievable
    (ALARA)
ASN
    American Society of Neuroradiology
ASNase
    Escherichia coli ASNase
    polyethylene glycol-modified *E. coli*
        ASNase
ASO
    AIDS service organization
    allele-specific oligonucleotide
    antistreptolysin O
    ASO assay
    ASO titer
AsO$_3$
    arsenic trioxide
L-**asparaginase**
    ara-C, Oncovin, prednisone, L-a.
        (AOPA)
    L-a., BCNU, hydroxyurea
    cyclophosphamide, rubidazone,
        Oncovin, prednisone, L-a.

NOTES

L-**asparaginase** *(continued)*
 daunorubicin, vincristine,
  prednisone, L-a. (DVPL-ASP)
 dexamethasone, etoposide, cisplatin,
  ara-C, L-a. (DECAL)
 Erwinia L-a.
 Escherichia coli L-a.
 L-a., ifosfamide, methotrexate (AIM)
 L-a. and methotrexate (LAM)
 native L-a.
 Oncovin and L-a.
 Oncovin, prednisone, L-a. (OPAL)
 polyethylene glycol-conjugated L-a.
  (PEG-L-ASP)
 porton L-a.
 L-a., prednisone, Oncovin,
  cytarabine, Adriamycin (LAPOCA)
 prednisone, vincristine, L-a. (PVA)
 prednisone, vincristine,
  daunorubicin, L-a. (PVDA)
 vincristine, daunorubicin, L-a.
  (VDA)
 vincristine, prednisone, L-a. (VP+A)
aspargine-glycine-arginine sequence
aspartate
 a. aminotransferase (AST)
 a. target
 a. transaminase
aspartic
 a. acid
 a. proteinase
aspartyl protease class
aspect
 dorsal a.
Aspen ultrasound system
aspergilloma
aspergillosis
 allergic bronchopulmonary a.
 bronchopulmonary a.
 invasive a. (IA)
 invasive pulmonary a. (IPA)
 pleural a.
 primary a.
 pulmonary a.
 semiinvasive a.
Aspergillus
 A. endocarditis
 A. *flavus*
 A. *fumigatus*
 A. *galactomannan*
 A. *niger*
 A. *terreus*
Aspergum
aspirate
 bone marrow a.
aspirated foreign body (AFB)
aspiration
 a. biopsy
 bone marrow a.

breast cyst a.
continuous ultrasonic surgical a.
 (CUSA)
CT-guided needle a.
cyst a.
a. cytology
fine-needle a. (FNA)
a. needle
percutaneous fine-needle a. (PFNA)
a. pneumonia
transbronchial needle a.
transthoracic needle a. (TTNA)
ultrasound-guided needle a.
aspirational biopsy
aspirator
 Cavitron ultrasonic surgical a.
  (CUSA)
 FirstCyte A.
 InDuct breast a.
 Vabra a.
aspirin
 Bayer A.
 a. and codeine
 hydrocodone and a.
 oxycodone and a.
 propoxyphene and a.
 a. tolerance test
aspirin-like disorder
asplenia
 functional a.
 a. syndrome R
ASPO
 American Society of Preventive
  Oncology
ASPS
 alveolar soft part sarcoma
ASR
 aldosterone secretion rate
 atrial septal resection
ASS
 argininosuccinate synthetase
assay
 Abbot a.
 activated protein C resistance a.
 adenomatous polyposis coli gene
  mutation a.
 agglutination a.
 alkali denaturation a.
 allele-specific oligonucleotide a.
 anti-cathepsin D autoantibody a.
 anti-cytochrome P4502D6 a.
 antigen capture a.
 antiplatelet antibody a.
 APC gene mutation a.
 apoptosis a.
 Architect CA125 II tumor
  marker a.
 Architect CA 15-3 tumor
  marker a.

ASO a.
ATX a.
automated LCx factor V Leiden a.
autotaxin a.
Bax a.
bcr/abl multiplex reverse
  transcriptase polymerase chain
  reaciton a.
BFU-E bone marrow stem cell a.
binding a.
Bioclot protein S a.
bladder tumor a.
bone marrow granulocyte reserve a.
branched chain DNA
  amplification a.
breast cancer candidate of
  metastasis-1 a.
CA125 antigen a.
Campylobacter 16S-23S rRNA
  internal spacer region length a.
CA-1 prothrombin a.
carinactivase-1 prothrombin a.
cathepsin D a.
CD-117 a.
CEA-Roche a.
c-erbB2 p185 tumor marker a.
CFU-Dexter bone marrow stem
  cell a.
CFU-F bone marrow stem cell a.
CFU-GEMM bone marrow stem
  cell a.
CFU-GM bone marrow stem
  cell a.
chromium release a.
clinical a.
clonogenic a.
Coamate antithrombin a.
colony-forming a. (CFA)
comet a.
complement a.
Coulter HIV-1p24 antigen a.
CYP2D6 antibody a.
differential staining cytotoxicity a.
DiSC a.
DNA transfection a.
dye exclusion a.
EAC rosette a.
EDR a.
ELISPOT a.
endostatin a.
enzymatically recycling a.

enzyme-linked
  immunoelectrodiffusion a.
  (ELIEDA)
enzyme-linked immunosorbent a.
  (ELISA)
enzyme-linked immunospot a.
E rosette a.
Escherichia coli O157:H7
  fluorescent bacteriophage a.
estrogen receptor a. (ERA)
excision a.
ex vivo aortic ring sprouting a.
factor a.
fibrinogen a.
firefly luciferase a.
fluorescent bacteriophage a. (FBA)
fluorescent cytoprint a.
fluorescent multiplex polymerase
  chain reaction a.
galactomannan a.
gel-shift a.
GeneSeq HIV a.
gene transfer transcription a.
genomic a.
Guthrie bacterial inhibition a.
Hemochron Jr. Citrate PT a.
hemolytic complement a.
hemolytic plaque a.
HER-2 a.
HER-3 a.
HER-4 a.
histoculture drug response a.
  (HDRA)
HIV p25 antigen a.
HIV PCR a.
HIV-RNA PCR a.
hollow fiber a.
hormonal a.
HPP-CFC bone marrow stem
  cell a.
hybridization protection a.
Immulite PSA a.
immunocytochemical a. (ICA)
immunofluorescence antibody a.
immunoradiometric a. (IRMA)
in situ a.
insulin-like growth factor binding
  protein-3 a.
InSure a.
intracellular cytokine staining a.
Invader a.
in vitro antibody production a.
in vitro flow cytometric a.

NOTES

assay *(continued)*
in vitro transcription a.
ISET a.
Jerne plaque a.
laboratory a.
limulus amoebocyte lysate a.
liver-kidney microsomal type 1
   antibody target a.
LKM1 a.
LTC-IC bone marrow stem cell a.
lymphocyte proliferation a.
matrix metalloproteinase-2 a.
method clotting a.
a. methodology
microculture tetrazolium dye a.
microcytotoxicity a.
microencapsulation a.
microhemagglutination assay-
   Treponema pallidum a. (MHA-
   TPA)
microplate plasma methotrexate a.
microplate plasma MTX a.
mobility shift a.
multiple marker reverse
   transcriptase-polymerase chain
   reaction a.
mutagenesis a.
myelin basic protein a.
neuropilin 1, 2 a.
a. normalization
Oncotech a.
oxidized lipoprotein(a) a.
parvovirus B19 neutralizing
   antibody a.
PEG r-hirudin a.
PhenoSense GT Combination HIV
   Drug Resistance A.
plasmoid reactivation a.
4-point a.
polyethylene glycol r-hirudin
   mutein a.
predictive a.
proliferation a.
quantitative polymerase chain
   reaction a.
radioimmune a.
radioimmunoprecipitation a. (RIPA)
radioreceptor a.
Raji cell a.
reverse transcriptase-polymerase
   chain reaction a.
RHD pseudogene a.
SCGE a.
secreted motility-stimulating
   factor a.
serum folic acid a.
serum-induced platelet procoagulant
   activity a.
single-cell gel electrophoresis a.

specific factor a.
spleen colony a.
standardized CFU a.
standardized CFU-GM a.
standardized colony-forming unit a.
standardized progenitor a.
a. target
tartrate-resistant acid phosphatase a.
a. technique
telomerase activity a.
tissue inhibitor of metalloproteinase-
   2 a.
TRAP a.
triple-color flow cytometric a.
tube formation a.
tumor M2-pyruvate kinase a.
urinary catecholamine a.
virus-neutralization laboratory a.
Vysis UroVysion DNA probe a.
assembly
microtubule a.
posttranslation viral a.
Assera
A. AT-III
A. vWF
Asserachrom
A. APA
A. beta-TG
A. D-Di ELISA
A. FPA
A. PF4
A. thrombospondin
A. VII:Ag10000
A. vWF
A. X:Ag
assessment
arterial noninvasive vascular a.
biomarker risk a.
cell viability a.
Diagnostic and Therapeutic
   Technology A. (DATTA)
individualized functional status a.
   (IFSA)
Multicenter Oral Carvedilol Heart
   Failure A. (MOCHA)
neurologic a.
noninvasive vascular a. (NIVA)
nutritional a.
pretreatment a.
QOL a.
quality of life a.
venous noninvasive vascular a.
volume imaging for breast a.
   (VIBRANT)
weight estimation and a.
ASSIST
American Stop Smoking Intervention
   Study for Cancer Prevention
assist/control (A/C)

association

American Brain Tumor A. (ABTA)
American College of
Cardiology/American Heart A.
(ACC/AHA)
American Lung A. (ALA)
American Urological A. (AUA)
A. of Community Cancer Centers
A. for the Cure of Cancer of the
Prostate
cyclopia-astomia-agnathia-
holoprosencephaly a.
a. fiber
National Lung Transplant
Patient A.
noncausal a.
Oncology Nurses A.
telomeric a.
tibia aplasia a.
a. tract
VATER a.

AST

androgen suppression therapy
aspartate aminotransferase

astatine-211 (^{211}At)
astemizole
asterixis
asteroid body
asteroides

Nocardia a.

asthma

acute bronchopulmonary a.
atopic a.
bronchial a.
bronchopulmonary a.
extrinsic a.

asthma-related death
asthmatic bronchitis
Astler-Coller

A.-C. modification of Dukes
classification
A.-C. staging system

astragalocalcanean
astragaloscaphoid
astragalotibial
astragalus
Astramorph PF Injection
astringent soak
ASTRO

American Society for Therapeutic
Radiology and Oncology

astroblastoma

astrocyte

subpial a.

astrocytic hamartoma
astrocytoma

anaplastic a. (AA)
calcified a.
cerebellar a.
cerebral a.
chiasmatic-hypothalamic pilocytic a.
cystic pilocytic a.
desmoplastic cerebral a.
desmoplastic infantile a. (DIA)
diffuse fibrillary a.
fibrillary a.
gemistocytic a.
a. gene
giant cell a.
grade I–IV a.
hemispheral a.
infantile a.
infiltrative a.
juvenile pilocytic a. (JPA)
low-grade a.
malignant a.
nonpilocytic a.
pilocytic a.
piloid a.
protoplasmic a.
recurrent high-grade a.
solid pilocytic a.
subependymal giant cell a. (SEGA)
supratentorial pilocytic a.
temporoinsular a.

asymmetric

a. bile duct
a. data sampling
a. echo
a. jaws
a. septal hypertrophy

asymmetry
asymptomatic

A. Cardiac Ischemia Pilot (ACIP)
a. hyperamylasemia
a. hyperlactemia
a. lactic acidemia
a. metastatic hormone-refractory
prostate cancer
a. neurosyphilis

asynchrony
asynergy
AT

antithrombin
autologous transplant

NOTES

AT *(continued)*
    AT mutation (ATM)
    AT mutation gene
²¹¹At
    astatine-211
AT-III
    angiotensin III
    Assera AT-III
    AT-III concentrate
    AT-III deficiency
    Liatest AT-III
    lyophilized human AT-III
    purified human AT-III
    Stachrom AT-III
ATAC
    Arimidex, Tamoxifen, Alone or in
    Combination
    ATAC trial
Atasol
ataxia
    cerebellar a.
    Friedreich a.
    a. telangiectasia
ataxia-hemiparesis syndrome
ataxia-telangiectasia
atazanavir/ritonavir (ATV/r)
ATBC
    alpha-tocopherol beta-carotene
ATCL
    angioimmunoblastic T-cell lymphoma
Atec Trimark marker system
atelectasis
    adhesive a.
atelectatic asbestos pseudotumor
ATG
    antithymocyte globulin
Atgam
atherectomy
    a. device
    directional a.
    percutaneous a.
atheroembolic renal disease
atheroembolus
atherogenesis
atherolysis
atherolytic
    a. reperfusion wire
    a. reperfusion wire device
atheroma
atheromatous plaque
atherosclerosis obliterans
atherosclerotic
    a. change
    a. disease
    a. lesion
    a. plaque
    a. ulcer
athrombia
    essential a.

athyreotic thyroglobulin
AT-II-induced intraarterial
    chemotherapy
Ativan, Benadryl, Haldol (ABH)
Atkin epiphysial fracture
Atkinson
    A. Life Happiness (ATKLH)
    A. Life Happiness Rating
    A. tube
ATKLH
    Atkinson Life Happiness
ATL
    acute tumor lysis
    adult T-cell leukemia
    adult T-cell lymphoma
    ATL syndrome
atlantoaxial
    a. joint
    a. subluxation
atlantodental
atlantooccipital dislocation
atlas fracture
ATLL
    adult T-cell leukemia/lymphoma
ATM
    AT mutation
    ATM gene
ATO
    arsenic trioxide
Atolone Oral
atomic
    a. absorption spectrophotometry
    a. absorption spectroscopy
    a. mass
atonia, atony
atonic urinary bladder
atopic
    a. asthma
    a. dermatitis
    a. diathesis
    a. eczema
atopy
atorvastatin
atovaquone suspension
ATP
    adenosine 5′-triphosphate
    ATP binding site
ATPase locus
ATP-binding cassette transporter
    (ABCT)
ATPsynthase
ATRA
    all-*trans*-retinoic acid
Atragen
atrasentan
atraumatic
    a., multidirectional, bilateral
        instability
    a. needle

atresia
>   anorectal a.
>   aortic arch a.
>   aortic valve a.
>   biliary a.
>   bronchial a.
>   duodenal a.
>   esophageal a.

atretic segment

atria (*pl. of* atrium)

atrial
>   a. appendage
>   a. circumflex artery
>   a. fibrillation
>   a. flutter
>   a. mesenchymoma
>   a. myxoma
>   a. natriuretic factor receptor
>   a. natriuretic peptide
>   a. septal defect
>   a. septal resection (ASR)
>   a. septostomy
>   a. septum
>   a. situs
>   a. thrombosis

Atrigel drug delivery system

A TriMark marker system

atrioventricular (A-V)
>   a. block
>   a. bundle
>   a. canal
>   a. connection
>   a. discordance
>   a. junction
>   a. junction anomaly
>   a. node
>   a. node mesothelioma
>   a. septal defect
>   a. valve

atrium, pl. **atria**

atrophic
>   a. candidiasis
>   a. fracture
>   a. gastritis
>   a. pyelonephritis

atrophie blanche

atrophy
>   brain a.
>   bulbar muscular a.
>   cerebellar a.
>   cerebral a.
>   cortical a.
>   disuse a.

>   essential iris a.
>   optic a.
>   spinal muscular a. (SMA)
>   vaginal a.
>   vulvar a.

atropine
>   difenoxin and a.
>   diphenoxylate and a.

ATRT
>   atypical teratoid rhabdoid tumor

ATS
>   American Thoracic Society

ATT
>   alternating triple therapy

attachment
>   biopsy-guided a.

attapulgite

attenuant

attenuate

attenuated
>   a. adenomatous polyposis
>   a. bacterial vector
>   a. familial adenomatous polyposis
>   (AFAP)

attenuation
>   beam a.
>   a. coefficient
>   a. compensation
>   a. correction
>   differential a.
>   lesion a.
>   a. level
>   a. valve

attenuator

ATV/r
>   atazanavir/ritonavir

ATX
>   autotaxin
>   ATX assay

atypia
>   cellular a.
>   cytologic a.
>   inflammation/reactive a.
>   nuclear a.

atypical
>   a. angiomyolipoma (AA, AAML)
>   a. angiomyolipoma of kidney
>   a. cell
>   a. cell of undetermined significance
>   a. ductal hyperplasia (ADH)
>   a. epithelium
>   a. fibroxanthoma (AFX)

NOTES

atypical *(continued)*
- a. glandular cell of unknown significance (AGCUS, AGUS)
- a. leiomyoma
- a. lobular hyperplasia
- a. lymphoproliferative disorder
- a. measles pneumonia
- a. meningioma
- a. mycobacteriosis
- a. nevus
- a. regenerative hyperplasia
- a. squamous cells of undetermined significance (ASCUS)
- a. teratoid rhabdoid tumor (ATRT)
- a. thymoma
- a. tuberculosis
- a. vessel colposcopic pattern

Atzpodien
- A. regimen
- A. regimen for renal cell carcinoma

Au
- gold

^{198}Au
- gold-198

AUA
- American Urological Association
- AUA classification

Auberger blood group

AuBMT
- autologous bone marrow transplantation

AUC
- area under the curve

audiometry
- brainstem-evoked response a. (BSERA)

auditory
- a. canal
- a. tube

Auer
- A. body
- A. rods

Auerbach plexus

auger electron

augmentation
- bladder a.
- breast a.
- a. mammoplasty

augmented breast

Augmentin

augmerosen

AUL
- acute undifferentiated leukemia

AuraTek rapid cancer test

aureus
- *Staphylococcus a.*

auricle

auricular
- a. artery
- a. tachycardia

Aurora MR breast imaging system

aurotherapy

auscultation

Austrian Breast Cancer Study Group

autoanalyzer
- Kodak Ektachem a.
- technetium H2 a.

autoantibody
- anticytoplasmic a. (ACPA)
- anti-Hu antineuronal a.
- platelet-derived a.
- thyroid-peroxidase a. (TPO.Ab)

autoantigen

autochthonous
- a. neoplasm
- a. tumor

Auto-Crane device

autocrine
- a. effect
- a. growth factor
- a. mechanism
- a. motility factor receptor

AutoCyte PREP System

autoerythrocyte sensitization syndrome

autofluorescence

autogenous

autograft
- stem cell a.

autografting
- peripheral blood stem cell a.

autohemotherapy

autoimmune
- a. condition
- a. disease
- a. hemolytic anemia (AHA, AIHA)
- a. hemolytic disease (AHD)
- a. inflammatory demyelination
- a. leukopenia
- a. lymphoproliferative disorder
- a. neonatal thrombocytopenia
- a. neutropenia
- a. phenomenon
- a. polyendocrine-candidiasis syndrome
- a. response
- a. sialadenitis
- a. thrombocytopenic purpura (AITP)

autoimmunization

autologous
- a. and allogeneic marrow transplantation
- a. antibody
- a. blood
- a. blood clot
- A. Blood and Marrow Transplant Registry (ABMTR)

a. blood stem cell transplantation
a. bone graft
a. bone marrow cell
a. bone marrow rescue (ABMR)
a. bone marrow support (ABMS)
a. bone marrow transplant (ABMT)
a. bone marrow transplantation
  (ABMT, AuBMT)
a. cellular therapy
a. cell vaccine
a. donor
a. fat
a. hematopoietic cell
a. hematopoietic progenitor cell
  transplantation (AHPCT)
a. hematopoietic stem cell support
a. hematopoietic stem cell
  transplantation (AHSCT)
a. leukapheresis, processing, storage
  (ALPS)
a. ovarian transplantation
a. peripheral blood stem cell
  transplantation (APBSCT)
a. peripheral hematopoietic stem
  cell support (APHSCS)
a. red blood cell
a. red cell salvage
a. stem (AS)
a. stem cell
a. stem cell rescue (ASCR)
a. stem cell support (ASCS)
a. T lymphocyte
a. T lymphocytes stimulated with
  the patient's tumor-specific
  mutated RAS peptides
a. transplant (AT)
a. tumor
a. tumor cell immunization
a. tumor rejection antigen
autolymphocyte-based
  a.-b. treatment
  a.-b. treatment for renal cell
    carcinoma (ALT-RCC)
autolymphocyte therapy
autolysin
automated
  a. cardiac flow measurement
    (ACFM)
  a. cellular imaging system (ACIS)
  A. Central Tumor Registry
    (ACTUR)
  a. complete blood test

a. computerized axial tomography
  (ACAT)
a. enzyme immunoassay for
  antinuclear antibody
a. factor V Leiden mutation test
a. hematology analysis
a. large-core breast biopsy
a. laser-fluorescence sequencer
a. LCx factor V Leiden assay
a. method
a. white blood cell differential
automation
automotility factor
autonephrectomy
autonomic
  a. nerve block
  a. pathway
  a. sympathetic ganglion
autonomous adenoma
AutoPap
  A. 300 QC automatic Pap screener
  A. 300 QC System
autophosphorylation
Autoplex T
autoradiography
  quantitative track etch a.
autoregressive moving average (AMA)
autoreinfusion
autosomal
  a. dominant (AD)
  a. gene
  a. recessive inheritance
autosomal-dominant polycystic kidney
  disease
autosomal-recessive
  a.-r. polycystic kidney disease
  a.-r. SCID
autotaxin (ATX)
  a. assay
autotoxic
autotransfusion
autotransplant
autotransplantation
  a. O
  tissue a.
autovaccination
Autovac needle
AV
  Adriamycin and vincristine
A-V
  arteriovenous
  atrioventricular

NOTES

A-V *(continued)*
A-V fistula
A-V node
AVAD
Adriamycin, vincristine, cytarabine, dexamethasone
avascular necrosis (AVN)
Avastin
AVC cream
AVCF
Adriamycin, vincristine, cyclophosphamide, 5-fluorouracil
AVEG
AIDS Vaccine Evaluation Group
Avelox
average
autoregressive moving a. (AMA)
a. gradient number
a. peak velocity (APV)
a. radiation dose
AVEU
AIDS Vaccine Evaluation Unit
AVEU research program
AVF
arteriovenous fistula
avian
a. E26 virus
a. leukemia-sarcoma complex
a. leukosis-sarcoma complex
a. leukosis-sarcoma virus
a. sarcoma virus
Avicidin
Avicine
avidin-biotin complex
avidin-biotin-peroxidase
a.-b.-p. complex method
a.-b.-p. reagent
avidity
Avinza capsule
Avirax
avirulent
Avitene
avium-intracellulare
Mycobacterium a.-i. (MAI)
Aviva mammography system
AVM
Adriamycin, vinblastine, methotrexate
Adriamycin, vincristine, mitomycin C
AVN
avascular necrosis
AvocetPT rapid prothrombin time meter
Avonex
AVP
actinomycin D, vincristine, Platinol
Adriamycin, vincristine, procarbazine

avulsion
anterior labroligamentous periosteal sleeve a.
a. stress fracture
avulsive cortical irregularity
AvWD
acquired von Willebrand disease
Aware AccuMeter rapid HIV test
axes (*pl. of* axis)
axetil
cefuroxime a.
axial
a. angiography
a. cineangiography
a. hernia
a. image
a. plane
a. radiograph
a. resolution
a. section
a. skeleton
a. view
axilla, pl. **axillae**
axillary
a. adenopathy
a. artery
a. hematoma
a. irradiation
a. lymphadenopathy
a. lymph node (ALN)
a. lymph node dissection (ALND)
a. node involvement
a. node metastasis
a. region
a. sentinel lymph node (ASLN)
a. sheath
a. skin lesion
a. tail
a. tumor downstaging
a. ultrasonography
a. vein
a. vessel
a. view
axillobifemoral bypass graft
axillosubclavian vein thrombosis
axis, pl. **axes**
beam a.
celiac a.
couch a.
craniospinal a.
a. fracture
hypothalamic-pituitary-adrenal a.
Ayercillin
Ayurvedic medicine
AZA
azelaic acid
5-AZA
5-azacytidine

Azactam
5-azacytidine (5-AZA, 5-AZC)
azacytosine arabinoside (ara-AC)
azapropazone
azathioprine sodium
5-AZC
    5-azacytidine
AZdU
    3′-azido-2′,3′-dideoxyurine
azelaic acid (AZA)
azelastine
3′-azido-2′,3′-dideoxyurine (AZdU)
azidothymidine (AZT)
    a. erosion
    lamivudine triphosphate and a.
      (3TC/AZT)
    a. myopathy
azidouridine
aziridine
aziridinylbenzoquinone (AZQ)
azithromycin
azlocillin
    polymyxin B, amphotericin B,
      nalidixic acid, trimethoprim, a.
      (PANTA)
azocarbonamide
azole-resistant *Candida albicans*

azoospermia
azotemia
azovan blue
AZQ
    aziridinylbenzoquinone
AZT
    azidothymidine
      AZT failure
      AZT ineligibility
      AZT intolerance
      AZT myopathy
AZT-induced erosion
aztreonam
azurophilia
azurophilic granule
azygoesophageal
    a. line
    a. recess
azygos
    a. anterior cerebral artery
    a. continuation
    a. fissure
    a. lobe
    a. lymph node
    a. vein
    a. vein enlargement
Azzopardi tumor

NOTES

β (*var. of* beta)

B
 B cell
 cyclin B
 didemnin B
 erb B
 B lineage
 B lymphocyte
 solitary osteochondroma B
 B symptom
 B virus

B₁
 Fumonisin B_1

B1 therapy

B7
 B-cell surface antigen B7
 B7 CD28 T cell costimulatory pathway

B19 parvovirus

B42 RNA polymerase activation domain

Babesia microti

babesiosis

Babinski sign

BAC
 bronchoalveolar carcinoma

bacampicillin

baccatin III

Bacid

bacillary
 b. angiomatosis
 b. dysentery
 b. epithelioid angiomatosis (BEA)
 b. peliosis hepatis

bacille
 b. Calmette-Guérin (BCG)
 b. Calmette-Guérin vaccine

bacilliformis
 Bartonella b.

bacillus, pl. bacilli
 acid-fast b. (AFB)
 b. anthracis pneumonia
 Calmette-Guérin b.

backbone
 GeneVax DNA plasmid b.
 oligolysine b.

backflow

background equivalent radiation time

backprojection

backscatter

backwash ileitis

BACOD
 bleomycin, Adriamycin, CCNU,
 Oncovin, dexamethasone

BACON
 bleomycin, Adriamycin, CCNU,
 Oncovin, nitrogen mustard

BACOP
 bleomycin, Adriamycin,
 cyclophosphamide, Oncovin,
 prednisone

BACT
 BCNU, ara-C, cyclophosphamide, 6-
 thioguanine

bacteremia
 catheter-associated b.
 clostridial b.

bacteria (*pl. of* bacterium)

bacterial
 b. aneurysm
 b. aortitis
 b. endocarditis
 b. ependymitis
 b. epiglottitis
 b. filtration-capture immunoassay
 b. infection
 b. keratitis
 b. meningitis
 b. nephritis
 b. osteomyelitis
 b. pneumonia
 b. pneumonitis
 b. septicemia
 b. sinusitis
 b. toxin
 b. translocation
 b. vaginosis
 b. vasculitis
 b. vector

bactericidal

bactericide

bacteriobilia

bacteriohemolysin

bacteriohemolysin

bacteriolytic

bacteriophage

bacteriosis

bacteriostasis

bacteriostat

bacteriostatic activity

bacteriotoxic

bacterium, pl. bacteria
 antibiotic-resistant bacteria
 endogenous bacteria
 Gram-negative bacteria
 Gram-negative enteric bacteria
 Gram-positive bacteria

bacteriuria

Bacteroides fragilis

Bactrim DS
baculovirus
    B. Expression Vector System
      (BEVS)
    b. transfected cell
b-adaptin gene family
bag
    Belly Bag urine storage b.
    EndoCatch b.
Baghdad Spring anemia
Bair Hugger warming blanket
baked talc
baker
    B. Antifol, cyclophosphamide,
      Adriamycin, Platinol
    b. cyst
BAL
    British anti-Lewisite
    bronchoalveolar lavage
    BAL in Oil
Balamuthia mandrillaris
balance
    hemostatic b.
balanitis xerotica obliterans
balanopreputial region
Balb/C sarcoma virus
Balkan nephropathy
ball
    fungus b.
    b. thrombus
ball-and-socket
    b.-a.-s. epiphysis
    b.-a.-s. joint
    b.-a.-s. prosthesis
ball-in-hand appearance
ballistic material
balloon
    b. atrial septostomy
    Balt b.
    Bardex b.
    Brandt cytology b.
    b. bronchoplasty
    b. catheter
    b. catheter technique
    b. cell
    b. counterpulsation
    b. dilatation
    b. dilation angioplasty
    b. dilation valvuloplasty
    b. dilator
    b. embolotherapy
    b. epiphysis
    b. occlusion pulmonary angiography
    b. pericardiotomy
    b. pump
    Schwarten Microglide LP b.
    b. tamponade
    b. test occlusion
balloon-cell melanoma

balloon-expandable tantalum stent
balloon-occluded arterial infusion
balloon-on-a-wire
BALT
    bronchial-associated lymphoid tissue
    bronchus-associated lymphoid tissue
Baltaxe-Mitty-Pollack needle
Balt balloon
BAM22
    chromosome 22q region BAM22
Bamberger hematogenic albuminuria
BAMON
    bleomycin, Adriamycin, methotrexate,
      Oncovin, nitrogen mustard
Bancap HC
bancrofti
    Wuchereria b.
band
    dense metaphysial b.'s
    germline b.
    Ladd b.
    lucent b.
    metaphysial lucent b.
    monoclonal b.
    oligoclonal b.
bandemia
banding procedure
bank
    AIDS and Cancer Specimen B.
      (ACSB)
    gene b.
    tissue b.
banking
    preoperative sperm b.
    sperm b.
Banti splenic anemia
Barbados leg
Barbilixir
barbiturate
bard
    B. absorption dressing
    B. syndrome
Bardex
    B. balloon
    B. catheter
bare lymphocyte syndrome
baritosis
barium
    b. artifact
    b. bolus
    b. enema
    b. enema with air contrast
    b. examination
    b. meal
    b. mixture
    b. pneumoconiosis
    b. study
    b. sulfate

b. suspension
b. swallow
barium-filled colon
barium-water esophagram
bark
cinchona b.
baroreceptor
Barosperse
barotrauma
barrel-shaped lesion
Barrett
B. epithelium (BE)
B. esophagus
B. esophagus-associated
adenocarcinoma (BEAC)
B. metaplasia
barrier
anatomic b.
blood-tumor b. (BTB)
cerebrospinal fluid-brain b.
endothelial b.
facial b.
genetic b.
integumentary b.
mucosal b.
b. protection
Barron pump
Bartholin
B. duct
B. gland carcinoma
Bartl grade
Bartonella
B. anemia
B. *bacilliformis*
B. *henselae*
B. *quintana*
bartonellosis
Barton fracture
Barton-Smith fracture
basal
b. angle
b. cell adenocarcinoma
b. cell adenoma
b. cell carcinoma (BCC)
b. cell nevus syndrome
b. cell papilloma
b. cerebral artery
b. cistern
b. cytoplasmic vacuolization
b. descent
b. ganglia calcification
b. ganglia hematoma
b. ganglia infarct

b. lamella
b. lamina
b. neck fracture
b. nucleus
b. vein of Rosenthal
Basaljel
basaloid
b. nonkeratinizing carcinoma
b. squamous cell carcinoma
base
pyramidine b.
Schiff b.
skull b.
tongue b.
baseline
pretherapy b.
basement membrane
basic fibroblast growth factor (bFGF)
basilar
b. angiography
b. artery
b. femoral neck fracture
b. impression
b. invagination
basilic vein
basin
jugulodigastric b.
lymph node b.
nodal b.
basion-axial interval
basion-dens interval
basivertebral vein
basket
Amplatz through-and-through b.
basocytopenia
basocytosis
basopenia
basophil
b. chemotactic factor
b. count
basophilia
paraneoplastic b.
basophilic
b. adenoma
b. erythroblast
b. erythrocyte
b. granule
b. leukemia
b. leukocyte
b. normoblast
b. stippling
b. structure

NOTES

basophilism
Cushing b.
basophil/lobularity channel
basophilocytic leukemia
basosquamous
b. cell acanthoma
b. cell carcinoma
b. nonkeratinizing carcinoma
Bassen-Kornzweig
B.-K. disease
B.-K. syndrome
BAT
B-mode acquisition and targeting
BAT radiation therapy technique
BAT system
Bateman
B. disease
B. purpura
B. syndrome
batimastat
Batson vertebral venous plexus
Bauermeister scale
Bauer Temno biopsy needle
bauxite pneumoconiosis
BAVIP
bleomycin, Adriamycin, vinblastine, imidazole carboxamide, prednisone
bax
B. assay
b. expression level
b. gene
B. protein
Baxter
B. Infusor
B. pump
Baycol
Bayer
B. Aspirin
B. HER-2/neu serum test
Bayesian pharmacokinetic
Bazex
B. disease
B. syndrome
BB
both bones
BBVP-M
BCNU, bleomycin, VePesid, prednisone, methotrexate
BCAP
BCNU, cyclophosphamide, Adriamycin, prednisone
b-catenin expression
BCAVe, B-CAVe
bleomycin, CCNU, Adriamycin, Velban
BCC
basal cell carcinoma
BCD
bleomycin, cyclophosphamide, dactinomycin

B-cell
B-c. acute lymphoblastic leukemia
B-c. acute lymphocytic leukemia
B-c. chronic lymphocytic leukemia
B-c. differentiation
B-c. differentiation factor
B-c. epitope protein
B-c. help
B-c. lineage antigen
B-c. lymphoma
B-c. lymphoplasmacytic tumor
B-c. malignancy
B-c. marker
B-c. neoplasia
B-c. neoplasm
B-c. non-Hodgkin lymphoma (B-NHL)
B-c. stimulating factor
B-c. surface antigen B7
B-c. surface immunoglobulin
BCG
bacille Calmette-Guérin
bronchocentric granulomatosis
ftorafur, Adriamycin, cyclophosphamide, BCG (FAC-BCG)
BCG live product
BCG osteomyelitis
Pacis BCG
scarification of BCG
TICE BCG
BCG vaccine
B-CHOP
bleomycin, Cytoxan, hydroxydaunomycin, Oncovin, prednisone
BCI-Immune activator
BCIS
breast carcinoma in situ
bcl-2
bcl-2 antisense
bcl-2 antisense molecule G3139
bcl-2 family protein
bcl-2 gene
bcl-2/Ig fusion gene
bcl-2 oncogene
bcl-2 protooncogene/oncogene
bcl-2 and P-glycoprotein coexpression
bcl-2 protooncogene translocation product
bcl-1 oncogene
bcl-3 oncogene
bcl-10 gene testing
bcl-x gene
BCMF
bleomycin, cyclophosphamide, methotrexate, 5-fluorouracil

BCNU
- bischloroethylnitrosourea
- bischloronitrosourea
- carmustine
    - Adriamycin plus BCNU
    - BCNU, ara-C, cyclophosphamide, 6-thioguanine (BACT)
    - BCNU, bleomycin, VePesid, prednisone, methotrexate (BBVP-M)
    - CPT-11 plus BCNU
    - BCNU, cyclophosphamide, Adriamycin, prednisone (BCAP)
    - BCNU, cyclophosphamide, Oncovin, prednisone (BCOP)
    - cyclophosphamide, Platinol, BCNU (CPB)
    - BCNU, cyclophosphamide, prednisone (BCP)
    - BCNU, cyclophosphamide, vinblastine, procarbazine, prednisone (BCVPP)
    - BCNU, cyclophosphamide, vincristine, prednisone (BCVP)
    - BCNU, etoposide, ara-C, cyclophosphamide (BEAC)
    - BCNU, etoposide, ara-C, melphalan (BEAM, mini-BEAM)
    - 5-fluorouracil, imidazole, vincristine, BCNU (FIVB)
    - BCNU, hydroxyurea, dacarbazine (BHD)
    - BCNU, hydroxyurea, dacarbazine, vincristine (BHD-V)
    - interstitial BCNU
    - BCNU, methotrexate, procarbazine (BMP)
    - BCNU, Oncovin, prednisone (BOP)
    - BCNU, Oncovin, procarbazine, prednisone (BOPP)
    - BCNU and thalidomide
    - topotecan plus BCNU
    - BCNU, vinblastine, cyclophosphamide, procarbazine, prednisone (BVCPP)
    - BCNU, vincristine, Adriamycin, prednisone (BVAP)
    - BCNU, vincristine, procarbazine, prednisone (BVPP)

BCNU-impregnated wafer

BCOP
- BCNU, cyclophosphamide, Oncovin, prednisone

BCP
- BCNU, cyclophosphamide, prednisone

BCPT
- Breast Cancer Prevention Trial

BCR
- breakpoint cluster region

bcr/abl
- *bcr/abl* DNA probe
- *bcr/abl* fusion gene
- *bcr/abl* kinase
- *bcr/abl* multiplex reverse transcriptase polymerase chain reaction assay
- *bcr/abl* multiplex RT-PCR
- *bcr/abl* protein test
- *bcr/abl* transcript
- *bcr/abl* tyrosine kinase inhibitor

BCR-negative
- breakpoint cluster region-negative

BCRP
- breast cancer resistance protein

BCR-positive
- breakpoint cluster region-positive

BCS
- breast conservation surgery
- breast-conserving surgery

BCT
- breast-conserving therapy

BCVP
- BCNU, cyclophosphamide, vincristine, prednisone

BCVPP
- BCNU, cyclophosphamide, vinblastine, procarbazine, prednisone
- bleomycin, cyclophosphamide, vincristine, procarbazine, prednisone

BD
- Becton Dickinson
    - BD bone marrow biopsy needle
    - BD glucose tablet

B7-DC antigen

B-DOPA
- bleomycin, DTIC, Oncovin, prednisone, Adriamycin

B/D recombinant

BE
- Barrett epithelium

BEA
- bacillary epithelioid angiomatosis

BEAC
- Barrett esophagus-associated adenocarcinoma

NOTES

BEAC *(continued)*
 BCNU, etoposide, ara-C,
  cyclophosphamide
  BEAC cell
BEACOPP
 bleomycin, etoposide, Adriamycin,
  cyclophosphamide, vincristine,
  procarbazine, prednisone
  BEACOPP regimen
bead
  B. Block polyvinyl alcohol embolic
   microsphere
  Dynal M450 magnetic b.
  magnetic b.
  polyacrylamide b.
  Sephadex b.
beaded
  b. appearance
  b. ductal dilatation
  b. pancreatic duct
  b. ureter
beak
  b. fracture
  b. sign
beaked appearance
beaking
  antral b.
BEAM
 BCNU, etoposide, ara-C, melphalan
beam
  b. angle
  b. aperture
  b. attenuation
  b. axis
  carbon-ion b.
  b. compensator
  coplanar b.
  b. definition
  electron b.
  b. energy
  equivalent b.
  b.'s eye view (BEV)
  b. filtration
  b. flattener
  b. hardening
  helium ion b.
  ipsilateral electron b.
  b. limitation
  b. modification
  neutron b.
  noncoplanar b.
  orthovoltage b.
  parallel-opposed b.'s
  b. pattern
  pencil electron b.
  b. penumbra
  proton b.
  b. shaper
  split b.

  b. splitter
  b. steering
  b. weighting
beam-hardening
  b.-h. artifact
  b.-h. effect
beam-modifying device
beam-splitting mirror
Beau line
becatecarin
Bechterew *(var. of* Bekhterev)
Becker
  B. melanosis
  B. pigmented hairy epidermal
   nevus
  B. tissue expander/breast prosthesis
Beck Hopelessness Scale (BHS)
Beckman UV spectrophotometer
Beckwith-Wiedemann syndrome (BWS)
Becotin Pulvules
becquerel (Bq)
Becton Dickinson (BD)
BED
 bioeffect dose
 biologically equivalent dose
 biologic effective dose
bed
  Advanta b.
  capillary b.
  Clinitron b.
  head of b. (HOB)
  KinAir b.
  prostatic b.
  tumor b.
Bednar tumor
bedroom fracture
bedside radiography
beef heart antigen
Béguez César disease
behavior
  addictive b.
  Michaelis-Menten
   pharmacokinetic b.
**Behavioral Risk Factor Surveillance
 System (BRFSS)**
Behring law
beigelii
  Trichosporon b.
Bekhterev, Bechterew
  erythrosis of B.
BELD
 bleomycin, Eldisine, lomustine,
  dacarbazine
belladonna
  b. and opium
  PMS-Opium & b.
bell-and-clapper deformity
Bellergal-S

belli
>   *Isospora b.*

Bellini duct carcinoma

Bell palsy

belly
>   B. Bag urine storage bag
>   b. bath chemotherapy
>   b. board

BEMP
>   bleomycin, Eldisine, mitomycin, Platinol

Benadryl

Bence
>   B. Jones albumin
>   B. Jones body
>   B. Jones myeloma
>   B. Jones protein
>   B. Jones proteinuria

bendamustine/prednisone

bendroflumethiazide

beneficence

beneficial
>   antidotally b.

BeneFin

benefit
>   maximum cytoreductive b.

BeneFix hemophilia B blood clotting factor

benign
>   b. acini prostate gland
>   b. bone lesion
>   b. breast disease
>   b. cyst
>   b. duct ectasia
>   b. ethnic neutropenia
>   b. fetal hamartoma
>   b. fibrous histiocytoma
>   b. gastric ulcer
>   b. glioma
>   b. infiltrate
>   b. intracranial hypertension
>   b. juvenile melanoma
>   b. lymphadenopathy
>   b. lymphadenosis
>   b. lymphocytoma cutis
>   b. lymphoepithelial lesion (BLL)
>   b. lymphoepithelial parotid tumor
>   b. lymphoma
>   b. lymphoma of rectum
>   b. lymphoproliferative lesion
>   b. mass
>   b. meningeal fibrosis
>   b. metastasizing chondroblastoma

>   b. metastasizing leiomyomatosis (BML)
>   b. mixed oligoastrocytoma
>   b. nevus
>   b. ovarian tumor
>   b. pheochromocytoma
>   b. proliferation
>   b. proliferative disorder
>   b. prostate condition
>   b. prostatic hyperplasia (BPH)
>   b. prostatic hypertrophy (BPH)
>   b. pulmonary and esophageal tumors
>   b. salivary gland tumor
>   b. vascular lesion

benignity

benignum
>   lymphogranuloma b.

Bennett
>   B. classification
>   B. classification of lymphoma
>   B. comminuted fracture

Bentley-Milan approach

Benuryl

benzamide
>   disulfide b.
>   disulfide-substituted b.
>   substituted b.

benzathine
>   penicillin G b.

benzbromarone

benzene-induced hyperdiploidy

benzisothiazolone

benzoate
>   methyl b.
>   sodium phenylacetate and sodium b.

benzocaine
>   b., gelatin, pectin, sodium carboxymethylcellulose
>   Orabase with B.

Benzodent

benzodiazepine receptor

benzoic acid

benzoporphyrin

benzothiazine dioxide

benzquinamide

benzthiazide

benztropine

benzydamine

BEP
>   bleomycin, etoposide, Platinol

bepridil

NOTES

Berard
   B. classification
   B. classification for follicular lymphoma
bereavement services
Berger point kernel method
Berkson bias
Berkson-Gage method
Berlin-Frankfurt-Munster therapy
Berlix Oncology Foundation
Bernard-Soulier syndrome
berry
   b. aneurysm
   b. cell
   chaste tree b.
beryllium granuloma
besudotox
   cintredekin b.
beta, β
   b. alethine
   b. carotene
   epoetin b.
   fibroblast-derived interferon b.
   interferon b. (IFN-beta)
   B. LT
   nuclear factor kappa b. (NF-κB, NF-kB)
   b. ray
   recombinant human interferon b.
   b. thalassemia
   transforming growth factor b. (TGF-beta)
beta-4
   transforming growth factor b.-4
beta-1a
   interferon b.-1a
beta-adrenergic receptor
beta-alethine
beta-carotene
   alpha-tocopherol b.-c. (Alpha-Beta, ATBC)
beta-catenin
beta-chain variable region (V-beta)
beta-emitting isotope
2′beta-fluoro-2′,3′-dideoxyadenosine (FddA)
beta-hairpin structure
beta-hCG test
beta-hemolytic *Streptococcus*
beta-ionone
BetaKine
betamethasone
beta₂-microglobulin level
beta-propiolactone
beta-ray ophthalmic plaque therapy
Betaseron
BetaSorb device

beta-TG
   beta-thromboglobulin
   Asserachrom beta-TG
Betathine
beta-thromboglobulin (beta-TG)
betatron
Betaxin
betel
   b. cancer
   b. nut
   b. quid
Bethesda
   B. classification
   B. criteria
   B. rating scale
   B. rating scale for Pap smears
   B. system
   B. unit
betulinic acid
BEV
   beam's eye view
bevacizumab
Bevalac system
Bevan procedure
beveled-tip needle
BEVS
   Baculovirus Expression Vector System
bexarotene gel
Bexidem
Bexxar
   B. radiolabeled monoclonal antibody
   B. therapy
bezafibrate
Bezalip
bFGF
   basic fibroblast growth factor
   bFGF and VEGF production
BFI
   Brief Fatigue Inventory
B/F recombinant
BFU-E bone marrow stem cell assay
BHC
   body habitus change
B-hCG tumor marker
BHD
   BCNU, hydroxyurea, dacarbazine
BHD-V
   BCNU, hydroxyurea, dacarbazine, vincristine
BHS
   Beck Hopelessness Scale
BIAcore system
Biafine wound dressing emulsion
bias
   Berkson b.
   lead time b.
Biaxin
bibasilar

bicalutamide
bicarbonate
    potassium b.
    sodium b.
biceps
    b. brachii
    b. brachii tendon
    b. brachii tendon reflex test
    b. femoris
biceps-labral complex
Bichat foramen
Bicillin L-A
bicipital
    b. groove
    b. tendon sheath
biclonal
    b. follicular lymphoma
    b. gammopathy
biclonality
BiCNU
    carmustine
bicondylar
    b. T-shaped fracture
    b. Y-shaped fracture
bicyclam
bidi cigarette
bidimensional tumor measurement
Bielschowsky stain
Bierman needle
Biermer anemia
bifemoral graft
bifid
    b. collecting system
    b. gallbladder
    b. renal pelvis
    b. ribs
    b. ureter
bifrontal
    b. index
    b. oligodendroglioma
bifunctional
    b. alkylating agent
    b. antibody
bifurcation
    b. aneurysm
    aortic b.
bilateral
    b. carotid arteriography
    b. ductal ectasia
    b. iliac crest
    b. infarction
    b. intrafacetal dislocation
    b. knee effusions

    b. locked facets
    b. lower lobe pneumonia
    b. lymphadenectomy
    b. myocutaneous graft
    b. percutaneous cervical cordotomy (BPCC)
    b. salpingo-oophorectomy (BSO)
    b. technique
    b. vestibular schwannomas
bile
    b. acid
    b. duct
    b. duct cancer
    b. duct carcinoma
    b. duct dilatation
    b. duct manipulation
    b. encrustation
    b. flow
    high-density b.
    b. leakage
    b. reflux gastritis
bilharzial granuloma
bilharziasis
biliary
    b. atresia
    b. calculus
    b. cirrhosis
    b. coaxial dilator
    b. colic
    b. cystadenoma
    b. decompression
    b. drainage
    b. drainage catheter
    b. duct
    b. endoprosthesis
    b. intervention
    b. lithotripsy
    b. manipulation catheter
    b. neoplasm
    b. obstruction syndrome
    b. radicle
    b. sepsis
    b. stent
    b. stone
    b. stricture
    b. system
    b. tract
    b. tract cancer
    b. tract disease
    b. tract obstruction
    b. tree
    b. tree obstruction

NOTES

biliary-enteric
  b.-e. anastomosis
  b.-e. anastomosis operation
  b.-e. bypass
  b.-e. fistula
bilirubin
  indirect b.
  b. test
  total b.
bilirubinemia
Billroth disease
biloba
  ginkgo b.
bilobed plasma cell
biloma
  intrahepatic b.
bimalleolar fracture
B-immunoblast
binary
  b. ascariasis
  b. digit
binding
  b. activity
  b. assay
  b. energy
  fragment antigen b. (Fab)
  Ig b.
  iron b.
  lentil agglutination b.
  protein b.
  proteoglycan b.
  b. site
  in vivo b.
Binet
  B. classification of chronic
    lymphocytic leukemia (stage A–C)
  B. modified cyclophosphamide
  B. staging system
  B. staging system for chronic
    lymphocytic leukemia
  B. system of classification
binucleated
  b. chondrocyte
  b. lymphocyte
bioaccumulator
bioadhesive
bioavailability
  oral b.
Biocef
biochemical
  b. epidemiology
  b. marker
  b. metastasis
  b. modulation
  b. recurrence-free survival (bRFS)
biochemistry
biochemopreventive therapy
biochemotherapy
biocidal

Bioclate
Bioclot protein S assay
Bioclusive TFD
bioeffect dose (BED)
bioelectromagnetics
biofeedback
Bioflex
  B. Rx222P tape
  B. Rx216V tape
  B. Rx232V tape
  B. 647 tape
  B. 648 tape
BioGlue adhesive/sealant
BioHepB recombinant hepatitis B
  vaccine
biologic
  b. effective dose (BED)
  b. effective dose formula
  b. half-life
  b. heterogeneity
  b. marker
  b. therapy
  b. window
biologically equivalent dose (BED)
BioLogic-HT system
biology
  cell b.
  molecular cell b.
  tumor b.
biomarker
  RECAF b.
  b. risk assessment
biomedical ethics
biopsy, pl. **biopsies**
  abdominal lymph node b.
  adrenal gland b.
  aspiration b.
  aspirational b.
  automated large-core breast b.
  blind b.
  bone marrow aspirate and b.
  brain b.
  breast b.
  cold b.
  core b. (Cbx)
  core needle b.
  CT-based stereotactic b.
  CT-guided b.
  CT- and MRI-based stereotactic b.
  cytobrush b.
  endobronchial b.
  endometrial b.
  endomyocardial b.
  endoscopic b.
  excisional b.
  fine-needle aspiration b. (FNAB)
  FNA b.
  hilar b.
  b. immunophenotype

incisional b.
intramedullary tumor b.
invasive b.
liver b.
lymph node b.
monoclonal antibody A103 fine-needle aspiration b.
MRI-based stereotactic b.
mucosal b.
multiple core biopsies
b. needle
needle b.
pancreatic b.
parathyroid b.
pelvic aspiration b.
percutaneous fine-needle aspiration b. (PFNAB)
percutaneous liver b.
percutaneous transthoracic needle aspiration b.
pleural b.
punch b.
scalene node b.
sentinel lymph node b. (SLNB)
sentinel lymph node mapping and b.
sentinel node b.
sextant b.
shave b.
skeletal b.
skin b.
stereotactic b.
stereotactically guided core needle b. (SCNB)
stereotactic core b.
stereotactic needle core b. (SNCB)
stereotactic vacuum-assisted b. (SVAB)
surgical excision b.
testicular b.
thyroid needle b.
b. tract
transbronchial b.
transbronchoscopic b.
b. transducer
transrectal ultrasound b.
transthoracic needle b.
transthoracic percutaneous fine-needle aspiration b.
trephine b.
Tru-Cut needle b.
TRUS b.

ultrasonographically guided core needle b. (USCNB)
ultrasound-guided needle core b. (UNCB)
vacuum-assisted breast b. (VAB)
b. volume index
vulvar b.
Wang needle b.
biopsy-guided attachment
biopsy-proven typical nephropathy
Biopsys mammotome
Biopty-Cut biopsy needle
Biopty gun
Bio-Rad
    B.-R. Model 5000 Titanium system
    B.-R. Sequi-Gen apparatus
bioreductive agent
biosynthesis
    pyrimidine nucleotide b.
Bio-Tab
biotherapy
biotransformation
BioVant
    CaP B.
BIP
    bleomycin, ifosfamide, Platinol
    bleomycin, ifosfamide with mesna rescue, Platinol
biparietal diameter
bipedal lymphangiography
biphasic
    b. malignant mesothelioma
    b. pulmonary blastoma
biphenotypic leukemia
biplane
    b. angiography
    b. method
bipotential precursor cell tumor
BI-RADS
    Breast Imaging Reporting and Data System
bird's nest filter
biricodar dicitrate
Birt-Hogg-Dubé syndrome
bisacetamide
    hexamethylene b. (HMBA)
Bisac-Evac
bisacodyl
Bisacodyl Uniserts
bisantrene hydrochloride
bischloroethylnitrosourea (BCNU)
bischloronitrosourea (BCNU)
Bisco-Lax

NOTES

bisexual
B-islet cell
Bismatrol
bismuth
    B. classification
    b. subgallate
    b. subsalicylate
bismuth-213-HuM195 anti-CD33
bispecific
    b. antibody
    b. T-cell engager
bisphosphonate
    oral b.
    synthetic b.
bisphosphonate-associated osteonecrosis
bispiperazinedione (ICRF)
bispivaloyloxymethyl
BiTE molecule
Bittner agent
bivalirudin
biweekly
bizarre leiomyoma
bizelesin
Bizzozero
    B. corpuscle
    B. platelet
    B. red cell
BK virus
Blac
    Linctus Codeine B.
black
    b. adenoma
    b. cohosh
    B. Draught
    B. nuclear grading system
    Sudan B. B (SBB)
    b. tobacco
Blackfan-Diamond anemia
blackwater fever
bladder
    atonic urinary b.
    b. augmentation
    b. cancer
    b. carcinoma
    b. catheterization
    b. congenital abnormality
    b. cuff
    b. diverticulitis
    b. diverticulum
    dome of b.
    b. dysfunction
    b. endometriosis
    b. exstrophy
    b. flap
    b. flap hematoma
    b. hemorrhage
    b. incontinence
    b. laceration
    b. map

OncoRad for b.
    b. outlet obstruction
    spastic urinary b.
    transurethral resection of b.
      (TURB)
    b. tumor (BT)
    b. tumor assay
    urinary b.
    b. wall
    b. wall thickening
    b. wall thickness
BladderScan test
bladder-within-bladder sign
blade catheter
blanc fixe
blanche
    atrophie b.
blanket
    Bair Hugger warming b.
blast
    B-lymphocyte b.
    b. cell
    b. cell leukemia
    b. colony-forming unit
    b. crisis
    excess b.'s
    extrafollicular b.
    leukemic b.
    b. phase
    refractory anemia with excess b.'s
blastema
    metanephric b.
blastic
    b. crisis
    b. lesion
    b. metastasis
    b. natural killer cell leukemia
    b. phase
    b. transformation
    b. variant
blastocyst
Blastocystis hominis
blastocytoma
blastogenesis
blastogenic factor
blastoma
    biphasic pulmonary b.
    parenchymal b.
    pleuropulmonary b.
    pulmonary b.
Blastomyces dermatitidis
blastomycosis
    European b.
bleb
    emphysematous b.
blebbing
bleeder in tumor mass
bleeding
    b. diathesis

b. disorder
gingival b.
intracranial b.
occult b.
packing for b.
b. point
b. site
splenic b.
b. time
b. time test
uterine b.
vaginal b.
variceal b.
blennorrhagicum
keratoderma b.
Blenoxane
BLEO
bleomycin
BLEO-COMF
bleomycin, cyclophosphamide, Oncovin,
methotrexate, 5-fluorouracil
bleomycin (BLEO)
b., Adriamycin, CCNU, Oncovin,
dexamethasone (BACOD)
b., Adriamycin, CCNU, Oncovin,
nitrogen mustard (BACON)
b., Adriamycin, cyclophosphamide,
Oncovin, prednisone (BACOP)
b., Adriamycin, methotrexate,
Oncovin, nitrogen mustard
(BAMON)
b., Adriamycin, vinblastine,
imidazole carboxamide, prednisone
(BAVIP)
carboplatin, etoposide, b. (CEB)
b., CCNU, Adriamycin, Velban
(BCAVe, B-CAVe)
CCNU, cyclophosphamide,
Oncovin, b. (CCOB)
CCNU, vinblastine, b. (CVB)
cisplatin, Oncovin, b. (COB)
cisplatin, Velban, etoposide, b.
(CVEB)
cisplatin, vinblastine, etoposide, b.
(CVEB)
cyclophosphamide, Adriamycin,
methotrexate, b. (CAMB)
b., cyclophosphamide, dactinomycin
(BCD)
cyclophosphamide, doxorubicin,
teniposide, prednisone,
vincristine, b.

cyclophosphamide, epirubicin,
Oncovin, prednisone, b.
cyclophosphamide,
hydroxydaunomycin, Oncovin, b.
(CHOB)
cyclophosphamide,
hydroxydaunomycin, Oncovin,
prednisone, b. (CHOP-BLEO)
cyclophosphamide,
hydroxydaunorubicin, Oncovin,
prednisone, b.
b., cyclophosphamide, methotrexate,
5-fluorouracil (BCMF)
cyclophosphamide, methotrexate, 5-
fluorouracil, b. (CMF-BLEO)
cyclophosphamide, Oncomycin,
prednisone, b. (CEOP-B)
cyclophosphamide, Oncovin, ara-C,
prednisone, b. (COAP-BLEO)
cyclophosphamide, Oncovin,
MeCCNU, b. (COMB)
cyclophosphamide, Oncovin,
methotrexate, b. (COMB)
b., cyclophosphamide, Oncovin,
methotrexate, 5-fluorouracil
(BLEO-COMF)
cyclophosphamide, Oncovin,
prednisone, b. (COPB, COP-B,
COP-BLEO)
cyclophosphamide, Oncovin,
prednisone, Adriamycin, b.
(COPA-BLEO)
cyclophosphamide, prednisone,
Oncovin, b. (CPOB)
cyclophosphamide, vincristine,
prednisone, b. (CVP-BLEO)
b., cyclophosphamide, vincristine,
procarbazine, prednisone (BCVPP)
Cytoxan, Adriamycin,
methotrexate, b. (CAMB)
b., Cytoxan, hydroxydaunomycin,
Oncovin, prednisone (B-CHOP)
DDP, vindesine, b. (DVB)
b., DTIC, Oncovin, prednisone,
Adriamycin (B-DOPA)
b., Eldisine, lomustine, dacarbazine
(BELD)
b., Eldisine, mitomycin, Platinol
(BEMP)
b., etoposide, Adriamycin,
cyclophosphamide, vincristine,
procarbazine, prednisone
(BEACOPP)

NOTES

73

bleomycin *(continued)*
    etoposide, doxorubicin,
      cyclophosphamide, vincristine,
      prednisone, b. (VALOP-B)
    b., etoposide, Platinol (BEP)
    b., etoposide, prednimustine,
      procarbazine, cyclophosphamide,
      doxorubicin, vincristine
    high-dose Platinol, etoposide, b.
      (HDPEB)
    hydroxydaunomycin, Oncovin, ara-
      C, prednisone plus b. (HOAP-
      BLEO)
    b., ifosfamide, carboplatin
    b., ifosfamide, Platinol (BIP)
    b., ifosfamide with mesna rescue,
      Platinol (BIP)
    intralesional b.
    mechlorethamine, Oncovin, b.
      (MOB)
    b., mechlorethamine, Oncovin,
      procarbazine, prednisone (B-
      MOPP)
    mechlorethamine, Oncovin,
      procarbazine, prednisone, b.
      (MOPP-BLEO)
    mechlorethamine, Oncovin,
      procarbazine, prednisone, high-
      dose b.
    mechlorethamine, Oncovin,
      procarbazine, prednisone, low-
      dose b.
    methotrexate, Adriamycin,
      cyclophosphamide, Oncovin, b.
      (MACOB)
    methotrexate, Adriamycin,
      cyclophosphamide, Oncovin,
      prednisone, b. (MACOP-B)
    methotrexate, leucovorin,
      Adriamycin, cyclophosphamide,
      Oncovin, prednisone, b.
    Mustargen, Oncovin, b. (MOB)
    b., Oncovin, Adriamycin,
      prednisone (BOAP)
    Oncovin, ara-C, prednisone, b.
      (OAP-BLEO)
    b., Oncovin, lomustine, dacarbazine
      (BOLD)
    b., Oncovin, Matulane, prednisone
      (BOMP)
    b., Oncovin, methotrexate
    b., Oncovin, mitomycin, Platinol
      (BOMP)
    b., Oncovin, Platinol (BOP)
    b., Oncovin, prednisone,
      Adriamycin, mechlorethamine,
      methotrexate (BOPAM)
    b., Oncovin, streptozocin, etoposide
    Platinol, etoposide, b. (PEB)

Platinol, methotrexate, b. (PMB)
Platinol, vinblastine, b. (PVB)
streptozocin, CCNU, Adriamycin, b.
    (SCAB)
b. sulfate
b., Velban, doxorubicin,
    streptozocin (BVDS)
vinblastine and b. (VB)
vinblastine, actinomycin D, b.
    (VAB)
b., vinblastine, DTIC
vinblastine, Platinol, b. (VPB)
VP-16, ifosfamide, mitoxantrone, b.
    (VIMB)
VP-16, ifosfamide, Platinol, b.
    (VIP-B)
blighted ovum
blind
    b. biopsy
    b. endosonography probe
    b. spot
B-lineage acute lymphoblastic cell
blister cell
BLL
    benign lymphoepithelial lesion
bloc
    en b.
Bloch-Sulzberger syndrome
block
    alcohol subarachnoid b.
    atrioventricular b.
    autonomic nerve b.
    celiac plexus b. (CPB)
    Cerrobend trim b.
    epidural b.
    full-thickness kidney b.
    ganglion neurolytic b.
    hand b.
    heart b. (HB)
    intrathecal b.
    kidney and cord b.
    lung b.
    missing b.
    myelographic b.
    nerve b.
    neurolytic nerve b.
    peripheral nerve b.
    RadiaCare Sun B.
    regional neurolytic b.
    shadowing of b.
    shielding b.
    spinal b.
    splanchnic nerve b.
    split-beam b.
    tissue b.
blockade
    androgen b.
    celiac plexus b.
    combined androgen b. (CAB)

B

intermittent androgen b. (IAB)
maximal androgen b. (MAB)
peripheral androgen b. (PAB)
receptor b.
sequential androgen b. (SAB)
serotonergic b.
total androgen b.
virus b.
blocked beam algorithm
Blocked-Beam-Generator integration
blocker
adrenergic b.
alpha-adrenergic b.
calcium channel b.
VEGF receptor signal b.
blocking
b. antibody
conformal b.
customized b.
b. factor
tissue b.
Bloedorn applicator
blond tobacco
blood
b. agar plate
arterial b.
autologous b.
b. calculus
b. cancer
b. cell
b. cell allogeneic transplantation
b. cell antigen
b. cell aplasia
citrated b.
b. clot
b. clotting factor
b. coagulation factor
b. component
b. component support
b. component therapy
cord b.
b. crisis
b. culture
defibrinated b.
b. derivative
b. donation
fetoplacental b.
b. fluke
b. gas
b. group
b. group antigen
b. group oligosaccharide
determinant

b. group system (A, AB, B, O)
irradiated b.
lactescent b.
b. lake
laked b.
occult b.
b. oxygenation level-dependent (BOLD)
b. oxygenation level-dependent contrast
peripheral b. (PB)
platelet-poor b. (PPB)
platelet-rich b.
b. pressure
b. product
rheology of b.
b. sample
b. sampling
b. smear
stagnant b.
subacute b.
b. substitute
b. sugar
b. supply
transfused b.
b. transfusion
b. transfusion reaction
b. tumor
b. type
b. typing
b. typing system
umbilical cord b.
umbilical human cord b.
b. urea nitrogen (BUN)
b. urea nitrogen test
b. velocity
venous b.
b. vessel
b. vessel invasion (BVI)
b. warmer
whole b.
bloodborne
blood-brain barrier disruption
bloodstream
blood-tumor barrier (BTB)
Bloom-Richardson classification
Bloom syndrome
blot
MTN b.
Northern b.
Southern b.
Western ligand b. (WLB)

NOTES

blotting
> ligand b.

blue
> azovan b.
> b. cell tumor
> b. dye
> gentian b.
> high-iron diamine/Alcian b. (HID/AB)
> methylene b.
> b. nail pigmentation
> Prussian b.
> toluidine b.
> Urolene B.

blueberry muffin syndrome

Blumer shelf

blush
> choroid plexus b.
> papillary b.
> tumor b.

B-ly-7 antigen

B-lym oncogene

B-lymphocyte
> B-l. blast
> B-l. differentiation
> B-l. proliferation
> B-l. stimulator (BLyS)
> B-l. stimulatory factor

BLyS
> B-lymphocyte stimulator

BM
> bone marrow

BMD
> bone mineral density

BMI
> body mass index

BML
> benign metastasizing leiomyomatosis

BMMP
> bone marrow myeloid precursor

B-mode
> B-m. acquisition and targeting (BAT)
> B-m. echocardiography
> B-m. ultrasonography

B-MOPP
> bleomycin, mechlorethamine, Oncovin, procarbazine, prednisone

BMP
> BCNU, methotrexate, procarbazine

BMT
> bone marrow transplant
> bone marrow transplantation

BN
> brown Norwegian
> BN acute myelocytic leukemia
> BN ProSpec testing reagent

BNCT
> boron neutron capture therapy

B-NHL
> B-cell non-Hodgkin lymphoma

BNML
> brown Norwegian rat acute myelocytic leukemia

BOAP
> bleomycin, Oncovin, Adriamycin, prednisone

board
> belly b.
> institutional review b. (IRB)

Bochdalek
> B. foramen
> B. hernia

Bocking classification

bodily fluid

Bodin-Gibb staging system

body
> Arnold b.
> Aschoff b.
> aspirated foreign b. (AFB)
> asteroid b.
> Auer b.
> Bence Jones b.
> brassy b.
> Cabot ring b.
> Call-Exner b.
> cancer b.
> b. cavity non-Hodgkin lymphoma
> ciliary b.
> Councilman b.
> crescent b.
> Deetjen b.
> demilune b.
> Dohle b.
> Donovan b.
> Dutcher b.
> Ehrlich hemoglobinemia b.
> elementary b.
> embryonal tumor of ciliary b.
> fibrin b.
> b. fluid
> Gamna-Favre b.
> Guarnieri b.
> b. habitus
> b. habitus change (BHC)
> Hamazaki-Wesenberg b.
> Harting b.
> Heinz b.
> Heinz-Ehrlich b.
> hematoxylin b.
> Howell-Jolly b.
> Jaworski b.
> Jolly b.
> ketone b.
> Lallemand b.
> Lallemand-Trousseau b.
> Leishman-Donovan b.
> Lipschütz b.

Luse b.
lyssa b.
b. mass index (BMI)
Mott b.
Müller duct b.
Negri b.
Neill-Mooser b.
owl's eye inclusion b.
b. of pancreas
Pappenheimer b.
paranuclear b.
psammoma b.
b. scanning
Schaumann b.
Schiller-Duval b.
b. of stomach
b. surface area calculation
b. surface normogram
tympanic b.
b. of uterus
Virchow-Hassall b.
Boeck sarcoid
BOLD
  bleomycin, Oncovin, lomustine,
    dacarbazine
  blood oxygenation level-dependent
    BOLD contrast
Bolton-Hunter technique
bolus
  b. administration
  b. administration of intravenous
    contrast medium
  barium b.
  daily b.
  b. injection
  b. material
  nose b.
  b. tagging
  tissue-equivalent b.
  b. tracking
Bombriski melanoma
BOMP
  bleomycin, Oncovin, Matulane,
    prednisone
  bleomycin, Oncovin, mitomycin, Platinol
    BOMP chemotherapy regimen
bond
  phosphodiester b.
Bondronat
bone
  b. abnormality
  b. age
  b. algorithm

both b.'s (BB)
bowed long b.
cancellous b.
b. cancer
carpal b.
b. center
chondrosarcoma of b.
cortical b.
b. cyst
b. demineralization
b. densitometer
b. destruction
b. dysplasia
ethmoid b.
b. flap
giant cell sarcoma of b.
b. graft
haversian canal of b.
b. imaging
b. infarct
b. infarction
b. island
lamellated b.
b. length study
malignant fibrous histiocytoma
  of b.
b. marrow (BM)
b. marrow aplasia
b. marrow aspirate
b. marrow aspirate and biopsy
b. marrow aspiration
b. marrow cellularity
b. marrow depression
b. marrow donor
b. marrow dose
b. marrow failure state
b. marrow failure syndrome
b. marrow fibroblast
b. marrow fibrosis
b. marrow granulocyte reserve
  assay
b. marrow harvesting
b. marrow histochemistry
b. marrow hypocellularity
b. marrow hypoplasia
b. marrow immunohistology
b. marrow infiltration
b. marrow involvement
b. marrow lesion
b. marrow lymphoid hyperplasia
b. marrow microenvironment
b. marrow myeloid precursor
  (BMMP)

NOTES

bone *(continued)*
    b. marrow neoangiogenesis
    b. marrow purging
    b. marrow relapse
    b. marrow rescue
    b. marrow scintigraphy
    b. marrow staining
    b. marrow stem cell
    b. marrow stroma
    b. marrow suppression
    b. marrow toxicity
    b. marrow transplant (BMT)
    b. marrow transplantation (BMT)
    medullary b.
    b. metastasis
    b. mineral accrual
    b. mineral content
    b. mineral density (BMD)
    b. morphogenetic activity
    b. neoplasm
    osteosarcoma of b.
    b. overdevelopment
    b. pain
    parallel b.'s
    periosteal b.
    b. plug
    primary lymphoma of b. (PLB)
    b. quantitative CT (BQCT)
    b. reabsorption
    b. resorption marker
    b. sarcoma
    B. Sarcoma Registry
    b. scan
    b. sclerosis
    solitary plasmacytoma of b. (SPB)
    b. spiculation
    b. spicule
    b. spur
    b. strut
    b. tumor
bone-air interface
bone-chip allograft
bone-forming tumor
Bonefos
bone-hardening artifact
bone-on-bone contact
bone-targeted therapy
bone-tendon-bone graft
bone-within-bone
    b.-w.-b. appearance
    b.-w.-b. vertebra
Bonferroni
    B. procedure
    B. test
Bonviva
bony
    b. alignment
    b. ankylosis

    b. bridging
    b. contusion
    b. erosion
    b. hyperostosis
    b. labyrinth
    b. metastasis
    b. nonunion
    b. pelvis
    b. projection
    b. resorption
    b. semicircular canal
    b. thorax
    b. trabecular pattern
boost
    breast b.
    concomitant b.
    coned-down b.
    cone electron b.
    b. dose
    endoluminal b.
    local b.
    posterior fossa b.
    prime b.
    radiation b.
    stereotactic b.
    b. technique
    b. therapy
    whole brain radiation therapy
      without stereotactic b.
    whole brain radiation therapy with
      stereotactic b.
bootstrap analysis
BOP
    BCNU, Oncovin, prednisone
    bleomycin, Oncovin, Platinol
BOPAM
    bleomycin, Oncovin, prednisone,
      Adriamycin, mechlorethamine,
      methotrexate
BOPP
    BCNU, Oncovin, procarbazine,
      prednisone
    boronated porphyrin
borderline
    b. malignant epithelial ovarian
      neoplasm
    b. ovarian tumor
Bordetella
    B. pertussis
    B. pertussis infection
Borocell
boron
    b. capture
    b. neutron capture therapy (BNCT)
boronated porphyrin (BOPP)
Borrelia burgdorferi
borreliosis
    Lyme b.

Borrmann
B. classification
B. gastric cancer typing system
bortezomib
Bosniak classification system
boss
carpal b.
bossing
frontal b.
Boston exanthem
B&O Supprettes
both-bone fracture
both bones (BB)
both-column fracture
botryoid
b. embryonal rhabdomyosarcoma
b. sarcoma
botryoides
sarcoma b.
bougie
bougienage technique
boundary
air-bone-tissue b.
b. layer
bound/free
bounding peripheral pulse
bovine
b. anticryptosporidium
b. immunoglobulin
pegademase b. (PEG-ADA)
bovis
Moraxella b.
Mycobacterium b.
bowed long bone
bowel
b. cancer
b. distention
b. gas artifact
b. incontinence
b. infarction
large b.
b. obstruction
b. preparation
small b.
b. sounds
b. wall
b. wall hematoma
b. wall penetration
Bowen disease
bowenoid
b. papulosis
b. papulosis of vulva

bowing
anterior tibial b.
b. fracture
box
isocentric 4-field b.
TATA b.
boydii
Pseudoallescheria b.
BPCC
bilateral percutaneous cervical cordotomy
BPH
benign prostatic hyperplasia
benign prostatic hypertrophy
BPI
brief pain inventory
Bq
becquerel
BQCT
bone quantitative CT
BR64 antibody
BR96 antibody
BRACAnalysis genetic susceptibility test for breast and ovarian cancer
brace
2-poster b.
SOMI b.
sternooccipital-mandibular immobilization b.
Yale b.
bracelet
alert b.
lymphedema alert b.
medical alert b.
brachial
b. artery
b. artery approach
b. plexopathy
b. plexus
b. plexus birth injury
b. plexus infiltration
b. vein
brachialis
brachii
biceps b.
brachiocephalic
b. artery
b. branch
b. trunk
b. vessel
brachioproctic eroticism
brachioradialis
b. tendon
b. tendon reflex test

B

NOTES

brachium pontis
brachycephaly
BrachySeed
    B. brachytherapy seed
    B. palladium-103 seed
    B. Pd-103 implant
brachytherapy
    b. balloon applicator
    3D-virtual b.
    endobronchial b. (EBB)
    endoluminal b.
    HDR b.
    high dose rate intracavitary b.
      (HDRIB)
    high dose rate remote b.
    interstitial b.
    intracavitary b. (IBT)
    intraductal b.
    intraluminal b.
    intravaginal b. (IVBT)
    intravascular b.
    magnetic resonance spectroscopic
      imaging-guided b.
    MammoSite b. (MSB)
    Manchester system for b.
    Paris system for b.
    PDR b.
    permanent seed implant b.
    prostate b.
    pulsed b.
    remote afterloading b. (RAB)
    stereotactic b.
    transcatheter b.
    transluminal b.
    transperineal prostate b.
    ULDR b.
    ultra-low dose rate b.
    vascular b.
BrachyVision 6.0 software
B-RAF oncogene
Bragg-Gray cavity
Bragg peak
brain
    b. abscess
    b. aneurysm
    b. atrophy
    b. biopsy
    b. cancer
    b. concussion
    b. cyst
    b. death
    b. disease
    b. dysfunction
    b. edema
    b. geography
    b. homeostasis
    b. imaging
    b. infection
    b. lesion

    b. mapping
    b. mass
    b. metastasis
    b. parenchyma
    b. perfusion
    b. perfusion reserve
    b. region vesicle
    b. scintigraphy
    b. substance
    b. tumor (BT)
    b. tumor therapy
    whole b.
brainstem
    b. edema
    b. encephalitis
    b. ependymoma
    b. glioma
    b. infarction
brainstem-evoked response audiometry
    (BSERA)
bran
    wheat b.
branch
    brachiocephalic b.
    b. pulmonary artery
    b. pulmonary artery stenosis
branched
    b. chain
    b. chain DNA amplification assay
    b. decay
branchial
    b. arch
    b. cleft cyst
    b. sinus
branching
    anomalous b.
branchiomeric paraganglia
Brandt cytology balloon
Brånemark implant
Branhamella catarrhalis
brassy
    b. body
    b. cough
braziliensis
    Paracoccidioides b.
BRCA1
    breast cancer 1 gene
    BRCA1 expression
    BRCA1 gene
    BRCA1 gene mutation
    BRCA1 genetic testing
    BRCA1 susceptibility gene
    BRCA1 susceptibility gene for
      breast cancer
BRCA2
    breast cancer 2 gene
    BRCA2 expression
    BRCA2 gene
BrE-1 antibody

BrE-2 antibody
BrE-3 antibody
breakdown
matrix b.
wound b.
breakpoint
b. cluster region (BCR)
b. cluster region-negative (BCR-negative)
b. cluster region-positive (BCR-positive)
breast
b. abnormality
b. abscess
adenoma of b.
adolescent b.
adult b.
b. augmentation
augmented b.
b. biopsy
b. boost
b. calcification
b. cancer
b. cancer antigen
b. cancer candidate of metastasis-1 assay
b. cancer during pregnancy
b. cancer epithelium
B. Cancer Family Registry
b. cancer 1 gene (*BRCA1*)
b. cancer 2 gene (*BRCA2*)
B. Cancer Prevention Trial (BCPT)
b. cancer resistance protein (BCRP)
b. cancer vaccine
b. carcinoma
b. carcinoma in situ (BCIS)
B. CFR
b. coil
b. conservation surgery (BCS)
b. cyst
b. cyst aspiration
cystic disease of b.
b. disease
b. dosimetry
b. edema
b. embryology
b. epithelial cell
fascia of b.
b. hyperplasia
B. Imaging Reporting and Data System (BI-RADS)
b. irradiation
b. lesion

b. metastasis
b. mucocele
B., Ovarian and Colorectal Cancer Family Registries
b. parenchyma
b. preservation
b. pump
b. reconstruction
b. self-examination (BSE)
b. sonography
tail of b.
b. tissue density
b. traction
BreastAlert
B. differential temperature sensor
B. test
BreastCheck
breast-conserving
b.-c. surgery (BCS)
b.-c. therapy (BCT)
breast-ovarian cancer syndrome
BreastScan IR system
breath
b. hold
b. sounds
breathing
carbogen b.
Brecher-Cronkite method
Breen and Tullis method
Breezee Mist Antifungal
bregma
Bremsstrahlung effect
Brenner tumor
brequinar sodium
Breslow
B. classification
B. classification for malignant melanoma
B. depth
B. microstaging method
B. microstaging system
B. staging
B. thickness
B. thickness in malignant melanoma
Brethine
Bretschneider HTK solution
Breus mole
BrevaRex
brevicollis
brevifolia
Taxus b.

NOTES

brevis
    adductor b.
    Demodex b.
    extensor carpi radialis b.
    extensor digitorum b.
    extensor tensor pollicis b.
bRFS
    biochemical recurrence-free survival
BRFSS
    Behavioral Risk Factor Surveillance
    System
Bricker procedure
bridge
    intercellular b.
bridging
    bony b.
    internuclear b.
brief
    B. Fatigue Inventory (BFI)
    b. pain inventory (BPI)
bright signal
brim
    pelvic b.
    b. of pelvis
British anti-Lewisite (BAL)
broad
    b. fuzzy penumbra
    b. ligament
broad-spectrum antibiotic
Broca
    B. area
    B. index
    B. region
Brochner-Mortensen method
Brocq
    erythrose péribuccale pigmentaire
    of B.
Broders
    B. classification
    B. grade
    B. index
    B. system
Brodie abscess
brodifacoum
bromfenac
bromide
    pancuronium b.
    tetrazolium b.
brominated oil
5-bromodeoxyuridine (BUdR)
5-bromouracil
Brompton cocktail
bronchi (*pl. of* bronchus)
bronchial
    b. adenoma
    b. angiography
    b. arteriography
    b. artery
    b. artery embolization

    b. asthma
    b. atresia
    b. brushing
    b. carcinoid tumor
    b. carcinoma
    b. duplication cyst
    b. epithelium
    b. fracture
    b. inflammation
    b. mucosal gland
    b. obstruction
    b. sinus
    b. spur
    b. stenosis
    b. tract
    b. tree
    b. washing
bronchial-associated lymphoid tissue (BALT)
bronchiectasis
    cystic b.
bronchiolar adenocarcinoma
bronchiolitis
    constrictive b.
bronchioloalveolar carcinoma
bronchitis
    asthmatic b.
    lymphocytic b.
bronchoalveolar
    b. carcinoma (BAC)
    b. cell adenoma
    b. lavage (BAL)
bronchocentric granulomatosis (BCG)
bronchoconstriction
bronchoesophageal fistula
bronchogenic
    b. carcinoma
    b. cyst
bronchogram
    air b.
bronchography
broncholithiasis
bronchoplasty
    balloon b.
bronchopleural fistula
bronchopneumonia
bronchopulmonary
    b. aspergillosis
    b. asthma
    b. dysplasia
    b. fibrosarcoma
    b. fistula
    b. foregut
    b. neoplasm
    b. segment
    b. sequestration
    b. toilet
bronchorrhea

bronchoscope
> flexible b.
> open-tube rigid b.
> rigid b.

bronchoscopy
> flexible fiberoptic b.
> laser-induced fluorescence
>   emission b.
> LIFE Imaging System and White
>   Light b.
> light-induced fluorescence
>   endoscopic b.
> therapeutic b.
> virtual b.

bronchospasm

bronchostenosis

bronchovascular pattern

bronchus, pl. **bronchi**
> carcinoma of b.
> ectatic b.
> b. intermedius
> lobar b.
> proximal segmental b.
> b. sign

bronchus-associated lymphoid tissue
  (BALT)

Brooke tumor

Brookmeyer-Crowley method

bropirimine (ABPP)

broth
> Middlebrook b.

brown
> b. cell cyst
> b. Norwegian (BN)
> b. Norwegian rat acute myelocytic
>   leukemia (BNML)
> B. University Oncology Group
>   (BrUOG)

Brown-Bovari machine

Brown-Roberts-Wells frame

Brown-Sequard syndrome

Broxine

broxuridine

Brucella abortus

brucellosis

Bruch membrane

Brunhilde virus

Brunner
> B. gland
> B. gland hyperplasia
> B. gland hypertrophy

BrUOG
> Brown University Oncology Group

brush cytology

brushing
> bronchial b.

Bruton sex-linked agammaglobulinemia

bryostatin 1

BSE
> breast self-examination

BSERA
> brainstem-evoked response audiometry

B-sitosterol

BSO
> bilateral salpingo-oophorectomy
> buthionine sulfoximine

BT
> bladder tumor
> brain tumor

BTA stat test

BTB
> blood-tumor barrier

B/T Blue Gene Rearrangement test

BU
> busulfan

bubble
> encapsulated gas b.

bubbly bone lesion

bucca, pl. **buccae**

buccal
> b. mucosa
> b. mucosal cancer
> Nitrogard B.
> b. space
> b. space infection

buccarum
> morsicatio b.

Buck fascia

buckled drainage catheter

buckle fracture

BU-CY
> busulfan-cyclophosphamide

budding yeast

Bud Percuflex catheter

BUdR
> 5-bromodeoxyuridine
> BUdR protocol

Buerger prostatic needle

buffalo hump

buffer
> D-Di b.
> Michaelis b.
> Owren-Koller b.
> Spli-Prest b.

Bufferin

NOTES

buffy
  b. coat
  b. coat component
  b. coat preparation
  b. coat smear
buffy-coated cell
bulb
  duodenal b.
  jugular b.
  sinovaginal b.
  tumor b.
bulbar
  b. muscular atrophy
  b. palsy
bulbi
  phthisis b.
  siderosis b.
bulbourethral
  b. artery
  b. gland
bulbous enlargement
bulge
  anular disc b.
bulging
  b. anulus
  b. disc
  b. fissure
bulk
  Modane B.
bulky
  b. Hodgkin disease
  b. lymphadenopathy
  b. mass
  b. mediastinal tumor
bulla, pl. **bullae**
  emphysematous b.
  ethmoidal b.
bullous
  b. disorder
  b. emphysema
  b. lung disease
  b. pemphigoid
bumetanide
Bumex
BUN
  blood urea nitrogen
bundle
  atrioventricular b.
  neurovascular b. (NVB)
Bunn-Lamberg classification
Bunyavirus
bupivacaine
Buprenex
buprenorphine
bupropion
burden
  cell b.
  leukemic b.
  plasma viral b.

  radiation b.
  symptom b.
  tumor b.
burdock
burgdorferi
  Borrelia b.
Burinex
Burkholderia
  B. aeruginosa
  B. cepacia
Burkitt
  B. leukemia
  B. lymphoma
  B. tumor
Burkitt-like lymphoma
burn
  caustic b.
  b. injury
burned-out tumor
Burnett cylinder
burnt-out colon
burr cell
bursa, pl. **bursae**
  b. of Fabricius
bursal
  b. calcification
  b. osteochondromatosis
bursitis
burst
  b. forming
  b. fracture
  macrophage oxidative b.
  oxidative b.
burst-forming
  b.-f. cell
  b.-f. unit
Buruli ulcer
Buschke-Löwenstein
  B.-L. condyloma
  B.-L. tumor
buserelin acetate
Busse-Buschke disease
busulfan (BU)
  b. alkylation
  b. conditioning
  b., melphalan, thiotepa
busulfan-cyclophosphamide (BU-CY)
Busulfex
butadienyl
butalbital compound and codeine
Butchart
  B. classification of malignant
    mesothelioma
  B. staging classification
buthionine sulfoximine (BSO)
butoconazole
butorphanol tartrate
butterfly
  b. coil

b. configuration
b. fracture
b. glioblastoma
b. glioma
b. needle
b. pattern
b. rash
buttockectomy
button
Panje voice b.
b. sequestrum
butyl
b. DNJ
b. nitrate inhalant
butyrophenone
buyo cheek cancer
BVAP
BCNU, vincristine, Adriamycin,
prednisone
BVCPP
BCNU, vinblastine, cyclophosphamide,
procarbazine, prednisone

BVDS
bleomycin, Velban, doxorubicin,
streptozocin
BVI
blood vessel invasion
BVPP
BCNU, vincristine, procarbazine,
prednisone
Bwamba virus
BWS
Beckwith-Wiedemann syndrome
bypass
aortobifemoral b.
aortofemoral b. (AFB)
aortovisceral b.
biliary-enteric b.
gastroenteric b.
V b.
B-zone small lymphocytic lymphoma

B

NOTES

C
   carboplatin

C-1000
   Revitalose C-1000

C$_{max}$
   maximal drug concentration

C1 inactivator

C3 receptor

CA15-3
   CA15-3 breast cancer tumor marker
   CA15-3 RIA serum tumor marker

CA125, CA-125
   cancer antigen 125
      CA125 antigen assay
      CA125 cross-reactivity
      CA125 ovarian tumor marker
      serum CA125

CA
   cancer
   cancer antigen
   capsid
   carcinoma
   cellulose acetate
   cyclophosphamide and Adriamycin
   cytosine arabinoside
      Calibrator CA
      CA M26 tumor marker
      CA M29 tumor marker
      CA virus

CA19-9
   CA19-9 tumor marker

C17-1A
   chimeric 17-1A

CA27.29
   CA27.29 tumor marker

CA125-11 tumor marker

CA15-2 RIA test

CA195 tumor marker

CA-1 prothrombin assay

CA50 tumor marker

CA549 breast cancer tumor marker

CA72-4 tumor marker

CAB
   combined androgen blockade

cabergoline

c-abl protooncogene/oncogene

CABOP, CA-BOP
   cyclophosphamide, Adriamycin, bleomycin, Oncovin, prednisone

Cabot ring body

CABS
   CCNU, Adriamycin, bleomycin, streptozocin

CAC
   cisplatin, ara-C, caffeine

CA/CAF
   cyclophosphamide and doxorubicin with or without 5-fluorouracil

cachectic

cachectin

Cache Valley virus

cachexia
   cancer c.
   paraneoplastic c.

CACP
   cisplatin

CACS
   cancer, anorexia, cachexia syndrome

cactinomycin

CAD
   cyclophosphamide, Adriamycin, dacarbazine
   cytosine arabinoside and daunorubicin
      CAD chemotherapy protocol
      RapidScreen digital CAD

CADD
   central-axis-depth-dose
      CADD value

CADD-PLUS external volumetric programmable pump

CADD-TPN
      CADD-TPN ambulatory infusion system
      CADD-TPN pump

cadherin
   skin c.

CADIC
   cyclophosphamide, Adriamycin, dacarbazine

cadmium

CAE
   cyclophosphamide, Adriamycin, etoposide

Caelyx

Caenorhabditis elegans

CAF
   Cytoxan, Adriamycin, 5-fluorouracil

café au lait spot

caffeic acid

caffeine
   acetaminophen, aspirin, c.
   cisplatin, ara-C, c. (CAC)
   5-fluorouracil, cisplatin, cytarabine, c. (PACE)
   orphenadrine, aspirin, c.

CAFFI
   cyclophosphamide, Adriamycin, 5-fluorouracil by continuous infusion

CAFP
cyclophosphamide, Adriamycin, 5-fluorouracil, prednisone
CAFTH
cyclophosphamide, Adriamycin, 5-fluorouracil, tamoxifen, Halotestin
CAFVP
cyclophosphamide, Adriamycin, 5-fluorouracil, vincristine, prednisone
CAG
CAG microsatellite of exon 1
CAG trinucleotide repeat
cage
antiprotrusio c.
CAI
carboxyamidotriazole
CAIDS
community-acquired immunodeficiency syndrome
cake
c. mix kit
c. of tumor
calcaneal spur
calcanei (*pl. of* calcaneus)
calcaneocuboid joint
calcaneofibular ligament
calcaneus, pl. **calcanei**
Cal Carb-HD
Calcibind
Calci-Chew
Calciday-667
calcifediol
calcification
abdominal diffuse c.
abdominal vascular c.
abdominal wall c.
adrenal c.
alimentary tract c.
anterior spinal ligament c.
anular c.
arachnoid granulation c.
arterial c.
arteriovascular c.
basal ganglia c.
breast c.
bursal c.
coarse c.
dermal c.
diffuse abdominal c.
dystrophic c.
ectopic c.
eggshell c.
c. of falx cerebri
focus of c.
granular c.
granulomatous c.
intraductal c.
pleural c.

popcorn c.
psammomatous c.
calcified
c. astrocytoma
c. cartilage
c. fibroadenoma
c. liver metastasis
c. renal mass
calcifying
c. epithelioma
c. epithelioma of Malherbe
c. metastasis
Calcijex
Calci-Mix
calcineurin
calcinosis
tumoral c.
calciphylaxis
Calcite 500
calcitonin
calcitriol
calcium
c. acetate
c. antagonist therapy
c. carbonate
c. carbonate and simethicone
c. channel blocker
c. chloride
c. citrate
cottage cheese c.
dietary c.
C. Disodium Versenate
c. folinate
c. glubionate
c. gluceptate
c. gluconate
c. heparin
c. hydroxyapatite crystal
c. influx inhibitor
c. lactate
leucovorin c.
methotrexate, Platinol, 5-fluorouracil, leucovorin, c. (MPFL)
Orzel UFT/leucovorin c.
c. phosphate (CaP)
c. phosphate, dibasic
PMS-Docusate C.
c. polycarbophil
c. pyrophosphate deposition disease
c. pyrophosphate dihydrate
c. soap
UFT/leucovorin c.
calcium-DTPA
yttrium-90 radiolabeled humanized anti-Tac and c.-DTPA
calculation
body surface area c.
c. of planes
calculus, pl. **calculi**

biliary c.
blood c.
fibrin c.
hemic c.
struvite c.
Calderol
caldesmon
high molecular weight c.
Caldwell-Luc resection
CALF
cyclophosphamide, Adriamycin,
leucovorin rescue, 5-fluorouracil
CALF chemotherapy protocol
calf
c. swelling
c. vein thrombosis
CALF-E
cyclophosphamide, Adriamycin,
leucovorin rescue, 5-fluorouracil,
ethinyl estradiol
Cytoxan, Adriamycin, leucovorin
calcium, 5-fluorouracil, ethinyl estradiol
CALGB
cancer and leukemia group B
CALGB study
calibrated leak
calibration failure artifact
calibrator
C. CA
dose c.
caliceal, calyceal
c. abnormality
c. diverticulum
c. nephrostolithotomy
calices (*pl. of* calyx)
calicheamicin
caliectasis
California
C. Verbal Learning Test (CVLT)
C. virus
californium-252 (^{252}Cf)
caliper
calix (*var. of* calyx)
CALLA
common acute lymphoblastic leukemia
antigen
CALLA negative
CALLA positive
CALLA-positive myeloma
Call-Exner body
CALLF
Cytoxan, Adriamycin, leucovorin
calcium, 5-fluorouracil

callosum
dysgenesis of corpus c.
callus formation
calm
C. Formula Sleep Aide
C. Forte Sleep Aide
Calmette-Guérin
bacille C.-G. (BCG)
C.-G. bacillus
C.-G. immunotherapy
calmodulin inhibitor
caloric intake
caloris
stadium c.
Calphron
Cal-Plus
Calsan
Caltine
Caltrate 600
calusterone
calvarial
c. marrow
c. metastasis
Calvert formula
calyceal (*var. of* caliceal)
Calymmatobacterium
Calypte HIV-1 urine EIA
calyx, calix, pl. **calices**
abortive c.
CAM
complementary and alternative medicine
cyclophosphamide, Adriamycin,
methotrexate
CAMB
cyclophosphamide, Adriamycin,
methotrexate, bleomycin
Cytoxan, Adriamycin, methotrexate,
bleomycin
Cambridge classification
CAMELEON
cytosine arabinoside, high-dose
methotrexate, leucovorin, Oncovin
cameloid
c. anemia
c. cell
CAMEO
cyclophosphamide, Adriamycin,
methotrexate, etoposide, Oncovin
Camey reservoir
CAMF
cyclophosphamide, Adriamycin,
methotrexate, 5-fluorouracil
Camino micromanometer catheter

NOTES

89

CAMLO
    cytosine arabinoside, methotrexate, leucovorin, Oncovin
CAMP
    cyclophosphamide, Adriamycin, methotrexate, procarbazine
campaign
    Cancer Research C. (CRC)
Campath
    C. II
    C. humanized monoclonal antibody
Camptosar injection
Camptotheca
    C. acuminata
    colony-stimulating factor *C.*
camptothecin analog
Campylobacter
    C. colitis
    C. fetus
    C. jejuni
    C. pylori
    C. 16S-23S rRNA internal spacer region length assay
    C. 16S-23S rRNA ISR test
can
    c. oncogene
    c. protooncogene/oncogene
Canadian
    C. Cancer Society
    C. National Breast Screening Study-2 (CNBSS-2)
canal
    acoustic c.
    adductor c.
    alveolar c.
    anal c.
    anterior condylar c.
    antropyloric c.
    atrioventricular c.
    auditory c.
    bony semicircular c.
    external auditory c. (EAC)
    haversian c.
    c. of Lambert
canalicular immunostaining pattern
canarypox
    recombinant c.
    c. vector
canarypox-HIV gp120
cancellous
    c. bone
    c. osteoma
Cancell therapy
cancer (CA)
    adolescent c.
    adrenal gland c.
    advanced epithelial ovarian c.
    aerodigestive c.

American Joint Committee on C. (AJCC)
anal region c.
androgen-dependent prostate c.
androgen-independent prostate c. (AIPC)
anogenital c.
c., anorexia, cachexia syndrome (CACS)
anthracycline-nave metastatic breast c.
c. antigen (CA)
c. antigen 125 (CA125, CA-125)
appendiceal c.
asymptomatic metastatic hormone-refractory prostate c.
betel c.
bile duct c.
biliary tract c.
bladder c.
blood c.
c. body
bone c.
bowel c.
BRACAnalysis genetic susceptibility test for breast and ovarian c.
brain c.
BRCA1 susceptibility gene for breast c.
breast c.
buccal mucosal c.
buyo cheek c.
c. cachexia
cardiovascular c.
cecal c.
c. cell
c. cell-derived blood coagulating activity 1 (CCA-1)
cervical stump c.
childhood c.
chimney sweep's c.
colloid c.
colon c.
colorectal c. (CRC)
C. Committee of College of American Pathologists
common epithelial ovarian c.
conjugal c.
contralateral breast c. (CLBC)
cutaneous metastatic breast c.
c. death
deleted in colon c. (DCC)
c. à deux
disseminated c.
distal gastric c.
drug-sensitive c.
early gastric c.
encephaloid c.
c. en cuirasse

endobronchial c.
endometrial c.
epithelial ovarian c. (EOC)
esophageal c.
European Organization for Research and Treatment of C. (EORTC)
extracapsular prostate c.
extrapulmonary small cell c.
fallopian tube c.
familial c.
C. Family Registry (CFR)
c. free (CF)
fulguration of bladder c.
gallbladder c.
gastric remnant c.
gastrointestinal c.
gender-limited c.
genitourinary c.
C. Genome Anatomy Project (CGAP)
gingival c.
glandular c.
GOG staging system for ovarian c.
green c.
Gynecologic Oncology Group staging system for ovarian c.
hard palate c.
head and neck c.
hepatic flexure c.
hepatobiliary c.
hepatocellular c.
hereditary c.
hereditary nonpolyposis colon c. (HNPCC)
hereditary nonpolyposis colorectal c. (HNPCC)
HER-2/*neu*-expressing c.
high-risk breast c. (HRBC)
high-risk primary breast c. (HRPBC)
HLA-A2.1-positive colorectal c.
hormone-dependent prostate c.
hormone-refractory breast c.
hormone-refractory prostate c. (HRPC)
hypopharyngeal c.
inflammatory breast c. (IBC)
International Union Against C. (UICC)
interval c.
intrahepatic biliary c.
invasive penile c.

iodine-131 antiferritin treatment for hepatocellular c.
Jackson staging system for penile c.
Jewett-Strong-Marshall staging of bladder c.
Jewett-Strong staging of bladder c.
c. juice
kangri c.
kidney c.
large cell lung c.
large operable breast c. (LOBC)
laryngeal c.
larynx c.
Laurén classification of stomach c.
leptomeningeal c.
c. and leukemia group B (CALGB)
c. and leukemia group B study
limited-stage small cell lung c. (LSSCLC)
lip c.
liver c.
localization of prostate c.
locally advanced breast c. (LABC)
locally advanced head and neck c. (LAHNC)
locally advanced nonsmall-cell lung c. (LAD-NSCLC)
locoregional breast c. (LBC)
lung c.
c. map
medullary thyroid c.
mesothelioma c.
metastatic breast c. (MBC)
metastatic lung c.
microinvasive cervical c. (MICA)
Muir-Torre syndrome of hereditary nonpolyposis colon c.
mule-spinners' c.
mutated in colon c. (MCC)
myelodysplastic c.
nasal cavity c.
nasal vestibule c.
nasopharyngeal c.
nasopharynx c.
natural-end c.
C. Needs Questionnaire (CNQ)
c. nest
neuroendocrine c.
nonmelanoma skin c. (NMSC)
nonpolyposis colorectal c.
nonsmall cell lung c. (NSCLC)

NOTES

cancer *(continued)*
    oat cell lung c.
    obstructive colorectal c.
    occult c.
    operable breast c. (OBC)
    oral cavity c.
    oropharyngeal c.
    ovarian c. (OVCA)
    palpatory T-stage prostate c.
    pancreas c.
    pancreatic c.
    paraffin c.
    paranasal sinus c.
    parotid c.
    c. patient
    pediatric c.
    penile c.
    perforating colorectal c.
    pericardial c.
    pharyngeal wall c.
    pipe-smokers' c.
    piriform sinus c.
    pitch-workers' c.
    platinum-resistant ovarian c.
    pleural c.
    postcricoid pharyngeal c.
    preadult c.
    primary c.
    c. procoagulant
    prostate c.
    c. of prostate and brain gene
    prostatic c.
    PSA-detected c.
    pulmonary c.
    radiation-induced c.
    radiogenic breast c.
    rectal c.
    rectosigmoid c.
    recurrent c.
    refractory bladder c.
    C. Rehabilitation Evaluation System (CARES)
    renal cell c.
    C. Research Campaign (CRC)
    resectable colorectal c.
    retromolar trigone c.
    c. risk
    Robson renal cell c. (stage I-IV)
    Royal Marsden Hospital staging system for testicular c.
    salivary gland c.
    c. salve
    sarcomatoid renal cell c.
    scar c.
    c. screening
    secondary c.
    second primary c. (SPC)
    sinus c.
    skin c.
    small bowel c.
    small cell lung c. (SCLC)
    small intestine c.
    soft palate c.
    somatic mutation theory of c.
    spider c.
    splenic flexure c.
    c. staging
    C. and Steroid Hormone (CASH)
    C. and Steroid Hormone Study
    stomach c.
    stump c.
    suboptimally debulked c.
    superficial bladder c.
    C. Surveillance Program (CSP)
    suture line c.
    synchronous colorectal c.
    synchronous ipsilateral breast c. (SIBC)
    taxane-resistant breast c.
    telangiectatic c.
    testicular c.
    testis c.
    C. Therapy Evaluation Program (CTEP)
    thoracic c.
    thymoma c.
    thyroid c.
    tonsil c.
    tonsillar area c.
    transitional cell c.
    c. treatment
    treatment-related secondary c.
    Union Internationale Contre le C. (UICC)
    unresectable colorectal c.
    urothelial c.
    uterine cervical c.
    vaginal c.
    Van Nuys Prognostic Index in breast c.
    varicoid esophageal c.
    vocal cord c.
    vulvar c.
    water c.

cancer-associated
    c.-a. anemia
    c.-a. serum antigen (CASA)

cancer-detection method

cancer-hemolytic uremic syndrome (C-HUS)

cancericidal dose

cancerization
    field c.

cancerophobia *(var. of* carcinophobia)

cancerous mutation

cancer-related
    c.-r. fatigue (CRF)
    c.-r. mutation

CancerVax
Cancidas
Candida
    C. albicans
    C. endocarditis
    C. fungemia
    C. glabrata
    C. guilliermondii
    C. krusei
    C. lusitaniae
    C. parapsilosis
    C. tropicalis
candidal
    c. endophthalmitis
    c. esophagitis
candidate
    allogeneic antigen c.
    c. of metastasis-1 gene detection
candidemia
candidiasis
    c. angular cheilitis
    atrophic c.
    chronic disseminated c. (CDC)
    chronic hyperplastic c.
    chronic mucocutaneous c.
    disseminated c.
    c. erythematous
    esophageal c. (EC)
    fluconazole-resistant esophageal c.
    c. of glabrous skin
    hyperplastic c.
    mucocutaneous c.
    oral c.
    pseudomembranous c.
    recurrent vulvovaginal c.
    refractory mucosal c.
Candistatin
candle
    c. drippings appearance
    c. guttering
Candlelighters Childhood Cancer Foundation (CCCF)
Canesten
    C. Topical
    C. Vaginal
canine kidney
canis
    Ehrlichia c.
    Microsporum c.
cannabinoid
cannula, pl. cannulas, cannulae
    Interlink c.
    Rutner c.

cannulation
    endoscopic retrograde c.
cannulization, cannulation
canstatin
canthaxanthin
Cantlie line
Canvaxin cancer vaccine
CAO
    cyclophosphamide, Adriamycin, Oncovin
CAP
    Children's Art Project
    community-acquired pneumonia
    cyclophosphamide, Adriamycin, Platinol
    cyclophosphamide, Adriamycin, prednisone
CA4P
    Combretastatin A4 Prodrug
CaP
    calcium phosphate
    CaP BioVant
cap
    cartilaginous c.
    Doxy C.'s
    Interlink injection c.
capacity
    clonogenic c.
    diffusing c.
    DNA repair c. (DRC)
    iron-binding c. (IBC)
    latent iron-binding c. (LIBC)
    myeloid colony-forming c.
    total iron-binding c. (TIBC)
    vital c. (VC)
CAPB gene
CAP-BOP
    cyclophosphamide, Adriamycin, procarbazine, bleomycin, Oncovin, prednisone
capecitabine and docetaxel
CAP-I
    cyclophosphamide, Adriamycin, Platinol
CAP-II
    cyclophosphamide, Adriamycin, high-dose Platinol
capillary
    c. angioma
    c. bed
    c. beds of organs
    c. electrophoresis
    c. endothelium
    c. hemangioblastoma
    c. hemangioma
    c. leak syndrome

NOTES

C

capillary *(continued)*
   c. lymphatic space (CLS)
   c. malformation
   c. tube plasma viscosimeter
Capintec instant gamma counter
Capital and Codeine
capitellum, pl. **capitella**
capitis
   tinea c.
capitulum radiale humeri fracture
Capizzi protocol
caplet
   Kaopectate Maximum Strength C.'s
CAPPR, CAPPr
   Cytoxan, Adriamycin, Platinol,
    prednisone
capravirine
Capridine-Beta
caproate
   hydroxyprogesterone c.
capromab pendetide
capsaicin
capsid (CA)
   p24 c.
Capsin
capsular
   c. involvement
   c. vessel
capsulatum
   Histoplasma c.
capsule
   Avinza c.
   Catrix c.
   Dialose Plus C.
   Heyman-Simon c.
   Invirase c.
   liver c.
   M2A C.
   morphine sulfate extended-release c.
   parotid c.
   prostate c.
   ruptured c.
   saquinavir hard-gel c.
   saquinavir soft-gel c.
   Targretin c.
   Temodar c.
   c. video endoscopy
capsulitis
   adhesive c.
capsulolabral complex
capture
   boron c.
   electron c. (EC)
   Hybrid C. 2 (HC2)
Capzasin-P
Carac
caracemide
Carafate slurry
Carazzi hematoxylin

carbamate
   chlorphenesin c.
   fluoropyrimidine c.
carbamazepine
carbenicillin
   Keflin, gentamicin, c. (KGC)
carbetimer
Carb-HD
   Cal C.-HD
carbogen breathing
carbohemoglobin
carbohydrate antigen 19-9
carbon
   c. dioxide ice
   c. dioxide tracer
   c. monoxide poisoning
carbonate
   aluminum c.
   calcium c.
   lithium c.
carbon-ion beam
CarboPEC
   carboplatin, etoposide, cyclophosphamide
carboplatin (C, Cb)
   bleomycin, ifosfamide, c.
   cyclophosphamide, Platinol, c.
    (CPC)
   cyclophosphamide, thiotepa, c.
    (CTCb)
   Cytoxan, thiotepa, c. (CTCb)
   c., doxorubicin, cyclophosphamide
    (CDC)
   c., epirubicin, vincristine,
    actinomycin D, ifosfamide,
    etoposide (CEVAIE)
   c., etoposide, bleomycin (CEB)
   c., etoposide, cyclophosphamide
    (CarboPEC)
   high-dose etoposide, thiotepa, dose-
    adjusted c. (TVCa)
   lobradimil and c.
   Platinol, methotrexate, vinblastine,
    Adriamycin, c. (P-MVAC)
   c. and thalidomide
   thiotepa and c.
   thiotepa, etoposide, c. (TEC)
   VePesid and c. (VC)
   c., VePesid, ifosfamide (CVI)
   VP-16, ifosfamide, c. (VIC)
carboplatin/docetaxel
carboprost tromethamine
carboquone (CQ)
carboxamide
   cyclophosphamide, vincristine,
    Adriamycin,
    dimethyltriazenoimidazole c.
   dacarbazine imidazole c.
   dimethyltriazenoimidazole c. (DTIC)
   imidazole c.

carboxorolone
    succinic acid ester c.
carboxyamidotriazole **(CAI)**
carboxyhemoglobin
carboxyimamidate
carboxylesterase
carboxymethylcellulose
    benzocaine, gelatin, pectin,
      sodium c.
carboxyphosphamide
carcinoembryonic
    c. antigen (CEA)
    c. antigen doubling time (CEA-DT)
carcinogen
    chemical c.
    complete c.
    heterocyclic amine c.
carcinogenesis
    chemical c.
    fiber c.
    field c.
    foreign body c.
    gastric c.
    radiation-induced c.
carcinogenic
carcinogenicity
    transplacental c.
carcinoid
    colorectal c.
    c. crisis
    c. embryonic antigen
    goblet cell c. (GCC)
    c. heart disease
    stromal c.
    c. syndrome
    thymic c.
    c. tumor
    typical c. (TC)
carcinolytic
carcinoma, pl. **carcinomata, carcinomas**
  (CA)
    acinar cell c.
    adenocystic c.
    adenoid cystic c. (ACC)
    adenoid squamous cell c.
    adenosquamous c.
    adnexal c.
    adrenal cortical c.
    adrenocortical c. (ACC)
    advanced hepatocellular c.
      (AdHCC)
    alveolar cell c. (ACC)
    alveolar mucosal c.

amphicrine cell c.
ampullary c.
anal gland c.
anal squamous cell c.
anaplastic thyroid c.
androgen-independent prostate c.
  (AICP, AIPC, AI-PCa)
aneuploid colorectal c.
anthracycline-refractory metastatic
  breast c.
apocrine c.
apple core c.
Atzpodien regimen for renal
  cell c.
autolymphocyte-based treatment for
  renal cell c. (ALT-RCC)
Bartholin gland c.
basal cell c. (BCC)
basaloid nonkeratinizing c.
basaloid squamous cell c.
basosquamous cell c.
basosquamous nonkeratinizing c.
Bellini duct c.
bile duct c.
bladder c.
breast c.
bronchial c.
bronchioloalveolar c.
bronchoalveolar c. (BAC)
bronchogenic c.
c. of bronchus
cecal c.
cecum c.
cervical c.
cholangiocellular c.
choroid plexus c.
chromophobe c.
chromophobe renal cell c. (CRCC)
classic large cell c. (CLCC)
clear cell c.
cloacogenic nonkeratinizing c.
collecting duct c. (CDC)
colloid c.
colonic c.
colorectal c. (CRC)
columnar cell c.
contralateral synchronous c.
cribriform salivary c.
crypt cell c.
cuboidal c.
c. cutaneum
cylindromatous c.
cystic c.

NOTES

C

carcinoma *(continued)*
    de novo c.
    differentiated c.
    distal bile duct c. (DBDC)
    ductal papillary c.
    Dunning prostate c.
    early advanced hepatocellular c.
      (eAdHCC)
    early hepatocellular c. (eHCC)
    eccrine c.
    Edmondson-Steiner histologic
      grading of hepatocellular c.
    Ehrlich ascites c. (EAC)
    embryonal c.
    endometrial c. (EC)
    endometrial adenosquamous c.
    endometrioid c.
    endometriosis-associated ovarian c.
      (EAOC)
    epidermoid c.
    esophageal c.
    ethmoid sinus c.
    c. ex pleomorphic adenoma
    extrahepatic bile duct c.
    extraovarian serous c.
    extrapulmonary small cell c.
    fallopian tube c.
    false cord c.
    fibrolamellar c.
    fibrolamellar hepatocellular c. (FL-
      HCC)
    fibrolamellar liver cell c.
    flat colorectal c.
    foamy gland c.
    focal lobular c.
    follicular c.
    follicular thyroid c. (FTC)
    gallbladder c. (GBCA)
    gastric c. (GC)
    gastric stump c.
    gastroesophageal junction c.
    genital c.
    giant pore-type basal cell c.
    glandular c.
    glassy cell c.
    glottic c.
    head and neck squamous cell c.
      (HNSCC)
    hepatocellular c. (HCC)
    hereditary clear cell renal c.
      (HCRC)
    hereditary nonpolyposis colorectal c.
      (HNPCC)
    hereditary papillary renal c.
      (HPRC)
    HER-2-overexpressing breast c.
    hormone-refractory prostate c.
    Hürthle cell c.
    infiltrating ductal c.

    infiltrating lobular c.
    infiltrating salivary duct c.
    inflammatory breast c.
    initially metastatic breast c.
      (IMBC)
    insular c.
    intensive ductal c.
    intermediate c.
    intracystic papillary c.
    intraductal c. (IDC)
    intraductal breast c.
    intraductal oncocytic papillary c.
      (IPOC)
    intraductal papillary c.
    intraepidermal c.
    intraepithelial c.
    intramucosal c.
    invasive ductal c. (IDC)
    invasive lobular c.
    invasive papillotubular c.
    invasive solid tubular c.
    invasive squamous cell c.
    Jewett classification of bladder c.
    juvenile c.
    kangri burn c.
    keratinizing squamous cell c.
    Krompecher c.
    large cell neuroendocrine c.
      (LCNEC)
    latent c.
    lateral aberrant thyroid c.
    leptomeningeal c.
    linitis plastica c.
    liver cell c.
    lobular c.
    localized prostate c. (LPC)
    low-grade c.
    lymphoepithelioma-like c. (LELC)
    macrofollicular thyroid papillary c.
    male breast c. (MBC)
    maxillary sinus c.
    medullary thyroid c. (MTC)
    meibomian gland c.
    melanotic c.
    meningeal c.
    Merkel cell c. (MCC)
    mesometanephric c.
    mesonephric c.
    metachronous c.
    metaplastic c.
    metastatic breast c. (MBC)
    metastatic renal cell c. (mRCC)
    metatypical c.
    microcystic eccrine c.
    microinvasive c.
    micropapillary serous c. (MPSC)
    micropapillary serous ovarian c.
    microtrabecular hepatocellular c.
    mixed-type c.

morpheaform basal cell c.
morphea-type basal cell c.
mucinous eccrine c.
mucoepidermoid c.
multicentric mammary c. (MMC)
c. myxomatodes
nasopharyngeal c. (NPC)
neuroendocrine c. (NEC)
neuroendocrine small cell c.
nevoid basal cell c. (NBCC)
noninfiltrating lobular c.
noninvasive tubular c.
nonsmall cell c. (NSCC)
nonsmall cell lung c. (NSCLC)
nonsquamous c.
oat cell c.
obstructing c.
occult papillary c.
oncoplastic c.
oral squamous cell c. (OSCC)
orofacial c.
ovarian c. (OVCA)
ovarian endometrioid c.
ovarian epithelial c.
Paget c.
pancreatic ductectatic-type c.
papillary serous c.
papillary squamotransitional cell c.
papillary thyroid c. (PTC)
c. paradoxicum
parathyroid c.
periampullary c.
peripheral c.
pharyngeal wall c.
pilomatrix c.
polymorphous low-grade c.
poorly differentiated endocrine c.
  (PDEC)
poorly differentiated infiltrating
  duct c.
postgastrectomy c.
primary hepatocellular c.
primary neuroendocrine small
  cell c.
prostatic c.
Protocol 99-052 Regimen A for
  nasopharyngeal c.
pulmonary cavitating squamous
  cell c.
rectal c.
recurrent c.
renal cell c. (RCC)
renal cortical c.

renal medullary c.
renal pelvis c.
salivary gland c.
sarcomatoid squamous cell c.
scar c.
schneiderian c.
scirrhous c.
sclerosing basal cell c.
sebaceous c.
secondary c.
secretory c.
serous c.
signet ring cell c.
c. simplex
sinonasal c.
sinonasal undifferentiated c.
  (SNUC)
c. in situ (CIS)
small cell neuroendocrine c.
small cell undifferentiated c.
spindle cell c.
sporadic clear cell c.
squamous cell c. (SCC)
superficial spreading c.
superficial transitional cell c.
  (sTCC)
supraglottic c.
sweat gland c. (SGC)
synchronous c.
c. syndrome
c. syndrome immunoblot
syringoid eccrine c.
taxane refractory non-small-cell
  lung c.
taxane resistant non-small-cell
  lung c.
testicular germ cell c. (TGCC)
thymic c. (TCA)
thyroid c.
TIS c.
trabecular c.
trabecular insular solid c.
transitional cell c. (TCC)
transverse colon c.
trichilemmoma c.
tripartite duodenal c.
tubular c.
c. of uncertain primary site
  (CUPS)
undifferentiated c. (UC)
undifferentiated nasopharyngeal c.
  (UNPC)
c. of unknown primary (CUP)

NOTES

carcinoma *(continued)*
    urachal c.
    ureteral c.
    uterine papillary serous c. (UPSC)
    V-2 c.
    vaginal c.
    varicoid c.
    verrucous squamous cell c.
    villous c.
    vulvar c.
    vulvovaginal c.
    Walker c.
    well-circumscribed c.
    widely invasive follicular c.
      (WIFC)
    Wolfe classification of breast c.
    wolffian duct c.
carcinomatosa
    lymphangitis c.
carcinomatosis
    leptomeningeal c.
    lymphangitic c.
    meningeal c.
    peritoneal c.
    c. peritonei
carcinomatosum
    coma c.
carcinomatous
    c. implant
    c. meningitis
    c. myelopathy
    c. myopathy
    c. neuromyopathy
    c. neuropathy
    c. subacute cerebellar degeneration
carcinophilia
carcinophilic
carcinophobia, cancerophobia
carcinosarcoma, pl. **carcinosarcomata,**
  carcinosarcomas
    embryonal c.
    Flexner-Jobling c.
    renal c.
    teratoid c.
    uterine c.
    Walker c.
carcinosis
carcinostatic
card
    ECT test c.
    Memorial Pain Assessment C.
      (MPAC)
Cardak introducer
cardiac
    c. arrest
    c. chamber
    c. drug
    c. failure (CF)

    c. fibroma
    c. tamponade
    c. tumor
cardiomegaly
cardiomyopathy
    alcoholic c.
    anthracycline c.
    degenerative c.
cardiomyoplasty
cardiophrenic
    c. angle
    c. angle mass
cardioprotectant
cardioprotective
    c. agent
    c. effect
cardiopulmonary
    c. abnormality
    c. disease
    c. manifestation
cardiospasm
cardiothoracic
cardiotocogram
cardiotoxicity
    doxorubicin-induced c.
    mitomycin c.
cardiovascular
    c. cancer
    c. disease (CD)
    c. syphilis
Cardioxane
carditis
    acute lethal c.
care
    AIDS patient c.
    comfort c.
    continuing c.
    end-of-life c.
    home health c.
    hospice c.
    international cancer c.
    K + C.
    Life After Cancer C. (LACC)
    palliative c.
    patient c.
    perineal c.
    skin c.
    supportive c.
    terminal c.
CARES
    Cancer Rehabilitation Evaluation System
Carey-Coons stent
carina, pl. **carinae**
carinactivase-1 prothrombin assay
carinal angle
carinii
    Pneumocystis c.
carious teeth

CARM1
> coactivator-associated arginine methyltransferase 1

C-arm
> DEC 9800 plus cardiac mobile C-a.

carmustine (BCNU, BiCNU)
> Adriamycin and c. (AC)
> c. in ethanol
> c. implant
> polifeprosan 20 and c.
> SU101 in combination with c.
> c. wafer

Carney
> C. complex
> C. syndrome
> C. triad

carnitine

carotene
> beta c.

carotenemia

carotenoid

carotid
> c. body tumor
> c. endarterectomy (CEA)
> c. sheath adenoma

carpal
> c. bone
> c. bone stress fracture
> c. boss
> c. tunnel

Carpenter syndrome

carpometacarpal joint fracture

carrier
> doxorubicin adsorbed to magnetic targeted c. (MTC-DOX)
> HNPCC c.
> reduced folate c. (RFC)

Carrington
> C. Dermal wound gel
> C. oral wound rinse

Carrion disease

Carrisyn

CART
> Classification and Regression Tree
> combined antiretroviral therapy

Carter's Little Pills

cartilage
> articular c.
> arytenoid c.
> calcified c.
> cricoid c.
> oral shark c.

> shark c.
> thyroid c.
> c. tumor

cartilage-containing giant cell tumor

cartilage-forming tumor

cartilage-hair hypoplasia

cartilaginous
> c. cap
> c. lesion
> c. node
> c. tumor

cartwheel fracture

Cartwright blood group

carubicin HCl

carzelesin

CAS-200
> morphology system CAS-200

CASA
> cancer-associated serum antigen
> CASA tumor marker

casanthranol
> docusate and c.

cascade
> caspase c.
> clotting c.
> coagulation c.
> metastatic c.
> pain c.

cascara sagrada

caseating

case-control study

casei
> *Lactobacillus c.*

caseous pneumonia

CASH
> Cancer and Steroid Hormone
> CASH Study

Casodex

Casoni skin test

caspase
> c. cascade
> c. cleavage

caspase-9 antibody

Caspersson type B cell

caspofungin

cassette
> adenosine triphosphate-binding c. (ABC)

Cassidy-Scholte syndrome

cast
> Aquaplast c.
> red blood cell c.

NOTES

cast *(continued)*
    renal c.
    urinary c.
Castle factor
Castleman
    C. disease
    C. tumor
castor oil
castration
    medical c.
CAT
    cyclophosphamide, cytosine arabinoside,
      topotecan
    cytarabine, Adriamycin, 6-thioguanine
    cytosine arabinoside, Adriamycin, 6-
      thioguanine
    cytosine arabinoside and 6-thioguanine
      CAT expression gene
CATA2 zinc protein
Cataflam Oral
catalysis
    antibody-directed c. (ADC)
cataract
    posterior capsular c.
catarrhalis
    Branhamella c.
    Moraxella c.
catastrophizing
CATCH 22
    chromosome 22q11 microdeletion
catecholamine metabolite
catharanthine
cathartic
    saline c.
cathepsin
    c. B, L marker
    c. D assay
catheter
    Abbokinase c.
    abdominal abscess drainage c.
    afterloading c.
    Amplatz dual-stiffness Malecot c.
    Amplatz mechanical thrombolysis c.
    angiography c.
    Anthron heparinized c.
    Argyle Ingram trocar c.
    balloon c.
    Bardex c.
    biliary drainage c.
    biliary manipulation c.
    blade c.
    buckled drainage c.
    Bud Percuflex c.
    Camino micromanometer c.
    central venous c. (CVC)
    central venous pressure c.
    C-Flex c.
    Chemo-Port c.
    chronic indwelling c.

    condom c.
    Cook c.
    Dome Port c.
    double-J polyethylene c.
    double-J silicone rubber urinary c.
    double-lumen c.
    drainage c.
    c. drainage
    c. embolism
    c. fixation
    c. flushing
    Groshong c.
    Hohn c.
    indwelling vascular access c.
    c. infection
    Infuse-A-Port c.
    c. insertion
    inside-the-needle infusion c.
    jugular c.
    large-bore c.
    midline c.
    Müller empyema c.
    c. obstruction
    over-the-needle infusion c.
    PAS Port Fluoro-Free c.
    percutaneous nephrostomy c.
    percutaneous transhepatic c.
    peripherally inserted central c.
      (PICC)
    peripheral vein c.
    Per-Q-Cath c.
    pigtail c.
    Pleurx indwelling pleural c.
    Polaris LE c.
    polyethylene balloon c.
    polyvinyl chloride balloon c.
    Port-A-Cath c.
    c. position
    quadripolar 6-French diagnostic
      electrophysiology c.
    Quinton central venous c.
    Raaf c.
    rheolytic thrombectomy c.
    Ring biliary drainage c.
    Sacks c.
    Sacks-Malecot c.
    sidewinder c.
    silastic hemodialysis c.
    silver-coated c.
    single-use c.
    Stamey suprapubic Malecot c.
    subclavian apheresis c.
    suction c.
    SureCath port access c.
    Teflon c.
    Tenckhoff c.
    Thermistor c.
    ThoraCath c.
    c. tip

Tonnesen c.
totally implantable c.
Trach-Eze closed suction c.
Tracker coaxial infusion c.
Tracker-18 Unibody c.
transnasal intraduodenal feeding c.
triple-lumen c.
trocar c.
tunneled c.
U-loop nephrostomy c.
catheter-associated bacteremia
catheter-directed
  c.-d. fenestration
  c.-d. interventional procedure
catheter-induced
  c.-i. pulmonary artery hemorrhage
  c.-i. subclavian vein thrombosis
catheterization
  antegrade c.
  bladder c.
  central venous c.
  cephalic vein c.
  chronic c.
  hemodynamic c.
  transfemoral venous c.
  transseptal c.
  urinary c.
catheterized barbotage specimen
catheter-related thrombosis
catheter-securing technique
Cathflo Activase
cation
  c. exchange resin
  paramagnetic c.
Catrix
  C. capsule
  C. Ointment
  C. wound dressing
cat's claw
cat-scratch
  c.-s. disease
  c.-s. fever
CA1-18 tumor marker
Catu virus
cauliflower-like mass
causalgia
causality
cause-specific survival (CSS)
caustic burn
CAV
  cyclophosphamide, Adriamycin, Velban
  cyclophosphamide, Adriamycin, vinblastine

cyclophosphamide, Adriamycin, vincristine
cava (*pl. of* cavum)
caval filter
CAVe, CA-Ve
  CCNU, Adriamycin, Velban
  CCNU, Adriamycin, vinblastine
caveolin-1 expression
caveolin protein
cavernoma
cavernosa
  corpora c.
cavernosometry
  dynamic c.
cavernous
  c. hemangioma
  c. sinus
CAVH
  continuous arteriovenous hemofiltration
cavitary
  c. lung lesion
  c. small bowel lesion
cavitating
  c. metastasis
  c. neoplasm
cavitation
Cavitron ultrasonic surgical aspirator (CUSA)
cavity
  abdominal c.
  abdominopelvic c.
  acetabular c.
  Bragg-Gray c.
  endometrial c.
  grape-skin thin-walled lung c.
  oral c.
  sinonasal c.
  surgically created resection c.
  tumor c.
cavogram
CAVP
  cyclophosphamide, Adriamycin, vincristine, prednisone
CAVP16
  cyclophosphamide, Adriamycin, VP-16
  Cytoxan, Adriamycin, VP-16
CAVP-I
  cyclophosphamide, Adriamycin, vincristine, prednisone
CAVPM
  cyclophosphamide, Adriamycin, VP-16, prednisone, methotrexate
cavum, pl. **cava**

NOTES

101

cayetanensis
　　Cyclospora c.
Cb
　　carboplatin
CBC
　　complete blood count
CBCTR
　　Cooperative Breast Cancer Tissue
　　Resource
CBDT
　　cisplatin, BCNU, dacarbazine, tamoxifen
CBE
　　clinical breast examination
CBT
　　childhood brain tumor
CBTR
　　contralateral breast tumor recurrence
CBV
　　cyclophosphamide, BCNU, VePesid
　　cyclophosphamide, BCNU, VP-16-213
　　Cytoxan, BCNU, VP-16
CBVD
　　CCNU, bleomycin, vinblastine,
　　dexamethasone
Cbx
　　core biopsy
CC
　　　Adalat CC
CC49 monoclonal antibody
CCA
　　cholangiocarcinoma
CCA-1
　　cancer cell-derived blood coagulating
　　activity 1
CCAVV
　　CCNU, cyclophosphamide, Adriamycin,
　　vincristine, VP-16
CCCF
　　Candlelighters Childhood Cancer
　　Foundation
C-C chemokine
CC-CKR-5
　　nonsyncytium-inducing chemokine
CCE
　　clear cell ependymoma
C-cell hyperplasia
C2-ceramide
CCFE
　　cyclophosphamide, cisplatin, 5-
　　fluorouracil, estramustine
CCG
　　Children's Cancer Group
CCI-79 rapamycin analog
c-cis protooncogene/oncogene
CCK
　　cholecystokinin
CCKR5 receptor
CCM
　　cyclophosphamide, CCNU, methotrexate

CCMA
　　CCNU, cyclophosphamide, methotrexate,
　　Adriamycin
CCNU
　　cyclohexylchloroethylnitrosurea
　　Adriamycin and CCNU (AC)
　　CCNU, Adriamycin, bleomycin,
　　streptozocin (CABS)
　　Adriamycin, DTIC, bleomycin,
　　CCNU (ADBC)
　　CCNU, Adriamycin, Velban
　　(CAVe, CA-Ve)
　　CCNU, Adriamycin, vinblastine
　　(CAVe, CA-Ve)
　　CCNU, bleomycin, vinblastine,
　　dexamethasone (CBVD)
　　CCNU, cyclophosphamide,
　　Adriamycin, vincristine, VP-16
　　(CCAVV, VP-16)
　　cyclophosphamide, methotrexate,
　　CCNU (CMC)
　　CCNU, cyclophosphamide,
　　methotrexate, Adriamycin (CCMA)
　　CCNU, cyclophosphamide, Oncovin,
　　bleomycin (CCOB)
　　CCNU, cyclophosphamide, Velban,
　　procarbazine, prednisone (CCVPP)
　　cyclophosphamide, vinblastine,
　　procarbazine, prednisone plus
　　CCNU (CVPP-CCNU)
　　CCNU, cyclophosphamide,
　　vincristine (CCV)
　　CCNU, etoposide, prednimustine
　　(CEP)
　　CCNU, ifosfamide, Adriamycin
　　(CIA)
　　methotrexate, Adriamycin,
　　cyclophosphamide, CCNU
　　(MACC)
　　methotrexate, ara-C,
　　cyclophosphamide, CCNU
　　(MACC)
　　CCNU, methotrexate, procarbazine
　　(CMP)
　　nitrogen mustard, Adriamycin,
　　CCNU (NAC)
　　CCNU, Oncovin, methotrexate,
　　procarbazine (COMP)
　　CCNU, Oncovin, prednisone
　　(CCNU-OP)
　　CCNU, Oncovin, prednisone,
　　Adriamycin, cyclophosphamide
　　(COPAC)
　　CCNU, Oncovin, procarbazine,
　　prednisone (COPP)
　　CCNU, procarbazine, methotrexate
　　(CPM)
　　procarbazine, Oncovin, CCNU
　　(POC)

procarbazine, Oncovin,
cyclophosphamide, CCNU (POCC)
procarbazine, Oncovin, Cytoxan,
CCNU (POCC)
CCNU, vinblastine, bleomycin
(CVB)
CCNU, vinblastine, bleomycin,
dexamethasone (CVBD)
vinblastine, ifosfamide, CCNU
(VIC)
CCNU, vinblastine, prednisone,
procarbazine (CVPP)

CCNU-OP
CCNU, Oncovin, prednisone

CCOB
CCNU, cyclophosphamide, Oncovin,
bleomycin

CCR1–11
chemokine receptor 1-11

CCR2 transmembrane domain

CCR5
chemokine receptor 5
CCR5 gene deletion
HIV-1 binding to CCR5

CCRT, CC-RT
computer-controlled conformal radiation
therapy
computer-controlled radiotherapy
concurrent chemoradiotherapy

C-Crystals

CCS
clear cell sarcoma

CCSG
Children's Cancer Study Group

CCSS
Childhood Cancer Survivor Study

CCT
composite cyclic therapy

CCV
CCNU, cyclophosphamide, vincristine

CCVPP
CCNU, cyclophosphamide, Velban,
procarbazine, prednisone

CD
cardiovascular disease
Clostridium difficile
cluster of differentiation
combination drug
Crohn disease
CD antigen
Ceclor CD

CD1–166
cluster of differentiation 1-166

CD3+ cell
CD3– cell
CD3 monoclonal antibody
CD4
cluster of differentiation 4
CD4 cell count
CD4 cell-surface receptor
CD4 lymphopenia
CD4 protein
recombinant soluble CD4 (rsCD4)
recombinant soluble human CD4
(rCD4)
CD4 recombinant soluble human
soluble CD4
soluble recombinant human CD4
(sCD4)

CD4+
CD4+ CTL
CD4+ response
CD4+ T cell
CD4+ T-cell loss

CD$_4$ cell

CD4-IgG
cluster of differentiation 4
immunoglobulin G

CD5
CD5 marker
CD5 protein
CD5 surface antigen

CD5+ monoclonal antibody
CD5-T lymphocyte immunotoxin
CD8
cluster of differentiation 8
CD8 AIS CELLector
CD8 cell count
vaccine-induced noncytolic CD8

CD8+
CD8+ cell
CD8+ CTL
CD8+ response
CD8+ T-cell count

CD$_8$ cell
CD18 antigen
CD20 B-lymphocyte surface
CD20-positive lymphoma
CD21 antigen
CD22+
CD22+ leukemia
CD22+ lymphoma

CD26
CD26 coreceptor
CD26 protease

CD30/KI-1 positive lymphoma of skin

NOTES

CD33 antigen
CD34+
    CD34+ cell
    CD34+ derived mast cell precursor
CD34
    CD34 antigen
    CD34 content
    CD34 selected peripheral blood
      stem cell
    CD34 staining
CD34+/38lo cell
CD34⁺ cell dose
CD38 expression
CD40
    CD40 gene
    CD40 ligand
CD44 expression
CD44H testing
CD44v6 isoform
CD45Ro antibody
CD52
    CD52 antigen
    free circulating soluble CD52
CD95 breast cancer testing
CD-117 assay
CD137 testing
CD33-positive acute myeloid leukemia
CD34-derived dendritic cell
  immunization
CD4-gp120 interaction
2CDA
    2-chlorodeoxyadenosine
CDC
    carboplatin, doxorubicin,
      cyclophosphamide
    chronic disseminated candidiasis
    collecting duct carcinoma
Cddp
    cisplatin
CDE
    cyclophosphamide, doxorubicin,
      etoposide
    Cytoxan, doxorubicin, etoposide
C2-dihydro-ceramide
CDK
    cyclin-dependent kinase
CDK4
    CDK4 oncogene
    CDK4 protein
CDKN2/p16 gene
cDNA
    complementary DNA
    cDNA cloning
    herpesvirus thymidine kinase cDNA
    cDNA library
    cDNA microarray gene expression
CDR
    complementarity determining region

3CDRT
    3-dimensional conformal radiotherapy
CEA
    carcinoembryonic antigen
    carotid endarterectomy
      pleural fluid CEA
      CEA titer
      CEA tumor marker
CEA-Cide
CEA-DT
    carcinoembryonic antigen doubling time
CEA-Roche assay
CEA-Scan
CEA-TPA-CA15.3 tumor marker panel
CeaVac
CEB
    carboplatin, etoposide, bleomycin
Cebid Timecelles
CECA
    cisplatin, etoposide, cyclophosphamide,
      Adriamycin
    cisplatin, etoposide, Cytoxan, Adriamycin
ceca (*pl. of* cecum)
cecal
    c. cancer
    c. carcinoma
    c. deformity
    c. filling defect
    c. ileus
    c. volvulus
cecitis
cecocutaneous fistula
Cecon
cecostomy
    percutaneous c.
CECT
    contrast-enhanced computed tomography
cecum, pl. **ceca**
    c. carcinoma
    c. mobile
CeeNU
CEF
    cyclophosphamide, epirubicin, 5-
      fluorouracil
    Cytoxan, epirubicin, 5-fluorouracil
cefaclor
cefadroxil
Cefadyl
cefamandole
Cefanex
cefazolin
cefdinir
cefepime hydrochloride
cefixime
Cefizox
Ceflatonin
cefmetazole
Cefobid
Cefol Filmtab

cefonicid
cefoperazone
Cefotan
cefotaxime
cefotetan
cefoxitin
cefpodoxime
cefprozil
ceftazidime
ceftibuten
Ceftin Oral
ceftizoxime
ceftriaxone
cefuroxime axetil
Cefzil
ceiling dose
celecoxib
Celestin tube
Celestone
    C. Phosphate Injection
    C. Soluspan
celiac
    c. artery
    c. axis
    c. disease
    c. ganglion
    c. lymph node
    c. lymph node metastasis
    c. nodal involvement
    c. plexus block (CPB)
    c. plexus blockade
    c. plexus neurolysis
    c. sprue
    c. trunk
celiotomy
cell
    aberrant c.
    acinar c.
    activated endothelial c.
    c. activation
    additive solution red c.
    c. adhesion molecule
    adventitial c.
    agger nasi air c.
    allogeneic bone marrow c.
    allogeneic stem c.
    angiogenic c.
    antigen-presenting c. (APC)
    antigen-pulsed autologous
      dendritic c.
    antigen-sensitive c.
    antigen-specific T c.
    anuclear c.

apoptotic c.
Aschoff c.
AS red c.
atypical c.
autologous bone marrow c.
autologous hematopoietic c.
autologous red blood c.
autologous stem c.
B c.
baculovirus transfected c.
balloon c.
BEAC c.
berry c.
bilobed plasma c.
c. biology
B-islet c.
Bizzozero red c.
blast c.
B-lineage acute lymphoblastic c.
blister c.
c. block analysis
blood c.
bone marrow stem c.
breast epithelial c.
buffy-coated c.
c. burden
burr c.
burst-forming c.
cameloid c.
cancer c.
c. carcinoma of cervix
Caspersson type B c.
CD3+ c.
CD3− c.
CD$_4$ c.
CD4+ T c.
CD8+ c.
CD$_8$ c.
CD34+ c.
CD34+/38lo c.
CD34 selected peripheral blood
  stem c.
central neuroepithelial c.
centrocyte-like c.
cerebriform c.
CHO c.
choroidal c.
chromaffin c.
Clara c.
clonogenic lymphoma c.
clonogenic myeloma c.
clonogenic tumor c.

NOTES

105

cell *(continued)*

clusters of pancreatic acinar c.'s (CPAC)
c. collection
contaminating tumor c. (CTC)
contrasuppressor c.
Cos-1 c.
c. count
c. crenation
cryopreserved stem c.
CTCb supported by autologous bone marrow stem c.'s
c. cycle
c. cycle control
c. cycle kinetic analysis
c. cycle-regulating protein
c. cycle regulatory protein
c. cycle stage
c. cycling
c. cycling in chemotherapy
cytokeratin-positive c.
cytolytic T c.
cytotoxic T c.
c. death
dendritic c. (DC)
dermal dendric c.
dermal microvascular endothelial c. (DMVEC)
dormant c.
Downey c.
EBER-positive c.
Edelmann c.
effector c.
effusion-associated mononuclear c.
electroporation of c.'s
embryonic c.
endothelial c. (EC)
end-stage c.
enterochromaffin c. (ECC)
epithelial c. (EC)
Epstein-Barr early region-positive c.
estrogen-dependent cancer c.
ethmoid air c.
exfoliative c.
faggot c.
FAMPAC c.
Ferrata c.
fetal liver c.
fixed c.
flame c.
flower c.
foam c.
follicular dendritic c. (FDC)
follicular predominantly large c.
follicular predominantly small cleaved c.
formin c.
frozen red c.
fusiform c.

c. fusion
G c.
gastric enterochromaffin c.
gastrointestinal epithelial c.
G-CSF mobilized peripheral blood stem c.
ghost c.
giant c.
glandular c.
glioma c.
glitter c.
goblet c.
granulocyte, erythrocyte, monocyte, megakaryocyte colony-forming c. (GEMM-CFC)
grape c.
growth factor mobilized autologous peripheral blood stem c.
H9 c.
hairy c.
c. harvesting
HeLa c.
helmet c.
helper c.
hematopoietic progenitor c.
hematopoietic stem c. (HSC)
hematopoietic target c.
hemopoietic stem c.
hereditary mucolipid storage c.
hobnail c.
Hodgkin c.
Hofbauer c.
horse red blood c.
host c.
HRS c.
human dermal microvascular endothelial c.
human umbilical vein endothelial c. (HUVEC)
hybridoma c.
hyperchromatic spindle c.
c. imaging technology
immortal c.
immune c.
immunoblastic sarcoma of B and T c.'s
immunocompetent c.
immunohematopoietic stem c.
inclusion c.
indeterminate c.
c. infusion
c. interaction gene
interdigitating dendritic c. (IDC)
interstitial dendritic c.
intraepithelial c.
iodine ^{131}I murine MAb IgG2a to B c.
irreversible sickled c. (ISC)
c. island

C

isolated tumor c. (ITC)
isolation by size of epithelial
  tumor c.'s (ISET)
Jurkat c.
karyorrhectic c.
KG-1 c.
c. kill
killer c.
koilocytotic c.
Kulchitsky c.
Kupffer c.
lacunar c.
LAK c.
Langerhans dendritic c. (L-DC)
Langhans giant c.
large noncleaved follicular center c.
Leishman chrome c.
lepra c.
leukemic c.
leukocyte-poor red blood c.
leukopoor red blood c.
Leydig c.
L/H c.
linker for activation of T c.'s
  (LAT)
littoral c.
Loevit c.
low columnar c.
lyl B c.
lymphadenoma c.
lymphoid stem c.
lymphokine-activated killer c.
lymphoplasmacytoid c.
lymphoreticular c.
c. lysate
malignant c.
mammalian c.
mantle c.
marchalko c.
Marchand c.
marginal zone c.
marrow c.
Marschalko-type plasma c.
mast c.
mediator c.
melanoma antigen recognized by
  T c. (MART-1)
memory T c.
Merkel c.
mesenchymal stromal c.
mesothelial c.
Mexican hat c.
MHC-restricted cytotoxic T c.

microglial c.
c. migration
monocytoid B c.
mononuclear c.
Mooser c.
morular c.
mother c.
Mott c.
MT-2 c.
multinucleated osteoclastic giant c.
mummified c.
murine tumor c.
mutant c.
myeloid precursor c.
myeloma c.
myocardial c.
myoid c.
Nageotte c.
naive T c.
natural killer c.
neoplastic c.
Neumann c.
neuroendocrine c.
neutrophilic c.
NK c.
nonangiogenic c.
nonhematopoietic stem c.
nonimmunogenic murine tumor c.
nonneoplastic T c.
nonsmall c.
normal clonal CD4+ T c.
normal hematopoietic c.
nuclear c.
nuclear factor of activated T c.
  (NFAT)
nucleated red blood c.
null c.
nurse c.
oat c.
occult tumor c.
OKT4 c.
OKT8 c.
ox red blood c.
packed red blood c.'s
pancreatic acinar c.
Paneth c.
parafollicular C c.
paroxysmal nocturnal
  hemoglobinuria c.
peg c.
Pelger-Huët c.
peptide-pulsed c.

NOTES

cell *(continued)*

peripheral blood mononuclear c. (PBMC)
peripheral blood progenitor c. (PBPC)
peripheral blood stem c. (PBSC)
peripheral lymphoid c.
perithelial c.
perivascular epithelioid c. (PEC)
c.'s per unit area
pessary c.
phagocytic c.
Philadelphia-positive acute lymphoblastic leukemia c.
photo c.
physaliferous c.
phytohemagglutinin-stimulated Jurkat T c.
Pinocchio c.
plaque-forming c.
pluripotential c.
pluripotent stem c.
PNH c.
polychromatic c.
polygonal c.
polylobulated c.
polysialic-neural c.
polyvalent melanoma c.
popcorn Reed-Sternberg c.
precursor B, T c.
preplasma c.
primitive stem c.
primordial germ c.
professional antigen-presenting c.
progenitor c.
c. proliferation
prolymphocytic T c.
prototypic antigen-presenting c.
pseudostratified c.
pseudoxanthoma c.
pulmonary endocrine c.
purged progenitor c.
quiescent c.
Raji c.
rare malignant c.
red blood c.
Reed c.
Reed-Sternberg c.
regulatory T c.
c. repair competent
reticuloendothelial c.
reticulum c.
retroviral transduction of *mdr-1* gene into peripheral blood progenitor c.
Rieder c.
Rindfleisch c.
rod c.
rosette c.

Rouget c.
scavenger c.
Schwann c.
Sertoli c.
Sézary lymphoma c.
shadow c.
sickle c. (SC)
signet ring c.
small c.
smooth muscle c.
smudge c.
spindle c.
spindle-shaped tumor c.
spontaneous immortalization of breast epithelial c.'s
spur c.
squamous c.
stab c.
staff c.
stave c.
stem c.
stipple c.
stomach c.
stromal c.
subependymal giant c.
suppressor T c.
c. surface marker
c. survival
syncytiotrophoblast c.
syncytiotrophoblastic giant c.
T4 c.
tanned red c.
target c.
tart c.
T-cell-rich B c.
T-cytotoxic c.
telomerase-active stem c.
telomerase-expressing cancer c.
T helper c. (Th)
T helper c. 1 (Th1)
T helper c. 2 (Th2)
T4 helper c.
T helper suppressor c. (Ts)
Thoma-Zeiss counting c.
Th1-type T c.
Th2-type T c.
thymic interdigitating dendritic c.
TIL c.
Touton giant c.
transduced c.
transfected c.
c. transfer
transfusion-dependent packed red blood c.'s
T suppressor c.
c. tumor
tumor
tumor-derived activated c.
tumorigenic c.

Türk c.
unmodified G-CSF mobilized
  peripheral blood stem c.
urothelial transitional c.
vaccinia/BHK-21 c.
vaccinia/vero c.
vacuolated-appearing c.
vascular endothelial c.
veiled c.
veto c.
c. viability assessment
Virchow c.
volume of packed c.'s (VPC)
wandering c.
Warthin c.
Warthin-Finkeldey giant c.
washed red c.
white blood c. (WBC)
wild-type c.
wtp53 c.
zellballen c.
Cellano phenotype
cell-bound
  c.-b. antibody
  c.-b. antigen
cell-cell
  c.-c. contact
  c.-c. cytoskeletal interaction
CellCept
cell-cycle
  c.-c. arrest
  c.-c. effect
  c.-c. kinetics
  c.-c. parameter
  c.-c. regulator
Cell-Dyn
  C.-D. Sapphire hematology
    instrument
  C.-D. Slidemarker/Stainer
  C.-D. SMS
Cellect graft preparation device
CELLector
  CD8 AIS C.
CellFIT acquisition system
cell-fixed antibody
Cellfree Interleukin-2 Receptor kit
cell-lineage marker
cell-matrix cytoskeletal interaction
cell-mediated
  c.-m. antibody
  c.-m. immunity (CMI)
CellQuest acquisition system
cell-to-cell interaction

cellular
  c. abnormality
  c. adhesion
  c. anoxia
  c. atypia
  c. blue nevus
  c. component
  c. debris
  c. enumeration
  c. identification
  c. immune therapy
  c. immunity
  c. immunity deficiency syndrome
    (CIDS)
  c. immunity theory
  c. immunodeficiency
  c. immunotherapy
  c. leiomyoma (CL)
  c. lymphokine
  c. marker
  c. pleomorphism
  c. proliferation
  c. resistance
  c. retinol-binding protein (CRBP)
  c. suppressor gene
  c. transfusion product
  c. tumor
  c. whorling
  c. xenotransplantation
cellularity
  bone marrow c.
cellulitis
  perirectal c.
cellulose
  c. acetate (CA)
  oxidized c.
  c. sodium phosphate
Celsite implanted port
Cel-U-Jec Injection
CEM
  cytosine arabinoside, etoposide,
    methotrexate
cementifying fibroma
cementinoma
cementoblastoma
cementoma
cementosis
cementum fracture
CEM/HIV-1 cell line
Cena-K
Cenestin
Centara

NOTES

center
  accessory ossification c.
  Association of Community
    Cancer C.'s
  bone c.
  C. for Epidemiologic Studies-
    Depression (CES-D)
  epiphysial ossification c.
  Fred Hutchinson Cancer
    Research C.
  germinal c.
  International Cancer Information C.
    (ICIC)
  Johns Hopkins Oncology C.
  M.D. Anderson Cancer C.
  Memorial Sloan-Kettering
    Cancer C.
  progressively transformed
    germinal c.
  pseudofollicular proliferation c.
  Samsung Medical C. (SMC)
centigray (cGy)
central
  c. axis dose
  c. axis value
  c. cementifying fibroma
  c. cord syndrome
  c. fracture
  c. lymphatic irradiation
  c. lymphoid tissue
  c. nervous system (CNS)
  c. nervous system lymphoma
  c. nervous system malformation
  c. nervous system-penetrating
    abacavir
  c. nervous system tumor
  c. neurocytoma
  c. neuroepithelial cell
  c. neuroepithelial cell-origin tumor
  c. neurologic adverse effect
  c. ossifying fibroma
  c. pontine
  c. pontine demyelinolysis
  c. pontine myelinolysis (CPM)
  c. sinus lipomatosis
  c. sulcus
  c. tendon
  c. thermal dysregulation
  c. venous access
  c. venous catheter (CVC)
  c. venous catheterization
  c. venous drainage
  c. venous pressure (CVP)
  c. venous pressure catheter
  c. venous pressure line
central-axis-depth-dose (CADD)
centrally ordered phase encoding
Centrica rotational core biopsy system
Centricon-10 filter

centrifugal filter
centrifugation
  discontinuous density gradient c.
  Ficoll-Conray density gradient c.
  Ficoll-Hypaque density gradient c.
centrifuge
  CritSpin microhematocrit c.
  MicroPrep 2 c.
  PK110 c.
  StatSpin Express 2 c.
  StatSpin MP multipurpose c.
centrifugum
  erythema annulare c. (EAC)
centrilobular lesion
centriole
centroblast
centroblastic follicular lymphoma
centrocyte
centrocyte-like
  c.-l. cell
  c.-l. type
centrocytic follicular lymphoma
centrocytoid centroblastic lymphoma
centromere
centrosome
CEOP
  cyclophosphamide, epirubicin, Oncovin,
    prednisone
  cyclophosphamide, epirubicin,
    vincristine, prednisolone
CEOP-B
  cyclophosphamide, Oncomycin,
    prednisone, bleomycin
CEP
  CCNU, etoposide, prednimustine
  chronic eosinophilic pneumonia
  congenital erythropoietic porphyria
  cyclophosphamide, etoposide, Platinol
cepacia
  Burkholderia c.
cephalexin
cephalgia, cephalalgia
cephalhematoma
cephalic
  c. vein
  c. vein catheterization
cephalin
cephalosporin
Cephalosporium granulomatis
cephalothin
cephapirin
cephradine
Cephulac
Ceplene
Ceporacin
Ceprate SC Instrument II
Ceptaz
ceramidase

ceramide
    c. cell signaling
    c. synthase activity
    c. synthesis
c-erbB1 gene
c-erbB2
    c-erbB2 amplification
    c-erbB2 gene product
    c-erbB2 oncogene
    c-erbB2 overexpression
    c-erbB2 protein
    c-erbB2 p185 test
    c-erbB2 p185 tumor marker assay
c-erbB2/neu gene
cerebella (*pl. of* cerebellum)
cerebellar
    c. anaplastic
    c. artery
    c. astrocytoma
    c. ataxia
    c. atrophy
    c. degeneration
    c. ectopia
    c. epidermoid
    c. gliosarcoma
    c. hemangioblastoma
    c. hemisphere
    c. hemorrhage
    c. hypoplasia
    c. peduncle
    c. peg
    c. tonsil
cerebelli
    falx c.
    tentorium c.
cerebellolabyrinthine artery
cerebellopontine
    c. angle
    c. angle mass
    c. angle meningioma
    c. angle tumor
    c. recess
cerebelloretinal
    c. hemangioblastoma
    c. hemangioblastomatosis
cerebellum, pl. cerebella
cerebral
    c. amyloid angiopathy
    c. aneurysm
    c. angiography
    c. anoxia
    c. aqueduct
    c. arteriovenous malformation

    c. artery
    c. astrocytoma
    c. atrophy
    c. blood flow
    c. blood vessel
    c. blood volume
    c. blood volume map
    c. circulation
    c. circulation time
    c. contusion
    c. convexity
    c. cortex
    c. death
    c. edema
    c. embolism
    c. gumma
    c. hemisphere
    c. hemorrhage
    c. hypoperfusion
    c. infarction
    c. ischemia
    c. lymphoma
    c. mantle
    c. metastasis
    c. neuroblastoma
    c. nodule
    c. palsy
    c. palsy pathological fracture
    c. parenchyma
    c. peduncle
    c. reticulum cell sarcoma
    c. sinovenous occlusion
    c. sulcus
    c. toxoplasmosis
    c. vasculature
    c. vasoreactivity
    c. vein
    c. ventricle
    c. ventricular shunt connector
    c. ventriculography
    c. white matter hypoplasia
cerebri
    calcification of falx c.
    falx c.
    gliomatosis c. (GC)
cerebriform
    c. cell
    c. pattern
cerebritis
cerebrohepatorenal syndrome
cerebroside
cerebrospinal
    c. fever

NOTES

cerebrospinal *(continued)*
    c. fluid (CSF)
    c. fluid-brain barrier
    c. fluid cryptococcal antigen titer
    c. fluid pleocytosis
    c. fluid Venereal Disease Research
      Laboratory test
    c. fluid volume
cerebrovascular
    c. disease
    c. malformation
cerebrum semiovale
Cereport
Cerepro
Ceretec technetium-99m exametazime agent white blood cell scanning
cerevisiae
    Saccharomyces c.
cerium
cerivastatin
Cernevit-12
Cerrobend trim block
Cerubidine
ceruloplasmin
ceruminoma
cervical
    c. adenocarcinoma
    c. adenopathy
    c. artery
    c. cancer screening
    c. cap delivery system
    c. carcinoma
    c. carcinoma in situ
    c. conization
    c. cord
    c. disc
    c. disc herniation
    c. disc syndrome
    c. dysplasia
    c. enlargement
    c. esophagostomy
    c. eversion
    c. fascia
    c. injury
    c. intraepithelial neoplasia (CIN)
    c. intraepithelial neoplasia classification
    c. intraepithelial neoplasm (CIN)
    c. lymph node
    c. meningocele
    c. myelogram
    c. neural foramen
    c. os
    c. pain syndrome
    c. plexus
    c. sarcoma
    c. spine
    c. spine fracture
    c. spine fusion
    c. spine spondylosis
    c. stroma
    c. structure
    c. stump
    c. stump cancer
    c. triangle
    c. tumor
    c. vertebra
cervices (*pl. of* cervix)
cervicis (*gen. of* cervix)
cervicitis
cervicography
cervicomedullary kink
cervicotrochanteric fracture
cervix, gen. cervicis, pl. cervices
    cell carcinoma of c.
    international classification of cancer of c.
    malignant tumor of c.
    c. sign
    uterine c.
CES
    clinical estimation of survival
CES-D
    Center for Epidemiologic Studies-Depression
    CES-D Scale
cesium
    c. implant
    c. needle
    c. therapy
cesium-137 (^{137}Cs)
cessation
    smoking c.
cestode
cetiedil citrate
c-ets oncogene
Cetus trial
cetuximab
CEV
    cyclophosphamide, etoposide, vincristine
CEVAIE
    carboplatin, epirubicin, vincristine, actinomycin D, ifosfamide, etoposide
    CEVAIE regimen
Cevalin
CEVD
    cyclophosphamide, etoposide, vincristine, dexamethasone
    CEVD regimen
Cevi-Bid
cevimeline
CF
    cancer free
    cardiac failure
    chemotactic factor
    Christmas factor
    citrovorum factor
    complement factor

complement fixation
cystic fibrosis
²⁵²Cf
californium-252
CFA
colony-forming assay
complement-fixing antibody
complete Freund adjuvant
CFEV
cyclophosphamide, 5-fluorouracil,
epirubicin, vincristine
CFIDS
chronic fatigue and immune dysfunction
syndrome
CFL
cisplatin, 5-fluorouracil, leucovorin
C-Flex
C-F. catheter
C-F. double-J stent
c-fms
c-fms oncogene
c-fms protooncogene/oncogene
c-fos
c-fos gene
c-fos oncogene
c-fos-**dependent pathway**
c-fos-**independent pathway**
CFOV
circular field of view
CFP
cyclophosphamide, 5-fluorouracil,
prednisone
CFR
Cancer Family Registry
Breast CFR
Colon CFR
CFRBCS
Cooperative Family Registry for Breast
Cancer Studies
CFS
chronic fatigue syndrome
CFT
Complex Figure Test
CFU
colony-forming unit
CFU-C
colony-forming unit-culture
**CFU-Dexter bone marrow stem cell
assay**
CFU-E
colony-forming unit-erythrocyte
CFU_EOS
colony-forming unit-eosinophil

CFU-F
colony-forming unit-fibroblast
CFU-F bone marrow stem cell
assay
CFU-GEMM
colony-forming unit–granulocyte,
erythrocyte, megakaryocyte,
macrophage
CFU-GEMM bone marrow stem
cell assay
CFU-GM
colony-forming unit-granulocyte-
macrophage
colony-forming unit–granulocyte-
macrophage
CFU-GM bone marrow stem cell
assay
CgA
chromogranin A
CGAP
Cancer Genome Anatomy Project
CGCT
combined germ cell tumor
CGH
comparative genomic hybridization
CGL
chronic granulocytic leukemia
cGMP
cyclic guanosine monophosphate
cGVHD
chronic graft-versus-host disease
cGy
centigray
CH-296
human fibronectin fragment CH-296
CHA
chronic hemolytic anemia
congenital hypoplastic anemia
Chachoua staging system
CHAD
cyclophosphamide, hexamethylmelamine,
Adriamycin, DDP
CHAD protocol
Chagas disease
chain
amyloid light c.
branched c.
closed c.
extracellular immunoglobulin
light c.
gamma c.
globin c.
immunoglobulin alpha c.

NOTES

113

chain *(continued)*
  immunoglobulin delta c.
  immunoglobulin epsilon c.
  immunoglobulin gamma c.
  immunoglobulin heavy c.
  immunoglobulin kappa c.
  immunoglobulin lambda c.
  immunoglobulin mu c.
  internal mammary c.
  internal mammary lymph node c.
    (IMN)
  inverse polymerase c.
  J c.
  joining c.
  jugular c.
  kappa light c.
  paratracheal node c.
  periesophageal nodal c.
  polymorphic class I c.
  posterior nodal c.
  ricin A c.
chain-terminating inhibitor
chalasia, chalasis
chalazion, pl. **chalazia**
chamber
  cardiac c.
  farmer c.
  Fuchs-Rosenthal c.
  reentrant well c.
chamberlain
  C. line
  C. procedure
CHAM-OCA, CHAMOCA
  cyclophosphamide, hydroxyurea,
    actinomycin D, methotrexate, Oncovin,
    citrovorum factor, Adriamycin
chamomile mouthwash
chancre
chancroid
change
  atherosclerotic c.
  body habitus c. (BHC)
  cystic c.
  degenerative c.
  E:A c.
  epithelial degenerative c.
  histologic c.
  pigment c.
  polyneuropathy, organomegaly,
    endocrine abnormalities, M
    protein, skin c.'s (POEMS)
  polyneuropathy, organomegaly,
    endocrinopathy, monoclonal
    gammopathy, skin c.'s (POEMS)
  postbiopsy c.
  posttherapy c.
  precancerous c.
  pseudo-Pelger-Hüet c.

  radiation-related ischemic c.
  redox c.
  signal c.
Chang staging system
channel
  basophil/lobularity c.
  lymph c.
  surface epithelium vascular c.
CHAP
  cyclophosphamide, Hexalen, Adriamycin,
    Platinol
  cyclophosphamide, hexamethylmelamine,
    Adriamycin, Platinol
chaparral tea
chaperone
  molecular c.
characteristic
  c. radiation
  transfer c.
characterization
  immunologic c.
charbon
Charcot-Bottcher filament
Charcot-Marie-Tooth disease
charged-particle
  c.-p. equilibrium
  c.-p. irradiation
Charles procedure
CHART
  continuous hyperfractionated accelerated
    radiation therapy
chart
  Levy-Jennings c.
chaste tree berry
Chaussier
  C. areola
  C. line
  C. sign
chaw *(var. of* chew)
Chealamide
check
  delta c.
  c. film
  Hepatitis C C.
checklist
  Rotterdam Symptom C.
Chédiak-Higashi
  C.-H. disease
  C.-H. syndrome
cheek advancement flap
cheilitis
  candidiasis angular c.
  c. granulomatosa
chelated
  c. antibody
  c. immunoglobulin
chelate immunoconjugate
chelating agent

chelation
  c. therapy
  zinc c.
chelonae
  Mycobacterium c.
Chemet
chemical
  c. arachnoiditis
  c. carcinogen
  c. carcinogenesis
  c. exchange
  c. linkage
  c. mediator
  c. pneumonitis
  pteridine c.
  c. rhizotomy
  c. shift imaging (CSI)
  c. shift imaging technique
  small molecular weight c.
  c. splanchnicectomy
  sulforaphane c.
chemically modified protein
chemiluminescence
chemiluminescent substrate kit
chemistry
  anomalous serum c.
  combinatorial c.
  computational c.
  radiopharmaceutical c.
  serum c.
chemoattractant cytokine
ChemoBloc vial venting system
chemobrain
chemodectoma
chemoembolization
  intrahepatic arterial c.
  transcatheter arterial c.
chemoembolotherapy
chemoendocrine therapy
chemofiltration
  extracorporeal c.
chemohormonal therapy
chemohormonotherapy
chemoimmunology
chemoirradiation
  concomitant c.
chemokine
  C-C c.
  c. coreceptor
  CXC c.
  CX3C c.
  c. inhibition
  macrophage-derived c. (CXCR4)

nonsyncytium-inducing c. (CC-CKR-5)
  c. receptor 1-11 (CCR1–11)
  c. receptor 5 (CCR5)
  c. receptor-mediated viral entry
  c. receptor-related strategy
  c. related
  c. with CC sequence
chemokine-related receptor (CXCR4)
chemolitholysis
chemolysis
chemonucleolysis
chemoperfusion
Chemo-Port catheter
chemopotentiator
chemoprevention
  hormonal c.
chemopreventive agent
chemoprophylaxis
  postexposure c.
chemoprotector
chemoradiation
  adjuvant c.
  concomitant c.
  5-fluorouracil/mitomycin c.
  marrow-ablative c.
  c. therapy
chemoradiotherapy
  concurrent c. (CCRT, CC-RT)
  high-dose c.
  myeloablative c.
chemoreceptor
  c. trigger zone (CTZ)
  c. tumor
chemoresistance
chemoresistant tumor
chemosensitive brain tumor
chemosensitizer
chemoserotherapy
chemosuppression
chemotactic
  c. factor (CF)
  c. peptide
chemotaxis
chemotherapeutic
  c. agent
  c. cycle
  c. drug
  c. index
chemotherapy (CTx)
  adjuvant c.
  anthracycline-based induction c.
  AT-II-induced intraarterial c.

NOTES

C

115

chemotherapy *(continued)*
    belly bath c.
    cell cycling in c.
    cisplatin-based combination c.
    combination c.
    consolidation c.
    continuous intravenous infusion c.
    conventional dose c.
    curative c.
    cytostatic c.
    cytotoxic c.
    DACE c.
    dexamethasone, ara-C, carboplatin, etoposide c.
    dose-adjusted EPOCH c.
    dose-intensive induction c.
    double high-dose c.
    c. enteritis
    experimental c.
    F/CDDP/VP16 combination c.
    first-line c.
    fotemustine/cisplatin/etoposide combination c.
    heated intraoperative intraperitoneal c. (HIIC)
    hepatic arterial c.
    hepatic infusion c.
    high-dose c. (HDC, HDCh, HDCT, HD-CT)
    high-dose ECV consolidation c.
    highly emetogenic c. (HEC)
    hypertensive intraarterial c.
    hyperthermic intraperitoneal intraoperative c. (HIIC)
    induction and consolidation c.
    induction-remission c.
    infusion c.
    intensification c.
    intensive consolidation c.
    interleukin-12 and EPOCH c.
    internal iliac arterial infusion c.
    intraarterial c. (IAC)
    intraarterial cisplatin c.
    intracavitary c.
    intracerebral spinal fluid c.
    intra-CSF c.
    intrahepatic artery c. (IHAC)
    intramuscular c.
    intraperitoneal hyperthermic c. (IPHC)
    intrapleural c.
    intrathecal c.
    intravenous infusion c.
    intraventricular c.
    intravesical c.
    in vitro induction-remission c.
    LOPP c.
    low-dose c.
    MADDOC c.

    maintenance c.
    mechlorethamine, Adriamycin, dacarbazine, DDP, Oncovin, cyclophosphamide c.
    metabolism in intraperitoneal c.
    metronomic c.
    moderately emetogenic c. (MEC)
    multiagent c.
    multitargeted c.
    myeloablative c.
    myelosuppression c.
    myelosuppressive c.
    neoadjuvant c. (NACT, NCT)
    novel form of consolidation c.
    palliative c.
    parenteral c.
    platinum-based c.
    platinum-taxane c.
    postoperative c.
    preoperative c.
    presurgical c.
    primary c. (CT1)
    prophylactic c.
    c. protocol
    radiolabeled antibody and VP-16 and cyclophosphamide systemic c.
    random high-dose c.
    c. regimen
    regional c.
    reinduction c.
    remission-induction c.
    Revici-guided c.
    Rituxan and fludarabine c.
    salvage c.
    sandwich c.
    second-line c.
    sequential postremission c.
    single-agent high-dose c.
    standard-dose c. (SD-CT)
    sterilizing c.
    systemic c.
    tandem high-dose c.
    topical c.
    c. wafer
chemotherapy-hemolytic uremic syndrome (C-HUS)
chemotherapy-induced
    c.-i. diarrhea (CID)
    c.-i. gastritis
    c.-i. ischemia
    c.-i. myelotoxicity
    c.-i. nausea and vomiting (CINV)
    c.-i. pericarditis
    c.-i. peripheral neuropathy
    c.-i. pulmonary toxicity
chemotherapy-related
    c.-r. amenorrhea (CRA)
    c.-r. mucositis
chemotherapy-responsive patient

Chernobyl nuclear accident
cherry
    c. angioma
    c. red endobronchial lesion
Chesapeake
    hemoglobin C.
CHESS
    comprehensive health enhancement
    support system
chest
    c. film
    c. mass
    pneumonectomy c.
    c. radiograph
    c. radiology
    c. tube
    c. wall
    c. wall and sternal tumor
    c. x-ray
chew, chaw
chewable
    E.E.S. C.
ChexUP
    cyclophosphamide, hexamethylmelamine,
    5-fluorouracil, Platinol
CHF
    cyclophosphamide, hexamethylmelamine,
    5-fluorouracil
chiasmatic-hypothalamic
    c.-h. glioma
    c.-h. pilocytic astrocytoma
Chiba needle
chick-cell agglutination
chicken fat clot
chickenpox
child
    C. cirrhosis
    C. classification
    c. lymphoblastic leukemia
childhood
    c. brain tumor (CBT)
    C. Brain Tumor Foundation
    c. cancer
    C. Cancer Survivor Study (CCSS)
    c. granulomatous disease
    non-T, non-B acute lymphocytic
    leukemia of c.
    c. polycystic disease
Child-Pugh score
children
    C.'s Advil Suspension
    C.'s Art Project (CAP)
    C.'s Cancer Group (CCG)

    C.'s Cancer Group criteria
    C.'s Cancer Study Group (CCSG)
    C.'s Hospital Medical Center
    sarcoma chemotherapy protocol
    C.'s Motrin Suspension
Child-Turcott classification
chimera
chimeric
    c. 17-1A (C17-1A)
    c. anti-GD3 antibody
    c. antigen receptor gene
    c. bcr/abl gene
    c. L6 monoclonal antibody
    c. protein
    c. virus
chimerism
    all-donor c.
    hematopoietic c.
    mixed donor-host hematopoietic c.
chimney sweep's cancer
Chinese
    C. cucumber
    C. hamster ovary (CHO)
    C. liver fluke
CHIP
    cis-dichlorotransdihydroxy-bis-
    isoprophylamine platinum IV
chiropractice
CHK
    Csk homologous kinase
Chlamydia
    C. pneumoniae
    C. psittaci
    C. trachomatis
chlorambucil
    AMSA, prednisone, c. (APC)
    methotrexate, actinomycin D, c.
    (MAC)
    c. and prednisone (CP)
    pulse c.
    vinblastine, actinomycin D,
    bleomycin, cisplatin,
    cyclophosphamide, c. (VAB 3,
    VAB-III)
    c., vinblastine, procarbazine,
    prednisone (ChlVPP, CH1-VPP)
    c., vinblastine, procarbazine,
    prednisone, etoposide, vincristine,
    Adriamycin (ChlVPP/EVA)
    c., vincristine, procarbazine,
    prednisone (LOPP)
chloramine T
chloramphenicol acetyltransferase

NOTES

Chloraseptic
  Vicks Children's C.
chlorbutin
chlordiazepoxide
  amitriptyline and c.
Chloresium
  C. ointment
  C. solution
chlorhexidine
  c. digluconate
  c. mouthwash
chloride
  ammonium c.
  calcium c.
  magnesium c.
  potassium c.
  c. shift
  sodium c.
  zinc c.
chlormadinone
chlormethine HCl
chloroacetaldehyde
chloroacetate esterase-butyrate esterase stain
8-chloro-cAMP
2-chlorodeoxyadenosine (2CDA)
chloroethylnitrosourea (CNU)
  sarcosinamide c. (SarCNU)
chloroma
chloromatous sarcoma
chloromyeloma
chloroquine
  c. phosphate
  c. and primaquine
chlorothiazide
chlorotic anemia
chlorotrianisene
chlorozotocin
chlorphenesin carbamate
Chlorpromanyl
chlorpromazine
chlorthalidone
ChlVPP
  chlorambucil, vinblastine, procarbazine, prednisone
ChlVPP/EVA
  chlorambucil, vinblastine, procarbazine, prednisone, etoposide, vincristine, Adriamycin
CHM
  complete hydatidiform mole
CHO
  Chinese hamster ovary
  cyclophosphamide, hydroxydaunomycin, Oncovin
  CHO cell
choanal polyp

CHOB
  cyclophosphamide, hydroxydaunomycin, Oncovin, bleomycin
chocolate
  c. cyst
  c. joint effusion
  c. sauce abscess
CHOD
  cyclophosphamide, hydroxydaunomycin, Oncovin, dexamethasone
Cholac
cholangiectasis
  extrahepatic c.
cholangiocarcinoma (CCA)
  extrahepatic c.
  hepatocellular c.
  hilar c. (HCCA)
  intrahepatic c. (ICC)
  Klatskin c.
  oncocytic c.
  peripheral c.
cholangiocellular carcinoma
cholangiodrainage
cholangiogram
cholangiography
  fine-needle transhepatic c.
  percutaneous transhepatic c. (PTC)
cholangiohepatitis
cholangiolithiasis
cholangiopancreatography
  endoscopic retrograde c. (ERCP)
cholangitis
  acute nonsuppurative ascending c.
  acute suppurative ascending c.
  chronic nonsuppurative
    destructive c.
  sclerosing c.
cholecystectomy
cholecystitis
  acute c.
  chronic c.
  emphysematous c.
cholecystocholangiography
cholecystocholangitis
cholecystocolic fistula
cholecystocolonic fistula
cholecystoduodenal fistula
cholecystogram
cholecystography
cholecystojejunostomy
cholecystokinin (CCK)
cholecystolithiasis
cholecystomegaly
cholecystosis
  hyperplastic c.
cholecystostomy
choledochal cyst
choledochocele
choledochocholedochostomy

choledochoduodenal fistula
choledochojejunostomy
    Roux-en-Y c.
    c. stricture
choledocholithiasis
choledochoscope
cholelithiasis
cholera
    pancreatic c.
cholerae
    Vibrio c.
cholestasis, cholestasia
    intrahepatic c.
cholesteatoma
    inflammatory c.
cholesterol cleft
cholesterosis
cholestyramine resin
choline
    c. magnesium trisalicylate
    c. salicylate
cholinergic drug
chondramide
chondritis
chondroblastic
    c. osteosarcoma
    c. sarcoma
chondroblastoma
    benign metastasizing c.
chondrocalcinosis
chondrocyte
    binucleated c.
chondrodermatitis nodularis helicis
chondrodysplasia
    Jansen-type metaphysial c.
    metaphysial c.
    c. punctata
chondrodystrophia calcificans congenita
chondrofibroma
chondroid
    c. chordoma
    c. hamartoma
    c. syringoma
chondroma
    soft tissue c.
chondromatous element
chondromyxoid fibroma (CMF)
chondrosarcoma
    c. of bone
    clear cell c.
    dedifferentiated c.
    endosteal c.
    exostotic c.

    extraskeletal myxoid c. (EMC)
    laryngeal c.
    mesenchymal c.
    peripheral c.
    postirradiation c.
    skeletal myxoid c. (SMC)
    uterine c.
Chooz
CHOP
    cyclophosphamide, Halotestin, Oncovin, prednisone
    cyclophosphamide, hydroxydaunomycin, Oncovin, prednisone
    cyclophosphamide, hydroxydaunorubicin, Oncovin, prednisone
CHOP-BLEO
    cyclophosphamide, hydroxydaunomycin, Oncovin, prednisone, bleomycin
CHOPE
    cyclophosphamide, Halotestin, Oncovin, prednisone, etoposide
    cyclophosphamide, hydroxydaunomycin, Oncovin, prednisone, etoposide
    Cytoxan, Halotestin, Oncovin, prednisone, etoposide
CHOP/GADD153 oncogene
CHOR
    cyclophosphamide, hydroxydaunomycin, Oncovin, radiotherapy
chordoid sarcoma
chordoma
    chondroid c.
    nonskull base c. (NSBC)
    sacral c.
    c. of sacrum
    skull base c. (SBC)
chorea
    Huntington c.
    Sydenham c.
chorioadenoma destruens
choriocapillaris
choriocarcinoma
    esophageal c.
    gestational c.
    ovarian c.
    pure c.
choriomeningitis
    lymphocytic c.
chorion frondosum
chorionic
    c. gonadotropin
    c. villus sampling (CVS)

NOTES

choroid
  c. plexus
  c. plexus blush
  c. plexus carcinoma
  c. plexus cyst
  c. plexus neoplasm
  c. plexus papilloma
  c. point
choroidal
  c. artery
  c. cell
  c. fissure
  c. hemangioma
  c. melanoma
  c. nevus
  c. osteoma
choroidal-hippocampal fissure complex
choroidea
choroideum
  glomus c.
choroidopathy
  Pneumocystis c.
CHPP
  continuous hyperthermic peritoneal
  perfusion
CHR
  complete hematologic response
Christmas
  C. disease
  C. factor (CF)
chromaffin
  c. cell
  c. lineage
  c. staining
  c. tumor
Chromagen OB
Chroma-Pak
chromatid
chromatin
  condensed c.
  pyknotic c.
chromatography
  antiidiotypic affinity c.
  heparin affinity c.
  high-performance liquid c. (HPLC)
  high-performance size-exclusion c.
    (HPSEC)
  high-pressure liquid c. (HPLC)
  lentil lectin affinity c.
  micellar electrokinetic capillary c.
    (MECC)
chromic
  c. phosphate
  c. phosphate ^{32}P
  c. phosphate ^{32}P colloidal
    suspension
chromium release assay
chromogranin A (CgA)
chromophilic adenoma

chromophobe
  c. adenoma
  c. carcinoma
  c. renal cell carcinoma (CRCC)
chromoscopy
chromosomal
  c. sex marker
  c. translocation
chromosome
  c. 9, 10
  c. analysis
  c. 13 deletion
  dicentric c.
  double minute c. (DMC)
  i(12p) marker c.
  long arm of c. (q)
  c. 3p
  c. 9p
  c. 16p
  c. 17p
  Philadelphia c.
  phosphatase and tensin homologue
    deleted on c. (PTEN)
  c. 1p and 19q loss
  c. 5q
  c. 13q
  c. 17q
  c. 22q
  c. 19q locus
  c. 22q11 microdeletion (CATCH
    22)
  c. 22q region BAM22
  c. 14q tumor marker
  short arm of c. (p)
  yeast artificial c. (YAC)
chromosome-negative
chromosome-positive
chronic
  c. acquired hepatic failure
  c. active hepatitis
  c. allograft rejection
  c. ambulatory peritoneal dialysis
  c. antimicrobial prophylaxis
  c. atrophic gastritis
  c. breast abscess
  c. catheterization
  c. cholecystitis
  c. communicating hydrocephalus
  c. demyelinating disease
  c. diffuse sclerosing alveolitis
  c. disseminated candidiasis (CDC)
  c. eosinophilic pneumonia (CEP)
  c. fatigue and immune dysfunction
    syndrome (CFIDS)
  c. fatigue syndrome (CFS)
  c. fibrosing alveolitis
  c. graft-versus-host disease
    (cGVHD)
  c. granulocytic leukemia (CGL)

c. granulomatous disease
c. hemolytic anemia (CHA)
c. hyperplastic candidiasis
c. indwelling catheter
c. inflammatory demyelinating polyneuropathy
c. intestinal isosporiasis
c. lymphocytic leukemia (stage A-C) (CLL)
c. lymphocytic lymphoma
c. lymphoid leukemia (stage A-C)
c. megakaryocytic myelosis
c. monocytic leukemia
c. mucocutaneous candidiasis
c. myelocytic leukemia (CML)
c. myelogenous leukemia (CML)
c. myelogenous leukemia blast crisis (CML-BC)
c. myelogenous leukemia blastic phase (CML-BP)
c. myeloid leukemia (CML)
c. myeloid leukemia blast phase (CML-BP)
c. myelomonocytic leukemia (CMML)
c. nephritis
c. neutrophilic leukemia
c. nonleukemic myelosis
c. nonsuppurative destructive cholangitis
c. obstructive pulmonary disease (COPD)
c. obstructive uropathy
c. pain
c. pain syndrome
c. pancreatitis
c. phase
c. phase chronic myelogenous leukemia (CP-CML)
c. pluripotential immunoproliferative syndrome
c. PTSD
c. renal failure (CRF)
c. venous stasis
c. venous statis syndrome

chronomodulation
chronotherapy
adjuvant c.
Chronulac
Churg-Strauss syndrome
C-HUS
cancer-hemolytic uremic syndrome

chemotherapy-hemolytic uremic syndrome
Chvostek
C. anemia
C. sign
CHVP
cyclophosphamide, hydroxydaunomycin, VM-26, prednisone
CH1-VPP
chlorambucil, vinblastine, procarbazine, prednisone
chyli
cisterna c.
chylomicron, pl. **chylomicra, chylomicrons**
chylous ascites
Chymar
Alpha C.
chymopapain
CI
confidence interval
CIA
CCNU, ifosfamide, Adriamycin
CIC
circulating immune complex
ciclopirox
CID
chemotherapy-induced diarrhea
cytomegalic inclusion disease
cidofovir
Cidomycin
CIDS
cellular immunity deficiency syndrome
Ciel
Kay C.
cigarette
bidi c.
c. smoking
CIITA
class II transcriptional activator
cilastatin
imipenem and c.
Cilengitide
ciliary
c. body
c. body melanoma
c. function
c. ganglion
c. muscle
c. neurotrophic factor
ciliated cell adenocarcinoma
cimetidine hydrochloride
Cimicifuga racemosa

NOTES

121

CIN
cervical intraepithelial neoplasia
cervical intraepithelial neoplasm
CIN classification
cinchona bark
cineangiography
axial c.
cingulate gyrus
cingulotomy
Cinobac Pulvules
cinoxacin
cintredekin besudotox
CINV
chemotherapy-induced nausea and
vomiting
Cipro
ciprofloxacin
circadian-modified floxuridine
circadian rhythm
circinate erythema
circle
anastomotic arterial c.
circle-to-W flap
circular
c. collimator
c. field of view (CFOV)
circulating
c. free virus
c. immune complex (CIC)
c. recombinant form
circulation
cerebral c.
extracorporeal c.
extracranial carotid c.
c. time
circulator
circulatory overload
circumcision
circumference
middle upper arm c. (MUAC)
circumferential venous stenosis
circumoral paresthesia
circumscribe
**circumscribed cerebellar arachnoid
sarcoma**
circumvallate papilla
cirrhosis
alcoholic c. (AC)
antihepatitis C virus-positive c.
biliary c.
Child c.
diffuse c.
Laënnec c.
macronodular c.
progressive familial cholestatic c.
CIS
carcinoma in situ
cisapride

CisCA
cisplatin, cyclophosphamide, Adriamycin
cis-**diamminedichloroplatinum (DDP)**
cis-**dichlorotransdihydroxy-bis-
isoprophylamine**
c.-d.-b.-i. platinum
c.-d.-b.-i. platinum IV (CHIP)
cisplatin (CACP, Cddp, CPT)
Adriamycin and c. (AC)
c. analog
c., ara-C, caffeine (CAC)
c., BCNU, dacarbazine, tamoxifen
(CBDT)
continuous infusion paclitaxel
plus c.
c., cyclophosphamide, Adriamycin
(CisCA)
c., cyclophosphamide, doxorubicin,
vincristine, prednisone (P-CHOP)
dexamethasone, cyclophosphamide,
etoposide, c. (DCEP)
c., doxorubicin, mitomycin C
c. and epinephrine
c., epirubicin, folinic acid, 5-
fluorouracil (PELF)
escalated methotrexate, vinblastine,
Adriamycin, c. (E-MVAC)
etoposide and c.
c., etoposide, cyclophosphamide,
Adriamycin (CECA)
c., etoposide, Cytoxan, Adriamycin
(CECA)
c. and 5-fluorouracil
c., 5-fluorouracil, leucovorin (CFL)
c., 5-fluorouracil, leucovorin,
interferon alfa-2b (PFL-IFN)
high-dose methotrexate, vinblastine,
Adriamycin, c. (HD-VAC)
methotrexate, bleomycin, c. (MBC)
c., methotrexate, vinblastine (CMV)
methotrexate, vinblastine,
Adriamycin, c. (MVAC)
mitomycin C, Oncovin,
bleomycin, c. (MOB-III)
c. nephrotoxicity
c. neutralization
c., Oncovin, bleomycin (COB)
c., Oncovin, doxorubicin, etoposide
(CODE)
recombinant interleukin-2,
dacarbazine, c. (RIDD)
c., Velban, etoposide, bleomycin
(CVEB)
c. and VePesid (CV)
vinblastine, actinomycin D,
bleomycin, c. (VAB 2, VAB-II)
vinblastine, actinomycin D,
bleomycin, cyclophosphamide, c.

(VAB 5, VAB-V, VAB 6, VAB-VI)
vinblastine, bleomycin, c. (VBC)
c., vinblastine, dacarbazine (CVD)
c., vinblastine, etoposide, bleomycin (CVEB)
vinblastine, ifosfamide, c.
vincristine, Adriamycin, c.
vinorelbine and c. (VC)
c. and VP-16 (CV)
cisplatin-based combination chemotherapy
cisplatin/collagen matrix
cisplatin/epinephrine
cisplatin-induced ototoxicity
cis-**platinum**
c.-p. diammine dichloride (CPDD)
mesna, ifosfamide, Novantrone, etoposide plus etoposide, methylprednisolone, high-dose ara-C, c.-p. (MINE/ESHAP)
cis-**retinoic acid (CRA)**
9-*cis*-**retinoic acid**
13-*cis*-**retinoic acid (13-CRA)**
cistern
ambient wing of quadrigeminal c.
basal c.
pontine c.
quadrigeminal c.
cisterna chyli
Citracal
citrate
c. agar electrophoresis
calcium c.
cetiedil c.
daunorubicin c.
fentanyl c.
ferric ammonium c.
liposomal daunorubicin c.
magnesium c.
potassium acetate, potassium bicarbonate, potassium c.
potassium bicarbonate, potassium chloride, potassium c.
c. reaction
tamoxifen c.
toremifene c.
citrated
c. blood
c. plasma
citrate-phosphate vehicle

citrovorum
c. factor (CF)
c. rescue factor
Citrucel
citrulline
CIVIC chemotherapy regimen
CJD
Creutzfeldt-Jakob disease
CK
creatine kinase
CK20
cytokeratin 20
CK-BB
creatine kinase-BB isoenzyme
CK-BB tumor marker
c/kg
coulombs per kilogram
c-kit
c-kit enzyme
c-kit gene
c-kit inhibitor
c-kit ligand
CKR5 receptor
CKS
classical Kaposi sarcoma
CL
cellular leiomyoma
clade B HIV
clade-specific clinical entity
cladribine
Claforan
Clara
C. cell
C. cell adenocarcinoma
C. hematoxylin
Claripex
clarithromycin
Clark
C. classification system
C. level
C. level of invasion
C. microstaging method
C. staging system
C. staging system for malignant melanoma
Clark-Elder malignant melanoma classification
Clarkson
C. integration
C. scatter-summation algorithm
clasmatocyte
class
aspartyl protease c.

NOTES

class *(continued)*
- c. II gene product HLA-DP
- c. II gene product HLA-DQ
- c. II gene product HLA-DR
- c. II histocompatibility antigen
- c. I, II allele
- c. II transcriptional activator (CIITA)
- c. switch

classical Kaposi sarcoma (CKS)
classic large cell carcinoma (CLCC)
classification
- AJCC/UICC c.
- American Urological Association c.
- Ann Arbor c.
- Ann Arbor/Cotswold staging c.
- Ashhurst-Bromer c.
- Astler-Coller modification of Dukes c.
- AUA c.
- Bennett c.
- Berard c.
- Bethesda c.
- Binet system of c.
- Bismuth c.
- Bloom-Richardson c.
- Bocking c.
- Borrmann c.
- Breslow c.
- Broders c.
- Bunn-Lamberg c.
- Butchart staging c.
- Cambridge c.
- cervical intraepithelial neoplasia c.
- Child c.
- Child-Turcott c.
- CIN c.
- Clark-Elder malignant melanoma c.
- Columbia Clinical Cancer c.
- Cotswolds staging c.
- Couinaud liver disease c.
- Dixon-Moore c.
- Dukes c.
- Dukes-Astler-Coller adenocarcinoma c.
- Durie-Salmon multiple myeloma c.
- Elder malignant melanoma c.
- FAB c.
- French-American-British c.
- Fuhrman c.
- Gaeta c.
- Gell-Coombs c.
- Glasscock-Jackson c.
- Goldman c.
- Haggitt c.
- histopathologic tumor c.
- Holland c.
- Ho staging c.
- IMIG c.
- immunologic c.
- Intergroup Rhabdomyosarcoma Study Group Presurgical Staging C.
- International Neuroblastoma Pathology C. (INPC)
- IRSG Presurgical Staging C.
- Jackson-Parker c.
- Jansky c.
- Jewett-Whitmore c.
- Kiel tumor cell c.
- Klatskin tumor c.
- Lancefield c.
- Laurén c.
- Lennert c.
- Linell-Ljungberg c.
- Lugano c.
- Lukes-Butler c.
- Lukes-Collins c.
- Magano c.
- Marshall-Jewett-Strong c.
- McCabe-Fletcher c.
- M.D. Anderson Hospital c.
- microinvasive carcinoma c.
- morphologic c.
- Mostofi c.
- Papavasiliou c.
- Rai c. (stage 0-IV)
- Rappaport c.
- REAL c.
- Reese-Ellsworth c.
- C. and Regression Tree (CART)
- C. and Regression Tree analysis
- Revised European-American Lymphoma c.
- Robson c.
- Russell c.
- Rutledge c.
- Rye c.
- Shimada system of c.
- Simpson c.
- SOMA c.
- subjective, objective, management, analytic c.
- TNM c.
- tumor, node, metastasis c.
- UICC c.
- Van Nuys c.
- Wolfe breast carcinoma c.
- Working Formula c.
- World Health Organization c.

clathrin protein
claudication
- intermittent c.

clavulanate
Clavulin
claw
- cat's c.

CLBC
contralateral breast cancer
CLCC
classic large cell carcinoma
cleanser
RadiaCare Klenz wound c.
Septi-Soft skin care c.
clear
c. cell adenocarcinoma
c. cell carcinoma
c. cell chondrosarcoma
c. cell ependymoma (CCE)
c. cell sarcoma (CCS)
c. cell tumor
c. space
clearance
immune c.
insulin c.
renal c.
c. test
cleavage
caspase c.
endoproteolytic c.
cleaved
c. polyprotein precursor molecule (p55)
c. polyprotein precursor molecule product (p7, p9, p24)
cleft
cholesterol c.
c. face syndrome
Cleocin
C. Phosphate Injection
C. T Topical
Climara Transdermal
Clinda-Derm Topical
clindamycin
clinical
c. assay
c. breast examination (CBE)
C. Cancer Genetics
c. cardioprotective effect
c. correlation
c. cross reactivity
c. disease expression
c. estimation of survival (CES)
c. feature
c. latency
c. partial response (CPR)
c. stage
c. staging
c. target volume (CTV)

c. trial
c. tumor volume (CTV)
clinically detectable liver disease
clinicopathologic
c. correlation
c. study
Clinitron bed
Clinoril
clip
aneurysmal c.
radiopaque c.
clitoris enlargement
clivus, pl. **clivi**
lower c.
c. meningioma
c. metastasis
upper c.
CLL
chronic lymphocytic leukemia (stage A-C)
CLND
complete lymph node dissection
cloacae
Enterobacter c.
cloacogenic
c. carcinoma of anorectum
c. nonkeratinizing carcinoma
clobetasol
clodronate
clofarabine
Clofarex
clofazimine
clofibrate
Clolar
clonal
c. B lymphocyte
c. cytogenetic abnormality
c. deletion
c. deletion theory
c. development
c. eosinophilic disorder
c. evolution
c. inhibitory factor
c. lesion
c. marker
c. remission
c. selection
c. selection theory
clonality study
clone
immortalized c.
leukemic c.
neoplastic c.

NOTES

C

cloned
    c. gene
    c. peripheral blood lymphocyte
clonidine transdermal tape
cloning
    cDNA c.
    gene c.
    molecular c.
    subtraction c.
clonogenic
    c. assay
    c. capacity
    c. lymphoma cell
    c. myeloma cell
    c. tumor cell
clonorchiasis, clonorchiosis
    C. sinensis
Cloquet node
clorazepate
Cloretazine
closed chain
close margins
clostridial
    c. bacteremia
    c. sepsis
Clostridium
    C. difficile (CD)
    C. difficile enterocolitis
    C. histolyticum
    C. perfringens
    C. septicum
closure
    c. time
    transcatheter c.
clot
    autologous blood c.
    blood c.
    chicken fat c.
    currant jelly c.
    fibrin c.
    fibrinous c.
    c. lysis
    plasma c.
    c. retraction time
    sentinel c.
clothing artifact
Clotrimaderm
clotrimazole
clotting
    c. cascade
    c. factor
    c. factor deficiency
    c. factor VIII
    c. time
Cloudman melanoma
cloxacillin
Cloxapen

CLRSS
    Composite Laryngeal Recurrence Staging
    System
CLS
    capillary lymphatic space
clubbing
    digital c.
clumping
    platelet c.
cluster
    c. designation
    c. of differentiation (CD)
    c. of differentiation 1-166
      (CD1–166)
    c. of differentiation 4 (CD4)
    c. of differentiation 8 (CD8)
    c. of differentiation 40 gene
    c. of differentiation 4
      immunoglobulin G (CD4-IgG)
    flocculent c.
    monophyletic c.
    c.'s of pancreatic acinar cells
      (CPAC)
    stippled c.
Clutton joint
CM
    cutaneous melanoma
CMC
    cyclophosphamide, methotrexate, CCNU
CMC-VAP
    cyclophosphamide, methotrexate, CCNU,
    vincristine, Adriamycin, procarbazine
CMED
    cyclophosphamide, methotrexate,
    etoposide, dexamethasone
c-met gene
C-methionine PET
CMEV
    cyclophosphamide, methotrexate,
    epirubicin, vincristine
CMF
    chondromyxoid fibroma
    cyclophosphamide, methotrexate, 5-
    fluorouracil
    Cytoxan, methotrexate, 5-fluorouracil
CMF-AV
    cyclophosphamide, methotrexate, 5-
    fluorouracil, Adriamycin, vincristine
CMFAVP
    cyclophosphamide, methotrexate, 5-
    fluorouracil, Adriamycin, vincristine,
    prednisone
CMF-BLEO
    cyclophosphamide, methotrexate, 5-
    fluorouracil, bleomycin
CMF-FLU
    cyclophosphamide, methotrexate, 5-
    fluorouracil, fluoxymesterone

CMFH
cyclophosphamide, methotrexate, 5-fluorouracil, hydroxyurea

CMFP
cyclophosphamide, methotrexate, 5-fluorouracil, prednisone

CMFPT
cyclophosphamide, methotrexate, 5-fluorouracil, prednisone, tamoxifen
Cytoxan, methotrexate, 5-fluorouracil, prednisone, tamoxifen

CMFPTH
cyclophosphamide, methotrexate, 5-fluorouracil, prednisone, tamoxifen, Halotestin

CMFP-VA
cyclophosphamide, methotrexate, 5-fluorouracil, prednisone, vincristine, Adriamycin

CMFT
cyclophosphamide, methotrexate, 5-fluorouracil, tamoxifen

CMF-TAM
cyclophosphamide, methotrexate, 5-fluorouracil, tamoxifen

CM-5-FU
cyclophosphamide, methotrexate, 5-fluorouracil

CMFV
cyclophosphamide, methotrexate, 5-fluorouracil, vincristine

CMFVAT
cyclophosphamide, methotrexate, 5-fluorouracil, vincristine, Adriamycin, testosterone

CMFVP
cyclophosphamide, methotrexate, 5-fluorouracil, vincristine, prednisone

CMH
cyclophosphamide, *m*-AMSA, hydroxyurea
Cytoxan, *m*-AMSA, hydroxyurea

CMI
cell-mediated immunity

CML
chronic myelocytic leukemia
chronic myelogenous leukemia
chronic myeloid leukemia
CML blast crisis

CML-BC
chronic myelogenous leukemia blast crisis

CML-BP
chronic myelogenous leukemia blastic phase
chronic myeloid leukemia blast phase

CMM
cutaneous malignant melanoma

CMML
chronic myelomonocytic leukemia
myelomonocytic leukemia, chronic

CMOPP, C-MOPP
cyclophosphamide, mechlorethamine, Oncovin, procarbazine, prednisone

CMOS
complementary metal oxide semiconductor

CMP
CCNU, methotrexate, procarbazine

CMP/dCMP-K
cytidylate/2′-deoxycytidylate kinase

CMPF
cyclophosphamide, methotrexate, prednisone, 5-fluorouracil

CMSI warming system

CMT
combined modality therapy

CMV
cisplatin, methotrexate, vinblastine
controlled mechanical ventilation
cytomegalovirus
CMV oophoritis

CMVIG
cytomegalovirus immune globulin

c-myb
c-myb oncogene
c-myb protooncogene/oncogene

c-myc
c-myc expression
c-myc gene rearrangement
c-myc oncogene
c-myc protein

CNBSS-2
Canadian National Breast Screening Study-2

CNF
cyclophosphamide, Novantrone, 5-fluorouracil

Cnidosporidia

CNOP, C-NOP
cyclophosphamide, Novantrone, Oncovin, prednisone
Cytoxan, Novantrone, Oncovin, prednisone

A1cNow glycemic monitoring device

NOTES

CNQ
Cancer Needs Questionnaire
CNS
central nervous system
CNS lymphoma
metastatic lymphoma of CNS
primary lymphoma of CNS
CNU
chloroethylnitrosourea
⁶⁰Co
cobalt-60
CoA
coenzyme A
coactivator-associated arginine methyltransferase 1 (CARM1)
coagglutination
CoaguChek
C. Pro/DM monitor
C. self-testing device
coagulation
c. analyzer
c. cascade
disseminated intravascular c. (DIC)
c. factor
c. factor disease
fulminant disseminated intravascular c.
laparoscopic microwave c.
laser c.
c. necrosis
c. pathway
phospholipid-dependent c.
c. profile
c. system
coagulative tumor cell necrosis
coagulator
cold c.
Coagulin-B
coagulopathy
consumption c.
intravascular consumption c.
co-alcohol fractionation
coalition
coal workers' pneumoconiosis
Coamate antithrombin assay
coanalgesic
COAP
Cytoxan, Oncovin, ara-C, prednisone
COAP-BLEO
cyclophosphamide, Oncovin, ara-C, prednisone, bleomycin
coaptation
coarctation
aortic c.
coarse
c. calcification
c. facies
c. reticulation

coast
c. of California café-au-lait spot
c. of Maine café-au-lait spot
coat
buffy c.
Coat-A-Count PSA IRMA test
CoA-transferase
COB
cisplatin, Oncovin, bleomycin
cobalt
c. megavoltage machine
c. pneumopathy
cobalt-60 (⁶⁰Co)
cobalt-bleomycin imaging agent
Cobas Mira analyzer
COBE
COBE 2991 Cell Processor
COBE Spectra apheresis system
Cobex
cocarcinogen
coccidia (*pl. of* coccidium)
coccidioidal granuloma
Coccidioides immitis
coccidioidin skin test
coccidioidomycosis arthritis
coccidiosis
coccidium, pl. **coccidia**
cochlear lesion
Cochran-Mantel-Haenszel test
Cockayne syndrome
Cockcroft-Gault formula
cocktail
Accutane/Rezulin c.
Brompton c.
MAK-6 c.
pain c.
Texas c.
coculturing
CODE
cisplatin, Oncovin, doxorubicin, etoposide
code
genetic c.
codeine
acetaminophen and c.
aspirin and c.
butalbital compound and c.
Capital and C.
Coryphen C.
Empirin with C.
Fiorinal with C.
Tylenol with C.
coding
gene c.
Codman
C. triangle
C. tumor
codominance

codominant
    c. epitope
    c. gene
codon
    c. mutation
    nonsense c.
CODOX-M/IVAC
    cyclophosphamide, doxorubicin, high-dose methotrexate/ifosfamide, etoposide, high-dose cytarabine
Codoxy
coefficient
    absorption c.
    apparent diffusion c.
    attenuation c.
    diffusion c.
    intraclass correlation c. (ICC)
    c. of variation
coelomic epithelium of ovary
coenzyme
    c. A (CoA)
    c. Q (CoQ)
Coe virus
coexpression
    bcl-2 and P-glycoprotein c.
    HER-3 c.
    HER-4 c.
cofactor
    heparin c.
    heparin c. II
    ristocetin von Willebrand c.
    Stachrom heparin c. II
CoFactor trial protocol
Cogentin
Co-Gesic
cognitive
    c. deficit
    c. distraction
    c. technique
    c. therapy
cognitive-behavioral therapy
coherent scattering
Cohn cold ethanol fractionation process
cohort
    c. effect
    c. study
cohosh
    black c.
coil
    breast c.
    butterfly c.
    endorectal c.
    field-profiling c.

    Gianturco steel c.
    intravascular c.
    phased-array c.
    radiofrequency c.
    surface c.
    thrombogenic c.
coimmunoprecipitation
coinfection
    viral hepatitis c.
Colace
Colaris genetic susceptibility test
colaspase
colchicine and probenecid
cold
    c. agglutinin
    c. agglutinin disease
    c. antibody
    c. antibody immune hemolysis
    c. biopsy
    c. coagulator
    c. conization
    c. hemagglutinin
    c. kit
    c. nodule
    c. spot
cold-knife conization
cold-type autoimmune hemolytic anemia
colectasia
colectomy
    laparoscopic c.
    laparoscopy-assisted c. (LAC)
Colestid
colestipol
Coley toxin
coli
    adenomatous polyposis c.
    Escherichia c. (EC)
    familial polyposis c. (FPC)
colic
    biliary c.
colistimethate
colistin
colitis
    adenovirus c.
    Campylobacter c.
    c. cystica profunda
    granulomatous c.
    mucous c.
    neutropenic c.
    spastic c.
    ulcerative c. (UC)
Collaborative Ocular Melanoma Study (COMS)

NOTES

collagen
- cross-linked C-terminal telopeptide of type 1 c.
- c. sponge
- c. synthesis
- c. turnover
- c. XVIII

collagenase

collagenous scar

collateral
- hemorrhoidal c.

collecting duct carcinoma (CDC)

collection
- abdominal air c.
- air c.
- cell c.
- crescentic c.
- extraaxial fluid c.
- extracerebral fluid c.
- periarticular fluid c.
- c. tube

colliculus, pl. **colliculi**

collimated SPECT

collimation
- c. aperture
- narrow c.

collimator
- circular c.
- c. cone
- forward segmental multileaf c.
- high-resolution multileaf c.
- inverse segmental multileaf c.
- c. jaw
- micromultileaf c.
- multileaf c. (MLC)
- c. rotation
- segmental multileaf c.

collision tumor

colloid
- c. adenoma
- c. cancer
- c. carcinoma
- c. cyst
- c. cyst of third ventricle
- c. goiter
- iron oxide dextran c.
- phytate c.
- c. shift
- sulfur c.

colloidal
- c. chromic phosphorus
- c. suspension

colloid-filled follicle

coloanal resection

coloboma, pl. **colobomas, colobomata**

colocolic fistula

colocolostomy

colon
- adenomatous polyposis of c. (APC)

- ascending c.
- barium-filled c.
- burnt-out c.
- c. cancer
- C. Cancer Alliance
- C. Cancer Family Registry
- C. CFR
- c. cutoff sign
- extrapelvic c.
- c. neoplasia
- c. perforation

colonic
- c. carcinoma
- c. diverticular hemorrhage
- c. diverticulitis
- c. diverticulosis
- c. diverticulum
- c. epithelium
- c. filling defect
- c. ileus
- c. narrowing
- c. neoplasm
- c. obstruction
- c. perforation
- c. polyp
- c. stricture
- c. ulcer
- c. varix
- c. volvulus

colonies (*pl. of* colony)

colonocyte

colonography
- computed tomographic c.
- CT c.

colonoscopic polypectomy

colonoscopy, coloscopy
- endocervical canal c.
- therapeutic c.
- virtual c.

colony, pl. **colonies**
- c. formation
- c. stimulating

colony-forming
- c.-f. assay (CFA)
- c.-f. unit (CFU)
- c.-f. unit-culture (CFU-C)
- c.-f. unit-eosinophil (CFU_{EOS})
- c.-f. unit-erythrocyte (CFU-E)
- c.-f. unit-fibroblast (CFU-F)
- c.-f. unit–granulocyte, erythrocyte, megakaryocyte, macrophage (CFU-GEMM)
- c.-f. unit-granulocyte-macrophage (CFU-GM)
- c.-f. unit–granulocyte-macrophage (CFU-GM)

colony-stimulating
- c.-s. factor (CSF)
- c.-s. factor *Camptotheca*

coloproctitis
color

    c. Doppler imaging
    c. Doppler ultrasound
    3-c. flow cytometry
    c. gain

Colorado tick fever virus
colorectal

    c. adenocarcinoma
    c. adenoma
    c. anastomosis
    c. cancer (CRC)
    c. cancer endoscopy
    c. cancer screening
    c. carcinoid
    c. carcinoma (CRC)
    c. hemorrhage
    c. lymphoma
    c. polyp

colorectal/ovarian (CR/OV)
color-flow

    c.-f. Doppler
    c.-f. Doppler imaging
    c.-f. Doppler sonography

colorimetric method
coloscopy (var. of colonoscopy)
colostomy

    diverting c.
    end c.
    fecal diversion c.
    temporary diverting c.

colostomy-related problem
colovaginal fistula
colovesical fistula
colpocephaly
colpocleisis
colpoperineoplasty
colposcopy
colpostat

    c. applicator
    dome c.
    FSD c.

Columbia Clinical Cancer classification
column

    acetabular c.
    c. or bead technology
    disposable PD-10 c.
    dye c.
    immunoadsorption c.
    NHS-activated HiTrap affinity c.
    PD-10 disposable Sephadex G-25 c.

    plasmapheresis through a Prosorba c.
    Prosorba c.
    Sephadex G-25 c.

columnar

    c. cell carcinoma
    c. cell type
    c. epithelium

columnar-lined esophagus
Coly-Mycin M Parenteral
COM

    cyclophosphamide, Oncovin, MeCCNU
    cyclophosphamide, Oncovin, methotrexate

COMA-A

    cyclophosphamide, Oncovin, methotrexate, Adriamycin, ara-C

coma carcinomatosum
Comalose-R
COMB

    cyclophosphamide, Oncovin, MeCCNU, bleomycin
    cyclophosphamide, Oncovin, methotrexate, bleomycin

COMBAP

    cyclophosphamide, Oncovin, methotrexate, bleomycin, Adriamycin, prednisone

Combidex MRI contrast agent
Combilight PDD 5133 laparoscope
combination

    AdV.RSV-TK and ganciclovir c.
    all-*trans*-retinoic acid/interferon-alfa 2a c.
    analog c.
    antineoplaston A10/low-dose methotrexate c.
    c. antiretroviral therapy
    Arimidex, Tamoxifen, Alone or in C. (ATAC)
    c. chemotherapy
    cyclophosphamide, mitoxantrone, Rituximab c.
    c. drug (CD)
    Epivir/Retrovir c.
    flavopiridol/3-hour paclitaxel infusion c.
    c. hormone therapy
    integrin-matrix c.
    c. nucleoside analogue antiviral regimen
    oxaliplatin/capecitabine c.
    sulfadoxine/pyrimethamine c.

NOTES

combinatorial
 C. Array Technology
 c. chemistry
combined
 c. androgen blockade (CAB)
 c. antiretroviral therapy (CART)
 c. germ cell tumor (CGCT)
 c. immunodeficiency
 c. modality staging
 c. modality therapy (CMT)
 c. modulators
 penicillin G benzathine and
  procaine c.
 c. proton-photon radiotherapy
combining-site antibody
Combitip Plus pipette tip
Combivir
Combretastatin A4 Prodrug (CA4P)
COMe
 cyclophosphamide, Oncovin,
  methotrexate
comedocarcinoma
 invasive c.
COMET-A
 cyclophosphamide, Oncovin,
  methotrexate, leucovorin, etoposide,
  ara-C
comet assay
COMF
 cyclophosphamide, Oncovin,
  methotrexate, 5-fluorouracil
Comfeel
 C. hydrocolloid dressing
 C. plus triangle dressing
comfort care
comfrey
COMLA
 cyclophosphamide, Oncovin,
  methotrexate, leucovorin,
  arabinosylcytosine
 cyclophosphamide, Oncovin,
  methotrexate, leucovorin, ara-C
commission
 Nuclear Regulatory C. (NRC)
commissural myelotomy
commissure
 anterior c. (AC)
committee
 Oncologic Drugs Advisory C.
  (ODAC)
common
 c. acquired nevus
 c. acute leukemia antigen
 c. acute lymphoblastic leukemia
  antigen (CALLA)
 c. bile duct obstruction
 c. epithelial ovarian cancer
 c. hereditary elliptocytosis
 c. iliac lymph node

 c. leukocyte antigen
 c. pathway
 C. Toxicity Criteria (CTC)
 c. variable agammaglobulinemia
 c. variable immunodeficiency
 c. variable immunodeficiency
  disease
Commonweal Cancer Help Program
community-acquired
 c.-a. immunodeficiency syndrome
  (CAIDS)
 c.-a. pneumonia (CAP)
 c.-a. respirator virus (CRV)
community immunity
comorbid disease
comorbidity
 illness c.
 psychiatric c.
COMP
 CCNU, Oncovin, methotrexate,
  procarbazine
 cyclophosphamide, Oncovin,
  methotrexate, prednisone
comparative genomic hybridization
 (CGH)
compartment
 extracellular c.
 extravascular c.
 intracellular c.
compartmental radioimmunoglobulin
 therapy
Compassionate Use Act
Compazine
compensated hypogonadism
compensation
 attenuation c.
 supratentorial flow c.
compensator
 beam c.
 Multivane Intensity Modulation C.
  (MIMIC)
 c. segment
compensatory
 c. emphysema
 c. hypertrophy
competence
 immunologic c.
competent
 cell repair c.
competition
 antigenic c.
complement
 c. assay
 erythrocyte, antibody, c.
 c. factor (CF)
 c. fixation (CF)
 c. fixation test
 c. 3 level
 c. 4 level

c. lysis
c. receptor
c. resistance
complementarity determining region (CDR)
complementary
c. and alternative cancer medicine
c. and alternative medicine (CAM)
c. DNA (cDNA)
c. gene
c. metal oxide semiconductor (CMOS)
complement-dependent cytotoxicity
complement-fixing antibody (CFA)
complement-mediated lysis
complete
c. blood count (CBC)
c. carcinogen
c. cytoreduction
c. decongestive physiotherapy
c. fracture
c. Freund adjuvant (CFA)
c. hematologic response (CHR)
c. hydatidiform mole (CHM)
c. lymphadenectomy
c. lymph node dissection (CLND)
c. remission (CR)
c. remission duration (CRD)
c. response (CR)
complex, pl. complexes
acyclic metal chelate c.
aggregation antibody-antigen c.
AIDS-dementia c. (ADC)
AIDS-related c. (ARC)
amphotericin B cholesteryl sulfate c.
amphotericin B lipid c. (ABLC)
antibody-antigen c.
antigen-antibody c.
antiinhibitor coagulant c.
arteriovenous glomus c.
avian leukemia-sarcoma c.
avian leukosis-sarcoma c.
avidin-biotin c.
biceps-labral c.
capsulolabral c.
Carney c.
c. chest mass
choroidal-hippocampal fissure c.
circulating immune c. (CIC)
c. cytogenetic abnormality
death-inducing signal c. (DISC)
c. decongestive physiotherapy

c. decongestive therapy
factor IX c.
ferrous sulfate, ascorbic acid, vitamin B c.
C. Figure Test (CFT)
Golgi c.
H-2 c.
histocompatibility c.
HLA c.
Humate-P antihemophilic factor/von Willebrand factor c.
immune c.
interstitial antigen-antibody c.
iron dextran c.
c. karyotype
labrum-ligament c. (LLC)
lipophilic cationic c.
c. lymphedema therapy
major histocompatibility c. (MHC)
Mega B C.
Michaelis c.
mitochondrial respiratory chain enzyme c.
Mycobacterium avium c. (MAC)
NeoVadrin B C.
peptide major histocompatibility c.
peptide-MHC c.
peptidomimetic inhibitor c.
phosphorus trihydrazide c.
polysaccharide-iron c.
c. PSA
Ranke c.
respiratory enzyme c.
ribosome-lamella c.
RT-DNA-Fab c.
synthetic HIV peptide c.
synthetic human immunodeficiency virus peptide c.
TAT III c.
thrombin-antithrombin III c.
thymidylate c.
tuberous sclerosis c. (TSC)
VATER c.
vitamin B c.
von Hippel-Lindau c.
zinc chelation c.
complexed prostate-specific antigen (cPSA)
compliance
pericardial c.
complicated
c. pneumoconiosis
c. silicosis

NOTES

complication
    gastrointestinal c.
    hematologic c.
    metabolic c.
    oral c.
    paraneoplastic c.
    postoperative c.
    pulmonary c.
    respiratory c.
component
    blood c.
    buffy coat c.
    cellular c.
    endometrioid adenocarcinomatous c.
    extensive intraductal c. (EIC)
    florid stromal spindle cell c.
    intraductal c.
    leukopoor blood c.
    plasma thromboplastin c. (PTC)
    secretory c.
    single-donor blood c.
    spindle cell stromal c.
    undifferentiated sarcomatous c.
composite
    c. cyclic therapy (CCT)
    C. Laryngeal Recurrence Staging System (CLRSS)
compound
    dihydrocodeine c. (DHC)
    disulfide-containing c.
    huC242 c.
    Hurler-Scheie c.
    isoprenoid plant c.
    macromolecular nonlipid c.
    macromolecular polar c.
    NeoLipid c.
    nitroimidazole c.
    N-nitroso c. (NOC)
    pentazocine c.
    platinum c.
    polar c.
    polyanionic sulfated c.
    polycyclic c.
    polyphenolic c.
    PSC-833 c.
    c. Q
    Talwin C.
    thiol c.
comprehensive
    c. care plan
    c. health enhancement support system (CHESS)
compressed lung
compression
    epidural spinal cord c. (ESCC)
    external pneumatic calf c.
    extrinsic bladder c.
    c. fracture
    intermittent pneumatic c. (IPC)

    c. neuropathy
    pneumatic c.
    spinal cord c.
    c. stockings
    superior vena caval c.
    c. ultrasound
Compton absorption
computational chemistry
computed
    c. radiography
    c. tomographic angiography
    c. tomographic colonography
    c. tomography (CT)
    c. tomography during arterial portography (CTAP)
    c. tomography laser mammography (CTLM)
    c. tomography scan
    c. tomography-single photon emission computed tomography (CT/SPECT)
computer-assisted controlled afterloading
computer-controlled
    c.-c. conformal radiation therapy (CCRT, CC-RT)
    c.-c. radiotherapy (CCRT, CC-RT)
computer-generated artifact
computerized
    c. axial tomography
    c. dosimetry
    c. patient record (CPR)
comring-enhancing lesion
COMS
    Collaborative Ocular Melanoma Study
concanavalin A
concavity
concentrate
    AT-III c.
    factor VIII c.
    M.V.I. C.
    platelet c.
concentration
    cytostatic c.
    hydrogen ion c. (pH)
    indinavir trough c.
    maximal drug c. (C_{max})
    mean corpuscular hemoglobin c. (MCHC)
    minimum inhibitory c. (MIC)
    nanomolar c.
    serum bilirubin c.
    serum p24 antigen c.
    serum transferrin receptor c.
    TfR c.
concentrator
    stem cell c.
concentric fibroma
concept
    growth fraction c.

halstedian c.
nonoverlapping toxicity c.
schedule dependency c.
self-care c.
total dose over time c.
concomitant
c. antiviral therapy
c. boost
c. chemoirradiation
c. chemoradiation
c. medication
c. pneumonia
c. triple antiretroviral therapy
concordance
HIV c.
human immunodeficiency virus c.
concretion
laminated calcified c.
concurrent
c. chemoradiotherapy (CCRT, CC-RT)
c. nephrotoxin
concussion
brain c.
condensation
nuclear c.
condensed chromatin
condition
autoimmune c.
benign prostate c.
genetic c.
precancerous c.
predisposing c.
premalignant c.
tumorlike bone c.
conditioning
busulfan c.
myeloablative c.
nonmyeloablative c.
condom
c. catheter
latex c.
conductive loop
conductivity
conductor resistivity
conduit
condylar fracture
condyle
condyloma, pl. **condylomata**
c. acuminatum
anal c.
Buschke-Löwenstein c.
condylomata lata

Condylox
cone
collimator c.
c. electron boost
Samsung Medical Center-type collimator c.
SMC-type collimator c.
cone-beam
c.-b. computed tomography
c.-b. CT
coned-down boost
conference
LENT Consensus C.
Confide HIV test kit
confidence interval (CI)
configuration
butterfly c.
Frank orthogonal c.
germline c.
keyhole c.
swallow-tail c.
confinement
regional tumor c.
confluence
confluent tumor
confocal
c. image
c. laser scanning
c. microscopy
conformal
c. blocking
c. proton therapy
c. radiation therapy (CRT)
Conforma 3000 Proton Beam Treatment System
conformational determinant
confounders
congenita
chondrodystrophia calcificans c.
dyskeratosis c.
macrocephaly-cutis marmorata telangiectatica c. (M-CMTC)
pachyonychia c.
congenital
c. agammaglobulinemia
c. anomaly
c. aplastic anemia
c. AT-III deficiency
c. cardiac tumor
c. dyserythropoietic anemia
c. erythropoietic porphyria (CEP)
c. hypercoagulable state
c. hypoplastic anemia (CHA)

NOTES

C

congenital *(continued)*
c. immunity
c. immunodeficiency disease
c. infection
c. mesoblastic nephroma
c. methemoglobinemia
c. neutropenia
c. prothrombotic disorder
c. spherocytosis
c. syphilis
Congest
congestion index
conglomerate anthracosilicosis
conglutinating complement absorption test
conglutination factor
conglutinogen-activating factor
coni (*pl. of* conus)
conization
cervical c.
cold c.
cold-knife c.
hot c.
laser c.
LEEP c.
conjoined
conjugal cancer
conjugate
antibody radionucleotide c.
fluorescein isothiocyanate c. (FITC)
lipid c.
conjugated
c. antigen
c. estrogen
c. hapten
conjunctiva, pl. **conjunctivae**
conjunctival
c. melanoma
c. plethora
conjunctivitis
connatal neuroblastoma
connection
atrioventricular c.
connective
c. tissue
c. tissue disease
c. tissue neoplasm
c. tissue tumor
connector
cerebral ventricular shunt c.
Conn syndrome
Conrad-Crosby bone marrow biopsy needle
consensus interferon
consent
informed c.
conservation laryngeal surgery
conservative treatment
consolidated lung

consolidating infiltrate
consolidation
c. chemotherapy
c. therapy
c. with peripheral blood progenitor cell support
consolidative radiotherapy
consortium
Texas Cancer Genetics C.
constant
air-kerma rate c.
equilibrium dissociation c.
equilibrium dose c.
Michaelis c.
Constilac
constipation
opioid-induced c.
constitutional
c. aplastic anemia
c. bone marrow syndrome
constricting lesion
constrictive
c. bronchiolitis
c. remodeling
constrictor muscle
construct
anti-rev c.
hapten-chelate c.
nucleic acid c.
plasmid c.
construction
McIndoe-Hayes c.
Constulose
consumption coagulopathy
contact
bone-on-bone c.
cell-cell c.
contagiosum
molluscum c.
container
ALPS c.
contaminating tumor cell (CTC)
contamination
metastatic c.
white blood cell c.
content
bone mineral c.
CD34 c.
disc water c.
hepatic iron c.
total body bone mineral c. (TBBMC)
contiguous
c. extranodal extension
c. lysine
c. organ involvement
c. spinal fluid reservoir
Contin
MS C.

continuation
    azygos c.
continuing care
continuous
    c. arteriovenous hemofiltration
      (CAVH)
    c. 3-day flavopiridol infusion
    c. epitope
    c. hyperfractionated accelerated
      radiation therapy (CHART)
    c. hyperthermic peritoneal perfusion
      (CHPP)
    c. infusion paclitaxel plus cisplatin
    c. infusion phenylbutyrate
    c. intravenous infusion
      chemotherapy
    c. microinfusion device
    c. renal replacement therapy
    c. ultrasonic surgical aspiration
      (CUSA)
    c. venovenous hemofiltration
      (CVVH)
continuous-course radiotherapy
continuous-wave
    c.-w. Doppler imaging
    c.-w. Doppler ultrasonography
    c.-w. NMR
contortrostatin
contour
    prosthetic buttock c.
contraceptive
    oral c. (OC)
contractile apparatus
contraction
    esophageal c.
    premature atrial c. (PAC)
contraindication
contralateral
    c. breast cancer (CLBC)
    c. breast tumor recurrence (CBTR)
    c. synchronous adrenalectomy
    c. synchronous carcinoma
contrast
    air c.
    barium enema with air c.
    blood oxygenation level-
      dependent c.
    BOLD c.
    c. filling
    Teslascan c.
    c. venography

contrast-enhanced
    c.-e. computed tomography (CECT)
    c.-e. CT
contrasuppressor cell
contribution
    primary c.
    scatter c.
control
    cell cycle c.
    D-Di negative c.
    D-Di positive c.
    HepCheck whole blood c.
    Liquichek Hematology-16 C.
    local c.
    locoregional c.
    pelvic and periaortic c. (PPC)
    quality c.
    Spli-Prest negative c.
    Spli-Prest positive c.
    vector transfectant c.
controlled
    c. mechanical ventilation (CMV)
    c. release
controlled-release morphine suppository
controller
    Imed Gemini PC-2 volumetric c.
    Pepcid AC Acid C.
contusion
    bony c.
    cerebral c.
conus, pl. **coni**
    c. elasticus
convalescent phase
conventional
    c. dose chemotherapy
    c. provider
conversion
    hemorrhagic c.
converter
    analog-to-digital c. (ADC)
    digital-to-analog c. (DAC)
convexity
    cerebral c.
convolution
    nuclear c.
convulsion
Cook catheter
Cooley anemia
Coomassie protein assay reagent
Coombs-negative hemolytic anemia
Coombs test

NOTES

cooperative
> C. Breast Cancer Tissue Resource (CBCTR)
> C. Colorectal Cancer Combination Chemotherapy Clinical Trial
> C. Family Registry for Breast Cancer Studies (CFRBCS)
> C. Oncology Group
> C. Prostate Cancer Tissue Resource (CPCTR)

Cooper regimen

CO-Oximeter

COP
> cyclophosphamide, Oncovin, prednisone

COPA
> cyclophosphamide, Oncovin, prednisone, Adriamycin

COPA-BLEO
> cyclophosphamide, Oncovin, prednisone, Adriamycin, bleomycin

COPAC
> CCNU, Oncovin, prednisone, Adriamycin, cyclophosphamide

COPB, COP-B
> cyclophosphamide, Oncovin, prednisone, bleomycin

COP-BLAM
> cyclophosphamide, Oncovin, prednisone, bleomycin, Adriamycin, Matulane

COP-BLEO
> cyclophosphamide, Oncovin, prednisone, bleomycin

COPD
> chronic obstructive pulmonary disease

COPE
> cyclophosphamide, Oncovin, Platinol, etoposide
> Cytoxan, Oncovin, Platinol, etoposide

Cope biopsy needle

coping
> Ways of C. (WOC)

coplanar
> c. arc
> c. beam
> c. field

copolymer
> polylactide c.

COPP
> CCNU, Oncovin, procarbazine, prednisone
> cyclophosphamide, Oncovin, procarbazine, prednisone

COPPA
> cyclophosphamide, Oncovin, procarbazine, prednisone, Adriamycin

COPP/ABVD
> cyclophosphamide, Oncovin, procarbazine, prednisone plus

> Adriamycin, bleomycin, vincristine, dacarbazine

copper-67

coproporphyria
> hereditary c.

copulation
> oral c.

CoQ
> coenzyme Q

cord
> c. blood
> cervical c.
> true vocal c.
> vocal c.

cordectomy

cordis
> C. balloon expandable stent R
> C. coaxial microcatheter
> ectopia c.

cordotomy
> bilateral percutaneous cervical c. (BPCC)
> percutaneous cervical c. (PCC)

cordycepin

core
> c. binding factor
> c. binding protein
> c. biopsy (Cbx)
> electron-dense c.
> necrotic c.
> c. needle biopsy
> c. of tissue

coreceptor
> CD26 c.
> chemokine c.

coregistration
> positron emission tomography-magnetic resonance imaging c.

corepressor

corneae
> herpes c.

corneoscleroiridosclerectomy

cornu, pl. **cornua**

coronal mandibulectomy

coronary
> c. intervention
> c. occlusion
> c. sinus
> c. thrombosis

coronoid lamella

corpora (pl. of corpus)

corporis
> tinea c.

corpulence

corpus, pl. **corpora**
> corpora cavernosa
> uterine c.

corpuscle
> Bizzozero c.

Eichhorst c.
Hassall c.
Lostorfer c.
malpighian c.
molluscum c.
Negri c.
Norris c.
correction
adaptive c.
attenuation c.
Hendel c.
correlation
clinical c.
clinicopathologic c.
cytogenetic-pathologic c.
Cortef oral
Cortenema Rectal
cortex, pl. **cortices**
adrenal c.
cerebral c.
motor c.
thymic c.
Corticaine Topical
cortical
c. abrasion
c. artery
c. atrophy
c. bone
c. defect
c. destruction
c. dysgenesis
c. lesion
c. necrosis
c. thymoma
c. window
cortices (*pl. of* cortex)
corticosteroid
corticotropin
corticotropin-releasing
c.-r. factor (CRF)
c.-r. hormone (CRH)
Cortifoam Rectal
cortisol
free c.
cortisone acetate
Cortrosyn-stimulating test
Corynebacterium
C. infantisepticum
C. parvum
Coryphen Codeine
coryza
Coryzavirus
Corzyme kit

Cos-1 cell
cosegregate
cosegregation
Cosmegen
cosmesis
cosmid
c. cloning vector
c. cloning vector for DNA
Costello protocol
costimulation
SLAM c.
costimulatory
c. molecule
c. signals
costotransversectomy
Cotara
cotinine
salivary c.
Cotrel-Dubousset system
co-trimoxazole
Cotswolds staging classification
cottage cheese calcium
cotton-wool
c.-w. sign
c.-w. spot
couch, pl. **couches**
c. axis
C. model
rotated collimators and couches
c. vernier
cough
brassy c.
Couinaud liver disease classification
coulombs per kilogram (c/kg)
Coulter
C. HIV-1p24 antigen assay
C. S-plus analyzer
coumarin
c. analog
c. treatment
council
Medical Research C. (MRC)
Councilman body
counseling
directive c.
genetic c.
posttest c.
risk-reduction c.
count
absolute cell c.
absolute granulocyte c. (ACG)
absolute neutrophil c. (ANC)
absolute reticulocyte c.

NOTES

count *(continued)*
    Addis c.
    Arneth c.
    basophil c.
    CD4 cell c.
    CD8 cell c.
    CD8+ T-cell c.
    cell c.
    complete blood c. (CBC)
    differential c.
    granulocyte c.
    interfollicular mitotic c.
    leukocyte differential c.
    lymphocyte c.
    nadir blood c.
    neutrophil lobe c.
    nucleated cell c.
    platelet c.
    c. rate
    red blood cell c.
    reticulocyte c.
    sperm c.
    total white cell c.
    WBC c.
    white blood cell c.
counter
    Capintec instant gamma c.
    Linson electronic cell c.
    LKB Wallac 1277 automatic
        gamma c.
countercurrent exchanger
  immunoelectrophoresis
counterelectrophoresis
counterimmunoelectrophoresis
counterpulsation
    balloon c.
countertransference
coupling
    dynamic c.
course
    disease c.
Courvoisier sign
covariate
coverslip method
Cowden
    C. disease
    C. syndrome
Cowper gland
COX
    cyclooxygenase
    COX pathway
Cox
    C. proportional hazard modeling
       technique
    C. regression analysis
COX-1 enzyme
COX-2
    COX-2 enzyme
    COX-2 upregulation

CP
    chlorambucil and prednisone
    cyclophosphamide and prednisone
    Cytoxan and Platinol
        Vancocin CP
CPA
    cyclophosphamide
    cyproterone acetate
CPAC
    clusters of pancreatic acinar cells
CPB
    celiac plexus block
    cyclophosphamide, Platinol, BCNU
CPC
    cyclophosphamide, Platinol, carboplatin
CP-CML
    chronic phase chronic myelogenous
       leukemia
CPCTR
    Cooperative Prostate Cancer Tissue
       Resource
CPDD
    cis-platinum diammine dichloride
CPK
    creatine phosphokinase
CPM
    CCNU, procarbazine, methotrexate
    central pontine myelinolysis
    cyclophosphamide
CPOB
    cyclophosphamide, prednisone, Oncovin,
       bleomycin
CPR
    clinical partial response
    computerized patient record
cPSA
    complexed prostate-specific antigen
CPT
    cisplatin
CPT-11 plus BCNU
CPTR
    cyproterone
CPV
    cyclophosphamide, Platinol, VP-16
CQ
    carboquone
CR
    complete remission
    complete response
CR49
    RIGScan CR49
CR103
    OncoScint CR103
CRA
    chemotherapy-related amenorrhea
    cis-retinoic acid
13-CRA
    13-*cis*-retinoic acid

cradle
  alpha c.
crania (*pl. of* cranium)
cranial
  c. fossa
  c. nerve neoplasm
  c. nerve palsy
  c. nerve rhizotomy
  c. neuropathy
craniectomy
  keyhole-shaped c.
craniocaudal mammogram
craniofacial resection
craniopharyngioma
  adamantinomatous c.
  ectopic c.
craniosacral therapy
craniospinal
  c. axis
  c. irradiation (CSI)
craniotomy
  c. defect
  endoscopic frontal c.
cranium, pl. **crania**
CRBP
  cellular retinol-binding protein
CRC
  Cancer Research Campaign
  colorectal cancer
  colorectal carcinoma
CRCC
  chromophobe renal cell carcinoma
CRD
  complete remission duration
CRE
  cumulative radiation effect
C-reactive protein (CRP)
cream
  allantoin vaginal c.
  AVC c.
  Dalacin C Vaginal C.
  EMLA c.
  eutectic mixture of local
    anesthetics c.
  Ogen Vaginal c.
  RadiaCare C.
  tretinoin emollient c.
creatine
  c. kinase (CK)
  c. kinase-BB isoenzyme (CK-BB)
  c. phosphokinase (CPK)
creatinine
  serum c.

Cremophor EL emulsifying agent
crenated erythrocyte
crenation
  cell c.
crenocytosis
crescent
  c. body
  c. cell anemia
  c. sign
crescentic collection
crest
  anterior iliac c.
  bilateral iliac c.
Cresyl violet stain
cretinism
  goitrous c.
Creutzfeldt-Jakob disease (CJD)
CRF
  cancer-related fatigue
  chronic renal failure
  corticotropin-releasing factor
CRH
  corticotropin-releasing hormone
criblé
  état c.
cribriform
  c. gland
  c. pattern
  c. plate
  c. salivary carcinoma
  c. salivary carcinoma of excretory
    duct
cricoid
  c. cartilage
  c. ring
cricopharyngeal dysphagia
cricothyroid
Crinone
crisis, pl. **crises**
  anaphylactoid c.
  aplastic c.
  blast c.
  blastic c.
  blood c.
  carcinoid c.
  chronic myelogenous leukemia
    blast c. (CML-BC)
  CML blast c.
  myelocytic c.
  oculogyric c.
  sickle cell c.
  transient aplastic c. (TAC)
  vasoocclusive c.

NOTES

C

crisnatol mesylate
crispatus
    Lactobacillus c.
criterion, pl. **criteria**
    Amsterdam Criteria
    Bethesda criteria
    Children's Cancer Group criteria
    Common Toxicity Criteria (CTC)
    Gainor criteria
    Jacobsson criteria
    Light c.
    Ming criteria
    National Cancer Institute Common Toxicity Criteria (NCI-CTC)
    National Prostatic Cancer Project criteria
    RECIST criteria
    response criteria (RC)
CritSpin microhematocrit centrifuge
Crixivan
crocetin
Crohn disease (CD)
Crolom
cromoglycate
    PMS-Sodium C.
cromolyn sodium
Cronkhite-Canada syndrome
CROP
    cyclophosphamide, rubidazone, Oncovin, prednisone
cross-agglutination
crossed immunoelectrophoresis
crossfire
    c. radiation therapy
    c. treatment
CrossLaps
    C. One Step ELISA
    Serum C.
cross-linked C-terminal telopeptide of type 1 collagen
crossmatch
crossover
    c. design
    c. trial
cross-reactive protein (CRP)
cross-reactivity
    CA125 c.-r.
cross-resistance pattern
cross-sectional imaging
cross-sensitization
croup-associated virus
CR/OV
    colorectal/ovarian
    OncoScint CR/OV
CRP
    C-reactive protein
    cross-reactive protein
CRT
    conformal radiation therapy

    3D CRT
    3-dimensional CRT
CRu
    unconfirmed/uncertain complete remission
cruciferous vegetable
cruris
    tinea c.
crus, pl. **crura**
    displaced c.
crutch
    Lofstrand c.
CRV
    community-acquired respirator virus
cryoablation
    Endocare renal c.
    office-based c.
    renal mass c.
    targeted c.
cryocrit
cryofibrinogen
cryoglobulin
    serum c.
cryoglobulinemia
    mixed c.
CryoGuide
    C. software-controlled ultrasound planning and guidance
    C. ultrasound guidance system
cryonecrosis
cryopoor plasma
cryoprecipitate
cryoprecipitate-depleted plasma
cryopreservation
cryopreserved stem cell
cryoprobe
cryoprostatectomy
cryosurgery
    nerve-sparing c.
    targeted c.
cryosurgical
    c. ablation
    c. ablation of prostate (CSAP)
cryotherapy system
cryotome
crypt
    c. cell carcinoma
    intestinal c.
Cryptaz
cryptococcal
    c. meningitis
    c. optic neuropathy
    c. spondylitis
cryptococcoma
cryptococcosis
Cryptococcus
    C. neoformans
    C. neoformans meningitis

cryptomeningitis
    neurosyphilis c.
cryptorchidism
cryptorchid testis
cryptorchism
cryptosporidiosis
    c. antibody
    c. enteritis
Cryptosporidium muris
crystal
    calcium hydroxyapatite c.
    leukocytic c.
    Reinke c.
    Teichmann c.
crystal-induced chemotactic factor
crystallizable fragment (Fc)
crystallography
    Laue x-ray c.
crystalloid
    intraluminal c.
crystalluria
Crystamine
^{137}**Cs**
    cesium-137
CS-5 cryosurgical system
CsA, CSA
    cyclosporin A
CSAP
    cryosurgical ablation of prostate
CSF
    cerebrospinal fluid
    colony-stimulating factor
        CSF cryptococcal antigen titer
        CSF cytology
        hematopoietic CSF
        human urinary CSF
        CSF pleocytosis
        recombinant methionyl human
          granulocyte CSF
        CSF VDRL
        CSF VDRL test
csf1R1 gene
CSI
    chemical shift imaging
    craniospinal irradiation
Csk homologous kinase (CHK)
CSLEX1 monoclonal antibody
CSP
    Cancer Surveillance Program
CSS
    cause-specific survival
CT
    computed tomography

    cytarabine and 6-thioguanine
        bone quantitative CT (BQCT)
        CT colonography
        cone-beam CT
        contrast-enhanced CT
        dynamic CT
        high-resolution CT
        CT laser mammography
        megavoltage CT
        portal phase contrast-enhanced
          spiral CT
        CT portography
        tomography cine CT
CT1
    primary chemotherapy
CTAP
    computed tomography during arterial
    portography
CT-based
    CT-b. stereotactic biopsy
    CT-b. volumetric imaging
CTC
    Common Toxicity Criteria
    contaminating tumor cell
CTCb
    cyclophosphamide, thiotepa, carboplatin
    Cytoxan, thiotepa, carboplatin
        CTCb supported by autologous
          bone marrow stem cells
CTCL
    cutaneous T-cell lymphoma
CTEP
    Cancer Therapy Evaluation Program
CT-guided
    CT-g. biopsy
    CT-g. needle aspiration
CTL
    cytotoxic T lymphocyte
        CD4+ CTL
        CD8+ CTL
        CTL epitope
        HIV-specific CTL
        CTL precursor
CTLA4Ig
    cytotoxic lymphocyte activation antigen 4
    immunoglobulin
CTLM
    computed tomography laser
    mammography
CTLp
    cytotoxic T lymphocyte precursor
CT- and MRI-based stereotactic biopsy
14C-Topotecan

NOTES

C

143

C-Trak hand-held gamma detector
CT/SPECT
    computed tomography-single photon
    emission computed tomography
        CT/SPECT fusion
CTV
    clinical target volume
    clinical tumor volume
CTX
    cyclophosphamide
    Cytoxan
        MTX, HiDAC, sequential CTX
CTx
    chemotherapy
CTX-Plat
    cyclophosphamide and Platinol
C-type retrovirus
CTZ
    chemoreceptor trigger zone
cuboidal carcinoma
cucumber
    Chinese c.
cuff
    bladder c.
    Dacron c.
    c. sphygmomanometer
    subcutaneous c.
    vaginal c.
    Vita c.
cuirasse
    cancer en c.
CuLCaSG
    Cuneo Lung Cancer Study Group
CultiSpher-G microcarrier
culture
    blood c.
    hanging-block c.
    hanging-drop c.
    mixed leukocyte c. (MLC)
    mixed lymphocyte c.
    positive cerebrospinal fluid c.
    positive CSF c.
    Rubacell II c.
    c. and sensitivity
cumulative
    c. dose
    c. radiation effect (CRE)
cumulus oophorus
Cuneo Lung Cancer Study Group
  (CuLCaSG)
cuniculatum
    epithelioma c.
cuniculi
    Encephalitozoon c.
CUP
    carcinoma of unknown primary
Cuprimine
CUPS
    carcinoma of uncertain primary site

curative
    c. chemotherapy
    c. intent
    c. resection
    c. surgery
    c. treatment
curcumin
cure
    C. for Lymphoma Foundation
    c. rate
cured patient
curettage
    endocervical c.
    intralesional c.
    suction c.
curettement
currant
    c. jelly clot
    c. jelly stool
curve
    area under the c. (AUC)
    dose-response c.
    dose-survival c.
    elimination c.
    fractionated dose-survival c.
    gompertzian growth c.
    H-D c.
    Hunter-Driffield c.
    isodose c.
    Kaplan-Meier survival c.
    planing c.
    radiation survival c.
    sensitometric c.
    sigmoid c.
    survival c.
curvilinear
Curvularia
CUSA
    Cavitron ultrasonic surgical aspirator
    continuous ultrasonic surgical aspiration
Cushing
    C. adenoma
    C. basophilism
    C. disease
    C. syndrome
    C. triad
    C. virilizing syndrome (CVS)
cushion
    EZ-Dish pressure relief c.
    Position Plus c.
    Xact positioning c.
customized blocking
custom tailoring
cutaneous
    c. adverse drug effect
    c. alternariosis
    c. angiocentric T-cell lymphoma
    c. immunocytoma
    c. lymphatic drainage

c. lymphocyte antigen
c. lymphoid hyperplasia
c. lymphoscintigraphy
c. malignant melanoma (CMM)
c. MBC
c. melanoma (CM)
c. Merkel cell tumor
c. metastasis
c. metastatic breast cancer
c. neoplasm
c. neurofibroma
c. pneumocystosis
c. T-cell lymphoma (CTCL)
c. viral infection

cutaneum
carcinoma c.
Trichosporon c.

cutdown
venous c.

cutis
aplasia c.
benign lymphocytoma c.
leiomyoma c.
leukemia c.

CV
cisplatin and VePesid
cisplatin and VP-16

CVA-BMP
cyclophosphamide, vincristine,
Adriamycin, BCNU, methotrexate,
procarbazine

CVAD, C-VAD
cyclophosphamide, vincristine,
Adriamycin, dexamethasone

CVB
CCNU, vinblastine, bleomycin

CVBD
CCNU, vinblastine, bleomycin,
dexamethasone

CVC
central venous catheter

CVD
cisplatin, vinblastine, dacarbazine

CVEB
cisplatin, Velban, etoposide, bleomycin
cisplatin, vinblastine, etoposide,
bleomycin

CVFVP
cyclophosphamide, methotrexate, 5-
fluorouracil, vincristine, prednisone

CVI
carboplatin, VePesid, ifosfamide

CVLT
California Verbal Learning Test

CVM
cyclophosphamide, vincristine,
methotrexate

CVP
central venous pressure
cyclophosphamide, vincristine,
prednisone

CVP-BLEO
cyclophosphamide, vincristine,
prednisone, bleomycin

CVPP
CCNU, vinblastine, prednisone,
procarbazine
cyclophosphamide, Velban, procarbazine,
prednisone

CVPP-CCNU
cyclophosphamide, vinblastine,
procarbazine, prednisone plus CCNU

CVS
chorionic villus sampling
Cushing virilizing syndrome

CVVH
continuous venovenous hemofiltration

CVXD
cyclophosphamide, vincristine,
DaunoXome, Decadron

CXC
CXC chemokine
CXC chemokine receptor

CX3C
CX3C chemokine
CX3C chemokine receptor

CXCR4
chemokine-related receptor
macrophage-derived chemokine
CXCR4 receptor

CY
cyclophosphamide
CY plus TBI preparative regimen

CyADIC
cyclophosphamide, Adriamycin,
dacarbazine

cyanhemoglobin
cyanmethemoglobin quantitative method
cyanmetmyoglobin
cyanoacrylate
isobutyl c. (IBCA)

cyanoborohydride
sodium c.

cyanocobalamin
Cyanoject

NOTES

145

cyanosis
cyanotic
CyberKnife
> C. SRS image-guided stereotactic radiosurgery precision radiotherapy
> C. SRS image-guided stereotactic radiosurgery precision radiotherapy system

CYC
> cyclophosphamide

cyclase
> soluble guanylate c. (sGC)

cycle
> cell c.
> chemotherapeutic c.
> division c.
> estrogen-progestin artificial c.
> futile c.
> HIV-1 replicative c.
> human immunodeficiency virus 1 replicative c.
> Krebs c.
> reticuloendothelial c.
> retroviral replication c.
> schizogonic c.
> c. time

cycle-nonspecific agent
cycle-specific agent
cyclic
> c. guanosine monophosphate (cGMP)
> c. urea-based inhibitor

cyclin
> c. A
> c. B
> c. D
> c. D1
> c. D2
> c. E

cyclin-dependent
> c.-d. kinase (CDK)
> c.-d. kinase 4
> c.-d. kinase inhibitor

cycling
> cell c.

cyclin-p34
cyclocreatine
cyclocytidine
cyclohexylchloroethylnitrosurea (CCNU)
cyclooxygenase (COX)
> c. pathway

cyclooxygenase-1 testing
cyclooxygenase-2 testing
cyclophilin A
cyclophosphamide (CPA, CPM, CTX, CY, CYC)
> actinomycin D, 5-fluorouracil, c. (AcFuCy)
> c. and Adriamycin (CA)

Adriamycin, BCNU, c. (ABC)
c., Adriamycin, bleomycin, Oncovin, prednisone (CABOP, CA-BOP)
c., Adriamycin, dacarbazine (CAD, CADIC, CyADIC)
Adriamycin, docetaxel, Oncovin, c. (ADOC)
c., Adriamycin, etoposide (CAE)
c., Adriamycin, 5-fluorouracil
c., Adriamycin, 5-fluorouracil by continuous infusion (CAFFI)
c., Adriamycin, 5-fluorouracil, prednisone (CAFP)
c., Adriamycin, 5-fluorouracil, tamoxifen, Halotestin (CAFTH)
c., Adriamycin, 5-fluorouracil, vincristine, prednisone (CAFVP)
c., Adriamycin, high-dose Platinol (CAP-II)
c., Adriamycin, leucovorin calcium, 5-fluorouracil
c., Adriamycin, leucovorin rescue, 5-fluorouracil (CALF)
c., Adriamycin, leucovorin rescue, 5-fluorouracil, ethinyl estradiol (CALF-E)
c., Adriamycin, methotrexate (CAM)
c., Adriamycin, methotrexate, bleomycin (CAMB)
c., Adriamycin, methotrexate, etoposide, Oncovin (CAMEO)
c., Adriamycin, methotrexate, 5-fluorouracil (CAMF)
c., Adriamycin, methotrexate, procarbazine (CAMP)
c., Adriamycin, Oncovin (CAO)
c., Adriamycin, Platinol (CAP, CAP-I)
c., Adriamycin, Platinol, prednisone (CAPPr)
c., Adriamycin, prednisone (CAP)
c., Adriamycin, procarbazine, bleomycin, Oncovin, prednisone (CAP-BOP)
c., Adriamycin, Velban (CAV)
c., Adriamycin, vinblastine (CAV)
c., Adriamycin, vincristine (CAV)
c., Adriamycin, vincristine, prednisone (CAVP, CAVP-I)
c., Adriamycin, vincristine, VP-16
c., Adriamycin, VM-26, prednisone
c., Adriamycin, VP-16 (CAVP16)
c., Adriamycin, VP-16, prednisone, methotrexate (CAVPM)
BCNU, etoposide, ara-C, c. (BEAC)
c., BCNU, VePesid (CBV)

c., BCNU, VP-16-213 (CBV)
Binet modified c.
carboplatin, doxorubicin, c. (CDC)
carboplatin, etoposide, c.
(CarboPEC)
c., CCNU, methotrexate (CCM)
CCNU, Oncovin, prednisone,
Adriamycin, c. (COPAC)
c., cisplatin, 5-fluorouracil,
estramustine (CCFE)
c., cytosine arabinoside, topotecan
(CAT)
dactinomycin, methotrexate, c.
(DMC)
c., doxorubicin, etoposide (CDE)
c., doxorubicin, high-dose
methotrexate/ifosfamide, etoposide,
high-dose cytarabine (CODOX-
M/IVAC)
c., doxorubicin, teniposide,
prednisone, vincristine, bleomycin
c., doxorubicin, vindesine,
bleomycin, and prednisone
c. and doxorubicin with or without
5-fluorouracil (CA/CAF)
c., epirubicin, 5-fluorouracil (CEF)
c., epirubicin, Oncovin, prednisone
(CEOP)
c., epirubicin, Oncovin, prednisone,
bleomycin
c., epirubicin, vincristine,
prednisolone (CEOP)
c., etoposide, Platinol (CEP)
c., etoposide, vincristine (CEV)
c., etoposide, vincristine,
dexamethasone (CEVD)
5-fluorouracil, Adriamycin, c.
(FAC)
5-fluorouracil, epirubicin, c. (FEC)
c., 5-fluorouracil, epirubicin,
vincristine (CFEV)
5-fluorouracil, Novantrone, c.
(FNC)
c., 5-fluorouracil, prednisone (CFP)
c., Halotestin, Oncovin, prednisone
(CHOP, CyHOP)
c., Halotestin, Oncovin, prednisone,
etoposide (CHOPE)
c., Hexalen, Adriamycin, Platinol
(CHAP)
c., hexamethylmelamine,
Adriamycin, DDP (CHAD)

c., hexamethylmelamine,
Adriamycin, Platinol (CHAP)
c., hexamethylmelamine, 5-
fluorouracil (CHF)
c., hexamethylmelamine, 5-
fluorouracil, Platinol (ChexUP)
c., hydroxydaunomycin, Oncovin
(CHO)
c., hydroxydaunomycin, Oncovin,
bleomycin (CHOB)
c., hydroxydaunomycin, Oncovin,
dexamethasone (CHOD)
c., hydroxydaunomycin, Oncovin,
prednisone (CHOP)
c., hydroxydaunomycin, Oncovin,
prednisone, bleomycin (CHOP-
BLEO)
c., hydroxydaunomycin, Oncovin,
prednisone, etoposide (CHOPE)
c., hydroxydaunomycin, Oncovin,
radiotherapy (CHOR)
c., hydroxydaunomycin, VM-26,
prednisone (CHVP)
c., hydroxydaunorubicin, Oncovin,
prednisone (CHOP)
c., hydroxydaunorubicin, Oncovin,
prednisone, bleomycin
c., hydroxyurea, actinomycin D,
methotrexate, Oncovin, citrovorum
factor, Adriamycin (CHAM-OCA,
CHAMOCA)
leucovorin, Oncovin, methotrexate,
Adriamycin, c. (LOMAC)
c., m-AMSA, hydroxyurea (CMH)
mechlorethamine, Adriamycin,
dacarbazine, DDP, Oncovin, c.
(MADDOC)
c., mechlorethamine, Oncovin,
procarbazine, prednisone (CMOPP,
C-MOPP)
methotrexate and c. (MeCy)
methotrexate, actinomycin D, c.
(MAC)
methotrexate, Adriamycin, c.
(MAC)
c., methotrexate, CCNU (CMC)
c., methotrexate, CCNU, vincristine,
Adriamycin, procarbazine (CMC-
VAP)
c., methotrexate, epirubicin,
vincristine (CMEV)
c., methotrexate, etoposide,
dexamethasone (CMED)

NOTES

cyclophosphamide *(continued)*

c., methotrexate, 5-fluorouracil
(CMF, CM-5-FU)

c., methotrexate, 5-fluorouracil,
Adriamycin, Oncovin

c., methotrexate, 5-fluorouracil,
Adriamycin, vincristine (CMF-AV)

c., methotrexate, 5-fluorouracil,
Adriamycin, vincristine, prednisone
(CMFAVP)

c., methotrexate, 5-fluorouracil,
bleomycin (CMF-BLEO)

c., methotrexate, 5-fluorouracil,
fluoxymesterone (CMF-FLU)

c., methotrexate, 5-fluorouracil,
hydroxyurea (CMFH)

c., methotrexate, 5-fluorouracil,
prednisone (CMFP)

c., methotrexate, 5-fluorouracil,
prednisone, tamoxifen (CMFPT)

c., methotrexate, 5-fluorouracil,
prednisone, tamoxifen, Halotestin
(CMFPTH)

c., methotrexate, 5-fluorouracil,
prednisone, vincristine, Adriamycin
(CMFP-VA)

c., methotrexate, 5-fluorouracil,
tamoxifen (CMFT, CMF-TAM)

c., methotrexate, 5-fluorouracil,
vincristine (CMFV)

c., methotrexate, 5-fluorouracil,
vincristine, Adriamycin,
testosterone (CMFVAT)

c., methotrexate, 5-fluorouracil,
vincristine, prednisone (CMFVP,
CVFVP)

c., methotrexate, prednisone, 5-
fluorouracil (CMPF)

mitomycin C, Adriamycin, c.
(MAC)

c., mitoxantrone, Rituximab
combination

mitoxantrone, vinblastine, c. (MVC)

c., Novantrone, 5-fluorouracil
(CNF)

c., Novantrone, Oncovin, prednisone
(CNOP, C-NOP)

c., Oncomycin, prednisone,
bleomycin (CEOP-B)

c., Oncovin, ara-C, prednisone,
bleomycin (COAP-BLEO)

c., Oncovin, bleomycin,
methotrexate, Adriamycin,
MeCCNU

c., Oncovin, 5-
fluorouracil/cyclophosphamide,
Oncovin, methotrexate

c., Oncovin, MeCCNU (COM)

c., Oncovin, MeCCNU, bleomycin
(COMB)

c., Oncovin, methotrexate (COM,
COMe)

c., Oncovin, methotrexate,
Adriamycin, ara-C (COMA-A)

c., Oncovin, methotrexate,
bleomycin (COMB)

c., Oncovin, methotrexate,
bleomycin, Adriamycin, prednisone
(COMBAP)

c., Oncovin, methotrexate, 5-
fluorouracil (COMF)

c., Oncovin, methotrexate,
leucovorin, arabinosylcytosine
(COMLA)

c., Oncovin, methotrexate,
leucovorin, ara-C (COMLA)

c., Oncovin, methotrexate,
leucovorin, etoposide, ara-C
(COMET-A)

c., Oncovin, methotrexate,
prednisone (COMP)

c., Oncovin, Platinol, etoposide
(COPE)

c., Oncovin, prednisone (COP)

c., Oncovin, prednisone,
Adriamycin (COPA)

c., Oncovin, prednisone,
Adriamycin, bleomycin (COPA-
BLEO)

c., Oncovin, prednisone, bleomycin
(COPB, COP-B, COP-BLEO)

c., Oncovin, prednisone, bleomycin,
Adriamycin, Matulane (COP-
BLAM)

c., Oncovin, procarbazine,
prednisone (COPP)

c., Oncovin, procarbazine,
prednisone, Adriamycin (COPPA)

Oncovin, procarbazine, prednisone,
Adriamycin, c.

c., Oncovin, procarbazine,
prednisone/Adriamycin, bleomycin,
vinblastine

c., Oncovin, procarbazine,
prednisone plus Adriamycin,
bleomycin, vincristine, dacarbazine
(COPP/ABVD)

c. and Platinol (CTX-Plat)

Platinol, Adriamycin, c. (PAC,
PAC-1)

c., Platinol, BCNU (CPB)

c., Platinol, carboplatin (CPC)

Platinol, etoposide, c. (PEC)

c., Platinol, VP-16 (CPV)

c. and prednisone (CP)

c., prednisone, Oncovin, bleomycin
(CPOB)

pulse vincristine, actinomycin D, c.
radiolabeled antibody with systemic
chemotherapy using VP-16 and c.
c., rubidazone, Oncovin, prednisone
(CROP)
c., rubidazone, Oncovin, prednisone,
L-asparaginase
c., thiotepa, carboplatin (CTCb)
c., total body irradiation,
monoclonal antibodies
c., Velban, procarbazine, prednisone
(CVPP)
VePesid, BCNU, c. (VBC)
vinblastine, actinomycin D, c.
vinblastine, actinomycin D,
bleomycin, cisplatin, c. (VAB 4,
VAB-IV)
vinblastine, actinomycin D,
bleomycin, cisplatin,
chlorambucil, c.
c., vinblastine, procarbazine,
prednisone plus CCNU (CVPP-
CCNU)
vincristine, actinomycin D, c.
(VAC)
vincristine, Adriamycin, c. (VAC)
c., vincristine, Adriamycin, BCNU,
methotrexate, procarbazine (CVA-
BMP)
c., vincristine, Adriamycin,
dactinomycin (CyVADACT, CY-
VA-DACT)
c., vincristine, Adriamycin,
dexamethasone (CVAD, C-VAD)
c., vincristine, Adriamycin,
dimethyltriazenoimidazole
carboxamide
c., vincristine, Adriamycin, DTIC
(CyVADIC, CyVMAD)
vincristine, amethopterin, 5-
fluorouracil, Adriamycin, c.
(VAFAC)
vincristine, dactinomycin, bleomycin,
cisplatin, c. (VDBCC)
c., vincristine, DaunoXome,
Decadron (CVXD)
c., vincristine, methotrexate (CVM)
c., vincristine, prednisone (CVP)
c., vincristine, prednisone,
bleomycin (CVP-BLEO)
c., vincristine, prednisone,
daunomycin, methotrexate,
cytarabine, 6-thioguanine

**cyclopia-astomia-agnathia-
holoprosencephaly association**
cyclopropylbenzindole
cyclosaligenyl prodrug
cycloserine
Cyclospora cayetanensis
cyclosporin A (CsA, CSA)
cyclosporine
　　c. analog
　　c. immunoassay
　　c. prophylaxis
　　c. therapy
　　c. toxicity
cyclotron
Cyd/dCyd-D
　　cytidine/2′deoxycytidine deaminase
CYFRA 21-1 tumor marker
CyHOP
　　cyclophosphamide, Halotestin, Oncovin,
　　prednisone
Cyklokapron
Cylex
cylinder
　　Burnett c.
　　dome c.
　　vaginal c.
cylindroma
cylindromatous carcinoma
cylindrosarcoma
Cyomin
CYP
　　cytochrome P450 enzyme
CYP1A2 gene
CYP2B6 gene
CYP2C9 gene
CYP3A4 enzyme system
CyPat
CYP2D6
　　CYP2D6 antibody assay
　　CYP2D6 gene
cypionate
　　testosterone c.
cyproheptadine
cyproterone (CPTR)
　　c. acetate (CPA)
cyst
　　adnexal c.
　　adrenal c.
　　ampulla of Vater c.
　　aneurysmal bone c.
　　apocrine c.
　　arachnoid c.
　　aryepiglottic c.

NOTES

cyst *(continued)*
   c. aspiration
   Baker c.
   benign c.
   bone c.
   brain c.
   branchial cleft c.
   breast c.
   bronchial duplication c.
   bronchogenic c.
   brown cell c.
   chocolate c.
   choledochal c.
   choroid plexus c.
   colloid c.
   cysticercus c.
   dermoid ovarian c.
   c. drainage
   duodenal duplication c.
   ejaculatory duct c.
   encapsulated c.
   endometriotic c.
   enteric c.
   enterogenous c.
   ependymal c.
   epidermoid inclusion c.
   epididymal c.
   epidural arachnoid c.
   epithelial c.
   esophageal duplication c.
   horn c.
   hydatid c.
   inclusion c.
   intraosseous keratin c.
   intrapulmonary bronchogenic c.
   leptomeningeal c.
   lipid c.
   lung c.
   lymphoepithelial c.
   medullary c.
   mesenteric c.
   Monro foramen colloid c.
   multilocular peritoneal inclusion c.
   ovarian c.
   pancreatic c.
   parovarian c.
   peritoneal mesothelial c.
   pilar c.
   pineal c.
   postmenopausal adnexal c.
   primordial c.
   Rathke cleft c.
   reactive c.
   solitary bone c.
   tailgut c.
   testicular c.
   traumatic bone c.
   traumatic lipid c.
   traumatic lung c.
   trichilemmal c.
   umbilical cord c.
   unicameral bone c.
   utricle c.

cystadenocarcinoma
   mucinous c.
   parovarian c.
   pseudomucinous c.
   serous c.

cystadenofibroma

cystadenoma
   apocrine c.
   biliary c.
   ductectatic mucinous c.
   glycogen-rich c.
   c. lymphomatosum
   mucinous c.
   ovarian proliferative c.
   papillary epididymal c.
   serous c.
   thyroid c.

Cystagon

cystectomy
   ovarian c.
   radical c.

cysteine
   c. precursor
   secreted protein acidic and rich in c. (SPARC)
   secreted protein, acidic and rich in c.

cysteinylglycine

cystic
   c. adenocarcinoma
   c. adenomatoid malformation
   c. adrenal mass
   c. adrenal neoplasm
   c. angiomatosis
   c. appearance
   c. arachnoiditis
   c. artery
   c. bronchiectasis
   c. carcinoma
   c. change
   c. chest mass
   c. dilatation
   c. disease of breast
   c. duct
   c. duct remnant
   c. duct stone
   c. dysplasia
   c. dysplasia disease
   c. fibrosis (CF)
   c. fluid
   c. ganglioglioma
   c. glandular hyperplasia
   c. glioma
   c. hemangioblastoma
   c. hygroma

c. hyperplasia photomicrograph
c. intraparenchymal meningioma
c. kidney disease
c. lesion
c. lymphangioma
c. mastitis
c. medial necrosis
c. mesothelioma
c. metastasis
c. myelomalacia
c. myelopathy
c. nephroma
c. ovarian disease
c. partially differentiated
    nephroblastoma
c. pelvic mass
c. pilocytic astrocytoma
c. pituitary adenoma
c. process
c. renal disease
c. structure
c. teratoma
c. tumor
cysticercosis
cysticercus cyst
cysticus
    Echinococcus c.
cystinosis
    nephropathic c.
cystinotic leukocyte
cystitis
    emphysematous c.
    eosinophilic c.
    c. glandularis
    granulomatous c.
    hemorrhagic c.
    radiation c.
cystocarcinoma
cystocele
cystofibroma
cystometrography
cystomyoma
cystoprostatectomy
    radical c.
cystosarcoma phyllodes
Cyt
    cytosine
CytaBOM
    cytarabine, bleomycin, Oncovin,
        mechlorethamine
Cytadren
cytapheresis
cytarabine (ara-C)

c., Adriamycin, 6-thioguanine
    (CAT)
c., bleomycin, Oncovin,
    mechlorethamine (CytaBOM)
c., bleomycin, Oncovin,
    methotrexate
cyclophosphamide, doxorubicin,
    high-dose methotrexate/ifosfamide,
    etoposide, high-dose c. (CODOX-
    M/IVAC)
daunorubicin and c. (DC)
c. and daunorubicin
c., daunorubicin, prednisolone,
    mercaptopurine
Depofoam encapsulated c.
high-dose c.
c. hydrochloride
liposomal c.
mitoxantrone and c.
c. plus Adriamycin
c. plus 6-thioguanine
prednisone, methotrexate, leucovorin,
    Adriamycin, cyclophosphamide,
    etoposide, c.
6-thioguanine and c. (TC)
c. and 6-thioguanine (CT)
**cytidine/2′deoxycytidine deaminase
(Cyd/dCyd-D)**
**cytidylate/2′-deoxycytidylate kinase
(CMP/dCMP-K)**
cytobrush biopsy
cytocentrifuge method
cytochemical staining method
cytochrome
    c. enzyme
    c. enzyme system
    hepatic c.
    c. P450 2D6 genotype
    c. P450 enzyme (CYP)
    c. P450 system
cytocidal
cytocide
cytocrit
cytodiagnosis
cytodifferentiation
cytofluorimetric analysis
CytoGam
cytogenetic
    c. abnormality
    c. analysis
    c. remission
cytogenetic-pathologic correlation

NOTES

cytogenetics
>favorable or intermediate
> prognosis c. (FIPC)
>interphase c.

cytogenic anemia

cytokeratin
>c. 20 (CK20)
>immunoperoxidase staining for c.
>c. membrane antigen
>c. subtype

cytokeratin-positive cell

cytokine
>chemoattractant c.
>diffusable inflammatory c.
>c. disease
>c. homolog
>inflammatory c.
>c. interleukin
>c. network
>pleiotropic c.
>c. polymorphism
>proinflammatory c.
>c. secretion
>Th1-associated c.
>c. therapy

cytokine-based approach

cytokine-mobilized
>c.-m. blood product
>c.-m. peripheral blood graft

cytokinesis

cytologic
>c. atypia
>c. screening

cytology
>aspiration c.
>brush c.
>CSF c.
>exfoliative c.
>fine-needle aspiration c. (FNAC)
>c. and histology
>histology and c.
>imprint c.
>LBP c.
>liquid-based Papanicolaou c.
>nipple aspiration c.
>pancreatoscopic c.
>peritoneal c.
>scrape c.
>sputum c.
>tumor imprint c.

cytolysin

cytolysis
>lymphocyte-mediated c.

cytolytic
>c. activity
>c. T cell

cytoma

cytomegalic inclusion disease (CID)

cytomegalovirus (CMV)

>c. disease
>c. encephalitis
>human c. (HCMV)
>human IgM monoclonal antibody
> to c.
>c. immune globulin (CMVIG)
>c. infection
>c. interstitial pneumonitis
>c. pneumonia
>c. retinitis
>c. ventriculitis
>c. with microcephaly

cytometer
>FACScan flow c.
>HmX Hematology Flow C.
>image c.

cytometry
>3-color flow c.
>DNA flow c.
>flow c.
>image c. (ICM)
>immune flow c.
>Krishan procedure for DNA
> analysis by flow c.
>multidimensional flow c.
>triple-color flow c.

cytomorphology

cytopathic effect

cytopathicity

cytopathogenicity

cytopathologist

cytopenia

cytophagy

cytophilic antibody

cytophotometry
>DNA c.

cytoplasm
>acidophilic c.
>Purkinje cell c.

cytoplasmic
>c. accumulation
>c. carboxy terminus
>c. CD3 antigen
>c. domain
>c. Ig
>c. immunoglobulin
>c. pleomorphism
>c. tail

cytopreparatory technique

cytoproliferation

cytoprotection

cytoprotector

cytoreduce

cytoreduction
>complete c.
>optimal c.
>pleural c.
>primary surgical c.
>tumor c.

cytoreductive
    c. regimen
    c. surgery
Cytosar
Cytosar-U
cytosine (Cyt)
    c. arabinoside (ara-C, CA)
    c. arabinoside, Adriamycin, 6-thioguanine (CAT)
    c. arabinoside and daunorubicin (CAD)
    c. arabinoside, etoposide, methotrexate (CEM)
    c. arabinoside, high-dose methotrexate, leucovorin, Oncovin (CAMELEON)
    c. arabinoside-liposome
    c. arabinoside, methotrexate, leucovorin, Oncovin (CAMLO)
    c. arabinoside and 6-thioguanine (CAT)
    c. arabinosine hydrochloride 3-hydroxy-2-phosphono-methoxypropyl c. (HPMPC)
cytoskeletal antigen
cytosolic
    c. thymidine kinase
    c. volume
cytospin smear
cytostatic
    c. chemotherapy
    c. concentration
CytoTAb polyclonal antibody
Cytotec
cytotoxic
    c. antibody
    c. antibody-mediated disease
    c. chemotherapeutic agent
    c. chemotherapy
    c. drug
    c. edema
    c. effect
    c. factor
    c. lymphocyte activation antigen 4 immunoglobulin (CTLA4Ig)
    c. reaction
    c. T cell
    c. T-cell lymphocyte response
    c. T lymphocyte (CTL)
    c. T lymphocyte precursor (CTLp)
cytotoxicity
    antibody-dependent cell c. (ADCC)

antibody-dependent cell-mediated c. (ADCC)
antibody-dependent cellular c. (ADCC)
complement-dependent c.
differential staining c. (DiSC)
immunotoxin-mediated c.
synergistic c.
cytotoxin
cytotrophoblast
cytotropic
cytotropism
Cytovene
Cytoxan (CTX)
    C., Adriamycin, 5-fluorouracil (CAF)
    C., Adriamycin, leucovorin calcium, 5-fluorouracil (CALLF)
    C., Adriamycin, leucovorin calcium, 5-fluorouracil, ethinyl estradiol (CALF-E)
    C., Adriamycin, methotrexate, bleomycin (CAMB)
    C., Adriamycin, Platinol, prednisone (CAPPR, CAPPr)
    C., Adriamycin, VP-16 (CAVP16)
    C., BCNU, VP-16 (CBV)
    C., doxorubicin, etoposide (CDE)
    C., epirubicin, 5-fluorouracil (CEF)
    5-fluorouracil, epirubicin, C. (FEC)
    5-fluorouracil, leucovorin calcium, Adriamycin, C.
    5-fluorouracil, vinblastine, Adriamycin, C. (FUVAC)
    C., Halotestin, Oncovin, prednisone, etoposide (CHOPE)
    C., hydroxyurea, actinomycin D, methotrexate, Oncovin, calcium folinate, Adriamycin (CHAMOCA)
    lyophilized C.
    C., *m*-AMSA, hydroxyurea (CMH)
    C., methotrexate, 5-fluorouracil (CMF)
    C., methotrexate, 5-fluorouracil, prednisone, tamoxifen (CMFPT)
    C., Novantrone, Oncovin, prednisone (CNOP, C-NOP)
    C., Oncovin, ara-C, prednisone (COAP, mini-COAP)
    C., Oncovin, 5-fluorouracil plus Cytoxan, Oncovin, methotrexate
    C., Oncovin, Platinol, etoposide (COPE)

C

NOTES

Cytoxan *(continued)*
    C. and Platinol (CP)
    Platinol, Adriamycin, bleomycin,
       escalating doses of C. (PAB-Esc-
       C)
    C., thiotepa, carboplatin (CTCb)
    vinblastine, BCNU, melphalan,
       prednisone, C. (VBMPC)
CyVADACT, CY-VA-DACT
    cyclophosphamide, vincristine,
       Adriamycin, dactinomycin

CyVADIC
    cyclophosphamide, vincristine,
       Adriamycin, DTIC
CyVMAD
    cyclophosphamide, vincristine,
       Adriamycin, DTIC
Czerny anemia

δ (*var. of* delta)

D

    cyclin D
    immunoglobulin D (IgD)
    vincristine, methotrexate,
      Adriamycin, actinomycin D
      (VMAD)

D1

    cyclin D1

2D

    2-dimensional
      2D PAGE

D2

    cyclin D2

3D

    3-dimensional
      3D conformal dose escalation
        radiotherapy
      3D conformal radiation
      3D CRT
      3D proton MR spectroscopic
        imaging
      3D radiation treatment planning
      3D RTP

2000D

    Senographe 2000D

D_{max}

    maximum depth

D5 half normal saline

DA

    daunorubicin and ara-C

DAB

    3,3′-diaminobenzidine tetrahydrochloride
    dihydrate

DAB389

    DAB389 antibody
    DAB389 IL-2

DABIL-2 toxin

DAC

    digital-to-analog converter

dacarbazine (DTIC)

    Adriamycin and d. (ADIC, A-DIC)
    Adriamycin, bleomycin, CCNU, d.
      (ABCD)
    Adriamycin, bleomycin,
      vinblastine, d. (ABVD)
    Adriamycin, bleomycin,
      vincristine, d. (ABVD)
    Adriamycin, Leukeran, Oncovin,
      methotrexate, actinomycin D, d.
      (ALOMAD)
    BCNU, hydroxyurea, d. (BHD)
    d., BCNU, vincristine (DBV)
    bleomycin, Eldisine, lomustine, d.
      (BELD)
    bleomycin, Oncovin, lomustine, d.
      (BOLD)
    d., CCNU, vincristine (DCV)
    cisplatin, vinblastine, d. (CVD)
    cyclophosphamide, Adriamycin, d.
      (CAD, CADIC, CyADIC)
    cyclophosphamide, Oncovin,
      procarbazine, prednisone plus
      Adriamycin, bleomycin,
      vincristine, d. (COPP/ABVD)
    doxorubicin and d.
    d. imidazole carboxamide
    mechlorethamine, Oncovin,
      procarbazine, prednisone plus
      Adriamycin, bleomycin,
      vinblastine, d. (MOPP/ABVD)
    mesna, Adriamycin, ifosfamide, d.
      (MAID)
    mesna, Adriamycin, interleukin-3, d.
      (MAID)
    Mesnex, Adriamycin, Ifex, d.
      (MAID)
    vinblastine and d.
    vinblastine, Adriamycin, Cytoxan,
      actinomycin D, d. (VACAD)
    vincristine, actinomycin D,
      cyclophosphamide, Adriamycin, d.
      (VACAD)

DACE

    dexamethasone, ara-C, carboplatin,
    etoposide
    DACE chemotherapy

DA-cell

    human interleukin for DA-c.

Dacie method

dacliximab

Dacodyl

Dacogen

Dacplat

Dacron cuff

DACT

    dactinomycin

dactinomycin (DACT)

    Adriamycin, cyclophosphamide,
      imidazole, d. (ACID)
    d., Adriamycin, vincristine,
      cyclophosphamide, radiation
    bleomycin, cyclophosphamide, d.
      (BCD)
    cyclophosphamide, vincristine,
      Adriamycin, d. (CyVADACT,
      CY-VA-DACT)
    methotrexate, calcium leucovorin
      rescue, Adriamycin, cisplatin,
      bleomycin, cyclophosphamide, d.

D

dactinomycin *(continued)*
   d., methotrexate, cyclophosphamide (DMC)
   Oncovin, methotrexate, Adriamycin, d. (OMAD)
dactinomycin-loaded liposome
dactylitis
DADAG
   diacetyldianhydrogalactitol
dAdo
   deoxyadenosine
dADP
   deoxyadenosine diphosphate
DAG
   diacylglycerol
dai
   qing d.
daily
   d. bolus
   d. fraction
   d. fractionation
   d. triangulation
Dakin solution
Dako HercepTest immunohistochemical test
Dalacin
   D. C Topical
   D. C Vaginal Cream
Dale gastrostomy tube holder
Dale-Laidlaw clotting time
DALM
   dysplasia-associated lesion or mass
dalteparin sodium
dam
   latex d.
damage
   adipocyte d.
   endothelial d.
   genetic d.
   potentially lethal d. (PLD)
   d. response gene
   U fiber d.
Damason-P
dammini
   Ixodes d.
dAMP
   deoxyadenosine monophosphate
Dana-Farber Cancer Institute (DFCI)
danaparoid
danazol
dandelion
Dane particle
Danggui Longhui Wan
daniplestim
DAP
   death-associated protein
   dianhydrogalactitol, Adriamycin, Platinol

DAPD
   diaminopurine dioxolane
dapsone and trimethoprim (DAP/TMP)
DAP/TMP
   dapsone and trimethoprim
da qing ye
Daraprim
darbepoetin alfa
Darier
   D. disease
   D. sign
dark signal
Darvocet-N 100
Darvon Compound-65 Pulvule
Darvon-N
darwinian theory
dasatinib molecule
DAT
   daunorubicin, ara-C, 6-thioguanine
data (*pl. of* datum)
datelliptium
dATP
   deoxyadenosine triphosphate
DATTA
   Diagnostic and Therapeutic Technology Assessment
datum, pl. **data**
   data acquisition
   data dredging
   epidemiological data
   data evaluation strategy
   FINE Storage of Measured Beam Data
   measured beam data
   data sampling
DATVP
   daunorubicin, ara-C, 6-thioguanine, vincristine, prednisone
daunomycin (DNM)
   d., ara-C, thioguanine, vincristine, prednisone
   d., cytarabine, 6-thioguanine
   d., cytosine, arabinoside, VP-16
   d. hydrochloride
   6-thioguanine, ara-C, d. (TAD)
daunorubicin (DNR)
   d. and ara-C (DA)
   d., ara-C, 6-thioguanine (DAT)
   d., ara-C, 6-thioguanine, vincristine, prednisone (DATVP)
   d., ara-C, VP-16 (DAV)
   d., azacitidine, ara-C, prednisone, Oncovin (DZAPO)
   d. citrate
   d., cyclocytidine, 6-mercaptopurine, prednisone (DCCMP)
   cytarabine and d.
   d. and cytarabine (DC)

d., cytarabine, 6-mercaptopurine, prednisone (DCMP)

d., cytarabine, prednisone, mercaptopurine (DCPM)

d., cytarabine, 6-thioguanine (DCT)

cytosine arabinoside and d. (CAD)

dexrazoxane in combination with idarubicin and/or d.

d. hydrochloride

liposomal d.

liposomally encapsulated d.

d., Oncovin, ara-C, prednisone (DOAP)

6-thioguanine, ara-C, d. (TAD)

vaccine-induced noncytolic cytarabine d.

VePesid, 6-thioguanine, ara-C, d. (V-TAD)

vincristine, ara-C, 6-thioguanine, d. (VATD)

d., vincristine, prednisone (DVP)

d., vincristine, prednisone, L-asparaginase (DVPL-ASP)

DaunoXome

DAV

daunorubicin, ara-C, VP-16

dibromodulcitol, Adriamycin, vincristine

DAVA

desacetyl vinblastine amide

Davanat

Davanat-1

DAVH

dibromodulcitol, Adriamycin, vincristine, Halotestin

DAVTH

dibromodulcitol, Adriamycin, vincristine, tamoxifen, Halotestin

dawn phenomenon

dAXP

total adenine deoxyribonucleotide

Day factor

Daypro

DBD

dibromodulcitol

DBDC

distal bile duct carcinoma

DBPT

dimethyltriazenoimidazole carboxamide, bischloroethylnitrosourea, Platinol, tamoxifen

DBV

dacarbazine, BCNU, vincristine

DC

daunorubicin and cytarabine

dendritic cell

DC anti-tumor vaccine

DC injection

DC 240 Softgel

DCAI

desmoplastic cerebral astrocytoma of infancy

DCBE

double-contrast barium enema

dual-contrast barium enema

DCC

deleted in colon cancer

DCC gene

DCCMP

daunorubicin, cyclocytidine, 6-mercaptopurine, prednisone

DCE-MRI

dynamic contrast-enhanced magnetic resonance imaging

DCEP

dexamethasone, cyclophosphamide, etoposide, cisplatin

DCF

2-deoxycoformycin

DCIS

ductal carcinoma in situ

dCK

2′-deoxycytidine kinase

DCM

dichloromethotrexate

DCMP

daunorubicin, cytarabine, 6-mercaptopurine, prednisone

dCMP-D

2′-deoxycytidylate deaminase

DCP

des-carboxy prothrombin

des-gamma-carboxy prothrombin

DCPM

daunorubicin, cytarabine, prednisone, mercaptopurine

DCT

daunorubicin, cytarabine, 6-thioguanine

dynamic computed tomography

dCTP

deoxycytidine triphosphate

DCV

dacarbazine, CCNU, vincristine

DTIC, CCNU, vincristine

dCYD

2′-deoxycytidine

NOTES

D

DD
    death domain
        Fas-associated DD
ddA
    dideoxyadenosine
ddAdo
    2′,3′-dideoxyadenosine
DDAVP
    1-deamino-8-ᴅ-arginine-vasopressin
DDC
    dideoxycytidine
ddC
    zalcitabine
ddCIAdo
    2′,3′-dideoxy-2-chloroadenosine
ddCMP
    2′,3′-dideoxycytidine 5′-monophosphate
ddCyd
    2′,3′-dideoxycytidine
DDFS
    distant disease-free survival
ddG
    dideoxyguanosine
DDI
    dideoxyinosine
    drug dose intensity
D-Di
    D-Di buffer
    D-Di negative control
    D-Di positive control
    D-Di test
ddI
    didanosine
    ddI monotherapy
D-dimer testing
DDL
    dideoxyinosine
ddlno
    2′,3′-dideoxyininosine
ddN
    2′,3′-dideoxynucleoside
DdNTP
    2′,3′-dideoxynucleoside-5′-triphosphate
DDP
    cis-diamminedichloroplatinum
    cyclophosphamide,
      hexamethylmelamine, Adriamycin,
      DDP (CHAD)
    5-fluorouracil, etoposide, DDP
      (FED)
    DDP, 5-fluorouracil, VePesid
      (DFV)
    hexamethylmelamine, Adriamycin,
      DDP (HAD)
    mechlorethamine, Adriamycin,
      dacarbazine, DDP
    methotrexate, bleomycin, DDP
    vinblastine, bleomycin, DDP (VBD)
    DDP, vindesine, bleomycin (DVB)

DDS
    Denys-Drash syndrome
    diaminodiphenylsulfone
de
    de novo
    de novo acute myeloid leukemia
    de novo carcinoma
    de novo generation
    de novo glioblastoma
    de novo myelodysplasia
    de Quervain disease
    de Quervain fracture
    de Quervain tenosynovitis
    de Quervain thyroiditis
deactivating reaction
DEAE
    diethylaminoethyl
deafness
    eighth cranial nerve d.
deaminase
    adenosine d. (ADA)
    cytidine/2′deoxycytidine d.
      (Cyd/dCyd-D)
    2′-deoxycytidylate d. (dCMP-D)
    polyethylene glycol-modified
      adenosine d. (PEG-ADA)
    porphobilinogen d.
deamination
1-deamino-8-ᴅ-arginine-vasopressin
    (DDAVP)
death
    activation-induced cell d. (AICD)
    apoptotic cell d.
    asthma-related d.
    brain d.
    cancer d.
    cell d.
    cerebral d.
    d. domain (DD)
    mediated cell d.
    necrotic cell d.
    pathologic cell d.
    physiologic cell d.
    programmed cell d.
    d. wish
death-associated protein (DAP)
death-inducing signal complex (DISC)
3-deazaguanine
3-deazauridine
DebioClip single-dose delivery system
Debré-De Toni-Fanconi syndrome
debris
    cellular d.
Debrisan
debulking
    d. surgery
    surgical d.
    d. of tumor

Decadron
cyclophosphamide, vincristine, DaunoXome, D. (CVXD)
D. Injection
vincristine, doxorubicin, D. (VAD)
Decadron-LA
Deca-Durabolin
Decaject
Decaject-LA
DECAL
dexamethasone, etoposide, cisplatin, ara-C, L-asparaginase
DECAL chemotherapy protocol
decalcified bone marrow sample
decanoate
Hybolin D.
decaptyl
decarboxylase
glutamic acid d.
histidine d.
ornithine d.
decarboxylation
amine precursor uptake and d. (APUD)
decay
branched d.
decidua
deciduocellular sarcoma
decision
d. analysis
d. theory
d. tree
decitabine-mediated induction
declopramide
decompensation
decomposition
decompression
biliary d.
endoscopic d.
d. sickness
surgical d.
deconditioned exercise response
decongestive
d. lymphatic therapy (DLT)
d. physiotherapy
deconvolution
decoupling
heteronuclear d.
DEC 9800 plus cardiac mobile C-arm
decreased myeloid/erythroid ratio
decrementi
stadium d.
dedicated push enteroscope

dedifferentiated
d. chondrosarcoma
d. tumor
dedifferentiation
Dedo laryngoscope
deendothelialized artery
deep
d. exposure
d. invasion
d. to nipple
d. tumor
d. vein thrombophlebitis
d. venous thrombosis (DVT)
deep-seated infection
Deetjen body
defect
abdominal wall d.
atrial septal d.
atrioventricular septal d.
cecal filling d.
colonic filling d.
cortical d.
craniotomy d.
dehalogenase d.
duodenal filling d.
electron transport chain d.
endocardial cushion d.
endocardial cushion-type ventricular septal d.
esophageal filling d.
extrinsic filling d.
extrinsic ureteral d.
hereditary storage pool d.
intraluminal filling d.
intravascular filling d.
slash d.
tumor d.
defective DNA repair disease
defense
host d.
phagocytic d.
deferoxamine
defervescentiae
stadium d.
defibrinated blood
defibrination syndrome
defibrotide
deficiency
acquired factor d.
acquired immune d.
adenosine deaminase d.
alpha-1 antitrypsin d.
ankyrin d.

D

NOTES

159

deficiency *(continued)*
> antigen d.
> antitrypsin d.
> arylsulfatase A d.
> AT-III d.
> clotting factor d.
> congenital AT-III d.
> factor VIII d.
> factor IX d.
> factor XII d.
> factor XIII d.
> fatty acyl-Co-A synthetase d.
> fibrinogen d.
> fibrinolytic factor d.
> galactosylamide beta-galactosidase d.
> gay-related immune d. (GRID)
> GdA d.
> glucose-6-phosphate
>   dehydrogenase d. (G6PD, G-6-PD)
> G6PD d.
> growth hormone d. (GHD)
> idiopathic growth hormone d.
> immune d.
> iron d.
> leukocyte adhesion d.
> nutritional d.
> ornithine transcarbamylase d.
> OTC d.
> prekallikrein d.
> primary immune d. (PID)
> pyridoxine d.
> pyruvate kinase d.
> selective immunoglobulin A d.
> specific granule d.
> spectrin d.
> thymic-dependent d.
> uridine 5′-diphosphate
>   glucuronosyltransferase d.
> vitamin B_{12} d.

deficit
> cognitive d.
> focal d.
> HIV-associated minor motor d.
> human immunodeficiency virus-
>   associated minor motor d.
> self-care d.

Deficol
defined
> lymphocyte d. (LD)

definition
> adolescent surveillance case d.
> beam d.

definitive
> d. diagnosis
> d. radiation therapy
> d. radiotherapy

deformity
> bell-and-clapper d.

> cecal d.
> gooseneck d.

degenerated fibroadenoma
degeneration
> acquired hepatocerebral d.
> carcinomatous subacute cerebellar d.
> cerebellar d.
> disc d.
> malignant d.
> paraneoplastic retinal d.
> peripheral disciform d.
> retinal pigmentary d.
> sarcomatous d.
> wallerian d.

degenerative
> d. arthritis
> d. brain disease
> d. cardiomyopathy
> d. change
> d. dementia
> d. disc
> d. disc disease
> d. joint disease
> d. microcystic formation
> d. narrowing
> d. nuclear pattern

deglutition
degradable starch microsphere
degradation
> d. of image
> tumor-matrix d.

degranulation
> histamine d.

degree of inspiration
dehalogenase defect
dehalogenation
dehiscence
DEHOP
> diethylhomospermine

dehydratase
> microassay for amino levulinate
>   acid d.

dehydration
dehydroascorbic acid
dehydrocholate (DHC)
dehydrocholesterol (DHC)
dehydrocholic acid
dehydroemetine
dehydroepiandrosterone (DHEA)
> d. sulfate (DHEAS)

dehydrogenase
> dihydropyrimidine d. (DPD)
> elevated serum lactate d.
> glyceraldehyde phosphate d.
>   (GAPDH)
> lactate d.
> lactic d. (LD, LDH)

DEI
> diffraction-enhanced imaging

dek
- dek oncogene
- dek protooncogene/oncogene

Delatest Injection
Delatestryl Injection
delavirdine (DLV)
delay
- d. time
- d. time selection

delayed
- d. acute radiation toxicity
- d. engraftment
- d. gastric emptying (DGE)
- d. healing
- d. hemolytic transfusion reaction
- d. hypersensitivity
- d. lymph node dissection
- d. small bowel transit
- d. vomiting

delayed-type
- d.-t. hypersensitivity (DTH)
- d.-t. hypersensitivity test

Delestrogen
deleted
- d. in colon cancer (DCC)
- d. in colon cancer gene

deletion
- CCR5 gene d.
- chromosome 13 d.
- clonal d.
- delta-32 d.
- DNA d.
- d. metagenesis
- polymerase chain reaction detection of haptoglobin gene d.
- T-cell d.

delirium, pl. **deliria**
- D. Rating Scale (DRS)

delitescence
delivered total dose (DTD)
delivery
- drug d.
- intracavitary d.
- intrahepatic d.
- intrapleural d.
- oxygen d.

dell'Adulto
- Gruppo Italiano Malattie Ematologiche Maligne d.'A. (GIMEMA)

Delrin applicator
delta, δ
- d. agent

- d. antigen
- d. check
- d. function
- d. granule
- d. protein

delta-32 deletion
delta-aminolevulinate dehydratase testing
deltacortisone
delta-heavy-chain disease
Deltasone
delta-9-tetrahydrocannabinol
Deltec-Pharmacia CADD pump
Deltec portable external infusion device
Del-Vi-A
DEM
- diethyl maleate

Demadex
demand
- oxygen d.

dematiaceous mold
d'emblée
- tumor mycosis fungoides d.

demeclocycline
dementia
- degenerative d.
- end-stage d.

Demerol
4-demethoxydaunorubicin
demethylase enzyme
demethylation test
demilune body
demineralization
- bone d.

Demodex
- *D. brevis*
- *D. folliculorum*

demographic determinant
Demser
demyelinating disease
demyelination
- autoimmune inflammatory d.
- focal d.
- white matter d.

demyelinolysis
- central pontine d.

denaturation
- alkaline d.

dendritic
- d. cell (DC)
- d. cell injection
- d. cell therapy
- d. cell vaccination

NOTES

dendritic *(continued)*
    d. sarcoma
    d. tumor cell vaccine
dendrocytoma
    dermal d.
    disseminated dermal d.
dengue
    d. fever
    d. virus
denileukin diftitox
Denny-Brown syndrome
dense
    d. brain mass
    d. granule
    d. metaphysial bands
    d. ribs
densitometer
    bone d.
    DPX Bravo bone d.
densitometry
density
    areal d.
    arterial linear d.
    bone mineral d. (BMD)
    breast tissue d.
    heterogenous d.
    linear d.
    mean optical d. (MOD)
    microvessel d. (MVD)
    nuclear spin d.
    prostate-specific antigen d. (PSAD)
    proton d.
    PSA d. (PSAD)
dental granuloma
dentate nucleus
dentinogenesis imperfecta
Denver
    D. chromosome identification
      system
    D. shunt
Denys-Drash syndrome (DDS)
Denys-Leclef phenomenon
deossification
deoxyadenosine (dAdo)
    d. diphosphate (dADP)
    d. monophosphate (dAMP)
    d. triphosphate (dATP)
5-deoxyazacytidine
deoxycholate
2-deoxycoformycin (DCF)
deoxycytidine
    fluoromethylene d. (FMdC)
    d. triphosphate (dCTP)
    2-d. 5′-triphosphate
2′-deoxycytidine (dCYD)
    2′-d. kinase (dCK)
deoxycytidylate
2′-deoxycytidylate deaminase (dCMP-D)

deoxy-D-glucose
5′-deoxy-5-fluorouridine (5-dFUR)
deoxyguanosine triphosphate (dGTP, GTP)
deoxyhemoglobin
2′-deoxy-2′-methyl-idenecytidine (DMDC)
deoxynojirimycin (DNJ)
deoxypyrimidine nucleoside analog
deoxyribonuclease (DNAse)
deoxyribonucleic
    d. acid (DNA)
    d. acid probe kit
deoxyribonucleoside
    5-FU d.
deoxyribonucleotide
    total adenine d. (dAXP)
deoxyriboside
    thymidine d. (TDR)
deoxyspergualin (DSG)
deoxythymidine (dTHd)
2′-deoxythymidine
    2′-d. 5′-triphosphate (dTTP)
    2′-d. kinase (dTK)
(2′-deoxy)thymidylate synthase (TS)
deoxythymidylic acid synthase
2′-deoxyuridine (dURD)
Depacon
Depakene
Depakote
deparaffinized
Depen
dependence
    nicotine d.
dependency
    schedule d.
dependent
    dose d.
depGynogen Injection
dephasing
    spin d.
depigmentation
depleted
    lymphocyte d.
depletion
    lymphocyte d.
    myeloid d.
    plasma d.
    superantigen-mediated d.
    white blood cell d.
depMedalone Injection
DepoCyt cytarabine liposomal injection
Depo-Estradiol Injection
Depofoam encapsulated cytarabine
Depogen Injection
depolymerization
    d. of microtubule
    d. of tubulin

Depo-Medrol Injection
depomedroxyprogesterone acetate (DMPA)
DepoMorphine
Deponit Patch
Depopred Injection
Depo-Provera Injection
deposit
  amyloid d.
  lipofuscin d.
  metastatic d.
  tumefactive amyloid d.
  tumorlike amyloid d.
deposition
  amyloid d.
  antibody d.
  fibrin d.
  iron d.
  reticulin d.
  d. of tracer
depot
  Androcur D.
  flutamide and Lupron D. (FL)
  Lupron D.
  Suprefact D.
  Trelstar D.
Depo-Testosterone Injection
Depot-Ped
  Lupron D.-P.
depression
  bone marrow d.
  Hamilton Rating Scale for D.
  rectilinear d.
deprivation
  androgen d.
  neoadjuvant androgen d. (NAAD)
depside
depsidone
depth
  Breslow d.
  maximum d. (D_{max})
  midplane d.
  skin d.
  target d.
DER
  dual-energy radiograph
deranged mucosa
derangement
derepressed gene
Derifil
derivation
  modeling d.

derivative
  blood d.
  diphenhydramine d.
  hematoporphyrin d. (HPD)
  muramyl dipeptide d.
  purified protein d. (PPD)
  valproic acid and d.'s
derm
  doobie d.
dermal
  d. calcification
  d. dendric cell
  d. dendrocytoma
  d. dendrocytome
  d. duct tumor
  d. microvascular endothelial cell (DMVEC)
  d. sinus tract
dermatitidis
  Blastomyces d.
dermatitis, pl. **dermatitides**
  allergic contact d.
  atopic d.
  exfoliative d.
  d. herpetiformis
  d. medicamentosa
  photosensitivity d.
  psoriasiform d.
  radiation d.
  seborrheic d. (SD)
Dermatobia hominis
dermatofibroma
dermatofibrosarcoma
  pigmented d.
  d. protuberans (DFSP)
dermatology
  general d.
dermatomal zoster
dermatome
dermatomyoma
dermatomyositis
  paraneoplastic d.
dermatopathic
  d. lymphadenitis
  d. lymphadenopathy
dermatophyte tinea infection
dermatosis, pl. **dermatoses**
  acantholytic d.
  d. papulosis nigra
  papulosquamous d.
Derma-Wand device
dermis

NOTES

dermoid
    d. ovarian cyst
    d. plug
    d. tumor
Dermoplast
dermoplastic trichoepithelioma
DES
    diethylstilbestrol
    DES task force
desacetyl vinblastine amide (DAVA)
DESAD
    National Collaborative Diethylstilbestrol
    Adenosis Project
des-carboxy prothrombin (DCP)
descent
    basal d.
    epididymal d.
desensitization
    systematic d.
desetope
desexualize
Desferal Mesylate
des-gamma-carboxy prothrombin (DCP)
desiccation
design
    crossover d.
    factorial d.
    kin-cohort d.
designation
    cluster d.
desipramine
desmethylmisonidazole (DMM)
desmin
desmoglein adhesion molecule
desmoid tumor
desmoplakin protein
desmoplasia
desmoplastic
    d. cerebral astrocytoma
    d. cerebral astrocytoma of infancy
    (DCAI)
    d. fibroma
    d. infantile astrocytoma (DIA)
    d. infantile ganglioglioma (DIG,
    DIGG)
    d. neurotropic melanoma (DNM)
    d. reaction
    d. small cell tumor
    d. small round-cell tumor (DSRCT)
desmopressin acetate
desmosome
    true d.
despeciated serum
desquamated epithelial hyperplasia
desquamation
    dry d.
    moist d.
desquamative
    d. fibrosing alveolitis

    d. interstitial pneumonia
    d. interstitial pneumonitis
destruction
    argon d.
    bone d.
    cortical d.
    immune-mediated d.
    laser d.
    periodontal bone d.
destructive bone lesion
destruens
    chorioadenoma d.
detachment
detection
    candidate of metastasis-1 gene d.
    early d.
    Escherichia coli strain O157:H7
      immunomagnetic separation and d.
    failed biopsy d. (FBD)
    gene d.
    HCV-RNA high-throughput
      extraction amplification and d.
    high-throughput extraction
      amplification and d. (HEAD)
    indirect d.
    SYT-SSX fusion gene d.
detector
    C-Trak hand-held gamma d.
    fluorescence d.
    Geiger-Muller d.
    Innova 4100 flat-panel d.
    mass spectrophotometric d.
    Navigator gamma ray d.
    nitrogen-phosphorus d.
    Revolution XR/d digital d.
    ultraviolet d.
    Waters M-440 fixed wavelength d.
Detensol
determinant
    antigen d.
    antigenic d.
    blood group oligosaccharide d.
    conformational d.
    demographic d.
    d. group
    immunogenic d.
    isoallotypic d.
    isotypic d.
determination
    immunoglobulin clonality d.
    protein level d.
De Toni-Debré-Fanconi syndrome
detorubicin
Detox
    D. adjuvant
    D. adjuvant vaccination
detoxification
    multidrug resistance d.

detrusor
    d. hyperreflexia
    d. muscle
deuterium-tritium generator
deuteron
deux
    cancer à d.
development
    clonal d.
    drug d.
    endocardial cushion d.
    pubertal d.
deviation
    genetic d.
    tracheal d.
Devic disease
device
    Accuray robotic d.
    A1cNow glycemic monitoring d.
    AIS CELLector CD8 Cell
      Culture D.
    Alexa 1000 breast lesion
      diagnostic d.
    Arnoff external fixation d.
    atherectomy d.
    atherolytic reperfusion wire d.
    Auto-Crane d.
    beam-modifying d.
    BetaSorb d.
    Cellect graft preparation d.
    CoaguChek self-testing d.
    continuous microinfusion d.
    Deltec portable external infusion d.
    Derma-Wand d.
    electronic portal imaging d.
    electrooptical d.
    electrovibratory d.
    expanded foam immobilization d.
    iFind handheld d.
    implantable vascular access d.
    InPath cervical cancer screening d.
    LifeSpex d.
    magnetic induction d.
    MammoSite RTS balloon
      interstitial d.
    Mammotome core biopsy d.
    prosthetic d.
    radiative hyperthermia d.
    Rashkind ductus occluder d.
    ReliefBand d.
    stereotactic vacuum-assisted
      biopsy d.
    d. success

    suction d.
    SVAB d.
    targeted cryoablation d.
    T-bar immobilization d.
    T-Scan 2000 breast imaging d.
    vacuum constriction d. (VCD)
    vacuum erection d.
    venous access d.
DeVilbiss nebulizer
Devine antral exclusion procedure
Devrom
DEXA, DXA
    dual-energy x-ray absorptiometry
dexamethasone (DM)
    Adriamycin, vincristine,
      cytarabine, d. (AVAD)
    d., ara-C, carboplatin, etoposide
      (DACE)
    d., ara-C, carboplatin, etoposide
      chemotherapy
    bleomycin, Adriamycin, CCNU,
      Oncovin, d. (BACOD)
    CCNU, bleomycin, vinblastine, d.
      (CBVD)
    CCNU, vinblastine, bleomycin, d.
      (CVBD)
    d., cyclophosphamide, etoposide,
      cisplatin (DCEP)
    cyclophosphamide, etoposide,
      vincristine, d. (CEVD)
    cyclophosphamide,
      hydroxydaunomycin, Oncovin, d.
      (CHOD)
    cyclophosphamide, methotrexate,
      etoposide, d. (CMED)
    cyclophosphamide, vincristine,
      Adriamycin, d. (CVAD, C-VAD)
    Doxil, vincristine, d.
    d., etoposide, cisplatin, ara-C, L-
      asparaginase (DECAL)
    fludarabine, mitoxantrone, d. (FMD)
    fludarabine, Novantrone, d. (FND)
    d., high-dose ara-C, Platinol
    high-dose methotrexate, bleomycin,
      Adriamycin, cyclophosphamide,
      Oncovin, d.
    hyperfractionated cyclophosphamide,
      vincristine, doxorubicin, d. (hyper-
      CVAD)
    methotrexate, bleomycin,
      Adriamycin, cyclophosphamide,
      Oncovin, d. (M-BACOD)

D

NOTES

dexamethasone *(continued)*
    methotrexate, leucovorin, bleomycin, Adriamycin, cyclophosphamide, Oncovin, d.
    methotrexate, Oncovin, L-asparaginase, d. (MOAD)
    moderate-dose methotrexate, bleomycin, Adriamycin, cyclophosphamide, Oncovin, d. (m-BACOD)
    d. suppression test
    d., thalidomide plus Adriamycin, cyclophosphamide, etoposide (DT-PACE)
    vincristine, Adriamycin, d. (VAD)
    vincristine, doxorubicin, d. (VDD)
Dexasone L.A.
Dexferrum
Dexone LA
Dexon mesh
dexormaplatin
dexrazoxane in combination with idarubicin and/or daunorubicin
dextran
dextranomer
dextranomer
dextrin sulfate
dextroamphetamine
dextrothyroxine
dexverapamil
dezaguanine mesylate
dezocine
DF3 antigen
DFA
    direct fluorescent antibody
DFA-TP
    direct fluorescent antibody staining for *Treponema pallidum*
DFCI
    Dana-Farber Cancer Institute
DFDC
    gemcitabine
DFI
    disease-free interval
DFMO
    difluoromethylornithine
DFS
    disease-free survival
DFSP
    dermatofibrosarcoma protuberans
5-dFUR
    5′-deoxy-5-fluorouridine
DFV
    DDP, 5-fluorouracil, VePesid
DGE
    delayed gastric emptying
dGTP
    deoxyguanosine triphosphate

DHAC
    dihydro-5-azacitidine
DHAD
    dihydroxyanthracenedione
    mitoxantrone
DHAP
    dihydroxyacetone phosphate
DHA-paclitaxel
    Taxoprexin DHA-p.
DHC
    dehydrocholate
    dehydrocholesterol
    dihydrocodeine compound
    DHC Plus
DHE
    dihematoporphyrin ether
    dihydroergocryptine
    dihydroergotamine
DHEA
    dehydroepiandrosterone
DHEAS
    dehydroepiandrosterone sulfate
DHFR
    dihydrofolate reductase
DHL
    diffuse histiocytic lymphoma
DHPG
    dihydroxypropoxymethylguanine
DI
    diabetes insipidus
    dose intensity
    double induction
Di
    Di Bella multitherapy
    Di Guglielmo disease
    Di Guglielmo syndrome
DIA
    desmoplastic infantile astrocytoma
diabetes
    d. inositus
    d. insipidus (DI)
    d. mellitus (type 1-3)
diacetyldianhydrogalactitol (DADAG)
diacetylmorphine
diacylglycerol (DAG)
diagnosis, pl. **diagnoses (DX)**
    definitive d.
    differential d.
    laparoscopic abdominal tumor d.
    near-UV excited autofluorescence d. (NEAD)
diagnostic
    d. contrast medicine
    d. imaging
    d. odd ratio (DOR)
    d. system
    D. and Therapeutic Technology Assessment (DATTA)
diagnostic-related group (DRG)

diagraph
Dialose
    D. Plus Capsule
    D. Tablet
Dialume
dialysis
    chronic ambulatory peritoneal d.
    peritoneal d.
    renal d.
dialyzer
    parallel plate d.
    Polyflux S d.
diameter
    anterior sagittal d.
    biparietal d.
diametric pelvic fracture
3,3'-diaminobenzidine tetrahydrochloride
   dihydrate (DAB)
diaminodiphenylsulfone (DDS)
diaminopurine dioxolane (DAPD)
diaminopyridine
diaminopyrimidine
Diamond-Blackfan
    D.-B. anemia
    D.-B. syndrome
Diamox Sequels
dianhydrogalactitol, Adriamycin, Platinol
   (DAP)
diapedesis
    leukocyte d.
diaphanoscope
diaphragm
    antral mucosal d.
    aperture d.
    duodenal d.
    eventration of d.
    excursion of d.
    muscular d.
    traumatic rupture of d. (TRD)
    urogenital d.
diaphragma sellae
diaphragmatic
    d. excursion
    d. hernia
    d. lymph node
    d. paralysis
    d. rupture
    d. slip
    d. sulcus
diaphysial, diaphyseal
    d. aclasis
    d. dysplasia
    d. fracture

    d. ossification
    d. periostitis
diaphysis, pl. diaphyses
    humeral d.
diaphysitis
diarrhea
    chemotherapy-induced d. (CID)
    irinotecan-induced d.
    malabsorptive d.
    secretory d.
    traveler's d.
diarrheogenic syndrome
diarthrodial joint
Diasorb
diastasis
diastole
diastolic velocity ratio
diathermy
    loop d.
diathesis
    atopic d.
    bleeding d.
diatrizoate
    d. meglumine
    d. meglumine radiopaque medium
diatrizoic acid
DiatxFe tablet
Diatx tablet
diazepam
diaziquone
diazohydroxide
    pyrazine d.
diazoxide
dibasic
    calcium phosphate, d.
dibenzamine
Dibenzyline
dibromodulcitol (DBD)
    d., Adriamycin, vincristine (DAV)
    d., Adriamycin, vincristine,
      Halotestin (DAVH)
    d., Adriamycin, vincristine,
      tamoxifen, Halotestin (DAVTH)
    d., doxorubicin, vincristine
dibromomannitol
dibucaine and hydrocortisone
DIC
    disseminated intravascular coagulation
Dicarbosil
dicentric chromosome
DICEP
    dose-interactive cyclophosphamide,
      etoposide, Platinol

D

NOTES

dichloride
> *cis*-platinum diammine d. (CPDD)
> platinum diammine d.

dichlorodiphenyltrichloroethane
dichloromethotrexate (DCM)
dichloromethylene diphosphonate
dichotomous
dicitrate
> biricodar d.

Dickinson
> Becton D. (BD)

Dick test
diclofenac
dicloxacillin
didanosine (ddI)
didehydrodeoxythymidine (d4T)
didehydrodideoxythymidine, stavudine, Zerit (d4T)
didemnin B
dideoxyadenosine (ddA)
2′,3′-dideoxyadenosine (ddAdo)
2′,3′-dideoxy-2-chloroadenosine (ddClAdo)
dideoxycytidine (DDC)
> 2′,3′-d. (ddCyd)
> 2′,3′-d. 5′-monophosphate (ddCMP)

2′,3′-dideoxy-2′-fluoro-9-beta-D-arabinofuranosyladenine (FddaraA)
dideoxyguanosine (ddG)
2′,3′-dideoxyininosine (ddIno)
dideoxyinosine (DDI, DDL)
2′,3′-dideoxynucleoside (ddN)
2′,3′-dideoxynucleoside-5′-triphosphate (DdNTP)
dideoxypurine analog
2′,3′-dideoxy-3′thiacytidine (3TC)
Di-dgA-RFB4 monoclonal antibody
Didronel
Diego blood group
diencephalic syndrome
diet
> high-fiber d.
> low-residue d.
> macrobiotic d.
> Minot-Murphy d.
> d. therapy
> Zen macrobiotic d.

dietary
> d. calcium
> d. fat
> d. fiber
> d. intervention
> d. therapy

diethylaminoethyl (DEAE)
diethyldithiocarbamate (DTC)
diethylenetriamine pentaacetic acid (DTPA)
diethylhomospermine (DEHOP)
diethyl maleate (DEM)

N,N-diethyl-2-[4-(phenylmethyl)phenoxy]ethanamine.HCl (DPPE)
diethylstilbestrol (DES)
> d. diphosphate

diet-induced coronary artery intimal hyperplasia
DIF
> DPD-inhibitory fluoropyrimidine

difenoxin and atropine
diferuloylmethane
difference
> field-echo d.

differential
> d. attenuation
> automated white blood cell d.
> d. CIITA expression
> d. count
> d. density sign
> d. diagnosis
> d. linearity
> manual d.
> d. staining cytotoxicity (DiSC)
> d. staining cytotoxicity assay
> d. temperature sensor
> d. uniformity

differentiated carcinoma
differentiation
> adenocarcinoma with squamous d.
> ameloblastomatous d.
> d. antigen
> B-cell d.
> B-lymphocyte d.
> cluster of d. (CD)
> cluster of d. 1-166 (CD1–166)
> cluster of d. 4 (CD4)
> cluster of d. 8 (CD8)
> ductal epithelial d.
> large cell carcinoma with neuroendocrine d. (LCCND)
> minimal d.
> myoepithelial d.
> neuroendocrine d.
> nonsmall cell lung carcinoma with neuroendocrine d. (NSCLC-ND)
> plasmablastic d.
> plasmacytoid d.
> sinonasal carcinoma with neuroendocrine d. (SNCD)
> squamous d.
> T-cell d.
> terminal d.

differentiation-inducing therapy
difficile
> *Clostridium d.* (CD)

Diff-Quik stain
diffraction-enhanced imaging (DEI)
diffusable inflammatory cytokine

diffuse
- d. abdominal calcification
- d. aggressive lymphoma
- d. air space disease
- d. bacterial nephritis
- d. cerebral histiocytosis
- d. cirrhosis
- d. fatty infiltration
- d. fibrillary astrocytoma
- d. fibrocystic disease
- d. fibrosis type
- d. fine reticulation
- d. hepatic enlargement
- d. histiocytic lymphoma (DHL)
- d. idiopathic skeletal hyperostosis
- d. intermediate lymphocytic lymphoma
- d. large B-cell lymphoma (DLBCL)
- d. large cell lymphoma (DLCL)
- d. lung disease
- d. malignant peritoneal mesothelioma
- d. mixed small and large cell lymphoma
- d. neuroendocrine system (DNES)
- d. osteosclerosis
- d. panbronchiolitis
- d. pancreatitis
- d. pattern
- d. pleural mesothelioma
- d. poorly differentiated lymphoma (DPDL)
- d. pulmonary alveolar hemorrhage
- d. reflectance spectroscopy (DRS)
- d. reflector
- d. sarcomatosis
- d. scleroderma
- d. sclerosing alveolitis
- d. sclerosis
- d. small cell lymphocytic lymphoma
- d. thickening
- d. thymic enlargement
- d. toxic goiter
- d. ulcerative lesion

diffusely swollen hemisphere
diffusible somatostatin analog
diffusing
- d. capacity
- d. capacity of lung for carbon monoxide (DLCO)

diffusion
- d. coefficient
- exchange d.
- d. factor
- d. imaging
- passive d.
- d. spectroscopy
- d. time (T_d)
- tumor water d.

diffusion-sensitive sequence
diffusion-weighted
- d.-w. imaging (DWI)
- d.-w. MR imaging
- d.-w. scanning

Diflucan
diflunisal
difluoride
- polyvinyldine d. (PVDF)

2′,2′-difluorodeoxycytidine
difluoromethylornithine (DFMO)
diftitox
- denileukin d.

DIG, DIGG
- desmoplastic infantile ganglioglioma

digastric muscle
Digene Cervical Sampler
DiGeorge syndrome
digestive system
DIGG (*var. of* DIG)
digiscope
digit
- binary d.
- D. Span of Wechsler Adult Intelligence Scale

digital
- d. clubbing
- d. mammography
- d. neuroma
- d. rectal examination (DRE)
- d. slide scanner
- d. subtraction angiography

digitalis
- herpes d.
- d. toxicity

digitally reconstructed radiograph (DRR)
digital-to-analog converter (DAC)
digitized chest radiography
digitorum
- extensor d.

digluconate
- chlorhexidine d.

digoxigenin-labeled oligonucleotide probe

NOTES

digoxin
dihematoporphyrin ether (DHE)
dihydrate
    calcium pyrophosphate d.
    3,3'-diaminobenzidine
      tetrahydrochloride d. (DAB)
    hydrochloride d.
dihydro-5-azacitidine (DHAC)
dihydrochloride
    histamine d.
    nolatrexed d.
    orthophenylenediamine d.
dihydrocodeine compound (DHC)
dihydroergocryptine (DHE)
dihydroergotamine (DHE)
dihydrofolate reductase (DHFR)
dihydropteroate synthesis
dihydropyrimidine dehydrogenase (DPD)
dihydrotachysterol
dihydrotestosterone
dihydroxyacetone phosphate (DHAP)
dihydroxyanthracenedione (DHAD)
4,4$^{\underline{1}}$dihydroxybenzophenone-2,4-
   dinitrophenylhydrazone
dihydroxypropoxymethylguanine (DHPG)
diiodohydroxyquin
dilatation, dilation
    aneurysmal d.
    balloon d.
    beaded ductal d.
    bile duct d.
    cystic d.
    ductal d.
    tract d.
    transurethral balloon d.
dilator
    Amplatz long tapered Teflon d.
    Amplatz renal d.
    Amplatz tapered-tip coaxial d.
    angiographic Teflon d.
    balloon d.
    biliary coaxial d.
    esophageal balloon d.
    fascial d.
    Jackson d.
    renal d.
    Savary d.
    Savary-Gilliard d.
    semirigid d.
    tapered-tip d.
    Teflon d.
Dilatrate-SR
Dilaudid
    D. Injection
    D. Oral
    D. Suppository
Dilaudid-HP Injection
diltiazem
diluent

dilutional hyponatremia
2-dimensional (2D)
    2-d. immunoelectrophoresis
    2-d. polyacrylamide gel
      electrophoresis
    2-d. structure analysis
3-dimensional (3D)
    3-d. assisted conformal treatment
    3-d. computed tomography
    3-d. conformal radiotherapy
      (3CDRT)
    3-d. conformal therapy
    3-d. CRT
    3-d. display of airways
    3-d. treatment planning
dimer
    thymine d.
dimercaprol
dimerization
    growth factor d.
Dimertest EIA
dimesna
dimethylbenzanthracene (DMBA)
dimethylhydrazine
dimethyl sulfoxide (DMSO)
dimethyltriazenoimidazole
    d. carboxamide (DTIC)
    d. carboxamide,
      bischloroethylnitrosourea, Platinol,
      tamoxifen (DBPT)
dimorphic anemia
dimple sign
1,2-dimyristyloxypropyl-3-
   dimethylhydroxyethyl ammonium
   bromide/dioleoylphosphatidylethano-
   lamine formulation (DMRIE/DOPE)
dinitrate
    glyceryl d. (GDN)
    isosorbide d.
dinitrochlorobenzene (DNCB)
dinoprostone
dinucleotide
    nicotinamide adenine d.
Diocto
Diocto-C
Diomycin
Dioval Injection
dioxide
    benzothiazine d.
    sulfur d.
dioxolane
    diaminopurine d. (DAPD)
    d. guanosine
dioxopiperazine inhibitor
dipalmitoyl
    disaccharide tripeptide glycerol d.
    d. phosphatidylethanolamine
dipeptide
    muramyl d.

diphenhydramine
    acetaminophen and d.
    d. derivative
    d. hydrochloride
diphenoxylate and atropine
diphenylhydantoin
diphosphate
    aminohydroxypropylidene d. (APD)
    deoxyadenosine d. (dADP)
    diethylstilbestrol d.
    guanosine d. (GDP)
5′-diphosphate
    adenosine 5′-d. (ADP)
    uridine 5′-d. (UDP)
diphosphonate
    dichloromethylene d.
diphtheria
    d. antigen
    d., tetanus, pertussis (DTP)
    d., tetanus, pertussis, *Haemophilus influenzae* type b vaccine
    d. and tetanus toxoid with acellular pertussis (DTaP)
Diplococcus pneumoniae
diploid
    DNA d.
    d. tumor
diplopia
dipping
    snuff d.
diprenorphine
dipyridamole
dipyridodiazepinone analog
direct
    d. coloanal anastomosis
    d. en face
    d. fluorescent antibody (DFA)
    d. fluorescent antibody staining
    d. fluorescent antibody staining for *Treponema pallidum* (DFA-TP)
    d. ray tracing
directional atherectomy
directive
    advance d.
    d. counseling
directly observed therapy (DOT)
directory
    AIDS/HIV Treatment D.
dirithromycin
disaccharide tripeptide glycerol dipalmitoyl
Disalcid
disarticulation

disassociation (*var. of* dissociation)
DISC
    death-inducing signal complex
DiSC
    differential staining cytotoxicity
    DiSC assay
disc, disk
    anular d.
    bulging d.
    cervical d.
    d. degeneration
    degenerative d.
    d. disease
    d. extrusion
    d. herniation
    d. margin
    d. protrusion
    d. sequestration
    d. space
    d. space infection
    d. space narrowing
    d. water content
discharge
    myokymic d.
    nipple d.
    d. planning
    vaginal d.
disciformis
    granulomatosis d.
discitis, diskitis
discodermolide
discography, diskography
discoloration
    skin d.
discontinuous density gradient centrifugation
discordance
    atrioventricular d.
    HIV d.
    human immunodeficiency virus d.
discounting
Discovery LS imaging system
Discrene breast form
discrete
    d. hyperintense focus
    d. lesion
disease
    acquired renal cystic d.
    acquired von Willebrand d. (AvWD)
    acute inflammatory d.
    acyanotic heart d.
    Addison d.

NOTES

disease *(continued)*
adrenal medullary d.
adrenocortical d.
adult polycystic kidney d.
air space d.
allergic d.
allogeneic d.
alloimmune d.
alpha-heavy-chain d.
alveolar d.
Alzheimer d. (AD)
amyloid oral cavity d.
anemia of chronic d.
angiomatous d.
anterior horn cell d.
aortic valvular d.
aortoiliac d.
apatite deposition d.
arterial d.
arteriosclerotic occlusive d.
arteriosclerotic renal d.
asbestos-related pleural d.
atheroembolic renal d.
atherosclerotic d.
autoimmune d.
autoimmune hemolytic d. (AHD)
autosomal-dominant polycystic
  kidney d.
autosomal-recessive polycystic
  kidney d.
Bassen-Kornzweig d.
Bateman d.
Bazex d.
Béguez César d.
benign breast d.
biliary tract d.
Billroth d.
Bowen d.
brain d.
breast d.
bulky Hodgkin d.
bullous lung d.
Busse-Buschke d.
calcium pyrophosphate deposition d.
carcinoid heart d.
cardiopulmonary d.
cardiovascular d. (CD)
Carrion d.
Castleman d.
cat-scratch d.
celiac d.
cerebrovascular d.
Chagas d.
Charcot-Marie-Tooth d.
Chédiak-Higashi d.
childhood granulomatous d.
childhood polycystic d.
Christmas d.
chronic demyelinating d.

chronic graft-versus-host d.
  (cGVHD)
chronic granulomatous d.
chronic obstructive pulmonary d.
  (COPD)
clinically detectable liver d.
coagulation factor d.
cold agglutinin d.
common variable
  immunodeficiency d.
comorbid d.
congenital immunodeficiency d.
connective tissue d.
d. course
Cowden d.
Creutzfeldt-Jakob d. (CJD)
Crohn d. (CD)
Cushing d.
cystic dysplasia d.
cystic kidney d.
cystic ovarian d.
cystic renal d.
cytokine d.
cytomegalic inclusion d. (CID)
cytomegalovirus d.
cytotoxic antibody-mediated d.
Darier d.
defective DNA repair d.
degenerative brain d.
degenerative disc d.
degenerative joint d.
delta-heavy-chain d.
demyelinating d.
de Quervain d.
Devic d.
diffuse air space d.
diffuse fibrocystic d.
diffuse lung d.
Di Guglielmo d.
disc d.
disseminated cryptococcal d.
diverticular d.
duodenal peptic ulcer d.
Dupont and Lachapelle d.
dysmyelinating d.
EBV-induced lymphoproliferative d.
embolic d.
end-stage renal d.
Epstein-Barr virus-induced
  lymphoproliferative d.
Evans stage IV-S d.
extensive-stage d.
extracranial carotid artery d.
extragenital Bowen d. (EBD)
extramammary Paget d.
extranodal Rosai-Dorfman d.
Fabry d.
Fallot d.
fibrocystic breast d.

field d.
fifth d.
Franklin d.
Gaisböck d.
gamma-heavy-chain d. (gamma-HCD)
Gaucher d.
gestational nonmetastatic trophoblastic d.
gestational trophoblastic d. (GTD)
glycogen storage d.
graft versus host d. (GVHD)
granulomatous d.
Graves d.
GVH d.
Hallervorden-Spatz d.
Hand-Schüller-Christian d.
Hansen d.
Hartnup d.
Hashimoto d.
heart d. (HD)
heavy-chain d.
hemoglobin S-C d.
hemoglobin S-O-Arab d.
hemoglobin S-thalassemia d.
hemolytic d.
hepatic venoocclusive d. (HVOD)
Hers d.
Hirschsprung d. (HD)
histiocytic nodular Hodgkin d.
HIV-induced d.
Hodgkin d. (HD)
homologous d.
Hong Kong d.
hormone-naive d.
hormone-refractory d.
Huntington d. (HD)
Hutchinson-Boeck d.
hyaline membrane d.
hyaline-vascular Castleman d.
hydatid d. (HD)
iatrogenic d.
immune complex d.
immunoproliferative small intestinal d. (IPSID)
index of coexistent d. (ICED)
indolent d.
infantile Refsum d.
inflammatory bowel d.
infradiaphragmatic Hodgkin d.
interfollicular Hodgkin d.
International Classification of D.'s (ICD)

Kahler d.
Kellgren d.
Kennedy d.
Kienböck d.
Krabbe d.
Kuru d.
Kyrle d.
Ledderhose d.
Legionnaires d.
Leiner d.
leptomeningeal d. (LMD)
Letterer-Siwe d.
Lhermitte-Duclos d.
lichenoid graft-versus-host d.
life-threatening d.
light chain deposition d. (LCDD)
limited-stage d.
Lobstein d.
locoregional d. (LR)
low volume d.
Lyme d.
lymphocyte-depletion Hodgkin d.
lymphocyte-predominant Hodgkin d. (LPHD)
lymphocytic nodular Hodgkin d.
lysosomal storage d.
macroscopic residual d.
Maffucci d.
d. management
March d.
Marchiafava-Micheli d.
Marek herpesvirus d.
mast cell d.
medullary cystic d.
Meige d.
metachronous d.
Meyer-Betz d.
Mikulicz d.
minimal residual d. (MRD)
mixed-cellularity Hodgkin d.
Mondor d.
Moschcowitz thrombotic thrombocytopenic purpura d.
Mucha-Habermann d.
mu-heavy-chain d. (mu-HCD)
multicentric Castleman d. (MCD)
Murri d.
myeloid d.
National Institute of Allergy and Infectious D. (NIAID)
natural d.
Newcastle d.
Niemann-Pick d.

NOTES

173

disease *(continued)*
  no active d. (NAD)
  no appreciable d. (NAD)
  node-negative d.
  node-positive d.
  nodular sclerosing Hodgkin d.
    (NSHD)
  no evidence of d. (NED)
  no evidence of disease-stationary d.
    (NED-SD)
  no evidence of recurrent d.
    (NERD)
  nonneoplastic d.
  Norrie d.
  obstructive lung d.
  Ollier d.
  optic chiasm d.
  Ormond d.
  Osler d.
  Owren d.
  Paget d.
  papulosquamous d.
  paranasopharyngeal d.
  paraneoplastic d.
  paraprotein d.
  Pel-Ebstein d.
  periodontal d.
  peripheral vascular d. (PVD)
  perirectal d.
  periureteral d.
  Peyronie d.
  Pick d.
  pigment stone d.
  Plummer d.
  polycystic ovarian d. (PCOD)
  polyvinylpyrrolidone storage d.
  precancerous d.
  preinvasive d.
  primary refractory Hodgkin d.
  progressive d.
  pseudo-Hodgkin d.
  Recklinghausen-Appelbaum d.
  Reed-Hodgkin d.
  Refsum d.
  relapsed chemosensitive Hodgkin d.
  Rendu-Osler-Weber d.
  renovascular d.
  residual d.
  reversible polyclonal posttransplant
    lymphoproliferative d.
  Rh(o) d.
  runt d.
  Schaumann d.
  Schüller d.
  Schüller-Christian d.
  sclerodermoid graft-versus-host d.
  secretory d.
  serious d.

  severe combined
    immunodeficiency d. (SCID)
  sickle cell d.
  sickle-Thal d.
  Simmond d.
  Sinding-Larsen-Johansson d.
  site of d.
  stable d.
  d. staging
  Sternberg d.
  Stokvis d.
  storage pool d.
  Sturge-Weber d.
  Symmers d.
  synchronous d.
  T-gamma proliferative d.
  thromboembolic d.
  transient myeloproliferative d.
  trophoblastic d.
  type I glycogen storage d.
  unilobar d.
  uremic medullary cystic d.
  Valsuani d.
  Vaquez-Osler d.
  venoocclusive d. (VOD)
  VHL d.
  von Hippel-Lindau d.
  von Recklinghausen d.
  von Willebrand d.
  Werlhof d.
  Whipple d.
  Winckel d.
  Wolman d.
  Woringer-Kolopp d.
disease-free
  d.-f. interval (DFI)
  d.-f. survival (DFS)
disease-modifying antirheumatic drug
  (DMARD)
disease-specific survival (DSS)
disharmonic delayed osseous maturation
disintegrin
disk *(var. of* disc)
diskectomy *(var. of* discectomy)
diskitis *(var. of* discitis)
diskography *(var. of* discography)
dislocation
  atlantooccipital d.
  bilateral intrafacetal d.
  dysplasia d.
  d. fracture
disodium
  d. clodronate tetrahydrate
  edetate calcium d.
  etidronate d.
  pamidronate d.
  pemetrexed d.
disorder
  acid-base d.

acquired prothrombotic d.
addiction d.
allergic lung d.
angiitis-granulomatosis d.
angiocentric immunoproliferative d.
architectural d.
articular d.
aspirin-like d.
atypical lymphoproliferative d.
autoimmune lymphoproliferative d.
benign proliferative d.
bleeding d.
bullous d.
clonal eosinophilic d.
congenital prothrombotic d.
drug-induced bullous d.
generalized anxiety d. (GAD)
granular lymphocyte-proliferative d.
  (GLPD)
granulomatous slack skin d.
hematologic d.
hematopoietic d.
hepatic coagulation protein d.
hereditary d.
ICE d.
immune complex d.
infiltrative d.
intrathoracic lymphoproliferative d.
lymphoproliferative d.
malignant lymphoproliferative d.
myeloproliferative d. (MPD)
nodular d.
nutritional d.
osteodysplastic slender-bone d.
platelet d.
posttransplant lymphoproliferative d.
  (PTLD)
posttraumatic stress d. (PTSD)
proliferative d.
prothrombotic d.
Quebec platelet d.
signal transduction d.
systemic lymphoproliferative d.
T-gamma lymphoproliferative d.
disparity
fetal-maternal HLA d.
HLA d.
dispersion
amphotericin B colloidal d.
  (ABCD)
displaced
d. crus
d. fracture

disposable PD-10 column
disruption
blood-brain barrier d.
dissection
aortic d.
arterial wall d.
axillary lymph node d. (ALND)
complete lymph node d. (CLND)
delayed lymph node d.
elective lymph node d. (ELND)
extraperitoneal endoscopic pelvic
  lymph node d. (EEPLND)
pelvic lymph node d. (PLND)
per anum intersphincteric rectal d.
radical axillary d.
radical neck d.
retroperitoneal lymph node d.
  (RPLND)
salvage neck d.
selective complete lymph node d.
  (SCLND)
sentinel node d.
supraomohyoid neck d.
therapeutic lymph node d. (TLND)
disseminata
leiomyomatosis peritonealis d.
disseminated
d. cancer
d. candidiasis
d. CNS histoplasmosis
d. cryptococcal disease
d. dermal dendrocytoma
d. fungal infection
d. herpes simplex
d. intravascular coagulation (DIC)
d. lipogranulomatosis
d. melanoma
d. necrotizing leukoencephalopathy
d. *Penicillium marneffei* infection
d. tuberculosis
dissemination
hematogenous d.
d. pattern
peritoneal d.
dissociation, disassociation
dissolution
distal
d. bile duct carcinoma (DBDC)
d. common bile duct obstruction
d. esophagus
d. femoral epiphysial fracture
d. femur
d. gastric cancer

NOTES

distal *(continued)*
  d. humoral fracture
  d. predominantly sensory
    polyneuropathy
  d. radial fracture
  d. rectal adenocarcinoma (DRA)
  d. shift
  d. splenorenal shunt
  d. symmetrical polyneuropathy
  d. symmetric polyneuropathy
    (DSPN)
distance
  focus-skin d. (FSD)
  interuncal d.
  source-film d.
  source-to-skin d. (SSD)
  source-tray d. (STD)
distant
  d. disease-free survival (DDFS)
  d. metastases failure-free survival
    (DMFFS)
  d. metastasis (DM)
  d. spread
distention, distension
  abdominal d.
  bowel d.
distinction
  distraction cognitive d.
  loss of d.
distraction
  cognitive d.
  d. cognitive distinction
  d. of fracture
Distress thermometer
distribution
  dose d.
  Gaussian d.
  intracerebral d.
  single-field isodose d.
  spherical dose d.
disulfide
  d. benzamide
  glutathione d.
disulfide-containing compound
disulfide-substituted benzamide
disulfiram
disuse
  d. atrophy
  d. syndrome
dithiocarbamate
Diucardin
diuretic
Diuril
divalproex sodium
diversion
  orthotopic d.
  urinary d.
diversity
  gene d.

diverticula (*pl. of* diverticulum)
diverticular
  d. abscess
  d. disease
  d. hemorrhage
diverticulation abnormality
diverticulitis
  acute d.
  bladder d.
  colonic d.
diverticulosis
  colonic d.
diverticulum, pl. **diverticula**
  bladder d.
  caliceal d.
  colonic d.
  ductus d.
  duodenal d.
  esophageal d.
diverting colostomy
division cycle
Dixon-Moore classification
Dixon technique
DL
  doxorubicin and lomustine
  ductal lavage
DLBCL
  diffuse large B-cell lymphoma
DLCL
  diffuse large cell lymphoma
DLCO
  diffusing capacity of lung for carbon
    monoxide
DL-lactide-coglycolide
D,L-leucovorin
DLT
  decongestive lymphatic therapy
  dose-limiting toxicity
DLV
  delavirdine
DM
  dexamethasone
  distant metastasis
DMA gene
DMARD
  disease-modifying antirheumatic drug
DMBA
  dimethylbenzanthracene
DMB gene
DMC
  dactinomycin, methotrexate,
    cyclophosphamide
  double minute chromosome
DMDC
  2′-deoxy-2′-methyl-idenecytidine
D-Med Injection
DMEM
  Dulbecco Modified Eagle Medium

DMFFS
    distant metastases failure-free survival
DMFO
    eflornithine
DMM
    desmethylmisonidazole
DMPA
    depomedroxyprogesterone acetate
DMRIE/DOPE
    1,2-dimyristyloxypropyl-3-
      dimethylhydroxyethyl ammonium
      bromide/dioleoylphosphatidylethano-
      lamine formulation
DMSO
    dimethyl sulfoxide
DMVEC
    dermal microvascular endothelial cell
DNA
    deoxyribonucleic acid
      acid labile DNA
      alkylate DNA
      DNA amplification procedure
      DNA aneuploidy
      DNA array
      DNA chain terminator
      complementary DNA (cDNA)
      DNA content analysis
      cosmid cloning vector for DNA
      DNA cytophotometry
      DNA deletion
      DNA diploid
      double-stranded proviral DNA
      DNA fingerprinting
      DNA flow cytometry
      DNA footprinting
      genomic DNA
      germline DNA
      DNA histogram
      DNA hybridization study
      DNA index
      DNA intercalator
      DNA library
      DNA methylation
      DNA microinjection technique
      minisatellite DNA
      mitochondrial DNA
      nuclear DNA
      DNA ploidy
      DNA polymerase
      DNA polymerase assay kit
      DNA probe kit
      recombinant DNA (rDNA)
      DNA repair capacity (DRC)

      DNA replication
      DNA sequencing
      DNA in situ hybridization
      telomeric DNA
      DNA topoisomerase type II
        enzyme
      DNA transfection
      DNA transfection assay
      DNA virus transforming gene
DNAse
    deoxyribonuclease
      DNAse footprinting
DNAzol kit
DNCB
    dinitrochlorobenzene
DNES
    diffuse neuroendocrine system
DNET
    dysembryoplastic neuroepithelial tumor
DNJ
    deoxynojirimycin
      butyl DNJ
DNM
    daunomycin
    desmoplastic neurotropic melanoma
DNR
    daunorubicin
    dose nonuniformity ratio
DNS
    dysplastic nevus syndrome
DNT
    dysembryoplastic neuroepithelial tumor
DOAP
    daunorubicin, Oncovin, ara-C, prednisone
Dobbhoff feeding tube
DOBI
    Dynamic Optical Breast Imaging
      DOBI system
docetaxel
      capecitabine and d.
      doxorubicin and d.
      German preoperative Adriamycin d.
        (GEPARDO)
      paclitaxel and d.
dock
      yellow d.
doctor-patient relationship
docusate and casanthranol
dogfish shark liver extract
Dohle body
Dolacet
dolasetron mesylate
dolastatin

NOTES

Dolobid
Dolophine
domain
  B42 RNA polymerase activation d.
  CCR2 transmembrane d.
  cytoplasmic d.
  death d. (DD)
  dose rate d.
  double zinc finger d.
  Fas-associated death d. (FADD)
  flexible loop d.
  HLH d.
  LexA DNA binding d.
  LIM d.
  Lin-11, Isl-1, Mec-3 gene d.
  TNF receptor-associated death d.
  transmembrane d.
  tumor necrosis factor receptor-
    associated death d. (TRADD)
  V3 d.
Dombrock blood group
dome
  d. of bladder
  d. colpostat
  d. cylinder
  D. Port catheter
dominant
  autosomal d. (AD)
  d. gene
  d. lethal mutation
  d. lump
  d. mass
Donath-Landsteiner antibody
donation
  blood d.
Donnagel-MB
donor
  allogeneic d.
  alternative d.
  autologous d.
  bone marrow d.
  d. bone marrow
  d. cell engraftment
  d. graft
  histocompatible d.
  HLA-identical d.
  HLA-nonidentical d.
  d. lymphocyte infusion
  matched related d.
  matched sibling d. (MSD)
  matched unrelated d. (MUD)
  mismatched related d.
  sibling bone marrow transplant d.
  d. site
  twin d.
  d. twin
  universal d.
  unrelated d. (URD)
  unrelated bone marrow d.

Donovan body
donovani
    Leishmania d.
doobie
    d. derm
    d. derm patch
dopamine agonist
Doppler
    color-flow D.
    pulsed D.
    D. sonography
    D. ultrasound
Dopram
DOR
    diagnostic odd ratio
d'orange
    peau d'o.
dormant cell
dorsal
    d. aspect
    d. column stimulation
    d. induction
    d. induction error
    d. intercalated segment instability
    d. interossei
    d. penile vein
    d. rim
    d. root entry zone lesion
    d. scapular
    d. spine
    d. tubercle
dorsalis
    d. pedis
    d. pedis pulse
Doryx
dose
    absorbed d.
    average radiation d.
    bioeffect d. (BED)
    biologically equivalent d. (BED)
    biologic effective d. (BED)
    bone marrow d.
    boost d.
    d. calibrator
    cancericidal d.
    CD34$^+$ cell d.
    ceiling d.
    central axis d.
    cumulative d.
    delivered total d. (DTD)
    d. dependent
    d. distribution
    effective d.
    d. equivalent
    equivalent d.
    d. escalated and tailored FEC
      therapy
    d. escalation
    exit d.

exposure d.
d. fractionation
integral d.
d. intensification
d. intensity (DI)
d. intensity analysis
isocenter d.
lethal d. (LD)
loading d.
matched peripheral d. (MPD)
maximum permissible d. (MPD)
maximum tolerated d. (MTD)
mean central d. (MCD)
medial lethal d.
medical internal radiation d. (MIRD)
midplane d.
minimal peripheral d. (MPD)
minimum effective d. (MED)
minimum tolerance d.
nominal standard d. (NSD)
d. nonuniformity ratio (DNR)
optimum biologic d. (OBD)
oral d.
organ tolerance d. (OTD)
percentage depth d. (PDD)
d. per fraction
planing curve d.
protocol-specified d.
radiation d.
rad surface d. (RSD)
d. rate
d. rate domain
d. rate effect
reference d.
d. response
scatter d.
single d. (SD)
skin erythema d.
subinfectious d.
tandem double d.
target d.
threshold d.
tumor lethal d. (TLD)
d. value
dose-adjusted EPOCH chemotherapy
dose-controlled phase
dose-delayed technique
dose-escalating study
dose-escalation BCNU therapy
dose-fraction schedule

dose-intensive
  d.-i. induction chemotherapy
  d.-i. regimen
dose-interactive cyclophosphamide, etoposide, Platinol (DICEP)
dose-limiting
  d.-l. factor
  d.-l. myelosuppression
  d.-l. neuropathy
  d.-l. toxicity (DLT)
Dosepak
  Medrol D.
dose-response
  d.-r. curve
  d.-r. relationship
dose-surface histogram
dose-survival curve
dose-time relationship
dose-volume histogram (DVH)
dose-wall histogram
dosimeter
  silicone diode d.
  thermoluminescence d.
  thermoluminescent d. (TLD)
dosimetrist
dosimetry
  breast d.
  computerized d.
  Fricke d.
  intravascular brachytherapy d.
  medical internal radiation d. (MIRD)
  penile bulb d.
  polymer d.
  radiation d.
dosing normogram
DOS Softgel
Dostinex
DOT
  directly observed therapy
dot
  d. blot analysis
  Maurer d.
  Schüffner d.
DOTA
  tetraazacyclododecanetetraacetic acid
DOTP
  tetraazacyclododecanetetraacetic tetramethylene phosphonate
double
  d. balloon method
  d. codon insertion
  d. dose-delayed technique

D

NOTES

double *(continued)*
    d. high-dose chemotherapy
    d. induction (DI)
    d. inversion recovery sequence
    d. Malecot prostatic stent
    d. minute
    d. minute chromosome (DMC)
    d. staining esterase
    d. strength (DS)
    d. transplant
    d. zinc finger domain
double-balloon applicator
double-contrast barium enema (DCBE)
double-immunofluorescence staining
double-J
    d.-J polyethylene catheter
    d.-J silicone rubber urinary catheter
    d.-J ureteral stent
double-lumen
    d.-l. catheter
    d.-l. endotracheal tube
double-peak-angle camera visualization
double-stranded
    d.-s. proviral deoxyribonucleic acid
    d.-s. proviral DNA
    d.-s. RNA-activated protein kinase
double-strand scission
down
    malignant d.
Downey cell
downstaging
    axillary tumor d.
    postirradiation d.
DOX
    doxorubicin
doxapram
doxazosin
doxepin
doxercalciferol
Doxil
    D. and Taxotere
    D., vincristine, dexamethasone
doxorubicin (DOX)
    d. adsorbed to magnetic targeted carrier (MTC-DOX)
    d., cyclophosphamide, 5-fluorouracil, methotrexate, vincristine
    d. and dacarbazine
    d. and docetaxel
    d. HCl
    d. hydrochloride
    liposomal d.
    liposome-encapsulated d. (LED)
    d. and lomustine (DL)
    d., methylprednisolone, cytosine arabinoside, and cisplatin alternating with methotrexate, bleomycin, cyclophosphamide,

    doxorubicin, vincristine, and methylprednisolone
    paclitaxel and d.
    pegylated liposomal d. (PEG-DOXO)
    topotecan, vincristine, d. (TVD)
    d., vinblastine, mechlorethamine, vincristine, bleomycin, etoposide, prednisone
doxorubicin-induced cardiotoxicity
Doxovir
Doxy Caps
Doxychel
Doxycin
doxycycline
Doxy-Tabs
Doxytec
DPD
    dihydropyrimidine dehydrogenase
DPD-inhibitory fluoropyrimidine (DIF)
DPDL
    diffuse poorly differentiated lymphoma
DPPE
    N,N-diethyl-2-[4-(phenylmethyl)phenoxy-]ethanamine.HCl
DPX Bravo bone densitometer
DQB1 allele
DQ gene
DR-70 tumor marker test
DRA
    distal rectal adenocarcinoma
Drabkin solution
dracunculosis, dracunculiasis
drain
    Penrose d.
    vacuum d.
drainage
    abscess d.
    afferent lymphatic d.
    biliary d.
    catheter d.
    d. catheter
    central venous d.
    cutaneous lymphatic d.
    cyst d.
    endoscopic retrograde biliary d. (ERBD)
    gravity d.
    lymphatic d.
    lymph node d.
    manual lymph d. (MLD)
    percussion and postural d. (PPD)
    percutaneous biliary d. (PBD)
    percutaneous catheter d.
    percutaneous transhepatic biliary d. (PTBD)
    pericardial d.

perinephric abscess d.
suction d.
Dramamine
draped
prepped and d.
Drash syndrome
draught
Black D.
DRB1 allele
DRC
DNA repair capacity
DRE
digital rectal examination
dredging
data d.
drepanocytemia
drepanocytic anemia
Dresbach
D. anemia
D. syndrome
Dreschlera
dressing
Acticoat composite d.
Acticoat foam d.
Bard absorption d.
Catrix wound d.
Comfeel hydrocolloid d.
Comfeel plus triangle d.
DuoDERM hydrocolloid d.
Geliperm gel d.
Hydragran absorption d.
hydrocolloid ulcer d.
Lipisorb d.
Mepilex foam d.
Nu-Derm foam island d.
Nu Gauze d.
OpSite d.
RadiaCare Hydrogel Wound D.
Restore hydrocolloid d.
Sorbex hydrocolloid wound d.
Tegaderm d.
thin film d. (TFD)
transparent film d.
ulcer d.
Uniflex d.
VigiFOAM d.
Vigilon gel d.
Dressler syndrome
DRG
diagnostic-related group
drift
antigenic d.
field d.

drink
effervescent d.
Drisdol
drive
sex d.
Drolban
droloxifene
dromostanolone propionate
dronabinol
drooped shoulder
drooping lily sign
drop
Fer-In-Sol D.'s
Lactaid d.'s
d. metastasis
vitamin C d.'s
droperidol and fentanyl
dropout
myofibrillar d.
drotrecogin alfa
drowning
dry d.
Droxia
DRR
digitally reconstructed radiograph
DRS
Delirium Rating Scale
diffuse reflectance spectroscopy
drug
d. absorption
d. action
adjuvant analgesic d.
d. administration
anticancer d.
anticholinergic d.
antimitotic d.
antineoplastic d.
antiretroviral d.
antisense d.
antitumor d.
3-d. antiviral therapy
cardiac d.
chemotherapeutic d.
cholinergic d.
combination d. (CD)
cytotoxic d.
d. delivery
d. delivery system
d. development
disease-modifying antirheumatic d.
(DMARD)
d. dose intensity (DDI)
d. formulation

NOTES

drug *(continued)*
 d. fraction
 d. handling
 d. holiday
 immune-enhancing d.
 immunosuppressive d.
 intravenous cytotoxic d.
 investigational new d. (IND)
 marrow toxic d.
 myelotoxic d.
 nonsaturable d.
 nonsteroidal antiinflammatory d.
  (NSAID)
 osteoporosis prevention d.
 parent d.
 psychomimetic d.
 d. pump
 d. rash
 d. reaction
 d. resistance
 d. resistance protein
 resistant-repellant d.
 Revlimid immunomodulatory d.
 selective apoptotic antineoplastic d.
  (SAAND)
 taxanes class of anticancer d.'s
 d. tolerance
 d. toxicity
drug-binding affinity
drug-induced
 d.-i. alopecia
 d.-i. bone marrow suppression
 d.-i. bullous disorder
 d.-i. drug resistance
 d.-i. immune hemolytic anemia
 d.-i. neutropenia
 d.-i. oxidant injury
 d.-i. SLE
 d.-i. systemic lupus erythematosus
drug-resistant tumor
drug-sensitive cancer
Drummond
 artery of D.
drusen
dry
 d. desquamation
 d. drowning
 d. ice
DS
 double strength
 Bactrim DS
 Septra DS
 Sulfatrim DS
 Tolectin DS
DSG
 deoxyspergualin
DSMC Plus
DSPN
 distal symmetric polyneuropathy

DSRCT
 desmoplastic small round-cell tumor
DSS
 disease-specific survival
D-S-S stool softener
D-Stat flowable hemostat
d4T
 didehydrodeoxythymidine
 didehydrodideoxythymidine, stavudine,
  Zerit
DTaP
 diphtheria and tetanus toxoid with
  acellular pertussis
DTC
 diethyldithiocarbamate
DTD
 delivered total dose
DTH
 delayed-type hypersensitivity
dTHd
 deoxythymidine
DTIC
 dacarbazine
 dimethyltriazenoimidazole carboxamide
  DTIC and actinomycin D (DTIC-
   ACTD)
  Adriamycin and DTIC (ADIC, A-
   DIC)
  bleomycin, vinblastine, DTIC
  DTIC, CCNU, vincristine (DCV)
  cyclophosphamide, vincristine,
   Adriamycin, DTIC (CyVADIC,
   CyVMAD)
  vinblastine, Adriamycin, bleomycin,
   CCNU, DTIC (VABCD)
DTIC-ACTD
 DTIC and actinomycin D
DTIC-Dome
dTK
 2′-deoxythymidine kinase
DTP
 diphtheria, tetanus, pertussis
DTPA
 diethylenetriamine pentaacetic acid
DT-PACE
 dexamethasone, thalidomide plus
  Adriamycin, cyclophosphamide,
  etoposide
DTP-Hib vaccine
dTTP
 2′-deoxythymidine 5′-triphosphate
dual-contrast barium enema (DCBE)
dual-diagnosis patient
dual-energy
 d.-e. radiograph (DER)
 d.-e. x-ray absorptiometry (DEXA,
  DXA)
dual-phase CT scan
duazomycin

Dubin-Johnson phenomenon
Dubreuilh precancerous melanosis
ducreyi
> *Haemophilus d.*

duct
> aberrant intrahepatic bile d.
> alveolar d.
> anicteric bile d.
> asymmetric bile d.
> Bartholin d.
> beaded pancreatic d.
> bile d.
> biliary d.
> d. cell adenocarcinoma
> cribriform salivary carcinoma of
> excretory d.
> cystic d.
> endolymphatic d.
> excretory d.
> extrahepatic bile d. (EHBD)
> intrahepatic bile d.
> main biliary d. (MBD)
> main pancreatic d. (MPD)
> main papillary d.
> mesonephric d.
> müllerian d.
> pancreaticobiliary d.
> subareolar d.
> Wharton d.
> wolffian d.

ductal
> d. adenoma
> d. carcinoma in situ (DCIS)
> d. dilatation
> d. ectasia
> d. epithelial differentiation
> d. hyperplasia
> d. lavage (DL)
> d. microcalcification
> d. papillary carcinoma
> d. papilloma

ductectatic
> d. mucinous cystadenoma
> d. mucinous cystic neoplasm
> d. mucinous tumor

ductectomy
ductography
ductoscopy
> fiberoptic d.

duct-to-mucosa pancreaticojejunostomy
ductule
ductus
> d. arch

d. arteriosus
d. diverticulum
d. infundibulum
silent d.
d. venosus

Duffy
> D. antibody
> D. antigen
> D. blood group

Duke bleeding time
Dukes-Astler-Coller adenocarcinoma
classification
Dukes classification
Dulbecco
> D. Modified Eagle Medium
> (DMEM)
> D. phosphate-buffered saline

Dulcolax
Dull-C
dumbbell
> d. mass
> d. needle
> d. tumor

dumbbell-shaped
> d.-s. spinal cavernous hemangioma
> d.-s. tumor

Dumdum fever
dummy source
dumping syndrome
Duncan syndrome
Dunning prostate carcinoma
duocarmycin antibiotic
Duocet
Duo-Cyp
duodenal
> d. artery
> d. atresia
> d. Brunner gland adenoma
> d. bulb
> d. diaphragm
> d. diverticulum
> d. duplication cyst
> d. filling defect
> d. hernia
> d. loop
> d. narrowing
> d. obstruction
> d. papilla
> d. peptic ulcer disease
> d. seromyectomy
> d. stricture
> d. sweep

D

NOTES

duodenal *(continued)*
    d. ulcer
    d. varix
duodenal-gastric outlet obstruction
duodenitis
    radiation d.
duodenogastroesophageal reflux
duodenography
duodenojejunitis
duodenopancreatectomy
    partial d.
duodenopancreatic fistula
duodenum
DuoDERM hydrocolloid dressing
DuP
    DuP 937 anthrapyrazole
    DuP 996 anthrapyrazole
Duphalac
duplex kidney
Dupont and Lachapelle disease
Durabolin
Duraclon
Duragesic
    D. Transdermal
    D. Transdermal patch
dural
    d. arachnoid lymphoma
    d. arteriovenous fistula
    d. sinus occlusion
    d. sinus thrombosis
    d. sinus thrombosis infarction
    d. tail
    d. venous sinus
Duralone injection
Duralutin
dura mater
Duramorph Injection
Duran-Reynals factor
Duratest Injection
duration
    complete remission d. (CRD)
dURD
    2′-deoxyuridine
Duret hemorrhage
Duricef
Durie-Salmon
    D.-S. classification of multiple myeloma
    D.-S. multiple myeloma classification
    D.-S. myeloma staging
    D.-S. staging system
Durie staging
Duros leuprolide implant
Durotep patch
Dutcher body
DVB
    DDP, vindesine, bleomycin

DVH
    dose-volume histogram
3D-virtual brachytherapy
DVP
    daunorubicin, vincristine, prednisone
    DVP chemotherapy protocol
DVPL-ASP
    daunorubicin, vincristine, prednisone, L-asparaginase
DVT
    deep venous thrombosis
dwell position
DWI
    diffusion-weighted imaging
DX
    diagnosis
DXA *(var. of* DEXA)
    dual-energy x-ray absorptiometry
Dyazide
Dyclone
dyclonine
dye
    ABI fluorescence d.
    blue d.
    d. column
    d. efflux
    Evans blue d.
    d. exclusion assay
    Hoechst d.
    indium-111 capromab pendetide d.
    isosulfan blue d.
    d. laser system
    patent blue V d.
    d. primer-based dideoxy sequencing
    d. reduction spot test
    d. terminator-based dideoxy sequencing
    d. terminator cycle sequencing core kit
    vital blue d.
dying trajectory
Dyke-Young syndrome
Dynabac
Dynabead
Dynal
    D. CELLection system
    D. M450 magnetic bead
dynamic
    d. acquisition
    d. bolus tracking technique
    d. bone scan
    d. cavernosometry
    d. computed tomography (DCT)
    d. contrast-enhanced magnetic resonance imaging (DCE-MRI)
    d. contrast-enhanced MRI
    d. coupling
    d. CT
    d. enhancement

d. image
d. magnetic resonance imaging
d. nuclear polarization
D. Optical Breast Imaging (DOBI)
D. Optical Breast Imaging System
pathogenesis d.
postural d.
d. range
d. stereotactic radiosurgery
d. volume imaging
d. wedge
dynamin protein
Dynapen
dynein protein
Dynepo
Dyrenium
dysadherin
dysarthria syndrome
dysautonomia
dysbaric osteonecrosis
dyschondroplasia
dyschondrosteosis
dyschromia
dyscrasia
dyscrasic fracture
dysdiadochokinesia
dysembryoma
dysembryoplastic neuroepithelial tumor
(DNET, DNT)
dysenteric illness
dysentery
amebic d.
bacillary d.
dysequilibrium
linkage d.
dyserythropoiesis
dyserythropoietic anemia
dysesthesia
dysesthetic pain
dysfibrinogenemia
dysfunction
bladder d.
brain d.
erectile d.
male sexual d.
mitochondrial d.
organic erectile d.
ovarian d.
platelet d.
postoperative bladder d.
qualitative platelet d.
renal d.
salivary gland d.

sexual d.
Trial on Reversing Endothelial D.
(TREND)
urinary d.
dysgenesis
d. of corpus callosum
cortical d.
epiphysial d.
ovarian d.
reticular d.
dysgenetic
dysgerminoma
d. germ cell tumor
ovarian d.
pineal d.
dysgeusia
dysglycemia
dysgranulocytopoiesis
dyshematopoiesis
dyshormonogenetic goiter
dysjunction
dyskaryosis
dyskeratoma
warty d.
dyskeratosis, pl. **dyskeratoses**
d. congenita
dyskeratotic keratinocyte
dyskinesis
dysmaturity
dysmegakaryocytopoiesis
dysmenorrhea
dysmorphism
dysmotility
esophageal d.
dysmyelinating disease
dysmyelination
dysmyelopoietic syndrome
dysontogenetic neoplasm
dysostosis, pl. **dysostoses**
epiphysial d.
dyspareunia
dysphagia
cricopharyngeal d.
dysplasia
acetabular residual d.
bone d.
bronchopulmonary d.
cervical d.
cystic d.
diaphysial d.
d. dislocation
ectodermal d.
d. epiphysealis hemimelica

D

NOTES

dysplasia *(continued)*
    d. epiphysealis multiplex
    epiphysial d.
    epithelial d.
    high-grade d. (HGD)
    low-grade d. (LGD)
    Meyer d.
    Mondini d.
    monostotic fibrous d.
    multiple epiphysial d. (MED)
    periapical cemental d.
    polyostotic fibrous d.
    postradiation d. (PRD)
dysplasia-associated lesion or mass (DALM)
dysplastic
    d. cerebellar gangliocytoma
    d. cortical hyperostosis
    d. leukoplakia lesion
    d. nevus

    d. nevus syndrome (DNS)
    d. nevus syndrome, familial type
dyspnea
dyspneic
dysproteinemia
    angioimmunoblastic
      lymphadenopathy with d. (AILD)
dysregulation
    central thermal d.
dysrhythmia
dyssynergia
dystonia
dystonic reaction
dystrophic calcification
dystrophy
    sympathetic d.
    twenty-nail d. (TND)
DZAPO
    daunorubicin, azacitidine, ara-C,
      prednisone, Oncovin

E

E antigen
cyclin E
immunoglobulin E (IgE)
E rosette
E rosette assay
E rosette negative
E rosette receptor
E subtype
E subtype of HIV

E₁

prostaglandin E_1

E1A gene
E1B gene
E2A

E2A oncogene
E2A protooncogene/oncogene

E5 protein
E6 protein
E7 protein
E-12

keratin 34 E-12

EA

ethacrynic acid

EAC

Ehrlich ascites carcinoma
erythema annulare centrifugum
external auditory canal
EAC rosette assay

E:A change
eAdHCC

early advanced hepatocellular carcinoma

eagle

E. basal medium
E. minimum essential medium

EAOC

endometriosis-associated ovarian
carcinoma

EAP

etoposide, Adriamycin, Platinol

ear

e. implant
middle e.
e. tumor

Earle L fibrosarcoma
early

e. advanced hepatocellular
carcinoma (eAdHCC)
e. antigen
E. Breast Cancer Trialists'
Collaborative Group (EBCTCG)
e. detection
E. Detection Research Network
(EDRN)
e. gastric cancer

e. gastric cancer of upper stomach
(EGCUS)
e. hepatocellular carcinoma (eHCC)
immediate e. (IE)
e. prostate cancer antigen (EPCA)
e. satiety
e. stromal invasion

Easprin
Eastern Cooperative Oncology Group
(ECOG)
EATL

enteropathy-associated T-cell lymphoma

Eaton agent
Eaton-Lambert

E.-L. muscular weakness
E.-L. myasthenic syndrome

ebaf protein
EBAP

Eldisine, BCNU, Adriamycin, prednisone

EBB

endobronchial brachytherapy

EBCTCG

Early Breast Cancer Trialists'
Collaborative Group

EBD

extragenital Bowen disease

EBER

Epstein-Barr early RNA

EBER-positive cell
EBF

erythroblastosis fetalis

EB-IORT

electron beam intraoperative radiation
therapy

EBNA

Epstein-Barr nuclear antigen
EBNA test

Ebola

E. fever
E. virus

Ebola-Marburg virus
EBRT

external beam radiation therapy

EBV

electron boost volume
epirubicin, bleomycin, vinblastine
Epstein-Barr virus

EBV-induced lymphoproliferative disease
EC

electron capture
endometrial carcinoma
endothelial cell
epithelial cell
Escherichia coli
esophageal candidiasis

EC *(continued)*
    extracellular
        Videx EC
E-cadherin
        E-c. adhesion molecule
        E-c. expression
        E-c. mutation
ECAM
    energy conservation and activity
      management
ECaP
    exceptional cancer patient
ecarin clotting time (ECT)
ECAT
    European Concerted Action on
      Thrombosis
ECBO
    enteric cytopathogenic bovine orphan
ECC
    enterochromaffin cell
ecchymosis, pl. **ecchymoses**
ecchymotic
eccrine
    e. carcinoma
    e. hidradenitis
    e. poroma
    e. sweat gland
ECG, EKG
    electrocardiogram
echinacea
echinocandin antifungal
echinococcosis
    alveolar e.
Echinococcus
    E. alveolaris
    E. cysticus
    E. granulosus
    E. multilocularis
echinocyte
echinomycin
ECHO
    enterocytopathogenic human orphan
      ECHO virus
echo
    asymmetric e.
    field e.
    gradient-recalled e. (GRE)
    magnitude preparation-rapid
      acquisition gradient e.
    e. planar imaging (EPI)
    e. planar MRI
echocardiography
    aortic valve e.
    B-mode e.
echoendoscope
    Olympus GF-UM30P e.
echogenic
    e. nodule
    e. plug

echogenicity
    high e.
echolalia
echolucent pattern
echonography
echopenic
    e. appearance
    e. liver metastasis
EchoSeed brachytherapy seed
echo-time (TE)
echovirus *(var. of* ECHO virus*)*
Eclipse blood collection needle
ECM
    extracellular matrix
ECMO
    enteric cytopathogenic monkey orphan
      ECMO virus
ECMV
    etoposide, Cytoxan, methotrexate,
      vincristine
ECOG
    Eastern Cooperative Oncology Group
ecology
    mucosal e.
econazole
Ecostatin
ecotaxis
Ecotrin
ECP
    extracorporeal photochemotherapy
ECRL
    extensor carpi radialis longus
ECT
    ecarin clotting time
    electrochemotherapy
    electroconvulsive therapy
    emission computed tomography
      ECT test card
ectasia
    benign duct e.
    bilateral ductal e.
    ductal e.
    gastric antral vascular e.
    mucinous duct e.
    scleral e.
ectatic
    e. bronchus
    e. carotid artery
ecteinascidin
ecthyma
ectoapyrases class of anticlotting agents
ectocervix
ectocyst
ectoderm
ectodermal dysplasia
ectoenzyme
ectomesenchyme
ectoparasitic infection

ectopia, ectopy
cerebellar e.
e. cordis
e. testis
ectopic
e. ACTH syndrome
e. anus
e. calcification
e. craniopharyngioma
e. Cushing syndrome
e. kidney
e. meningioma
e. nevus
e. ossification
e. pancreas
e. parathyroid
e. parathyroid adenoma
e. pinealoma
e. pregnancy
e. spleen
e. tissue
e. ureterocele
ectromelia
ectropion
eczema
atopic e.
ED
ethyldichloroarsine
EDAM
10-ethyl-10-deazaaminopterin
EDAP
etoposide, dexamethasone, ara-C, Platinol
edatrexate
Edecrin
Edelmann
E. anemia
E. cell
edema
alveolar pulmonary e.
arm e.
brain e.
brainstem e.
breast e.
cerebral e.
cytotoxic e.
macular e.
marrow e.
e. pattern
peritumoral brain e.
pulmonary e. (PE)
stromal e.
white matter e.
edematous pancreatitis

edentulous
edetate calcium disodium
EDL
extensor digitorum longus
Edman degradation procedure
Edmondson grade
Edmondson-Steiner
E.-S. grading system
E.-S. histologic grading
E.-S. histologic grading of
hepatocellular carcinoma
Edmonton
E. Staging System
E. Symptom Assessment Scale
(ESAS)
EDR
extreme drug resistance
EDR assay
edrecolomab
EDRN
Early Detection Research Network
EDTA
ethylene diamine tetraacetic acid
EDTMP
ethylene diamine tetramethylene
phosphonic acid
education
Alliance for Lung Cancer
Advocacy, Support, and E.
(ALCASE)
EEG
electroencephalogram
EEPLND
extraperitoneal endoscopic pelvic lymph
node dissection
E.E.S.
E.E.S. Chewable
E.E.S. Granules
efaproxiral
efavirenz
effect
abscopal e.
antiapoptotic e.
anticachectic e.
antiproliferative e.
antitumor e.
autocrine e.
beam-hardening e.
Bremsstrahlung e.
cardioprotective e.
cell-cycle e.
central neurologic adverse e.
clinical cardioprotective e.

E

NOTES

189

effect *(continued)*
    cohort e.
    cumulative radiation e. (CRE)
    cutaneous adverse drug e.
    cytopathic e.
    cytotoxic e.
    dose rate e.
    Fahraeus-Lindqvist e.
    genitourinary adverse e.
    graft versus immunocompetent
      cell e.
    graft versus leukemia e.
    graft versus lymphoma e.
    graft versus myeloma e.
    graft versus tumor e.
    granulocyte priming e.
    hematologic adverse e.
    HIV-1 cytopathic e.
    human immunodeficiency virus 1
      cytopathic e.
    immune anticancer e.
    immune-mediated antileukemia e.
    immunomodulating e.
    immunostimulatory e.
    isotope e.
    ladder e.
    log e.
    lymphangiography e.
    e. modifiers
    multilog e.
    neurologic adverse e.
    paracrine e.
    penumbral e.
    peripheral neurologic adverse e.
    physiochemical e.
    pulmonary adverse e.
    radiation e.
    sausage segment e.
    side e.
    skin-sparing e.
    stalk section e.
    teratogenic e.
    topical e.
    tumoricidal e.
    Venturi e.
effective
    e. dose
    e. half-life
    e. pathlength (EPL)
    e. renal plasma flow
    e. transverse relation time
effectiveness
    relative biological e. (RBE)
effector
    e. cell
    linkage e.
    e. mechanism
effector/target cell interaction

effeminate
efferent loop
Effer-K
Effer-Syllium
effervescent
    e. citrocarbonate granule
    e. drink
    K + Care E.
    K-Electrolyte E.
    K-Gen E.
    Klorvess E.
    K-Lyte E.
    potassium bicarbonate and
      potassium chloride e.
    potassium bicarbonate and
      potassium citrate e.
Effexor
Effexor-XR
efficacy study
efficient relaxation time
effluvium
    anagen e.
    telogen e.
efflux
    dye e.
effusion
    bilateral knee e.'s
    chocolate joint e.
    epidural e.
    exudative pleural e.
    joint e.
    knee e.
    e. lymphoma
    malignant e.
    pericardial e.
    pleural e.
    serous e.
effusion-associated mononuclear cell
effusive pericarditis
EFGR
    epidermal growth factor receptor
eflornithine (DMFO)
EFP
    etoposide, 5-fluorouracil, Platinol
EFS
    event-free survival
EFT
    Ewing family of tumors
Efudex Topical
EG
    esophagogastric
    EG junction
EGCg
    epigallocatechin gallate
EGCT
    extragonadal germ cell tumor
EGCUS
    early gastric cancer of upper stomach

EGF
    endothelial growth factor
    epidermal growth factor
EGFP
    enhanced green fluorescent protein
EGFR
    epidermal growth factor receptor
      EGFR gene
EGF-receptor specific monoclonal antibody
EGFR-TKI
    epidermal growth factor-tyrosine kinase inhibitor
eggshell calcification
egophony
EGP-2 glycoprotein
Egr-1 transcription factor
EGS
    extragonadal seminoma
EH
    endometrial hyperplasia
    epithelioid hemangioendothelioma
EHBD
    extrahepatic bile duct
eHCC
    early hepatocellular carcinoma
EHL
    electrohydraulic lithotripsy
    extensor hallucis longus
Ehrlich
    E. ascites carcinoma (EAC)
    E. hemoglobinemia body
    E. theory
    E. theory of antibody formation
Ehrlichia canis
ehrlichiosis
EIA
    enzyme immunoassay
    Calypte HIV-1 urine EIA
    Dimertest EIA
    Platelia Aspergillus EIA
EIC
    extensive intraductal component
Eichhorst corpuscle
eicosanoid fatty acid
eicosapentaenoic acid
eighth
    e. cranial nerve deafness
    e. cranial nerve tumor
EIN
    endometrial intraepithelial neoplasia
Eindhoven Cancer Registry

Einhorn regimen
einsteinium-255 (^{255}Es)
EIPV
    enhanced inactivated polio vaccine
EIS
    electrical impedance scanning
EIT
    electrical impedance tomography
ejaculate
ejaculation
    antegrade e.
    retrograde e.
ejaculatory duct cyst
EKG (*var. of* ECG)
Elase Ointment
elasticum
    pseudoxanthoma e.
elasticus
    conus e.
elastic van Gieson stain
elastofibroma
elastography
    magnetic resonance e. (MRE)
elastosis
    vascular e.
Elavil
elbow
    e. fracture
    e. joint
Eldercaps
Elder malignant melanoma classification
Eldisine
    E., BCNU, Adriamycin, prednisone (EBAP)
    Platinol, cyclophosphamide, E. (PCE)
elective
    e. lymphadenectomy
    e. lymph node dissection (ELND)
electric
    General E. (GE)
electrical
    e. impedance breast scanning
    e. impedance scanning (EIS)
    e. impedance tomography (EIT)
electrocardiography
electrocautery
    endoluminal radiofrequency e.
electrochemotherapy (ECT)
electrocoagulation
electroconvulsive therapy (ECT)

E

NOTES

electrode
    LeVeen radiofrequency ablation
      needle e.
    polarographic needle e.
electrodesiccation
    light e.
electroencephalogram (EEG)
electroencephalograph
electroencephalography
electrohydraulic lithotripsy (EHL)
electromagnet
electromagnetic (EM)
    e. absorption
    e. field (EMF)
    e. modeling
    e. radiation
    e. radiation exposure
    e. spectrum
    e. wave
electromotive force
electromyogram (EMG)
electromyography (EMG)
    perineal sphincter e.
electron
    e. arc technique
    auger e.
    e. beam
    e. beam boost field
    e. beam intraoperative radiation
      therapy (EB-IORT)
    e. beam radiation therapy
    e. boost volume (EBV)
    e. capture (EC)
    e. microscopy
    e. paramagnetic resonance (EPR)
    e. paramagnetic resonance
      spectroscopy
    e. spin
    e. spin resonance
    e. transport chain defect
    e. volt (eV)
electron-arc radiotherapy
electron-dense core
electron-denserex
electroneuromyography
electronic
    e. magnification
    e. portal imaging
    e. portal imaging device
electrooptical device
electropermeabilization
electropherogram
electrophile
    unstable e.
electrophilic species
electrophoresis
    agar gel e.
    alkaline e.
    capillary e.

    citrate agar e.
    2-dimensional polyacrylamide gel e.
    field inversion gel e.
    hemoglobin e.
    isoelectric focusing polyacrylamide
      gel in e. (IEF-PAGE)
    moving boundary e.
    Paragon immunofixation e.
    polyacrylamide gel e. (PAGE)
    protein e.
    serum protein e.
    single-cell gel e. (SCGE)
Electrophysiologic Study Versus
** Electrocardiographic Monitoring**
** (ESVEM)**
electroporation of cells
electrospray ionization mass
** spectroscopy**
electrostatic
    e. imaging
    e. imaging system
electrostimulation for nonunion of
** fracture**
electrovibratory device
elegans
    Caenorhabditis e.
element
    chondromatous e.
    estrogen-response e. (ERE)
    glandular e.
    human leukocyte antigen
      restriction e.
    myeloid blood e.
    nonhematopoietic e.
    promoter e.
    restriction e.
    REV response e. (RRE)
    Rex-responsive e. (RXRE)
    stromal e.
    tax-responsive e.
    volume e.
    voxel e.
elementary
    e. body
    e. fracture
elephantiasis neuromatosa
eleutherobin
elevated
    e. bilirubin level
    e. serum lactate dehydrogenase
    e. transaminase
elevation
    prolactin e.
ELF
    etoposide, leucovorin, 5-fluorouracil
elicited response
ELIEDA
    enzyme-linked immunoelectrodiffusion
    assay

Eligard
elimination
    e. curve
    e. half-life
ELISA
    enzyme-linked immunosorbent assay
    Asserachrom D-Di ELISA
    CrossLaps One Step ELISA
ELISPOT
    enzyme-linked immunospot
    ELISPOT assay
Elitek
ellagic acid
Ellence
Elliott's B solution
elliptical
ellipticine
elliptinium
elliptocyte
elliptocytosis
    common hereditary e.
    hereditary e. (HE)
elliptocytotic anemia
ELND
    elective lymph node dissection
Eloxatin
elsamitrucin
Elspar
El Tor vibrio
Eltroxin
elution
    acid e.
EM
    electromagnetic
    EM field
EMA
    epithelial membrane antigen
EMA-CO, EMACO
    etoposide, methotrexate, actinomycin D, cyclophosphamide, Oncovin
Embden-Meyerhof metabolic pathway
embedding
    paraffin block e.
    plastic block e.
embolectomy
emboli (*pl. of* embolus)
embolic
    e. disease
    e. infarction
    e. phenomenon
    e. reflux
    e. stroke

embolism
    air e.
    amniotic fluid e.
    catheter e.
    cerebral e.
    pulmonary e. (PE)
    tumor e.
embolization
    bronchial artery e.
    hepatic arterial e.
    particulate e.
    portal vein e. (PVE)
    renal artery e.
    transcatheter arterial e. (TAE)
    transcatheter splenic e.
    transcutaneous e.
embolize
embolotherapy
    balloon e.
embolus, pl. emboli
    intralymphatic emboli
    e. migration
    paradoxical e.
Embosphere microsphere
embryo
    adnexal e.
    e. transfer (ET)
embryology
    breast e.
    reproductive tract e.
    urogenital e.
embryonal
    e. adenoma
    e. carcinoma
    e. carcinosarcoma
    e. hematopoiesis
    e. leukemia
    e. remnant
    e. remnant of urachus
    e. rhabdomyosarcoma
    e. sarcoma
    e. teratoma
    e. tumor
    e. tumor of ciliary body
embryonic
    e. cell
    e. period
    e. tumor
embryopathy
EMC
    extraskeletal myxoid chondrosarcoma
Emcyt
emedullate

E

NOTES

Emend
emergency
    metabolic e.
    oncologic e.
    surgical e.
    urologic e.
Emerson-Segal Medimizer demand nebulizer
emesis
    Morrow Assessment of Nausea and E. (MANE)
emetic response
emetogenic
EMF
    electromagnetic field
EMG
    electromyogram
    electromyography
emissary sphenoidal foramen
emission
    e. computed tomography (ECT)
    e. range
EMIT
    enzyme-multiplied immunoassay technique
emitter
emivirine
EMLA
    eutectic mixture of local anesthetics
    EMLA cream
emotional
    e. functioning
    e. state
    e. support services
EMP
    estramustine phosphate
    extramedullary plasmacytoma
emperipolesis
emphysema
    bullous e.
    compensatory e.
    subcutaneous e.
emphysematous
    e. bleb
    e. bulla
    e. cholecystitis
    e. cystitis
    e. gastritis
    e. pyelonephritis
empiric therapy
Empirin with Codeine
Empracet
Empracet-30
Empracet-60
emptying
    delayed gastric e. (DGE)
empty sella syndrome

empyema
    epidural e.
    Müller e.
EMR
    endoscopic mucosal resection
Emtec
Emtec-30
emtricitabine
emulsion
    Biafine wound dressing e.
    magnesium hydroxide and mineral oil e.
    W/O/W e.
Emulsoil
E-MVAC
    escalated methotrexate, vinblastine, Adriamycin, cisplatin
E-Mycin
E-Mycin-E
en
    en bloc
    en bloc esophagectomy
    en bloc excision
    en bloc resection
    en face
enanthate
    testosterone e.
enantiomer
ENB
    esthesioneuroblastoma
Enbrel
Encap
    Novo-Rythro E.
encapsulated
    e. cyst
    e. fluid
    e. gas bubble
    T4 enolase V, liposome e.
encapsulation
encasement
    ventricular e.
    vessel e.
encephalic angioma
encephalitis, pl. **encephalitides**
    brainstem e.
    cytomegalovirus e.
    herpes simplex e.
    HIV e.
    limbic e.
    multifocal e.
    progressive multifocal e.
    subacute e.
    Toxoplasma e.
    Venezuelan equine e. (VEE)
Encephalitozoon cuniculi
encephalocele
encephalography
    air e.
encephaloid cancer

encephalomalacia
encephalomyelitis
    acute disseminated e.
    paraneoplastic e.
encephalomyelopathy
encephalomyopathy
    mitochondrial e.
encephalopathia subcorticalis progressiva
encephalopathy
    acute e.
    anoxic e.
    HIV e.
    ifosfamide e.
    Wernicke e.
encephalotrigeminal
    e. angiomatosis
    e. syndrome
enchondral ossification
enchondroma
enchondromatosis
enchondrosarcoma
encoding
    centrally ordered phase e.
encroachment
encrustation
    bile e.
end
    e. colostomy
    e. exhalation
    e. expiration
    e. inhalation
endarterectomy
    carotid e. (CEA)
endarteritis obliterans
end-diastolic
    e.-d. sphericity index
    e.-d. velocity measurement
endemic
    e. Burkitt lymphoma
    e. population
endemicum
    granuloma e.
end-labeling
    in situ DNA nick e.-l.
endobiliary stent
endobronchial
    e. biopsy
    e. brachytherapy (EBB)
    e. cancer
    e. lesion
    e. stent
    e. tuberculosis
endocardiac

endocardial
    e. cushion defect
    e. cushion development
    e. cushion-type ventricular septal
      defect
    e. fibroelastosis
endocarditis
    Aspergillus e.
    bacterial e.
    Candida e.
    Libman-Sacks e.
    marantic e.
    nonbacterial e.
    paraneoplastic e.
endocardium
Endocare renal cryoablation
EndoCatch bag
endocatheter ruler
endocavitary
    e. irradiation
    e. radiation
endocervical
    e. canal colonoscopy
    e. curettage
    e. interleukin
    e. mucosa
endocervix
Endocet
endochondral ossification
endochondroma
EndoCoil biliary stent
endocrine
    e. abnormality
    e. cell micronest
    e. exophthalmos
    e. imaging
    e. neoplasia
    e. pancreatic tumor (EPT)
    e. system
    e. therapy
    e. toxicity
endocrinoplasia
    multiple e.
endocyst
endocytic pathway
endocytosis
Endodan
endoderm
endodermal
    e. sinus
    e. sinus tumor
endoesophageal stent

E

NOTES

195

end-of-life
> e.-o.-l. care
> e.-o.-l. issues

endofluoroscopic technique

endofluoroscopy
> flexible e.

Endogen Human VEGF ELISA kit

endogenous
> e. antigen
> e. bacteria
> e. biotin activity
> e. flora
> e. GAD inhibitor
> e. hormone
> e. inhibitor of angiogenesis
> e. lipid pneumonia
> e. peroxidase activity
> e. retrovirus (ERV)
> e. retrovirus 3 (ERV3)

Endo-GIA stapler

endoglin

endoglycosidase

endoileostomy

endolarynx

endoluminal
> e. boost
> e. brachytherapy
> e. radiofrequency electrocautery
> e. sonography
> e. stent
> e. ultrasound

endolymphatic
> e. duct
> e. sac
> e. sac tumor
> e. stromal myosis

endometria (*pl. of* endometrium)

endometrial
> e. adenoacanthoma
> e. adenosquamous carcinoma
> e. biopsy
> e. cancer
> e. carcinoma (EC)
> e. cavity
> e. chemical shift imaging
> e. hyperplasia (EH)
> e. intraepithelial neoplasia (EIN)
> e. island
> e. jet washing
> e. polyp
> e. secretory adenocarcinoma
> e. stromal sarcoma (ESS)
> e. thickness

endometrioid
> e. adenocarcinoma
> e. adenocarcinomatous component
> e. carcinoma
> e. tumor

endometrioma

endometriosis
> bladder e.

endometriosis-associated ovarian carcinoma (EAOC)

endometriotic cyst

endometritis

endometrium, pl. **endometria**

endomyelography

endomyocardial
> e. biopsy
> e. fibroplasia
> e. fibrosis

endomysium

endoneural

endoneurium

endonuclease

endonucleolytic cleavage event

Endopap endometrial sampler

endopeptidase
> neutral e.

endophthalmitis
> candidal e.
> granulomatous e.

endophytic lesion

endophytum-type tumor

endoplasmic
> e. reticulum
> e. reticulum insertion signal sequence

endoprosthesis
> biliary e.
> endoscopic biliary e.
> Wallstent biliary e.

endoproteolytic cleavage

endopyelotomy

endorectal
> e. coil
> e. coil magnetic resonance imaging
> e. MR imaging
> e. ultrasonography (EUS)
> e. ultrasound

endoreduplication

end-organ resistance

endorphin

endosalpingosis

endoscope
> light-induced fluorescence e.
> lung imaging fluorescence e. (LIFE)
> Olympus GIF-2T20 end-viewing e.

endoscopic
> e. biliary endoprosthesis
> e. biopsy
> e. decompression
> e. frontal craniotomy
> e. laser
> e. mucosal resection (EMR)
> e. procedure
> e. removal

e. removal of duodenal Brunner gland adenoma
e. retrograde biliary drainage (ERBD)
e. retrograde cannulation
e. retrograde cholangiopancreatography (ERCP)
e. sinus surgery
e. sonography
e. surveillance
e. ultrasonography (EUS)
e. ultrasound (EUS)

endoscopy
5-aminolevulinic acid-induced fluorescence e. (AFE)
capsule video e.
colorectal cancer e.
intraoperative e. (IOE)
light-induced fluorescence e.
lung imaging fluorescent e. (LIFE)
percutaneous e.
video e.

endosonography
anal e.
e. probe
rectal e.

endostatin
e. assay
e. protein

endosteal
e. chondrosarcoma
e. scalloping

endosteum
endothelia (*pl. of* endothelium)
endothelial
e. barrier
e. cell (EC)
e. cell growth inhibitor
e. damage
e. growth factor (EGF)
e. injury
e. leukocyte
e. localization of antigen
e. myeloma

endothelialization
endothelin-receptor antagonist
endothelium, pl. **endothelia**
capillary e.

endothelium-derived relaxing factor
endothorax
endotoxin
endotracheal (ET)

e. intubation
e. tube

endourological therapy
endovaginal
e. sonography
e. ultrasonography

endovascular
e. proliferation
e. technique

Endoxan
Endoxan-Asta
endplate sclerosis
endpoint
multiple e.'s

Endrate
end-stage
e.-s. cell
e.-s. dementia
e.-s. renal disease

end-to-end anastomosis
end-to-side
e.-t.-s. anastomosis
e.-t.-s. portacaval shunt

Enduron
enema
air contrast barium e.
barium e.
double-contrast barium e. (DCBE)
dual-contrast barium e. (DCBE)
Fleet E.
Rowasa e.

Enemol
energy
beam e.
binding e.
e. conservation and activity management (ECAM)
e. level
e. pulsing
universal life e.

ENF
enfuvirtide

enflurane
enfuvirtide (ENF)
engager
bispecific T-cell e.

engineering
genetic e.

engrafted allogenic tissue
engraftment
allogeneic e.
delayed e.
donor cell e.

E

NOTES

engraftment *(continued)*
  hematologic e.
  hematopoietic e.
  myeloid e.
  neutrophil e.
  trilineage e.
  white blood cell e.
engulfment
enhanced
  e. green fluorescent protein (EGFP)
  e. inactivated polio vaccine (EIPV)
enhancement
  acoustic e.
  antibody-dependent e.
  dynamic e.
  evanescent e.
  hybrid rapid acquisition with
    relaxation e. (HRARE)
  immune e.
  immunologic e.
  leptomeningeal e.
  paramagnetic e.
  peripheral e.
  pharmacokinetic e.
  punctate e.
  radiation e.
  ring of e.
  e. ring
enhancing brain lesion
eniluracil
  5-fluorouracil plus e.
  e. inhibitor
enisoprost
enlarged placenta
enlargement
  adenomyosis in uterine e.
  air space e.
  apical cardiac nodal e.
  azygos vein e.
  bulbous e.
  cervical e.
  clitoris e.
  diffuse hepatic e.
  diffuse thymic e.
  epiglottic e.
  extraocular muscle e.
  gland e.
  heptic e.
  hilar e.
  nodal e.
  parathyroid gland e.
  parotid gland e.
  salivary gland e.
  thymic e.
  uterine e.
enloplatin
Enneking
  E. stage of bone tumors (I–III)

  E. stage I–III
  E. staging I–III
enocitabine
enolase
  neuron-specific e. (NSE)
enostosis
enoxacin
enpromate
ensiform process
Ensure nutritional supplement
Entamoeba histolytica
enteral
  e. feeding
  e. feeding tube
  e. nutrition
  e. nutritional supplement
enteric
  e. cyst
  e. cytopathogenic,
    enterocytopathogenic
  e. cytopathogenic bovine orphan
    (ECBO)
  e. cytopathogenic human orphan
  e. cytopathogenic monkey orphan
    (ECMO)
  e. fistula
  e. pathogen
  e. stricture
enteritidis
  Salmonella e.
enteritis
  chemotherapy e.
  cryptosporidiosis e.
  e. follicularis
  granulomatous e.
  radiation e.
Enterobacter
  E. aerogenes
  E. agglomerans
  E. cloacae
  E. gergoviae
  E. liquefaciens
  E. vermicularis
Enterobacteriaceae
enterochromaffin cell (ECC)
enteroclysis
enterococcus, pl. **enterococci**
enterocolic fistula
enterocolitis
  Clostridium difficile e.
  neutropenic e. (NE)
enterocutaneous fistula
enterocyte
  transferase e.
enterocytopathogenic *(var. of* enteric
  cytopathogenic)
  e. human orphan (ECHO)
enteroenteric fistula
enterogenous cyst

enterolith
enteropancreatic malignancy
enteropathica
  acrodermatitis e.
enteropathy
  AIDS e.
  protein-losing e.
enteropathy-associated T-cell lymphoma (EATL)
enteroscope
  dedicated push e.
enteroscopy
  small bowel e.
enterospinal fistula
enterostomy
  percutaneous e.
enterovaginal fistula
enterovesical fistula
enthesis
entity
  clade-specific clinical e.
Entrophen
entry
  chemokine receptor-mediated viral e.
  portal of e.
enucleation
  tumor e.
Enulose
enumeration
  cellular e.
enuresis
env
  e. antigen
  e. glycoprotein
  e. protein
envelope
  e. antibody
  fascial e.
  e. glycoprotein B gene
  glycosylated protein spanning viral e. (gp41)
  gp160 e.
  isodose e.
  e. protein
env/gag/pol
  vaccinia-HIV e./g./p.
environment
  nurse cell e.
  social e.
environmental
  e. factor
  e. tobacco smoke (ETS)

Enzinger and Weiss system
Enzone
enzootic transmission
enzymatically recycling assay
enzyme
  angiotensin-converting e. (ACE)
  c-kit e.
  COX-1 e.
  COX-2 e.
  cytochrome e.
  cytochrome P450 e. (CYP)
  demethylase e.
  DNA topoisomerase type II e.
  hepatic microsomal e.
  e. immunoassay (EIA)
  immunoglobulin-complexed e. (ICE)
  key terminal e.
  metalloproteinase-proteolytic e.
  mitochondrial hydroxylase e.
  mitochondrial respiratory chain e.
  NADPH e.
  NOX e.
  O-glycanase e.
  proteolytic e.
  recombinant N-glycanase glycerol-free e.
  restriction e.
  stratum corneum chymotryptic e.
  e. telomerase
enzyme-linked
  e.-l. immunoelectrodiffusion assay (ELIEDA)
  e.-l. immunosorbent assay (ELISA)
  e.-l. immunospot (ELISPOT)
  e.-l. immunospot assay
enzyme-multiplied immunoassay technique (EMIT)
EOC
  epithelial ovarian cancer
EORTC
  European Organization for Research and Treatment of Cancer
  EORTC index
  EORTC QLQ-C30
eosin
  hematoxylin and e. (H&E)
  e. stain
eosinophil chemotactic factor
eosinophilia
  paraneoplastic e.
  pulmonary infiltration with e.
  tropical e.
  tumor-associated tissue e. (TATE)

E

NOTES

eosinophilic
    e. adenoma
    e. cystitis
    e. endomyocardial fibroplasia
    e. fibrohistiocytic lesion
    e. fibrohistiocytosis
    e. gastroenteritis
    e. granuloma
    e. leukemia
    e. leukocyte
    e. myelocyte
    e. pneumonia

EP
    etoposide and Platinol

EPCA
    early prostate cancer antigen
    ProstaMark EPCA

Ep-CAM glycoprotein

EPE
    extraprostatic extension

ependymal cyst

ependymitis
    bacterial e.
    e. granularis

ependymoblastoma

ependymoma
    anaplastic e.
    brainstem e.
    clear cell e. (CCE)
    extraventricular supratentorial e.
    intracranial e.
    myxopapillary e.
    sacrococcygeal myxopapillary e.
    subcutaneous sacrococcygeal
      myxopapillary e.

ephedra

ephedrine

EPI
    echo planar imaging

epi-ADR
    epinephrine and Adriamycin

epicardial system

epicenter

epicondylar fracture

epicondyle

epidemic parotitis

epidemiological
    e. data
    e. study
    e. surveillance strategy

epidemiology
    biochemical e.
    molecular e.

epidermal
    e. growth factor (EGF)
    e. growth factor receptor (EFGR, EGFR)
    e. growth factor receptor gene

    e. growth factor-tyrosine kinase inhibitor (EGFR-TKI)
    e. nevus

epidermic pearl

epidermidis
    Staphylococcus e.

epidermis, pl. epidermides

epidermitis

epidermodysplasia verruciformis

epidermoid
    e. carcinoma
    e. carcinoma of anal margin
    e. carcinoma of vulva
    cerebellar e.
    e. inclusion cyst
    e. tumor

epidermoidoma
    intradural e.
    prepontine white e.

epididymal
    e. cyst
    e. descent
    e. fibrosarcoma
    e. mesothelioma

epididymis, pl. epididymides
    e. lesion

epididymitis

epididymoorchitis

epidoxorubicin (EPIDX)

epidural
    e. abscess
    e. analgesia
    e. anesthesia
    e. anesthetic
    e. angiolipoma
    e. arachnoid cyst
    e. block
    e. cavernous hemangioma
    e. effusion
    e. empyema
    e. extramedullary lesion
    e. fibrosis
    e. hematoma
    e. infusion
    e. injection
    e. lipomatosis
    e. meningitis
    e. pneumatosis
    e. space
    e. spinal cord compression (ESCC)

EPIDX
    epidoxorubicin

epigallocatechin gallate (EGCg)

epigastric
    e. region
    e. vein

epigastrium

epigenetic mechanism

epiglottic
    e. enlargement
    e. fold
epiglottis
epiglottitis
    bacterial e.
epiglycanin
epilarynx
epilation
epiluminescence microscopy
Epimorph
epinephrine
    e. and Adriamycin (epi-ADR)
    cisplatin and e.
epipharynx
epiphenomena
epiphora
epiphysial
    e. dysgenesis
    e. dysostosis
    e. dysplasia
    e. growth plate
    e. line
    e. ossification center
    e. overgrowth
    e. plate fracture
    e. plate injury
    e. slip fracture
    e. tibial fracture
epiphysis, pl. **epiphyses**
    ball-and-socket e.
    balloon e.
epiphysitis
epiploia
epiploic, pl. **epiploicae**
    e. foramen
epipodophyllotoxin
epipropidine
epiroprim
epirubicin
    e., bleomycin, vinblastine (EBV)
    e. hydrochloride
    e. injection
epistaxis
    Gull renal e.
epithalamus
epithelia (*pl. of* epithelium)
epithelial
    e. cancer of ovary
    e. cell (EC)
    e. cell nevus
    e. colonic polyp
    e. cyst

    e. degenerative change
    e. dysplasia
    e. hyperplasia
    e. marker
    e. membrane antigen (EMA)
    e. metaplasia
    e. neoplasm
    e. ovarian cancer (EOC)
    e. pearl
    e. toxicity
    e. transcytosis
    e. tumor
epithelial-cell based posttransplant genotyping
epithelialization
epithelial-rich thymoma
epithelioglandular organ
epithelioid
    e. angiomatosis
    e. hemangioendothelioma (EH)
    e. hemangioma
    e. leiomyoma
    e. mesothelioma
    e. osteosarcoma
    e. sarcoma
epithelioma
    calcifying e.
    e. cuniculatum
    e. of Ferguson-Smith
epitheliotropism
epithelium, pl. **epithelia**
    ameloblastic e.
    atypical e.
    Barrett e. (BE)
    breast cancer e.
    bronchial e.
    colonic e.
    columnar e.
    germinal e.
    glandular e.
    medullary duct e.
    metaplastic e.
    odontogenic e.
    oral mucosal e.
    ovarian e.
    retinal pigment e. (RPE)
    specialized metaplastic e.
    squamous e.
    vaginal e.
Epitol
epitope
    codominant e.
    continuous e.

NOTES

epitope *(continued)*
    CTL e.
    gp41 e.
    linear e.
    minimal cytotoxic e. (MCE)
    myc e.
    neutralization e.
    e. retrieval method
Epivir
Epivir-HBV
Epivir/Retrovir combination
EPL
    effective pathlength
    extensor pollicis longus
        EPL algorithm
EPO
    erythropoietin
EPOCH
    etoposide, prednisone, Oncovin,
      cyclophosphamide, Halotestin
    etoposide, prednisone, Oncovin, Cytoxan,
      Halotestin
epoetin
    e. alfa
    e. beta
Epogen
Epomax
epothilone B analog
Eppendorf
    E. pO_2 histograph
    E. pO_2 microelectrode
    E. Repeater Pro pipette
    E. tube
EPR
    electron paramagnetic resonance
        EPR spectroscopy
epratuzumab
Eprex
EPS
    extrapyramidal syndrome
Epstein-Barr
    E.-B. early region
    E.-B. early region-positive cell
    E.-B. early RNA (EBER)
    E.-B. infection
    E.-B. mononucleosis
    E.-B. nuclear antigen (EBNA)
    E.-B. virus (EBV)
    E.-B. virus-associated
      lymphoproliferative syndrome
    E.-B. virus-induced
      lymphoproliferative disease
    E.-B. virus-positive sinonasal
      lymphoma
EPT
    endocrine pancreatic tumor
Equalactin Chewable Tablet
equalization

equation
    Harris-Benedict e.
    Larmor e.
    Ussing e.
equi
    Rhodococcus e.
equianalgesic
Equilet
equilibrium
    charged-particle e.
    e. dissociation constant
    e. dose constant
    e. magnetization
    transient e.
equinovarus
    talipes e. (TEV)
equipoise
equipotent
equivalent
    e. beam
    e. dose
    dose e.
    radiobiologic e. (RBE)
equivocal findings
ER
    estrogen receptor
ERA
    estrogen receptor assay
eradication
    leukemia e.
    e. of malignancy
erb
    erb A
    erb A protein
    erb A protooncogene/oncogene
    erb B
    erb B oncogene
    erb B protooncogene/oncogene
erbB2
    erbB2 blood fluorescent in situ
      hybridization
    erbB2 bone marrow fluorescent in
      situ hybridization
ERBD
    endoscopic retrograde biliary drainage
Erbitux
erbulozole
ERCP
    endoscopic retrograde
      cholangiopancreatography
Erdheim tumor
ERE
    estrogen-response element
E-receptor
    suppressive E-r. (SER)
erectile
    e. dysfunction
    e. function
Ergamisol

erg1 gene
ergocalciferol
ergometer
ergot alkaloid
ergotamine
erlotinib
erosion
    azidothymidine e.
    AZT-induced e.
    bony e.
    tumor e.
erosive
    e. gastritis
    e. gingivitis
    e. osteoarthritis
eroticism, erotism
    brachioproctic e.
error
    dorsal induction e.
    intraobserver e.
ERT
    estrogen replacement therapy
    external beam radiation therapy
eruption
    erythematous morbilliform e.
    Kaposi varicelliform e.
    lichenoid drug e.
    papular e.
eruptive
ERV
    endogenous retrovirus
ERV3
    endogenous retrovirus 3
Erwinase
Erwinia L-asparaginase
Erybid
Eryc
erysipeloid
Ery-Tab
erythema
    e. ab igne
    acral e.
    e. annulare centrifugum (EAC)
    circinate e.
    facial e.
    e. gyratum repens
    heliotrope e.
    linear gingival e. (LGE)
    e. multiforme
    necrolytic migratory e.
    palmar e.
    paraneoplastic e.

erythematosus
    drug-induced systemic lupus e.
    lupus e. (LE)
    systemic lupus e. (SLE)
erythematous
    candidiasis e.
    e. morbilliform eruption
erythremic myelosis
erythroblast
    basophilic e.
    orthochromatic e.
    polychromatophilic e.
erythroblastic leukemia
erythroblastopenia
    transient e.
erythroblastosis
    fetal e.
    e. fetalis (EBF)
erythrocatalysis
Erythrocin
erythrocytapheresis
erythrocyte
    achromic e.
    e. aggregation
    e. antibody
    e., antibody, complement
    basophilic e.
    crenated e.
    e. histogram
    hypochromic e.
    e. maturation factor
    Mexican hat e.
    normochromic e.
    nucleated e.
    orthochromic e.
    packed e.'s
    polychromic e.
    target e.
    e. transfusion
    e. volume
erythrocythemia
erythrocytic inclusion
erythrocytolysis
erythrocytopenia
erythrocytophagy
erythrocytorrhexis
erythrocytoschisis
erythrocytosis
    paraneoplastic e.
erythrodegenerative
erythroderma
erythrodysesthesia
    palmar-plantar e. (PPED)

NOTES

E

erythroleukemia
erythroleukoplakia
erythroleukothrombocythemia
erythrolysis
erythromycin and sulfisoxazole
erythromyeloblastosis
erythron
erythroneocytosis
erythronormoblastic anemia
erythropenia
erythrophagia
erythrophagocytic
    e. lymphohistiocytosis
    e. T-gamma lymphoma
erythrophagocytosis
erythroplakia
erythroplasia
    Queyrat e.
    e. of Queyrat
erythropoiesis
erythropoietic porphyria
erythropoietic-stimulating factor
erythropoietin (EPO)
    e. gene
    gene-activated e.
    recombinant human e.
    serum e.
erythrose péribuccale pigmentaire of
  Brocq
erythrosis of Bekhterev
Eryzole
ES
    extracapsular spread
    extra strength
    Vicodin ES
^{255}Es
    einsteinium-255
ESAP
    etoposide, Solu-Medrol, ara-C, Platinol
ESAS
    Edmonton Symptom Assessment Scale
escalated methotrexate, vinblastine,
  Adriamycin, cisplatin (E-MVAC)
escalation
    dose e.
escape
    phenotypic e.
ESCC
    epidural spinal cord compression
Escherichia
    E. coli (EC)
    E. coli ASNase
    E. coli L-asparaginase
    E. coli O157:H7 fluorescent
    bacteriophage assay
    E. coli strain O157:H7
    immunomagnetic separation and
    detection
Esclim Transdermal

ESD
    esterase D
ESFT
    Ewing sarcoma family of tumors
ESHAP
    etoposide, Solu-Medrol, high-dose ara-C,
    Platinol
Esidrix
Eskalith
EsophaCoil
esophageal
    e. achalasia
    e. atresia
    e. balloon dilator
    e. cancer
    e. candidiasis (EC)
    e. carcinoma
    e. choriocarcinoma
    e. contraction
    e. diverticulum
    e. duplication cyst
    e. dysmotility
    e. filling defect
    e. hiatus
    e. inflammation
    e. intramural pseudodiverticulosis
    e. leiomyosarcoma
    e. narrowing
    e. neoplasm
    e. opening
    e. perforation
    e. peristalsis
    e. reflux
    e. ring
    e. rupture
    e. stricture
    e. tear
    e. tumor
    e. ulcer
    e. ulceration
    e. varix
    e. vein
    e. vestibule
    e. web
    e. Z-stent with dual anti-reflux
    valve
    e. Z-stent with uncoated flanges
esophagectomy
    en bloc e.
    Ivor-Lewis e.
    radical en bloc e.
    thoracic e.
    total thoracic e. (TTE)
    transhiatal e. (THE)
    transthoracic e.
esophagi (*pl. of* esophagus)
esophagitis
    candidal e.
esophagogastric (EG)

e. junction
e. neoplasia
esophagogastrostomy
intrathoracic e.
esophagojejunostomy
esophagoscopy
Lugol dye e.
esophagostomy
cervical e.
palliative e.
esophagotracheal fistula
esophagram
air e.
barium-water e.
esophagus, pl. **esophagi**
adenocarcinoma of e.
Barrett e.
columnar-lined e.
distal e.
Esophotrast
esorubicin HCl
ESS
endometrial stromal sarcoma
essential
e. athrombia
e. iris atrophy
e. osteolysis
e. thrombocythemia
Essiac tea
estazolam
ester
glutathione monoethyl e.
phorbol e.
quinuclidinyl e.
esterase
alpha-naphthyl acetate e.
alpha-naphthyl butyrate e.
aminocaproate e.
e. D (ESD)
double staining e.
nonspecific e.
esterified estrogen
esthesioneuroblastoma (ENB)
Hyams grading system for e.
Kadish staging of e.
esthesioneurocytoma
esthesioneuroepithelioma
estimation
Estinyl
Estracyt
Estraderm Transdermal

estradiol
cyclophosphamide, Adriamycin, leucovorin rescue, 5-fluorouracil, ethinyl e. (CALF-E)
Cytoxan, Adriamycin, leucovorin calcium, 5-fluorouracil, ethinyl e. (CALF-E)
ethinyl e.
transdermal e.
e. valerate
Estra-L
E.-L 40
E.-L Injection
estramustine
cyclophosphamide, cisplatin, 5-fluorouracil, e. (CCFE)
e. phosphate (EMP)
e. phosphate sodium
e. plus paclitaxel
estrane
Estratab
Estratest HS
Estraval-PA
Estren-Dameshek anemia
Estring
Estro-Cyp Injection
estrogen
e. antagonist
conjugated e.
esterified e.
e. and methyltestosterone
e. rebound regression
e. receptor (ER)
e. receptor assay (ERA)
e. receptor modulator
e. replacement therapy (ERT)
estrogen-dependent cancer cell
estrogenic
e. activity
e. property
estrogen-progestin artificial cycle
estrogen-receptor positive tumor
estrogen-response element (ERE)
estrone aqueous
estropipate
ESVEM
Electrophysiologic Study Versus Electrocardiographic Monitoring
ET
embryo transfer
endotracheal
etiology
ET tube

NOTES

etanidazole
Platinol and e.
Etaproxyn
état criblé
ethacrynic acid (EA)
ethambutol-induced optic neuritis
ethambutol toxicity
ethanol
absolute e.
carmustine in e.
e. gelation test
e. usage
ethanolamine
ethaverine
ether
dihematoporphyrin e. (DHE)
methyl-*tert*-butyl e.
ethesioneuroblastoma
Ethezyme papain-urea debriding ointment
ethics
biomedical e.
ethidium bromide staining
ethinyl estradiol
Ethiodol
Ethiofos
ethionamide
ethisterone
ethmocephaly
ethmoid
e. air cell
e. bone
e. foramen
e. sinus
e. sinus carcinoma
ethmoidal
e. artery
e. bulla
ethnic
e. neutropenia
e. variation
ethoglucid (*var. of* etoglucid)
ethosuximide
ethotoin
Ethrane
10-ethyl-10-deazaaminopterin (EDAM)
ethyldichloroarsine (ED)
ethylene
e. diamine tetraacetate
e. diamine tetraacetic acid (EDTA)
e. diamine tetramethylene phosphonic acid (EDTMP)
ethylester
glutathione e.
5-ethynyluracil
Ethyol
Etibi
etidronate disodium
etiology (ET)

etiopurpurin
tin ethyl e.
etodolac
etoglucid, ethoglucid
Etopophos
etoposide (VePesid)
Adriamycin, bleomycin, vincristine, e. (ABVE)
Adriamycin, cyclophosphamide, e. (ACE)
Adriamycin, Oncovin, prednisone, e. (AOPE)
e., Adriamycin, Platinol (EAP)
Adriamycin, Platinol, e. (APE)
ara-C, daunorubicin, e. (ADE)
ara-C, Platinol, e. (APE)
bleomycin, Oncovin, streptozocin, e.
carboplatin, epirubicin, vincristine, actinomycin D, ifosfamide, e. (CEVAIE)
e. chemotherapy treatment
e. and cisplatin
cisplatin, Oncovin, doxorubicin, e. (CODE)
cyclophosphamide, Adriamycin, e. (CAE)
cyclophosphamide, doxorubicin, e. (CDE)
cyclophosphamide, Halotestin, Oncovin, prednisone, e. (CHOPE)
e., cyclophosphamide, hydroxydaunomycin, Oncovin
cyclophosphamide, hydroxydaunomycin, Oncovin, prednisone, e. (CHOPE)
cyclophosphamide, Oncovin, Platinol, e. (COPE)
Cytoxan, doxorubicin, e. (CDE)
Cytoxan, Halotestin, Oncovin, prednisone, e. (CHOPE)
e., Cytoxan, methotrexate, vincristine (ECMV)
Cytoxan, Oncovin, Platinol, e. (COPE)
dexamethasone, ara-C, carboplatin, e. (DACE)
e., dexamethasone, ara-C, Platinol (EDAP)
dexamethasone, thalidomide plus Adriamycin, cyclophosphamide, e. (DT-PACE)
e., doxorubicin, cyclophosphamide, vincristine, prednisone, bleomycin (VALOP-B)
e., doxorubicin, Platinol
e., 5-fluorouracil, Platinol (EFP)
ifosfamide, carboplatin, e. (ICE)
ifosfamide, mesna uroprotection, methotrexate, e. (IMVP-16)

e., leucovorin, 5-fluorouracil (ELF)
mAMSA, azacitidine, e. (MAZE)
mesna, ifosfamide, mitoxantrone, e.
(MIME)
mesna, ifosfamide, Novantrone, e.
(MINE)
mesna rescue, ifosfamide,
carboplatin, e. (MICE)
mesna uroprotection and e.
e., methotrexate, actinomycin D,
cyclophosphamide, Oncovin
(EMA-CO, EMACO)
e., methotrexate, actinomycin D,
cyclophosphamide, Oncovin
(EMA-CO, EMACO)
e., mitoxantrone, prednimustine
e. phosphate
e. and Platinol (EP)
Platinol, Adriamycin,
cyclophosphamide, e. (PACE)
Platinol, Cytoxan, e. (PCE)
Platinol, 5-fluorouracil, e. (PFE)
prednisone, methotrexate-leucovorin,
Adriamycin, cyclophosphamide, e.
(ProMACE)
e., prednisone, Oncovin,
cyclophosphamide, Halotestin
(EPOCH)
e., prednisone, Oncovin, Cytoxan,
Halotestin (EPOCH)
e., Solu-Medrol, ara-C, Platinol
(ESAP)
e., Solu-Medrol, high-dose ara-C,
Platinol (ESHAP)
uroprotection and e.
e., vinblastine, Adriamycin (EVA)
vinblastine, Adriamycin, mitomycin
e., vinblastine, Adriamycin,
prednisone (EVAP)
vinblastine, Adriamycin,
procarbazine, e.
vinblastine, ifosfamide, e. (VIE)
vincristine, Adriamycin,
procarbazine, e. (VAPE)
vincristine, ifosfamide, e. (VIE)
vincristine, ifosfamide,
carboplatin, e. (VICE)
etoprine
Etrafon
etretinate
ETS
environmental tobacco smoke
ets-1 protooncogene/oncogene

ets-2 protooncogene/oncogene
ETtopoTax
EU
excretory urography
euchromatin
Euflex
euglobulin
e. clot lysis
e. lysis time
e. plasma fraction
eugonadal man
Eulexin
euplastic lymph
Euro Collins solution
European
E. blastomycosis
E. Concerted Action on
Thrombosis (ECAT)
E. Organization for Research and
Treatment of Cancer (EORTC)
E. Organization for Research and
Treatment of Cancer Core Quality
of Life
E. Organization for Research and
Treatment of Cancer index
EUS
endorectal ultrasonography
endoscopic ultrasonography
endoscopic ultrasound
eustachian tube
eutectic
e. mixture of local anesthetics
(EMLA)
e. mixture of local anesthetics
cream
euthanasia
euthyroid-sick syndrome
euvolemia
eV
electron volt
EVA
etoposide, vinblastine, Adriamycin
Evacet
E. and Herceptin
E. and trastuzumab
evacuation
evaluation
Multiple Outcomes for
Raloxifene E. (MORE)
neurodiagnostic e.
pretreatment e.
psychosocial e.
Wright-Giemsa e.

E

NOTES

evanescent enhancement
Evans
    E. blue dye
    E. stage I–IV
    E. stage IV-S disease
    E. stages of neuroblastoma (I–IV)
    E. syndrome
Evans-D'Angio staging system
EVAP
    etoposide, vinblastine, Adriamycin,
      prednisone
event
    endonucleolytic cleavage e.
    late fatal e.'s
    life e.
event-free survival (EFS)
eventration of diaphragm
Everone
    E. 200
    E. Injection
eversion
    cervical e.
evidence
    scintigraphic e.
evisceration
Evista
E-Vitamin
evolution
    clonal e.
Ewing
    E. family of tumors (EFT)
    E. sarcoma
    E. sarcoma family of tumors
      (ESFT)
EWS gene
ex
    ex vivo aortic ring sprouting assay
    ex vivo expansion
    ex vivo gene therapy
    ex vivo marrow treatment
    ex vivo stimulation
ExAblate 2000 ultrasound system
exacerbation
examination, exam
    barium e.
    clinical breast e. (CBE)
    digital rectal e. (DRE)
    gray scale e.
    histopathologic e.
    neurologic e.
    physical e. (PE)
    proctoscopic e.
    ProstaScint e.
    prostate spectroscopy and
      imaging e. (PROSE)
    rectopelvic e.
    self-breast e. (SBE)
    small bowel follow-through e.

    suboptimal e.
    tomodensitometric e.
Exanta
exanthem, exanthema
    acute HIV e.
    Boston e.
exanthematous drug rash
exatecan mesylate
exceptional cancer patient (ECaP)
excess
    e. blasts
    psychoactive drug e.
exchange
    air e.
    chemical e.
    e. diffusion
    recombinase mediated cassette e.
      (RMCE)
    sister chromatid e.
exchanger
    heat e.
excision
    e. assay
    en bloc e.
    large loop e.
    local e.
    total mesorectal e. (TME)
    wide local e. (WLE)
excisional biopsy
excitation
    2-photon e. (TPE)
exclusion
    antral e.
excretion
    absorption, distribution,
      metabolism, e. (ADME)
excretory
    e. duct
    e. urography (EU)
excursion
    e. of diaphragm
    diaphragmatic e.
Exelderm Topical
exemestane
exenterated
exenteration
    anterior e.
    orbital e.
    pelvic e.
    total pelvic e. (TPE)
exercise
    Kegel e.
    e. radionuclide angiocardiography
exfoliative
    e. cell
    e. cytology
    e. dermatitis
exhalation
    end e.

Exherin
existential
    e. issue
    e. pain
exisulind
exit dose
exocytosis
exogenous
    e. antigen
    e. flora
    e. hormone
    e. immunosuppressant medication
exon
    polymorphic e.
exophthalmos, exophthalmus
    endocrine e.
exophytic
    e. glioblastoma
    e. gut mass
    e. lesion
exophytum-type tumor
exostosis, pl. **exostoses**
    hereditary multiple e. (HME)
    multiple hereditary e.
exostotic chondrosarcoma
expanded
    e. foam immobilization device
    e. plasma
expander
    plasma e.
expansile unilocular well-demarcated
  bone lesion
expansion
    ex vivo e.
    in vivo clonal e.
expectancy
    quality-adjusted life e. (QALE)
experience
    human immunodeficiency virus-
      patient-reported status and e.
      (HIV-PARSE)
experimental
    e. chemotherapy
    e. therapy
    e. treatment
expiration
    end e.
expiratory
    e. computed tomography
    e. view
explosion fracture
explosive follicular hyperplasia
exponential kinetics

exportin protein
exposure
    deep e.
    e. dose
    electromagnetic radiation e.
    intrauterine hormonal e.
    intrauterine hormone e.
    mucous membrane e.
    percutaneous e.
    radiation e.
    e. risk
exposure-prevention strategy
exposure-specific factor
expression
    anomalous antigen e.
    antigen e.
    aRb protein e.
    b-catenin e.
    BRCA1 e.
    BRCA2 e.
    caveolin-1 e.
    CD38 e.
    CD44 e.
    cDNA microarray gene e.
    clinical disease e.
    c-myc e.
    differential CIITA e.
    E-cadherin e.
    FHIT protein e.
    e. of fusion protein
    gene e.
    immunoregulatory factor e.
    MHC receptor e.
    MIB-1 e.
    nef e.
    oncogene e.
    P-cadherin e.
    PD-ECGF e.
    phospholipase cyl-1 e.
    PRAD-1 gene e.
    Rb protein e. (pRb)
    serological analysis of recombinant
      cDNA e. (SEREX)
    thymidylate synthase e.
    trkA e.
    trkC e.
    tumor-liberated particle antigen e.
    tumor-suppressor gene e.
    viral e.
    Wnt-1 e.
exsanguinating hemorrhage
exsanguination
Exserohilum

E

NOTES

exstrophy
    bladder e.
Extencaps
    Micro-K 10 E.
extended
    e. field
    e. field of view
    e. radical mastectomy
extended-field irradiation therapy
extension
    contiguous extranodal e.
    extracapsular prostate cancer e.
    extranodal tumor e.
    extraprostatic e. (EPE)
    extrascleral e.
    extrathyroidal e.
    e. teardrop fracture
    e. view
extensive
    e. bilateral pneumonia
    e. intraductal component (EIC)
extensive-stage disease
extensor
    e. carpi radialis brevis
    e. carpi radialis longus (ECRL)
    e. carpi ulnaris
    e. digitorum
    e. digitorum brevis
    e. digitorum longus (EDL)
    e. hallucis longus (EHL)
    e. indicis
    e. pollicis longus (EPL)
    e. retinaculum
    e. tendon
    e. tensor pollicis brevis
external
    e. acoustic foramen
    e. auditory canal (EAC)
    e. auditory meatus
    e. beam field
    e. beam photon irradiation
    e. beam radiation
    e. beam radiation therapy (EBRT, ERT)
    e. carotid artery
    e. ear neoplasm
    e. elastic lamina
    e. iliac artery
    e. looping technique
    e. oblique muscle
    e. orthovoltage irradiation
    e. os
    e. photon
    e. pneumatic calf compression
    e. rotation view
    e. scanning
    e. ultrasound hyperthermia
    e. urethral sphincter

    e. volumetric pump
    e. x-ray therapy
extirpation
extirpative surgery
extraadrenal pheochromocytoma
extraarachnoid
    e. injection
    e. myelography
extraaxial
    e. cavernous hemangioma
    e. fluid collection
    e. lesion
    e. tumor
extracapsular
    e. fracture
    e. metastasis
    e. prostate cancer
    e. prostate cancer extension
    e. spread (ES)
extracardiac mass
extracellular (EC)
    e. antioxidant
    e. compartment
    e. fluid
    e. immunoglobulin light chain
    e. matrix (ECM)
    e. matrix/basement membrane interaction
extracerebral
    e. cavernous angioma
    e. fluid collection
extrachorialis
extrachorial placenta
extracorporeal
    e. chemofiltration
    e. circulation
    e. irradiation
    e. membrane oxygenation
    e. membrane oxygenator
    e. photochemotherapy (ECP)
    e. photophoresis
    e. shock wave
extracranial
    e. carotid artery disease
    e. carotid circulation
    e. cerebral vasculature
    e. mass lesion
    e. nontesticular germ cell tumor
extract
    dogfish shark liver e.
    malt soup e.
    mistletoe e.
    pine cone e.
    sea algae e.
    Serratia marcescens e.
extractable nuclear antigen
extraction
    liquid e.

micro liquid e.
testicular sperm e. (TESE)
extradural
    e. hematoma
    e. space
extrafascial hysterectomy
extrafollicular blast
extragenital Bowen disease (EBD)
extragnathic ameloblastoma
extragonadal
    e. germ cell tumor (EGCT)
    e. seminoma (EGS)
extrahepatic
    e. bile duct (EHBD)
    e. bile duct carcinoma
    e. binary obstruction
    e. cholangiectasis
    e. cholangiocarcinoma
    e. lesion
    e. neoplasm
    e. portal hypertension
    e. primary malignant tumor
    e. stone
extralobar sequestration
extraluminal
    e. gas
    e. hemorrhage
extramammary Paget disease
extramedullary
    e. hematopoiesis
    e. involvement
    e. lesion
    e. leukemic plasmacytoma
    e. mass
    e. plasmacytoma (EMP)
    e. toxicity
extraneuraxis
extranodal
    e. follicular lymphoma
    e. hemangioendothelioma
    e. involvement
    e. Ki-1 anaplastic large cell
      lymphoma
    e. natural killer T-cell lymphoma
    e. proliferation
    e. Rosai-Dorfman disease
    e. site
    e. tumor extension
extraoctave fracture
extraocular
    e. muscle
    e. muscle enlargement

extraosseous
    e. Ewing sarcoma
    e. osteosarcoma
extraovarian serous carcinoma
extrapelvic
    e. colon
    e. malignancy
extraperitoneal endoscopic pelvic lymph
    node dissection (EEPLND)
extrapleural pneumonectomy
extrapolate
extrapontine myelinolysis
extraprostatic extension (EPE)
extrapulmonary
    e. histoplasmosis
    e. metastasis
    e. sequestration
    e. small cell cancer
    e. small cell carcinoma
extrapyramidal
    e. reaction
    e. symptom
    e. syndrome (EPS)
    e. system
extraregional metastasis
extrarenal pelvis
extrascleral extension
extraskeletal
    e. myxoid
    e. myxoid chondrosarcoma (EMC)
    e. osteosarcoma
extra-stiff guidewire
extra strength (ES)
extratesticular
    e. lesion
    e. tumor
extrathoracic metastasis
extrathyroidal
    e. extension
    e. invasion
extrauterine pelvic mass
extravaginal testicular torsion
extravasation
extravascular
    e. compartment
    e. hemolysis
    e. hemolytic anemia
    e. mass
extraventricular
    e. obstructive hydrocephalus
    e. supratentorial ependymoma

E

NOTES

extravesical infrasphincteric ectopic ureter
extreme drug resistance (EDR)
extremely low-frequency field
extremity
  e. abnormality
  e. hemangioma
  e. malformation
  e. osteosarcoma
  e. rhabdomyosarcoma
extrinsic
  e. allergic alveolitis
  e. asthma
  e. bladder compression
  e. cellular parameter
  e. coagulation pathway
  e. esophageal impression
  e. field uniformity

  e. filling defect
  e. hemolytic anemia
  e. impression
  e. tumor
  e. ureteral defect
extruded disc fragment
extrusion
  disc e.
exudate absorber
exudative
  e. pleural effusion
  e. tuberculosis
eyeball urodynamics
eye exposure limit
EZ-Dish pressure relief cushion
Ezide
ezrin protein
EZ::TN insertion kit

F18
   fludeoxyglucose F18
FA
   folinic acid
FAA
   flavone acetic acid
FAB
   French-American-British
   FAB classification
Fab
   fragment antigen binding
   Fab fragment
Faber
   F. anemia
   F. syndrome
Fabian prostatic stent
Fabricius
   bursa of F.
Fabry disease
FAC
   5-fluorouracil, Adriamycin,
   cyclophosphamide
   prednisone, methotrexate, FAC
   (PMFAC)
FAC-BCG
   ftorafur, Adriamycin, cyclophosphamide,
   BCG
face
   direct en f.
   en f.
facet
   articular f.
   bilateral locked f.'s
facial
   f. artery
   f. barrier
   f. erythema
   f. hemangioma
   f. hypoesthesia
   f. lymph node
   f. marrow
   f. nerve
   f. nerve paralysis
   f. neurofibroma
   f. neuroma
   f. palsy
   f. trichilemmoma
faciale
   granuloma f.
facialis
   herpes f.
facies, pl. **facies**
   coarse f.

FAC-M
   5-fluorouracil, Adriamycin,
   cyclophosphamide, methotrexate
   5-fluorouracil, Adriamycin, Cytoxan,
   methotrexate
FACP
   ftorafur, Adriamycin, cyclophosphamide,
   Platinol
FACS
   fluorescence-activated cell sorting
   5-fluorouracil, Adriamycin,
   cyclophosphamide, streptozocin
FACScan flow cytometer
FACSVantage cell sorter
FACT
   Functional Assessment of Cancer
   Therapy
FACT-BL
   Functional Assessment of Cancer
   Therapy-Bladder
FACT-F
   Functional Assessment of Cancer
   Therapy-Fatigue
factor
   f. VII antigen (VII:Ag)
   f. V Leiden (FVL)
   f. VIIIR
   f. IX antigen (IX:Ag)
   f. X antigen (X:Ag)
   f. XIIIa (FXIIIa)
   accelerator f.
   acidic fibroblast growth f. (aFGF)
   activation f.
   active transcription f.
   adiposis inhibitor f.
   angiogenic f.
   anisotropy f.
   antianemia f.
   antiangiogenesis f.
   antihemophilic f.
   antihemophilic f. A
   antihemorrhagic f.
   antinuclear f. (ANF)
   apoptosis activating f. (APAF)
   f. assay
   autocrine growth f.
   automotility f.
   basic fibroblast growth f. (bFGF)
   basophil chemotactic f.
   B-cell differentiation f.
   B-cell stimulating f.
   BeneFix hemophilia B blood
     clotting f.
   blastogenic f.
   blocking f.

F

factor *(continued)*
    blood clotting f.
    blood coagulation f.
    B-lymphocyte stimulatory f.
    Castle f.
    chemotactic f. (CF)
    Christmas f. (CF)
    ciliary neurotrophic f.
    citrovorum f. (CF)
    citrovorum rescue f.
    clonal inhibitory f.
    clotting f.
    clotting f. VIII
    coagulation f.
    colony-stimulating f. (CSF)
    complement f. (CF)
    conglutination f.
    conglutinogen-activating f.
    core binding f.
    corticotropin-releasing f. (CRF)
    crystal-induced chemotactic f.
    cytotoxic f.
    Day f.
    diffusion f.
    dose-limiting f.
    Duran-Reynals f.
    Egr-1 transcription f.
    endothelial growth f. (EGF)
    endothelium-derived relaxing f.
    environmental f.
    eosinophil chemotactic f.
    epidermal growth f. (EGF)
    erythrocyte maturation f.
    erythropoietic-stimulating f.
    exposure-specific f.
    factor VIII:C heat-treated
      antihemophilic f.
    fibrin-stabilizing f.
    fibroblast growth f. (FGF)
    Fitzgerald f.
    Fletcher f.
    5-fluorouracil, Adriamycin,
      mitomycin, citrovorum f. (FAM-
      CF)
    genetic f.
    glass f.
    granulocyte colony-stimulating f.
      (G-CSF)
    granulocyte-macrophage colony-
      stimulating f. (GM-CSF)
    growth hormone-releasing f.
      (GHRF, GH-RF)
    H f.
    Hageman f.
    helper f.
    hematologic f.
    hematopoietic colony-stimulating f.
    hematopoietic growth f.
    hematopoietic stem cell f.

    heparin-binding growth f.
    hepatocyte growth f. (HGF)
    hepatocyte stimulating f.
    hepatoma-derived growth f. (HDGF)
    high-dose methotrexate and
      citrovorum f. (HDMTX-CF)
    HIV-inducing f. (HIF)
    host f.
    host-related f.
    human granulocyte-stimulating f.
    human growth f.
    human macrophage-monocyte
      chemotactic and activating f.
      (hMCAF)
    human urinary colony-stimulating f.
      (HU-CSF)
    humoral f.
    f. II inhibitor
    insulin-like growth f. (IGF, ILGF)
    interferon regulatory f. (IRF)
    interferon regulatory f. 1 (IRF-1)
    interferon regulatory f. 2 (IRF-2)
    f. IX complex
    f. IX deficiency
    f. IX inhibitor
    f. IX, purified human
    keratinocyte growth f. (KGF)
    keratinocyte growth f. 2 (KGF-2)
    kerma-to-dose conversion f.
    Lactobacillus casei f.
    Lactobacillus lactis Dorner f.
    Laki-Lorand f.
    LE f.
    Leishmania elongation initiation f.
      (LeIF)
    leucovorin-citrovorum f. (L-CF)
    leucovorin rescue f.
    leukemia inhibitory f. (LIF)
    limulus anti-DPS f.
    luteinizing hormone-releasing f.
      (LHRF)
    lymph node permeability f. (LNPF)
    lymphocyte-activating f. (LAF)
    lymphocyte mitogenic f.
    macrophage-activating f. (MAF)
    macrophage chemotactic f.
    macrophage colony-stimulating f.
      (M-CSF)
    macrophage growth f.
    mast cell growth f.
    Mayneord F f.
    megakaryocyte colony-stimulating f.
      (MEG-CSF)
    megakaryocyte growth and
      development f. (MGDF)
    milk f.
    mitogenic f.
    monocyte chemotactic and
      activating f.

monocyte colony-stimulating f.
monocyte tissue f.
multicolony-stimulating f.
murine granulocyte-macrophage
  colony-stimulating growth f.
myeloid growth f.
myeloid progenitor f. 1
myeloid progenitor inhibitory f.
  (MPIF)
myelopoietin growth f.
negative f. (NEF)
nerve growth f.
neu differentiation f. (NDF)
neuron-restrictive silencing f.
neutralizing antibody to vascular
  endothelial growth f.
neutrophil migration-inhibition f.
nonhematopoietic growth f.
NovoSeven Coagulation F. VIIa
nuclear f.
off-axis f. (OAF)
osteoclast-activating f.
P f.
p40 T-cell growth f.
Passovoy f.
P-cell stimulating f.
peakscatter f.
plasmacytoma growth f.
platelet f. 4 (PF4)
platelet-activating f.
platelet-derived endothelial cell
  growth f. (PD-ECGF)
platelet-derived growth f. (PDGF)
platelet-derived growth f. A
  (PDGFA)
platelet-derived growth f. B
pre-B-cell growth f.
prognostic f.
protection f.
protein f.
Prower f.
psychological f.
Q f.
quality f.
radiation weighting f.
f. receptor keratinocyte
recombinant hematopoietic
  growth f.
recombinant human granulocyte
  colony-stimulating f. (rhGm-CSF,
  rHuG-CSF)

recombinant human granulocyte-
  macrophage colony-stimulating f.
  (rGM-CSF)
recombinant human growth f.
recombinant humanized monoclonal
  antibody to vascular endothelial
  cell growth f. (rhuMAb-VEGF)
recombinant human keratinocyte
  growth f. (rHuKGF)
recombinant human macrophage
  colony-stimulating f. (rHM-CSF)
recruitment f.
ReFacto hemophilia A blood
  clotting f.
releasing f.
replication inhibition f. (RIF)
Rh f.
Rhesus f. (Rh)
risk f.
scatter f.
serum f. (SF)
Simon septic f.
social f.
Steel f.
stem cell f. (SCF)
stromal-derived f. 1
Stuart f.
Stuart-Prower f.
sun protection f. (SPF)
T-cell stimulating f.
therapeutic gain f. (TGF)
thrombopoietin growth f.
thymic humoral f.
thyrotropin-releasing f.
tissue f.
transcription f.
transfer f.
transforming growth f. a (TGFa)
tumor angiogenesis f.
tumor angiogenic f.
tumor autocrine mobility f.
tumor cell migration-inhibition f.
  (TMIF)
tumor-limiting f.
tumor necrosis f. a (TNFa)
tumor necrosis f. (TNF)
tumor necrosis factor receptor-
  associated f. (TRAF)
V f.
vascular endothelial f.
vascular endothelial growth f.
  (VEFG, VEGF)
vascular permeability f. (VPF)

NOTES

F

factor *(continued)*
  f. VIIa, recombinant
  f. VIII coagulation function
  f. VIII concentrate
  f. VIII deficiency
  f. VII inhibitor
  f. VIII-related antigen
  f. V inhibitor
  f. V Leiden mutation test
  von Willebrand f. (vWF)
  VP-16, methotrexate, citrovorum f. (VMC)
  wedge f.
  Wills f.
  WT1 transcription f.
  X f.
  f. XII deficiency
  f. XIII deficiency
  f. XII inhibitor
  f. XI inhibitor
  f. X inhibitor
factor-1
  hypoxia-inducible f.-1 (HIF-1)
  insulin-like growth f.-1 (IGF-1)
  myeloid progenitor inhibitory f.-1 (MPIF-1)
factor-2
  insulin-like growth f.-2 (IGF-2)
factor-3
  fibroblast growth f.-3
factor-4
  recombinant platelet f.-4 (rPF4)
factor-acidic
  fibroblast growth f.-a.
factor-alpha
  tumor necrosis f.-a. (TNF-alpha)
Factorate
factor-basic
  fibroblast growth f.-b.
factor-beta
  tumor necrosis f.-b. (TNF-beta)
factor-beta-lymphotoxin
  tumor necrosis f.-b.-l.
factor-C
  vascular endothelial growth f.-C (VEGF-C)
factor-dependent mitogenic signaling
factorial design
Factrel
FACVP
  5-fluorouracil, Adriamycin, cyclophosphamide, VP-16
FADD
  Fas-associated death domain
fadrozole HCl
faggot cell
Fahraeus-Lindqvist effect
Fahraeus method

FAI
  Fatigue Assessment Instrument
failed biopsy detection (FBD)
failing ovary syndrome
failure
  adrenal f.
  AZT f.
  cardiac f. (CF)
  chronic acquired hepatic f.
  chronic renal f. (CRF)
  fulminant hepatic f.
  graft f.
  induction f.
  left ventricle f.
  leptomeningeal f.
  liver f.
  locoregional f. (LRF)
  multiple organ f.
  multisystem organ f.
  organ f.
  ovarian f.
  postrenal f.
  preadult bone marrow f.
  prerenal f.
  renal f.
  f. to thrive
  time-to-treatment f. (TTF)
failure-free survival
faith healing
FAK
  focal adhesion kinase
falces (*pl. of* falx)
falciparum
  Plasmodium f.
fallopian
  f. tube
  f. tube cancer
  f. tube carcinoma
  f. tube mass
Fallot
  F. disease
  F. syndrome
false cord carcinoma
falx, pl. **falces**
  f. cerebelli
  f. cerebri
FAM
  fludarabine, ara-C, mitoxantrone
  5-fluorouracil, Adriamycin, mitomycin
FAM-C
  5-fluorouracil, Adriamycin, methyl-CCNU
FAM-CF
  5-fluorouracil, Adriamycin, mitomycin, citrovorum factor
famciclovir
FAMe, FAME
  5-fluorouracil, Adriamycin, MeCCNU

Familial

    F. Hypercholesterolemia Regression Study (FHRS)

familial

    f. adenomatous polyposis (FAP)
    f. adenomatous polyposis syndrome
    f. aggregation
    f. amyloidosis
    f. atypical multiple mole melanoma (FAMMM)
    f. atypical multiple mole melanoma syndrome
    f. cancer
    f. combined hyperlipidemia (FCH)
    f. dysplastic nevus syndrome (FDNS)
    f. erythrophagocytic lymphohistiocytosis
    f. hemophagocytic lymphohistiocytosis
    f. hypercholesterolemia
    F. Hypercholesterolemia Regression Study (FHRS)
    f. hypophosphatemic rickets
    f. immunity
    f. juvenile polyposis
    f. Mediterranean fever
    f. multiple polyposis
    f. polycythemia
    f. polyposis coli (FPC)
    f. retinoblastoma
    f. Wilms tumor
    f. xanthomatosis

familial-type dysplastic nevus syndrome

family

    ABC drug transporter f.
    b-adaptin gene f.
    notch gene f.
    f. pedigree
    tumor necrosis factor receptor f.

FAMMe

    5-fluorouracil, Adriamycin, mitomycin C, MeCCNU

FAMMM

    familial atypical multiple mole melanoma
    FAMMM syndrome

famotidine

FAMP

    fludarabine monophosphate

FAMPAC

    FAMPAC cell
    FAMPAC cell line

FAM-S

    5-fluorouracil, Adriamycin, mitomycin C, streptozocin

FAMTX

    5-fluorouracil, Adriamycin, methotrexate
    sequential high-dose methotrexate followed by 5-FU in combination with Adriamycin

Famvir

FANA

    fluorescent antinuclear antibody

Fanconi

    F. anemia
    F. syndrome

fan flap

Fansidar

F$_2$ antibody

FAP

    familial adenomatous polyposis
    5-fluorouracil, Adriamycin, Platinol

Fap-1

    Fas-associated phosphatase-1

Fareston

far field

farmer chamber

farmorubicin

farnesyl

    f. protein transferase inhibitor
    f. transferase (FT)
    f. transferase inhibitor (FTI)

Farr test

Fas

    F. ligand (FasL)
    ligation of F.

Fas-associated

    F.-a. DD
    F.-a. death domain (FADD)
    F.-a. phosphatase-1 (Fap-1)

fascia, pl. **fasciae, fascias**

    f. of breast
    Buck f.
    cervical f.
    obturator f.
    rectal f.

fascial

    f. dilator
    f. envelope
    f. incisor
    f. plane
    f. sarcoma

fascicular

    f. proliferation
    f. sarcoma

NOTES

F

fasciculation
fasciculus, pl. **fasciculi**
fasciitis
>   necrotizing f.
>   nodular f.

fascin
Fas-Fas ligand pathway
FasL
>   Fas ligand

Fas-ligand-mediated cytotoxic activity
Faslodex injection
Fas-mediated apoptosis
fast
>   f. adiabatic trajectory in steady
>   state (FATS)
>   f. hemoglobin
>   f. necrosis
>   f. neutron
>   f. neutron radiation therapy
>   f. spin-echo pulse sequence

fast-breeder reactor
fast-neutron radiotherapy
FastPack system
FastPrep DNA kit
fat
>   autologous f.
>   dietary f.
>   intratumoral f.
>   periprostatic f.
>   tumoral f.
>   unsaturated f.

fatal hemangioma
fatigue
>   F. Assessment Instrument (FAI)
>   cancer-related f. (CRF)
>   F. Symptom Inventory (FSI)

FATS
>   fast adiabatic trajectory in steady state

fat-suppressed MRI
fatty
>   f. acid
>   f. acid synthase
>   f. acyl-Co-A synthetase
>   f. acyl-Co-A synthetase deficiency
>   f. dysplastic regenerative hepatic
>   nodule
>   f. marrow replacement
>   f. tumor

Favid
favorable
>   f. histology
>   f. or intermediate prognosis
>   cytogenetics (FIPC)

fazarabine
FBA
>   fluorescent bacteriophage assay

FBD
>   failed biopsy detection

FbDP
>   fibrin degradation product
>   Fibrinostika FbDP

FC
>   Apo-Dipyridamole FC

Fc
>   crystallizable fragment
>   Fc fragment
>   Fc portion
>   Fc receptor

FCA
>   Freund complete adjuvant

FCAP
>   5-fluorouracil, cyclophosphamide,
>   Adriamycin, Platinol
>   5-fluorouracil, Cytoxan, Adriamycin,
>   Platinol
>   FCAP chemotherapy protocol

F/CDDP/VP16 combination
chemotherapy
FCH
>   familial combined hyperlipidemia

FCP
>   5-fluorouracil, cyclophosphamide,
>   prednisone

FCRT
>   focal cranial radiation therapy

FDA
>   Food and Drug Administration

FDC
>   follicular dendritic cell

FddA
>   2′beta-fluoro-2′,3′-dideoxyadenosine

FddaraA
>   2′,3′-dideoxy-2′-fluoro-9-beta-D-
>   arabinofuranosyladenine

FDG
>   18-fluoro-2-deoxyglucose
>   freeze-dried gel

FDG-PET
>   F-fluorodeoxyglucose dual-head positron
>   emission tomography
>   fluorodeoxyglucose positron emission
>   tomography

FDNS
>   familial dysplastic nevus syndrome

FDP
>   fibrin degradation product
>   FDP plasma

Fe
>   iron
>   Slow Fe

feature
>   clinical f.
>   large cell carcinoma with
>   neuroendocrine f.'s (LCNF)
>   myofibroblastic f.
>   pathologic f.

rhabdoid f.
rhabdomyosarcoma with rhabdoid f.
febrile
f. neutropenia
f. patient
febrilis
herpes f.
FEC
5-fluorouracil, epirubicin,
cyclophosphamide
5-fluorouracil, epirubicin, Cytoxan
standard FEC
tailored FEC
fecal
f. carcinoembryonic antigen
f. diversion colostomy
f. impaction
f. occult blood test (FOBT)
f. occult blood testing
f. tumor
fecapentaene
FED
5-fluorouracil, etoposide, DDP
feedback
zidovudine phosphate secondary to
negative f.
feeding
enteral f.
nasogastric f.
f. tube
f. vessel
Fe-ethylenehydroxyphenylglycine
Feiba VH Immuno
felbamate
Felbatol
Feldene
Feldenkrais method
feline
f. AIDS
f. ataxia virus
f. immunodeficiency virus (FIV)
f. leukemia
f. leukemia-sarcoma virus
f. leukemia virus
felon
herpetic f.
Felty syndrome
Femara
feminization syndrome (FS)
Feminone
Femiron
Femizol-M
Femogen

femoris
biceps f.
femtomoles per milligram (fmol/mg)
femur
distal f.
fenestration
catheter-directed f.
fenfluramine
fenofibrate
fenoldopam
fenoprofen
fenretinide
fentanyl
f. citrate
droperidol and f.
F. Oralet
F. Taifun
Feosol
Feostat
Feratab
Fergon
Ferguson-Smith
epithelioma of F.-S.
Feridex
Fer-In-Sol Drops
Fer-Iron
Fermalac
fermium-255 (^{255}Fm)
Ferralyn Lanacaps
Ferrata cell
ferric
f. ammonium citrate
f. gluconate
f. subsulfate
Ferris bone marrow aspiration needle
ferritin
f. aggregate
rabbit antirat f.
serum f.
Ferrlecit sodium ferric gluconate
complex in sucrose injection
ferrohemoglobin
Ferro-Sequels
ferrotherapy
ferrous
f. fumarate
f. gluconate
f. iron
f. salt and ascorbic acid
f. sulfate
f. sulfate, ascorbic acid, vitamin B
complex

NOTES

F

ferrous *(continued)*
    f. sulfate, ascorbic acid, vitamin B complex, folic acid
fertilization
    in vitro f.
fes/fps protooncogene/oncogene
fes protooncogene/oncogene
fetal
    f. adenocarcinoma
    f. blood analysis
    f. erythroblastosis
    f. hamartoma
    f. hemoglobin
    f. liver cell
    f. tissue sampling
fetalis
    erythroblastosis f. (EBF)
    hydrops f.
    nonimmune hydrops f.
fetal-maternal HLA disparity
fetomaternal transfusion
fetoplacental blood
fetoprotein
    alpha f. (AFP)
    iodine ^{131}I murine MAb to alpha f.
    maternal serum alpha f. (MSAFP)
    urinary basic f. (U-BFP)
Fetty syndrome
fetus, pl. **fetuses**
    Campylobacter f.
FEU
    fibrinogen equivalent unit
Feulgen staining
fever
    African swine f.
    Argentinian hemorrhagic f.
    blackwater f.
    cat-scratch f.
    cerebrospinal f.
    dengue f.
    Dumdum f.
    Ebola f.
    familial Mediterranean f.
    granulocytopenic f.
    hemorrhagic f.
    infusion-related f.
    Katayama f.
    Lone Star f.
    Mediterranean f.
    9-mile f.
    neutropenic f.
    Pel-Ebstein f.
    Philippine dengue f.
    Q f.
    unexplained f.
    f. of unknown origin (FUO)
    yellow f.
Feverall

feverfew
FFDM
    free from distant metastasis
F-fluorodeoxyglucose dual-head positron emission tomography (FDG-PET)
^{18}F-fluorodeoxyglucose PET
FFP
    freedom from progression
FFR
    free from recurrence
F-FU
    F-labeled 5-fluorouracil
FGF
    fibroblast growth factor
FGFR
    fibroblast growth factor receptor
FGFR4
    fibroblast growth factor receptor 4
FGN-1
    sulindac sulfone, FGN-1
fgr protooncogene/oncogene
FHIT
    fragile histidine triad
        FHIT gene
        FHIT protein
        FHIT protein expression
FHL
    focal hypoechoic lesion
FHRS
    Familial Hypercholesterolemia Regression Study
FI
    fluorescence index
fiacitabine
fialuridine (FIAU)
FIAU
    fialuridine
fiber
    anular f.
    asbestos f.
    association f.
    f. carcinogenesis
    dietary f.
    mineral f.
    Nutren with f.
    Rosenthal f.
    U f.
fiberoptic ductoscopy
Fibrepur
fibrillary
    f. astrocytic neoplasm
    f. astrocytoma
fibrillation
    atrial f.
fibrin
    f. body
    f. calculus
    f. clot

f. degradation product (FbDP, FDP)
f. deposition
Henle f.
f. inhibitor
f. plate method

fibrinogen
f. assay
f. deficiency
f. degradation product
f. equivalent unit (FEU)
f. inhibitor
f. split products

fibrinogenemia
fibrinogenopenia
fibrinolysin
fibrinolysis
fibrinolytic
f. factor deficiency
f. system
f. therapy

fibrinopeptide A (FPA)
fibrinoplatelet aggregate
Fibrinostika FbDP
fibrinous clot
fibrin-stabilizing factor
fibroadenoma
calcified f.
degenerated f.
juvenile f.

fibroadenomatosis
fibroblast
bone marrow f.
f. growth factor (FGF)
f. growth factor-3
f. growth factor-acidic
f. growth factor-basic
f. growth factor receptor (FGFR)
f. growth factor receptor 4 (FGFR4)
stromal f.

fibroblast-derived
f.-d. IFN-beta
f.-d. interferon beta

fibroblastic
f. osteosarcoma
f. sarcoma
f. variant

fibrocarcinoma
fibrocystic breast disease
fibroelastosis
endocardial f.

fibroepithelioma of Pinkus

fibrofolliculoma
fibrohemosideric
fibrohistiocytic nodular lesion
fibrohistiocytosis
eosinophilic f.

fibrolamellar (FL)
f. carcinoma
f. hepatocellular carcinoma (FL-HCC)
f. liver cell carcinoma
f. variant

fibrolymphohistiocytoma
fibroma
ameloblastic f.
aponeurotic f.
cardiac f.
cementifying f.
central cementifying f.
central ossifying f.
chondromyxoid f. (CMF)
concentric f.
desmoplastic f.
juvenile aponeurotic f.
nonossifying f.
nonosteogenic f.
odontogenic f.
peripheral ossifying f.
polypoid f.
rabbit f.
Shope f.
submesothelial f.
telangiectatic f.
ungual f.

fibromatosis
abdominal f.
aggressive f. (AF)
aggressive infantile f.
juvenile hyalin f.
juvenile palmoplantar f.

fibrometer
fibromyxoid sarcoma
fibronectin
f. adhesion molecule
oncofetal f.

fibroplasia
adventitial f.
endomyocardial f.
eosinophilic endomyocardial f.
retrolental f.

fibrosa
area hepatica f.

fibrosarcoma
ameloblastic f.

NOTES

F

fibrosarcoma *(continued)*
    bronchopulmonary f.
    Earle L f.
    epididymal f.
    infantile f.
    inflammatory f.
    periosteal f.
    primary bronchopulmonary f.
      (PBPF)
    f. variant
fibrosis
    anular f.
    benign meningeal f.
    bone marrow f.
    cystic f. (CF)
    endomyocardial f.
    epidural f.
    idiopathic pulmonary f. (IPF)
    lymph node f.
    marrow f.
    mature f.
    meningeal f.
    myocardial f.
    pulmonary f.
    radiation f.
fibrosum
    adenoma f.
fibrous
    f. meningioma
    f. tumor
fibroxanthoma
    atypical f. (AFX)
    pediatric f.
Ficoll-Conray density gradient centrifugation
Ficoll-Hypaque density gradient centrifugation
Ficoll-Paque gradient
fidelity
    lineage f.
fiducial alignment system
field
    f. cancerization
    f. carcinogenesis
    coplanar f.
    f. disease
    f. drift
    f. echo
    electromagnetic f. (EMF)
    electron beam boost f.
    EM f.
    f. emission tube
    extended f.
    external beam f.
    extremely low-frequency f.
    far f.
    f. gradient
    helmet f.
    high-power f. (hpf)

    f. inversion gel electrophoresis
    irradiated f.
    lateral f.
    f. lock
    low-power f. (lpf)
    nonsplit supraclavicular f.
    parallel-opposed f.'s
    rotational f.
    shaped mediastinal f.
    shrinking f.
    spade f.
    split f.
    stationary f.
    f. strength
    tangent f.'s
    4-f. technique
    f. uniformity
    f. of view
    wedged f.
3-field
    3-f. arc technique
    3-f. isocentric technique
    3-f. lymphadenectomy
field-echo
    f.-e. difference
    f.-e. imaging
    f.-e. sum
field-profiling coil
fifth disease
FIGO
    International Federation of Gynecology and Obstetrics
    FIGO nomenclature
    FIGO staging system
figure
    mitotic f.
filaggrin
filament
    Charcot-Bottcher f.
    f. polymorphonuclear leukocyte
filamentous virion
filariasis
file transfer protocol
filgrastim
filiform verruca
filling
    contrast f.
film
    abdominal plain f.
    check f.
    chest f.
    PA chest f.
    port f.
    portal f.
    postvoiding f.
    radiochromic f.
    simulation f.
    simulator f.

Filmtab
  Cefol F.
Filoviridae
Filovirus
filter
  Amplatz-Lund retrievable f.
  bird's nest f.
  caval f.
  Centricon-10 f.
  centrifugal f.
  Hann f.
  inherent f.
  Kim-Ray Greenfield caval f.
  leukocyte removal f.
  leukodepletion f.
  LeukoNet f.
  leukoreduction f. (LRF)
  LGM f.
  Millipore ultrafree-CL centrifugal f.
  Mobin-Uddin f.
  f. mold
  Pall ELD-96 Set Saver f.
  Pall leukocyte removal f.
  Pall PL100 f.
  Pall RC100 f.
  Pall RC50 f.
  Pall transfusion f.
  retrievable f.
  Thoreus #3 f.
  Vena-Tech f.
  wedge f.
  Whatmann f.
  Wiener f.
filtering
filtration
  beam f.
  gel f.
  f. rate
finasteride
finding
  equivocal f.'s
  laboratory f.'s
  neuroradiological f.'s
fine azurophilic granule
fine-needle
  f.-n. aspiration (FNA)
  f.-n. aspiration biopsy (FNAB)
  f.-n. aspiration cytology (FNAC)
  f.-n. transhepatic cholangiography
FINE Storage of Measured Beam Data
finger
  oxidizing retroviral f.
fingerlike projection

fingerprinting
  DNA f.
  oral epithelial cell genetic f.
fingerstick blood sample
fingertapping task
Finzi-Harmer operation
Fiorinal with Codeine
FIPC
  favorable or intermediate prognosis cytogenetics
firefly luciferase assay
first
  F. Temp Genius tympanic thermometer
  F. Warning system
FirstCyte
  F. Aspirator
  F. MicroCatheter
first-echelon lymph node
first-generation regimen
first-line
  f.-l. chemotherapy
  f.-l. salvage therapy
  f.-l. treatment
FISH
  fluorescence in situ hybridization
  fluorescent in situ hybridization
Fisher-plus slide
Fisher-Race theory
Fiske and Subbarow method
Fisons nebulizer
fissure
  accessory f.
  azygos f.
  bulging f.
  choroidal f.
  intralobar f.
  perioral f.
fistula, pl. **fistulae, fistulas**
  anorectal f.
  aortoenteric f.
  arterial-arterial f.
  arteriobiliary f.
  arterioportal f.
  arterioportobiliary f.
  arteriosinusoidal penile f.
  arteriovenous f. (AVF)
  A-V f.
  biliary-enteric f.
  bronchoesophageal f.
  bronchopleural f.
  bronchopulmonary f.
  cecocutaneous f.

NOTES

223

fistula *(continued)*
    cholecystocolic f.
    cholecystocolonic f.
    cholecystoduodenal f.
    choledochoduodenal f.
    colocolic f.
    colovaginal f.
    colovesical f.
    duodenopancreatic f.
    dural arteriovenous f.
    enteric f.
    enterocolic f.
    enterocutaneous f.
    enteroenteric f.
    enterospinal f.
    enterovaginal f.
    enterovesical f.
    esophagotracheal f.
    f. formation
    gastrocolic f.
    iatrogenic arteriovenous f.
    intrahepatic arterioportal f.
    pharyngocutaneous f.
    postbiopsy renal AV f.
    salivary f.
    tracheoesophageal f. (TEF)
FITC
    fluorescein isothiocyanate conjugate
Fitzgerald factor
FIV
    feline immunodeficiency virus
FIVB
    5-fluorouracil, imidazole, vincristine,
       BCNU
fixation
    catheter f.
    complement f. (CF)
    microwave f.
    tumor f.
fixative
    tannic acid f.
fixe
    blanc f.
fixed
    f. cell
    f. dose rate
    f. macrophage
fixed-beam portal
fixed-schedule treatment
FL
    fibrolamellar
    flutamide and Lupron Depot
F-labeled 5-fluorouracil (F-FU)
FLAG
    fludarabine, ara-C, G-CSF
       FLAG regimen
flagellate pigmentation
flagellation pigmentation

FLAG-ida
    fludarabine, ara-C, G-CSF, idarubicin
flag sign
Flagyl
flail joint
FLAIR
    fluid-attenuated inversion recovery
       FLAIR pulse sequence
FLAM
    fludarabine, cytarabine, mitoxantrone
       FLAM regimen
flame cell
flammeus
    nevus f.
flange
    esophageal Z-stent with
      uncoated f.'s
flank pain
FLAP
    5-fluorouracil, leucovorin calcium,
      Adriamycin, Platinol
flap
    advancement f.
    bladder f.
    bone f.
    cheek advancement f.
    circle-to-W f.
    fan f.
    free filet f.
    Gillies f.
    Karapandzic advancement f.
    Limberg f.
    McFarlane skin f.
    musculocutaneous f.
    myocutaneous f.
    osteomyocutaneous free f.
    pedicle transposition f.
    rectus abdominis
      musculocutaneous f.
    rectus abdominis myocutaneous f.
    rectus abdominis transverse f.
    skin f.
    Soutar f.
    TRAM f.
    transposition f.
    transverse f.
    Webster cheek advancement f.
flare
    hormonal f.
    f. phenomenon
    tumor f.
flaring scapula
flash
    hot f.
flat colorectal carcinoma
flattener
    beam f.
flava (*pl. of* flavum)
flavone acetic acid (FAA)

flavonoid
flavopiridol/3-hour paclitaxel infusion combination
flavopiridol infusion
flavoprotein
flavum, pl. **flava**
flavus
    Aspergillus f.
flaxseed oil
fleet
    F. Babylax Rectal
    F. Enema
    F. Flavored Castor Oil
    F. Laxative
    F. Pain Relief
    F. Phospho-Soda
FLEP
    5-fluorouracil, leucovorin, etoposide, Platinol
fleroxacin
Fletcher
    F. afterloader
    F. factor
    F. rule
    F. rule of irradiation tolerance
Fletcher-Suit
    F.-S. system
    F.-S. system for radium therapy
Fletcher-Suit-Delclos
    F.-S.-D. system
    F.-S.-D. tandem
fleur-de-lis pattern
flexible
    f. biopsy needle
    f. bronchoscope
    f. endofluoroscopy
    f. endosonography probe
    f. fiberoptic bronchoscopy
    f. forceps
    f. loop domain
    f. nephroscope
    f. sigmoidoscope
    f. sigmoidoscopy
Flexner-Jobling carcinosarcoma
Flexner-Wintersteiner rosette
FlexSure OBT test
flexure
    splenic f.
FL-HCC
    fibrolamellar hepatocellular carcinoma
FLIC
    Functional Living Index-Cancer
flight

Flint Colon Injury Scale
flip-flop phenomenon
FLK-1
    FLK-1 receptor
    FLK-1 receptor for VEGF
flocculation
flocculent
    f. cluster
    f. ring
Flocks-Kadesky system
Flodine
Flomax
floor of mouth
flora
    endogenous f.
    exogenous f.
    microbial f.
Florical
florid stromal spindle cell component
FloSeal matrix hemostatic sealant
flow
    absolute blood f.
    antegrade f.
    bile f.
    cerebral blood f.
    f. cytometric DNA ploidy
    f. cytometry
    effective renal plasma f.
    helical blood f.
    hypothalamic blood f.
    intramyocardial coronary blood f. (ICBF)
    laminar air f.
    f. pattern
    peritrophoblastic f.
    pharmacologic maintenance erection f.
    f. rate
    f. void
flower cell
Floxin
floxuridine (FUDR, FUdR)
    circadian-modified f.
    f. in hepatic metastasis
    intraarterial f.
FLSA
    follicular lymphosarcoma
FLT1
    FLT1 receptor
    FLT1 receptor for VEGF
FLT3 ligand
fluasterone

F

NOTES

**fluconazole-resistant esophageal
    candidiasis**
flucytosine
Fludara
fludarabine
    f., ara-C, G-CSF (FLAG)
    f., ara-C, G-CSF, idarubicin
      (FLAG-ida)
    f., ara-C, mitoxantrone (FAM)
    f., cytarabine, mitoxantrone (FLAM)
    f., mitoxantrone, dexamethasone
      (FMD)
    f. monophosphate (FAMP)
    f., Novantrone, dexamethasone
      (FND)
    f. phosphate
    UCN-01 and f.
fludeoxyglucose F18
fluence profile
flufenamic acid
fluffy infiltrate
fluid
    ascitic f.
    bodily f.
    body f.
    cerebrospinal f. (CSF)
    cystic f.
    encapsulated f.
    extracellular f.
    intravenous f.
    loculated pleural f.
    f. mosaic model
    nipple aspirate f. (NAF)
    nipple aspiration f. (NAF)
    peritoneal f.
    pleural f.
    f. screening
    spinal f.
    straw-colored f.
    xanthochromic cerebrospinal f.
**fluid-attenuated inversion recovery
    (FLAIR)**
fluke
    blood f.
    Chinese liver f.
fluorescein
    f. isothiocyanate
    f. isothiocyanate conjugate (FITC)
    f. isothiocyanate-conjugated
      secondary antibody
fluorescence
    f. detector
    f. index (FI)
    f. polarization
    red f.
    f. in situ hybridization (FISH)
    f. spectroscopy
    f. yield

fluorescence-activated
    f.-a. cell sorter
    f.-a. cell sorting (FACS)
**fluorescence-based single strand
    conformation analysis**
fluorescent
    f. antibody technique
    f. antinuclear antibody (FANA)
    f. auramine-rhodamine stain
    f. bacteriophage assay (FBA)
    f. cytoprint assay
    f. dye efflux negative
    f. dye efflux positive
    f. multiplexed polymerase chain
      reaction
    f. multiplexed polymerase chain
      reaction analysis
    f. multiplex polymerase chain
      reaction assay
    f. shift
    f. signal intensity
    f. in situ hybridization (FISH)
    f. treponemal antibody absorption
      (FTA-ABS)
    f. treponemal antibody virus
fluorescentiae
    stadium f.
fluoride
    yttrium lithium f. (YLF)
2-fluoro-ara-AMP
18-fluoro-2-deoxyglucose (FDG)
**fluorodeoxyglucose positron emission
    tomography (FDG-PET)**
fluorodeoxyuridine (FUDR, FUdR)
5-fluoro-2-deoxyuridine (FUdR)
2-fluoromethylene-2$\underline{1}$deoxycytidine
fluoromethylene deoxycytidine (FMdC)
fluorophore-linked antibody
Fluoroplex Topical
fluoropyrimidine
    f. carbamate
    DPD-inhibitory f. (DIF)
fluoroquinolone
fluorouracil (FU, FUra)
5-fluorouracil (5-FU)
    5-f., Adriamycin, cyclophosphamide
      (FAC)
    5-f., Adriamycin, cyclophosphamide,
      methotrexate (FAC-M)
    5-f., Adriamycin, cyclophosphamide,
      streptozocin (FACS)
    5-f., Adriamycin, cyclophosphamide,
      VP-16 (FACVP)
    5-f., Adriamycin, Cytoxan,
      methotrexate (FAC-M)
    5-f., Adriamycin, MeCCNU (FAMe,
      FAME)
    5-f., Adriamycin, methotrexate
      (FAMTX)

5-f., Adriamycin, methyl-CCNU
(FAM-C)

5-f., Adriamycin, mitomycin (FAM)

5-f., Adriamycin, mitomycin,
citrovorum factor (FAM-CF)

5-f., Adriamycin, mitomycin C,
MeCCNU (FAMMe)

5-f., Adriamycin, mitomycin C,
streptozocin (FAM-S)

5-f., Adriamycin, Platinol (FAP)

bleomycin, cyclophosphamide,
methotrexate, 5-f. (BCMF)

bleomycin, cyclophosphamide,
Oncovin, methotrexate, 5-f.
(BLEO-COMF)

cisplatin and 5-f.

5-f., cisplatin, cytarabine, caffeine
(PACE)

cisplatin, epirubicin, folinic acid, 5-
f. (PELF)

cyclophosphamide, Adriamycin, 5-f.

cyclophosphamide, Adriamycin,
leucovorin calcium, 5-f.

cyclophosphamide, Adriamycin,
leucovorin rescue, 5-f. (CALF)

cyclophosphamide, Adriamycin,
methotrexate, 5-f. (CAMF)

5-f., cyclophosphamide, Adriamycin,
Platinol (FCAP)

cyclophosphamide and doxorubicin
with or without 5-f. (CA/CAF)

cyclophosphamide, epirubicin, 5-f.
(CEF)

cyclophosphamide,
hexamethylmelamine, 5-f. (CHF)

cyclophosphamide, methotrexate, 5-f.
(CMF, CM-5-FU)

cyclophosphamide, methotrexate,
prednisone, 5-f. (CMPF)

cyclophosphamide, Novantrone, 5-f.
(CNF)

cyclophosphamide, Oncovin,
methotrexate, 5-f. (COMF)

5-f., cyclophosphamide, prednisone
(FCP)

Cytoxan, Adriamycin, 5-f. (CAF)

Cytoxan, Adriamycin, leucovorin
calcium, 5-f. (CALLF)

5-f., Cytoxan, Adriamycin, Platinol
(FCAP)

Cytoxan, epirubicin, 5-f. (CEF)

Cytoxan, methotrexate, 5-f. (CMF)

5-f., doxorubicin, methotrexate

5-f., epirubicin, cyclophosphamide
(FEC)

5-f., epirubicin, Cytoxan (FEC)

5-f., etoposide, DDP (FED)

etoposide, leucovorin, 5-f. (ELF)

F-labeled 5-f. (F-FU)

5-f., folinic acid, oxaliplatin
(FOLFOX)

5-f. given with eniluracil and low-
dose leucovorin

hexamethylmelamine,
cyclophosphamide,
methotrexate, 5-f. (Hexa-CAF)

Ifex, mesna, Folex, 5-f.

5-f., imidazole, vincristine, BCNU
(FIVB)

irinotecan, folinic acid, 5-f.
(FOLFIRI)

leucovorin and 5-f. (LV5FU2)

5-f., leucovorin calcium,
Adriamycin, Cytoxan

5-f., leucovorin calcium,
Adriamycin, Platinol (FLAP)

5-f., leucovorin, etoposide, Platinol
(FLEP)

Leukeran, methotrexate, 5-f. (LMF)

MeCCNU, Oncovin, 5-f. (MOF)

5-f. and methotrexate (FUM)

methotrexate and 5-f. (MF)

5-f., methotrexate, ara-C,
cyclophosphamide, Adriamycin,
oncovin, prednisone (F-MACHOP)

methotrexate, Oncovin, 5-f. (MOF)

mitomycin and 5-f. (MF)

5-f., mitomycin C, streptozocin
(FMS)

mitoxantrone, vinblastine, 5-f.

mitoxantrone, vincristine, 5-f.
(MVF)

5-f., Novantrone, cyclophosphamide
(FNC)

5-f., Novantrone, methotrexate
(FNM)

5-f., Oncovin, Adriamycin,
mitomycin C (FOAM)

5-f., Oncovin, mitomycin C (FOM,
FOMi)

oxaliplatin with leucovorin and 5-f.
(FOLFOX)

phenylalanine mustard,
methotrexate, 5-f. (PMF)

Platinol, interferon alfa,
Adriamycin, 5-f. (PIAF)

NOTES

F

5-fluorouracil *(continued)*
    5-f. plus eniluracil
    streptozocin, mitomycin, 5-f. (SMF)
    Taxotere, Platinol, 5-f. (TPF)
    5-f., vinblastine, Adriamycin,
      Cytoxan (FUVAC)
    vinblastine, bleomycin,
      methotrexate, 5-f. (VBMF)
    vincristine, bleomycin,
      methotrexate, 5-f. (VBMF)
    vincristine, cyclophosphamide, 5-f.
      (VCF)
    vincristine, prednisone,
      cyclophosphamide,
      methotrexate, 5-f. (VPCMF)
5-fluorouracil/leucovorin (5-FU/LV)
5-fluorouracil/mitomycin chemoradiation
fluorouridine
Fluosol
Fluosol-DA
fluoxetine
fluoxymesterone (FXM)
    cyclophosphamide, methotrexate, 5-
      fluorouracil, f. (CMF-FLU)
fluphenazine
flurazepam
flurbiprofen
flurocitabine
flush
    serotonin f.
flushing
    catheter f.
    f. technique
flutamide
    f. and Lupron Depot (FL)
    f. and Zoladex (FZ)
flutter
    atrial f.
fluvastatin
fluvoxamine
^{255}Fm
    fermium-255
F-MACHOP
    5-fluorouracil, methotrexate, ara-C,
      cyclophosphamide, Adriamycin,
      oncovin, prednisone
FMD
    fludarabine, mitoxantrone,
      dexamethasone
FMdC
    fluoromethylene deoxycytidine
F-misonidazole
fmol/mg
    femtomoles per milligram
fMRI
    functional magnetic resonance imaging
FMS
    5-fluorouracil, mitomycin C, streptozocin

fms
    fms oncogene
    fms protooncogene/oncogene
FNA
    fine-needle aspiration
    FNA biopsy
FNAB
    fine-needle aspiration biopsy
FNAC
    fine-needle aspiration cytology
FNC
    5-fluorouracil, Novantrone,
      cyclophosphamide
FND
    fludarabine, Novantrone, dexamethasone
FNH
    focal nodular hyperplasia
FNM
    5-fluorouracil, Novantrone, methotrexate
FOAM
    5-fluorouracil, Oncovin, Adriamycin,
      mitomycin C
foam
    f. cell
    polyvinyl alcohol f.
foamy
    f. agent
    f. gland carcinoma
    f. histiocyte
    f. lipophage
FOBT
    fecal occult blood test
focal
    f. adhesion kinase (FAK)
    f. adhesion kinase protein
    f. cranial radiation therapy (FCRT)
    f. deficit
    f. demyelination
    f. epithelial hyperplasia
    f. fatty infiltration
    f. hypoechoic lesion (FHL)
    f. lobular carcinoma
    f. nodular hyperplasia (FNH)
    f. pathology
    f. squamous metaplasia
FocalSeal-L surgical sealant
focus, pl. **foci**
    aberrant crypt f.
    f. of calcification
    discrete hyperintense f.
    hyperintense f.
    keratinization f.
    nodular hyperintense f.
    punctate hyperintense f.
    satellite f.
    synovial cartilaginous f.
focused heat technology
focus-skin distance (FSD)

foil
  scattering f.
Foille Medicated First Aid
folate
  f. antagonist
  f. polyglutamylation system
  f. uptake pathway
folate-binding protein
fold
  aryepiglottic f.
  epiglottic f.
  glossoepiglottic f.
  gray matter f.
  pharyngoepiglottic f.
FOLFIRI
  irinotecan, folinic acid, 5-fluorouracil
  FOLFIRI regimen
FOLFOX
  5-fluorouracil, folinic acid, oxaliplatin
  oxaliplatin with leucovorin and 5-
    fluorouracil
  FOLFOX regimen
FOLFUGEM
  folinic acid, leucovorin, 5-fluorouracil,
    gemcitabine
  FOLFUGEM regimen
FOLFUGEM-OX
  folinic acid, leucovorin, 5-fluorouracil,
    gemcitabine, oxaliplatin
  FOLFUGEM-OX regimen
folia (*pl. of* folium)
foliaceus
  pemphigus f.
folic
  f. acid
  f. acid antagonist
folinate
  calcium f.
folinic
  f. acid (FA)
  f. acid, leucovorin, 5-fluorouracil,
    gemcitabine (FOLFUGEM)
  f. acid, leucovorin, 5-fluorouracil,
    gemcitabine, oxaliplatin
    (FOLFUGEM-OX)
Folin and Wu method
folium, pl. **folia**
follicle
  f. center lymphoma
  colloid-filled f.
  lollipop f.
  neoplastic f.
  ovarian f.

follicle-stimulating
  f.-s. hormone (FSH)
  f.-s. hormone-releasing hormone
    (FSH-RH)
follicular
  f. adenocarcinoma
  f. adenocarcinoma of thyroid
  f. basal cell hyperplasia
  f. carcinoma
  f. dendritic cell (FDC)
  f. dendritic cell tumor
  f. dendritic sarcoma
  f. hyperplasia
  f. infundibulum
  f. keratosis
  f. lymphosarcoma (FLSA)
  f. mantle zone
  f. mucinosis
  f. non-Hodgkin lymphoma
  f. poroma
  f. predominantly large cell
  f. predominantly small cleaved cell
  f. thyroid carcinoma (FTC)
follicularis
  enteritis f.
folliculitis
  staphylococcal f.
folliculorum
  Demodex f.
Folvite
folylpolyglutamate synthetase
FOM, FOMi
  5-fluorouracil, Oncovin, mitomycin C
fomivirsen
fondaparinux sodium
Fonio solution
Fontana-Masson stain
Food and Drug Administration (FDA)
footprinting
  DNA f.
  DNAse f.
foramen, pl. **foramina**
  alveolar f.
  anterior condyloid f.
  anterior palatine f.
  anterior sacral f.
  aortic f.
  Bichat f.
  Bochdalek f.
  cervical neural f.
  emissary sphenoidal f.
  epiploic f.
  ethmoid f.

F

foramen *(continued)*
    external acoustic f.
    intervertebral f.
    stylomastoid f.
    sublabral f.
force
    DES task f.
    electromotive f.
    repulsive f.
forceps
    flexible f.
    Randall f.
    rigid f.
Fordyce
    F. granule
    F. spot
forefoot compression sleeve
foregut
    bronchopulmonary f.
foreign
    f. body carcinogenesis
    f. genome
form
    Alibert-Bazin f.
    circulating recombinant f.
    Discrene breast f.
    Groninger Intelligence Test,
       short f. (GIT-V)
    Nearly Me breast f.
    novel f.
    time-release f.
formaldehyde
formalin-fixed tissue
format
    peer-to-peer discussion f.
formation
    antiantibody f.
    antibody f.
    callus f.
    colony f.
    degenerative microcystic f.
    Ehrlich theory of antibody f.
    fistula f.
    Jerne theory of antibody f.
    membrane bleb f.
    microcystic f.
    new bone f.
    Rouleaux f.
forme fruste
formestane
formin cell
forming
    burst f.
formula, pl. **formulae, formulas**
    biologic effective dose f.
    Calvert f.
    Cockcroft-Gault f.
    Greenwood f.
    Kaopectate Advanced F.

    multivitamin-mineral f.
    Ostofresh f.
    Peto f.
    F. Q
    rapid dissolution f. (RDF)
formulation
    1,2-dimyristyloxypropyl-3-
      dimethylhydroxyethyl ammonium
      bromide/dioleoylphosphatidylethano-
      lamine f. (DMRIE/DOPE)
    drug f.
    lyophilized recombinant interferon f.
formyl
forskolin
Forssman
    F. antibody
    F. antigen
Fortaz
forte
    Norgesic F.
    Prenavite F.
    Radiostol F.
    Spectrum F. 29
    Vicon F.
    Zone-A F.
Fortovase
fortuitum
    Mycobacterium f.
Forvade
forward segmental multileaf collimator
Fosamax
Foscan mediated photodynamic therapy
foscarnet
Foscavir
fosfestrol
fosphenytoin
fos protooncogene/oncogene
fosquidone
fossa, pl. **fossae**
    acetabular f.
    antecubital f.
    cranial f.
    infratemporal f.
    pterygoid f.
    pterygomaxillary f.
    pterygopalatine f.
    f. of Rosenmüller
    supratentorium f.
fostriecin sodium
fotemustine/cisplatin/etoposide
    combination chemotherapy
Fouchet test
foul taste
foundation
    Berlix Oncology F.
    Candlelighters Childhood Cancer F.
    (CCCF)
    Childhood Brain Tumor F.
    Cure for Lymphoma F.

International Myeloma F.
National Childhood Cancer F.
founder mutation
Fournier gangrene
foveolar
fowlpox
Fox-Fordyce anomaly
FPA
    fibrinopeptide A
    Asserachrom FPA
FPC
    familial polyposis coli
FRA3B gene
FRACON
    framycetin, colistin, nystatin
fraction
    daily f.
    dose per f.
    drug f.
    euglobulin plasma f.
    growth f.
    heavy membrane mitochondrial
      subcellular f.
    multiple daily f.
    plasma protein f.
    quiescent f.
    rad f.
    f.'s of radiation
    f. size
    S-phase f.
fractional cell kill
fractionated
    f. dose-survival curve
    f. external beam irradiation
    f. extracranial stereotactic
      radiotherapy
    f. radiation therapy
    f. stereotactic radiosurgery
    f. total body irradiation (FTBI)
fractionation
    accelerated f.
    co-alcohol f.
    daily f.
    dose f.
    radiation f.
    f. regimen
    f. schedule
fracture
    abduction-external rotation f.
    acetabular posterior wall f.
    acetabular rim f.
    acute f.
    agenetic f.

anatomic f.
ankle mortise f.
anterior column f.
anterolateral compression f.
apophysial f.
arch f.
articular mass separation f.
articular pillar f.
Ashhurst-Bromer classification of
    ankle f.'s
Atkin epiphysial f.
atlas f.
atrophic f.
avulsion stress f.
axis f.
Barton f.
Barton-Smith f.
basal neck f.
basilar femoral neck f.
beak f.
bedroom f.
Bennett comminuted f.
bicondylar T-shaped f.
bicondylar Y-shaped f.
bimalleolar f.
both-bone f.
both-column f.
bowing f.
bronchial f.
buckle f.
burst f.
butterfly f.
capitulum radiale humeri f.
carpal bone stress f.
carpometacarpal joint f.
cartwheel f.
cementum f.
central f.
cerebral palsy pathological f.
cervical spine f.
cervicotrochanteric f.
complete f.
compression f.
condylar f.
de Quervain f.
diametric pelvic f.
diaphysial f.
dislocation f.
displaced f.
distal femoral epiphysial f.
distal humoral f.
distal radial f.
distraction of f.

NOTES

F

fracture *(continued)*
    dyscrasic f.
    elbow f.
    electrostimulation for nonunion
      of f.
    elementary f.
    epicondylar f.
    epiphysial plate f.
    epiphysial slip f.
    epiphysial tibial f.
    explosion f.
    extension teardrop f.
    extracapsular f.
    extraoctave f.
    inflammatory f.
    laminar f.
    nonunion of f.
    olecranon f.
    Papavasiliou classification of
      olecranon f.'s
    pathologic f.
    periarticular f.
    postirradiation f.
    f. site
    threatened pathologic f.
    traction f.
fragile
    f. histidine triad (FHIT)
    f. histidine triad gene
fragilis
    Bacteroides f.
fragilocytosis
fragment
    f. antigen binding (Fab)
    crystallizable f. (Fc)
    extruded disc f.
    Fab f.
    Fc f.
    LymphoScan Tc99m-labeled murine
      antibody f.
    single-chain variable f. (scFv)
fragmentation
    internucleosomal DNA f.
    nuclear f.
Fragmin
frame
    Brown-Roberts-Wells f.
    nonferromagnetic MR-compatible f.
    open reading f. (ORF)
    f. of reference
    relocatable stereotactic f.
framework
    genetic f.
framycetin, colistin, nystatin (FRACON)
Frankfort horizontal plane
Franklin disease
Franklin-Silverman biopsy needle
Frank orthogonal configuration
Franseen needle

F reagent
freckle
    Hutchinson melanotic f.
fredericamycin
**Fred Hutchinson Cancer Research
  Center**
free
    cancer f. (CF)
    f. circulating soluble CD52
    f. cortisol
    f. filet flap
    f. from distant metastasis (FFDM)
    f. from recurrence (FFR)
    f. macrophage
    f. PSA
    f. radical
    f. radical scavenging system
    salt f. (SF)
    f. testosterone
    f. thyroxine index
    f. versus complexed PSA
    f. water
freedom from progression (FFP)
free/total PSA index
freeze-dried
    f.-d. gel (FDG)
    f.-d. paraffin-embedded tissue
freeze/thaw protocol
freezing process
Frei antigen
fremitus
French-American-British (FAB)
    F.-A.-B. classification
frequency
    Larmor f.
    somatic mutation f.
frequency-elective pulse
Frerich theory
fresh
    f. cell suspension
    f. thrombotic occlusion
    f. tissue allocation
fresh-frozen
    f.-f. plasma
    f.-f. tissue section
Freund complete adjuvant (FCA)
Frey syndrome
Fricke
    F. dosimetry
    F. gel
frictional keratosis
Friedreich ataxia
Friend leukemia virus
frigoris
    stadium f.
Froben
Froben-SR
Froin syndrome

frondosum
    chorion f.
frontal bossing
front loading
frosted branch angiitis
frozen
    f. red cell
    f. tissue section
fruste
    forme f.
FS
    feminization syndrome
    antihemophilic factor VIII FS
    Helixate FS
    FS unit test
FSD
    focus-skin distance
    FSD colpostat
FSH
    follicle-stimulating hormone
FSH-RH
    follicle-stimulating hormone-releasing
      hormone
FSI
    Fatigue Symptom Inventory
FSU
    functional subunit
FT
    farnesyl transferase
    FT tumor marker
FTA-ABS
    fluorescent treponemal antibody
      absorption
FTBI
    fractionated total body irradiation
FTC
    follicular thyroid carcinoma
FTI
    farnesyl transferase inhibitor
ftorafur
    f., Adriamycin, cyclophosphamide,
      BCG (FAC-BCG)
    f., Adriamycin, cyclophosphamide,
      Platinol (FACP)
    f., Adriamycin, mitomycin C
      (FURAM)
    uracil plus f. (UFT)
FU
    fluorouracil
5-FU
    5-fluorouracil
    5-FU deoxyribonucleoside
    intralesional 5-FU

    leucovorin-modulated 5-FU
    LV plus 5-FU
    topical 5-FU
fuchsin
    aniline f.
Fuchs-Rosenthal chamber
Fucidin
    F. I.V.
    F. Oral Suspension
    F. Tablet
fucosylation index
fucoxanthin
FUDR
    floxuridine
    fluorodeoxyuridine
FUdR
    floxuridine
    fluorodeoxyuridine
    5-fluoro-2-deoxyuridine
fugax
    amaurosis f.
Fuhrman
    F. classification
    F. grading system
    F. nuclear grade
fulguration of bladder cancer
full-length
    f.-l. genome sequencing
    f.-l. integrase
full-thickness kidney block
fully automated blood typing system
fulminant
    f. disseminated intravascular
      coagulation
    f. hepatic failure
    f. hepatitis
    f. pancreatitis
5-FU/LV
    5-fluorouracil/leucovorin
fulvestrant injection
FUM
    5-fluorouracil and methotrexate
fumagillin
    synthetic analogue of f.
fumarate
    ferrous f.
    liarozole f.
fumigatus
    Aspergillus f.
Fumonisin B$_1$
function
    ciliary f.
    delta f.

NOTES

function *(continued)*
    erectile f.
    factor VIII coagulation f.
    fusogenic domain f.
    hematopoietic f.
    International Index of Erectile f.
      (IIEF)
    MALT f.
    menstrual f.
    mucosa-associated lymphoid
      tissue f.
    myocardial f.
    neuromuscular f.
    ovarian f.
    power f.
    renal f.
    reproductive f.
    Salmon-Durie staging f.
    sexual f.
    survival f.
    thyroid f.
    white blood cell f.
functional
    f. activation
    f. asplenia
    F. Assessment of Cancer Therapy
      (FACT)
    F. Assessment of Cancer Therapy-
      Bladder (FACT-BL)
    F. Assessment of Cancer Therapy-
      Fatigue (FACT-F)
    f. genomics
    f. independent measurement score
    F. Living Index-Cancer (FLIC)
    f. magnetic resonance imaging
      (fMRI)
    f. mapping
    f. MRI
    f. subunit (FSU)
functioning
    emotional f.
    physical f.
    role f.
    social f.
    spiritual f.
fund
    Imperial Cancer Research F.
fungal
    f. immunodiffusion titer
    f. pneumonia
fungating tumor
fungemia
    Candida f.
fungemic shock
Fungizone
fungoides
    Alibert-Bazin form of mycosis f.

    mycosis f. (MF)
    treatment-resistant mycosis f.
Fungoid Tincture
fungus ball
funisitis
FUO
    fever of unknown origin
FUra
    fluorouracil
Furadantin
FURAM
    ftorafur, Adriamycin, mitomycin C
furazolidone
furfur
    Malassezia f.
furifosmin
furocoumarin
furosemide
Furoside
furuncle
furuncular myiasis
furunculosis
furunculus
fusariosis
Fusarium
fusidic acid
fusiform cell
fusin 29 (SI)
fusion
    cell f.
    cervical spine f.
    CT/SPECT f.
    f. gene
    image f.
    müllerian duct formation and f.
    f. oncoprotein
    f. peptide
    f. products
    f. protein
fusogenic domain function
futile cycle
FUVAC
    5-fluorouracil, vinblastine, Adriamycin,
      Cytoxan
Fuzeon
FVL
    factor V Leiden
FXIIIa
    factor XIIIa
FXM
    fluoxymesterone
Fy antigen
FZ
    flutamide and Zoladex

γ (*var. of* gamma)
G
>gauss
>gingiva
>gingival
>guanine
>>G cell
>>G phase
>>G protein
>>G protooncogene/oncogene

G1
>immunoglobulin G1

G3139
>*bcl*-2 antisense molecule G3139

G$_o$
>G$_o$ period
>G$_o$ phase

G25 monoclonal antibody
G/A
>globulin/albumin

Ga
>gallium

^{67}Ga
>gallium-67
>^{67}Ga scan

GA733-2 glycoprotein
GAD
>generalized anxiety disorder

gadolinium
>motexafin g.
>g. scan
>g. texaphyrin (Gd-Tex)

Gaeta classification
gag
>g. lipopeptide P3C541b

Gag-Pol precursor
Gag protein
Gail breast cancer risk model
gain
>accelerated phase g.
>color g.

gain-of-function mutation
Gainor criteria
Gaisböck disease
gait
>antalgic g.

galactemia
galactitol
galactoglycoprotein
galactomannan
>*Aspergillus* g.
>g. assay

galactose
>g. oxidase-Schiff (GOS)
>g. oxidase-Schiff reaction

galactosemia
galactosyl
galactosylamide beta-galactosidase deficiency
galactosylation
galamustine
galectin-3
>g.-3 isoform
>g.-3 protein

gallate
>epigallocatechin g. (EGCg)

gallbladder
>bifid g.
>g. cancer
>g. carcinoma (GBCA)
>g. florid pyloric gland metaplasia

gallinarum
>*Haemophilus* g.

gallium (Ga)
>g. nitrate
>g. scan

gallium-67 (^{67}Ga)
GALT
>gut-associated lymphoid tissue

GALV
>gibbon ape leukemia virus

gambiense
>*Trypanosoma* g.

gametocyte
gametogony
Gamimune N
gamma, γ
>adeno-interferon g.
>Ad-IFN g.
>g. chain
>g. detection probe
>g. globulin
>g. glutamyl
>interferon g. (IFN-G, IFN-g)
>g. interferon (IFN-G, IFN-g)
>g. irradiation
>g. knife radiation
>g. knife radiosurgery
>g. knife surgery (GKS)
>mitochondrial deoxyribonucleic acid polymerase g.
>mitochondrial DNA polymerase g.
>recombinant interferon g.

gamma-1b
>interferon g.-1b

gamma-benzene hexachloride
gamma-delta-TCR
gamma-detecting probe
Gammagard S/D
gamma-glutamyl transpeptidase

G

235

gamma-HCD
gamma-heavy-chain disease
gamma-heavy-chain disease (gamma-HCD)
gamma-methylene-10-deazaaminopterin
Gammar-P I.V.
gammopathy
biclonal g.
monoclonal g.
polyclonal g.
Gamna-Favre body
Gamulin Rh
ganciclovir (GCV)
intravitreal g.
g. therapy
ganglia (*pl. of* ganglion)
gangliocytoma
dysplastic cerebellar g.
ganglioglioma
cystic g.
desmoplastic infantile g. (DIG, DIGG)
infantile g.
intracerebral g.
ganglioma
intracerebral g.
ganglion, pl. ganglia
autonomic sympathetic g.
celiac g.
ciliary g.
gasserian g.
intestinal parasympathetic g.
intraosseous g.
g. neurolytic block
parasympathetic g.
stellate g.
sympathetic g.
Troisier g.
ganglioneuroblastoma
ganglioneuroma
ganglioside
GD2 g.
GD3 g.
gangliosidosis
gangrene
Fournier g.
gangrenescens
granuloma g.
Ganite
Ganoderma Lucidum Karst
gantry
LINAC g.
gap
air g.
GAPDH
glyceraldehyde phosphate dehydrogenase
Garamycin
Garatec
Gardnerella vaginalis

Gardner-Rasheed sarcoma virus
Gardner syndrome
gas
blood g.
extraluminal g.
growing neural g. (GNG)
radon g.
gasserian
g. ganglion
g. thermorhizotomy
Gasser syndrome
gastrectomy
partial g.
total g.
gastric
g. antral vascular ectasia
g. carcinogenesis
g. carcinoma (GC)
g. enterochromaffin cell
g. leiomyosarcoma
g. MALT lymphoma
g. mucin
g. outlet obstruction
g. oxyntic mucosa
g. pullup
g. remnant cancer
g. stump
g. stump carcinoma
g. tumor marker antibody
g. ulcer
gastricae
areae g.
Gastrimmune
gastrin-releasing
g.-r. peptide (GRP)
g.-r. peptide receptor (GRPR, GRP-R)
gastritis
alcoholic g.
atrophic g.
bile reflux g.
chemotherapy-induced g.
chronic atrophic g.
emphysematous g.
erosive g.
granulomatous g.
hemorrhagic g.
multifocal atrophic g. (MAG)
gastrocolic fistula
gastroenteric bypass
gastroenteritis
eosinophilic g.
gastroenterostomy
percutaneous g.
gastroesophageal
g. junction carcinoma
g. reflux
gastrohepatic ligament

gastrointestinal
  g. agent
  g. cancer
  g. complication
  g. epithelial cell
  g. lymphoma
  g. malignancy
  g. sarcoma
  g. stromal tumor (GIST)
  g. tract adenocarcinoma
  G. Tumor Study Group (GITSG, GTSG)
gastrojejunostomy
  palliative g.
GastroMARK
gastropathy
  hyperplastic g.
gastrostomy
  palliative g.
  percutaneous endoscopic g. (PEG)
  g. tube
GATA1 zinc protein
gated
  g. irradiation
  g. irradiation system
gatekeeper gene
gatifloxacin
Gaucher disease
gauss (G)
Gaussian distribution
gay-related immune deficiency (GRID)
gaze palsy
GBCA
  gallbladder carcinoma
GBM
  glioblastoma multiforme
  glomerular basement membrane
    GBM antibody
GBq
  gigabecquerel
GC
  gastric carcinoma
  gliomatosis cerebri
GCC
  goblet cell carcinoid
G-cell hyperplasia
G-CFU
  granulocyte colony-forming unit
G-CSF
  granulocyte colony-stimulating factor
    fludarabine, ara-C, G-CSF (FLAG)
    granulocyte recombinant G-CSF

  G-CSF mobilized peripheral blood stem cell
  G-CSF prophylaxis
  recombinant G-CSF
GCT
  germ cell tumor
GCV
  ganciclovir
GD2
  GD2 cancer-associated antigen
  GD2 ganglioside
GD2-KLH vaccination
GD3 ganglioside
GdA deficiency
GDN
  glyceryl dinitrate
GDP
  guanosine diphosphate
Gd-Tex
  gadolinium texaphyrin
  Gd-Tex radiation sensitizer
GE
  General Electric
  GE Quest 300-H scanner
gefitinib
Gehan-Gilbert modification
Geiger-Muller detector
gel
  acoustic g.
  acrylamide g.
  bexarotene g.
  Carrington Dermal wound g.
  g. filtration
  freeze-dried g. (FDG)
  Fricke g.
  H.P. Acthar G.
  IntraDose injectable g.
  Panretin topical g.
  polyacrylamide g.
  PRO 2000 G.
  Targretin g.
  topical 4,4′-dihydroxybenzophenone-2,4-dinitrophenylhydrazone (A-007) 0.25% g.
gelatin
  absorbable g.
  g. sphere
  g. sponge
  g. sponge pad
  g. zymography
gelatinase
gelatin-encapsulated nitrogen microsphere

NOTES

G

gelatinous
  g. ascites
  g. pseudocyst
geldanamycin
Gelfoam
  G. Topical
  G. torpedo
Geliperm
  G. agar
  G. gel dressing
Gell-Coombs classification
Gelpirin
gel-shift assay
gelsolin
gemcitabine (DFDC)
  g., cisplatin, ifosfamide (GIOP)
  folinic acid, leucovorin, 5-
    fluorouracil, g. (FOLFUGEM)
  g. HCl
  g. hydrochloride
  g. plus oxaliplatin (GEMOX)
  g. plus oxaliplatin regimen
  Taxol, cisplatin, g. (TCG)
gemfibrozil
gemistocyte
gemistocytic astrocytoma
gemistocytoma
GEMM-CFC
  granulocyte, erythrocyte, monocyte,
    megakaryocyte colony-forming cell
GEMOX
  gemcitabine plus oxaliplatin
    GEMOX regimen
gemtuzumab ozogamicin (GO)
Gemzar
Genapap
Genasense
Genasoft Plus
Genaspor
genavense
  Mycobacterium g.
Gencalc 600
gender-limited cancer
gene
  adenopolyposis coli g.
  g. amplification
  antigen-processing g. Ii
  antigen receptor g.
  APC g.
  astrocytoma g.
  ATM g.
  AT mutation g.
  autosomal g.
  g. bank
  bax g.
  bcl-2 g.
  bcl-2/Ig fusion g.
  bcl-x g.
  bcr/abl fusion g.

BRCA1 g.
BRCA2 g.
BRCA1 susceptibility g.
breast cancer 1 g. (*BRCA1*)
breast cancer 2 g. (*BRCA2*)
CAPB g.
CAT expression g.
CD40 g.
CDKN2/p16 g.
cell interaction g.
cellular suppressor g.
c-erbB1 g.
c-erbB2/neu g.
c-fos g.
chimeric antigen receptor g.
chimeric bcr/abl g.
c-kit g.
cloned g.
g. cloning
cluster of differentiation 40 g.
c-met g.
g. coding
codominant g.
complementary g.
g. construct RevM10
csf1R1 g.
CYP1A2 g.
CYP2D6 g.
CYP2B6 g.
CYP2C9 g.
damage response g.
DCC g.
deleted in colon cancer g.
g. delivery vector
derepressed g.
g. detection
g. diversity
DMA g.
DMB g.
DNA virus transforming g.
dominant g.
DQ g.
E1A g.
E1B g.
EGFR g.
envelope glycoprotein B g.
epidermal growth factor receptor g.
erg1 g.
erythropoietin g.
EWS g.
g. expression
FHIT g.
FRA3B g.
fragile histidine triad g.
fusion g.
gatekeeper g.
globin g.
glutathione-S-transferase g.
GSTM1 g.

GSTP1 g.
GSTT1 g.
H g.
hairy g.
HER-2/neu g.
histocompatibility g.
hMLH1 g.
hMSH2 g.
hMSH3 g.
holandric g.
homeobox g.
HOX11 g.
hPMS1 g.
hPMS2 g.
H-ras g.
HRC g.
hTERC g.
hTERT g.
hTR g.
human androgen receptor g.
 (HUMARA)
Ig g.
immune response g.
immune suppressor g.
immunoglobulin g.
g. induction
inhibiting g.
KAI1/CD82 g.
Ki-ras g.
K-ras g.
leaky g.
lethal g.
g. library
lineage-associated g.
Lin-11, Isl-1, Mec-3 g.'s (LIM)
major g.
g. mapping
mats g.
MCC g.
MDM2 g.
mdr1 g.
melanoma differentiation-
 associated g. (*mda*-7)
Melastatin g.
MEN1 g.
met g.
MICA g.
MICB g.
mismatch repair g.
MLH1 g.
MLL g.
MLM g.
MMR g.

modifying g.
MSH2 g.
MSH3 (hMSH3) g.
multiple-drug resistance g.
mutant g.
myoD g.
NA-MYCN g.
nef g.
neurofibromatosis 2 g.
NF-1 g.
NF-2 g.
nm23 g.
nonstructural g.
N-ras g.
oncosuppressor g.
operator g.
ornithine transcarbamylase
 deficiency g.
OTC g.
p53 g.
p53 adenoviral g.
PAX-5 g.
PAX-7 g.
PGY1 g.
PGY3 g.
pleiotropic g.
pol g.
g. pool
proapoptotic g.
g. product (gp)
g. promoter
proneural g.
protease g.
PTCH g.
PTEN g.
RAG-1 g.
RAG-2 g.
RASSF1A g.
Rb g.
RCC1 g.
rearrangement of g.'s
g. rearrangement
g. rearrangement study
recessive g.
reciprocal g.
regenerating g. I (REG)
g. regulation
regulatory g.
g. replacement
g. replacement therapy
reporter g.
repressed g.
repressor g.

NOTES

G

gene *(continued)*
    retinoblastoma g.
    RNASEL g.
    Rp53 g.
    R11 tumor suppressor g.
    g. sequence
    g. sequencing
    sex-linked g.
    SOD2 Val/Val g.
    g. splicing
    g. structure
    sublethal g.
    suicide g.
    suppressor g.
    survivin g.
    g. switching
    tal-1/SIL fusion g.
    tax g.
    g. transcription
    g. transfection
    g. transfer
    g. transfer therapy
    g. transfer transcription assay
    transforming g.
    TS g.
    TSC2 g.
    tumor-associated differentially expressed g. 15 (TADG-15)
    tumor suppressor g. (TSG)
    Turcot g.
    V g.
    vero vector with IL2 g.
    VH g.
    VHL tumor suppressor g.
    von Hippel-Lindau g.
    vpr g.
    wild-type g.
    WT1 g.
    X-linked g.
    XRCC1 g.
gene-activated erythropoietin
GeneAmp PCR test
gene-based product
Genebs
general
    g. anesthesia
    g. anesthetic
    g. dermatology
    G. Electric (GE)
generalized
    g. anxiety disorder (GAD)
    g. nephrographic phase imaging
generation
    de novo g.
generator
    deuterium-tritium g.
    RF2000 Radiofrequency G.
GenESA system
GeneSeq HIV assay

gene-silencing phenomenon
genetic
    g. algorithm
    g. approach
    g. archive
    g. barrier
    g. code
    g. condition
    g. counseling
    g. damage
    g. deviation
    g. engineering
    g. factor
    g. framework
    g. heterogeneity
    g. immunity
    g. inheritance
    g. knockout
    g. lability
    g. lesion
    g. level
    g. linkage map
    g. marker
    g. marking
    g. masking tape
    g. mutation
    g. polymorphism
    g. probe
    g. recombination
    g. screening
    g. subtype
    g. susceptibility
    g. switch
    g. test
    g. testing
    g. thrombophilia
    g. variability
genetics
    Clinical Cancer G.
    molecular g.
GeneVax DNA plasmid backbone
Gengou phenomenon
geniculate ganglion schwannoma
genioglossus muscle
geniohyoid muscle
genistein
genital
    g. carcinoma
    g. human papillomavirus infection
    g. self-examination (GSE)
genitalia
    lymphatic drainage of g.
genitalis
    herpes g.
genitourinary
    g. adverse effect
    g. cancer
    g. infection
    g. rhabdomyosarcoma

Gen-K
Gen-Nifedipine
genodermatosis
genome
>foreign g.
>helper g.
>mosaic g.

genomic
>g. assay
>g. disease management
>g. DNA
>g. imprinting
>g. sequence
>g. viral
>g. viral messenger ribonucleic acid transcript
>g. viral mRNA transcript

genomics
>functional g.

genotoxic
genotype
>cytochrome P450 2D6 g.
>SOD2 Val/Val g.

genotypic analysis
genotyping
>epithelial-cell based posttransplant g.
>oral epithelial cell g.
>VircoGEN g.

Genpril
Gen-Probe hybridization kit
GENS-S Cell hematology workstation
Gent-AK
gentamicin
gentian
>g. blue
>g. violet

Gentrasul
Geocillin
geographic pattern
geography
>brain g.

Geo-Matt therapeutic foam overlay
geometric optimization algorithm
geometry
>implant g.

Geopen
George and Desu method
geotrichosis
GEP
>granulin-epithelin precursor

GEPARDO
>German preoperative Adriamycin docetaxel

gergoviae
>*Enterobacter* g.

germ
>g. cell neoplasm
>g. cell testicular tumor
>g. cell tumor (GCT)
>g. tube test

German preoperative Adriamycin docetaxel (GEPARDO)
germinal
>g. aplasia
>g. center
>g. center pattern
>g. epithelium
>g. matrix hemorrhage
>g. matrix-related hemorrhage

germinolysis
germinoma
>pineal g.
>suprasellar hemorrhagic g.

Germiston virus
germline
>g. band
>g. configuration
>g. DNA
>g. mutation

Gerson therapy
gestational
>g. choriocarcinoma
>g. nonmetastatic trophoblastic disease
>g. trophoblastic disease (GTD)
>g. trophoblastic neoplasia
>g. trophoblastic neoplasm
>g. trophoblastic tumor

gestationis
>herpes g.

Gesterol
Gevrabon
GFAP
>glial fibrillary acidic protein

GFP
>green-fluorescent protein

GFR
>glomerular filtration rate

GF-UM3 scanner
G_1, G_2 subphase
GH
>growth hormone

NOTES

G

GHD
  growth hormone deficiency
ghost
  g. cell
  red cell g.
GHRF, GH-RF
  growth hormone-releasing factor
GHRH, GH-RH
  growth hormone-releasing hormone
GH-RIH
  growth hormone release-inhibiting
  hormone
Gianotti-Crosti syndrome
giant
  g. aggressive keratoacanthoma
  g. cell
  g. cell angiofibroma
  g. cell aortitis
  g. cell arteritis
  g. cell astrocytoma
  g. cell carcinoma of thyroid gland
  g. cell hepatitis
  g. cell hepatitis of infancy
  g. cell myeloma
  g. cell reaction
  g. cell reparative granuloma
  g. cell sarcoma
  g. cell sarcoma of bone
  g. cell tumor
  g. cell tumor of tendon sheath
  g. hemangioma
  g. lymph node hyperplasia
  g. melanocytic nevus
  g. pore type
  g. pore-type basal cell carcinoma
Gianturco steel coil
Giardia
  G. intestinalis
  G. lamblia
giardiasis
gibbon
  g. ape leukemia virus (GALV)
  g. ape lymphosarcoma virus
gibbus
  thoracic g.
Giemsa stain
Giemsa-trypsin banding procedure
gigabecquerel (GBq)
gigantism
Gigli saw
gill arch
Gillies flap
GIMEMA
  Gruppo Italiano Malattie Ematologiche
  Maligne dell'Adulto
  GIMEMA protocol
gingiva, pl. **gingivae (G)**
gingival (G)
  g. bleeding

  g. cancer
  g. mucosa
  g. recession
gingival-buccal sulcus
gingival-labial sulcus
gingivitis
  erosive g.
  HIV necrotizing g.
  human immunodeficiency
    necrotizing g.
  necrotizing ulcerative g.
gingivostomatitis
  herpetic g.
ginkgo biloba
ginseng
  Panax g.
  Siberian g.
GIOP
  gemcitabine, cisplatin, ifosfamide
gip2 protooncogene/oncogene
girdle
  pelvic g.
  shoulder g.
GIST
  gastrointestinal stromal tumor
GITSG, GTSG
  Gastrointestinal Tumor Study Group
GIT-V
  Groninger Intelligence Test, short form
GIVIO
  Gruppo Interdisciplinare Valutazione
    Interventi in Oncologia
GJT
  glomus jugulare tumor
GKS
  gamma knife surgery
glabrata
  Candida g.
glabrous skin
gladiatorum
  herpes g.
gland
  adrenal g.
  apocrine sweat g.
  benign acini prostate g.
  bronchial mucosal g.
  Brunner g.
  bulbourethral g.
  Cowper g.
  cribriform g.
  eccrine sweat g.
  g. enlargement
  giant cell carcinoma of thyroid g.
  infiltrating g.
  lymphoid g.
  malignant acini prostate g.
  metaplastic pyloric g.
  mixed tumor of salivary g.
  Montgomery g.

pancreatic g.
parathymus g.
parathyroid g.
parotid g.
periurethral g.
pineal g.
pituitary g.
primary lymphoma of lymphoid g.
prostate g.
salivary g.
sebaceous g.
sublingual g.
submaxillary g.
sweat g.
thyroid g.
g.'s of Zeis
Glandosane
glandular
   g. cancer
   g. carcinoma
   g. cell
   g. element
   g. epithelium
   g. hyperplasia
   g. parenchyma
   g. sarcoma
   g. structure
   g. tissue
glandularis
   cystitis g.
Glanzmann
   G. syndrome
   G. thrombasthenia
Glasscock-Jackson classification
glass factor
glassy cell carcinoma
Glazunov tumor
Gleason
   G. grade 1-5
   G. score
   G. sum 2-10
   G. tumor grading system
Gleevec, Glivec
Gliadel
   G. plus CPT-11 or Temodal
   G. wafer
   G. wafer therapy
glial
   g. brain tumor
   g. fibrillary acidic protein (GFAP)
   g. stranding
GliaSite
   G. radiation therapy system

G. RTS
G. RTS system
glioblastoma
   adeno p53 therapy of recurrent g.
   butterfly g.
   de novo g.
   exophytic g.
   herpes viral therapy of recurrent g.
   HSV-tk with ganciclovir therapy of
     recurrent g.
   irradiated g.
   g. multiforme (GBM)
   recurrent g.
gliofibrillary
gliofibroma
glioma
   anaplastic mixed g.
   benign g.
   brainstem g.
   butterfly g.
   g. cell
   chiasmatic-hypothalamic g.
   cystic g.
   hypothalamic g.
   infiltrating g.
   low-grade g. (LGG)
   malignant g.
   multicentric malignant g.
   optic pathway g.
   orthotopic g.
   pediatric brainstem g.
   pontine g.
   recurrent g.
   supratentorial g.
   tectal g.
   temporooccipital g.
   thalamic infiltrating g.
   visual pathway g.
gliomatosis cerebri (GC)
gli oncogene
glioneurocytoma
glioneuronal neoplasm
gliosarcoma
   cerebellar g.
gliosis
   isomorphic g.
glitter cell
Glivec (*var. of* Gleevec)
globe cell anemia
globin
   g. chain
   g. gene
globoid cell leukodystrophy

G

NOTES

globular
- g. leukocyte
- g. meningioma

globule
- human milk fat g. (HMFG)

globulin
- antihemophilic g. (AHG)
- anti-HIV immune serum g.
- anti-human g.
- antithymocyte g. (ATG)
- cytomegalovirus immune g. (CMVIG)
- gamma g.
- hepatitis B immune g.
- horse antihuman thymus g.
- hyperimmune cytomegalovirus g.
- hyperimmune intravenous gamma g.
- immune gamma g.
- lymphocyte immune g.
- rabies immune g.
- Rho(D) immune g.
- sex hormone-binding g. (SHBG)
- tetanus immune g.
- thyroxin-binding g.
- WinRho SDF immune g.

globulin/albumin (G/A)

glomangioma

glomera (*pl. of* glomus)

glomerular
- g. basement membrane (GBM)
- g. filtration rate (GFR)
- g. mesangial hyperplasia

glomerulonephritis
- membranoproliferative g. (MPGN)

glomerulopathy
- membranous g.

glomerulosclerosis

glomic cell line

glomus, pl. **glomera**
- g. caroticum tumor
- g. choroideum
- g. jugulare
- g. jugulare tumor (GJT)
- g. malignant tumor

glossectomy
- total g.

glossitis
- Hunter g.

glossoepiglottic fold

glossopalatine sulcus

glottic carcinoma

glove
- Sensi-Care synthetic powder-free surgical g.'s
- surgical g.'s

GLPD
- granular lymphocyte-proliferative disorder

glubionate
- calcium g.

glucagon

glucagonoma syndrome

glucarate

gluceptate
- calcium g.

glucocerebrosidase

glucocorticoid

gluconate
- Apo-Ferrous G.
- calcium g.
- ferric g.
- ferrous g.
- magnesium g.
- potassium chloride and potassium g.
- potassium citrate and potassium g.
- trimetrexate g.

glucoprotein
- transmembrane g.

glucopyranoside moiety

glucoraphanin

glucose
- hypertonic g.
- instant g.
- g. metabolism
- g. polymer
- g. transporter protein (GLUT)
- g. transporter protein 1 through 13 (GLUT1–13)

glucose-6-phosphate dehydrogenase deficiency (G6PD, G-6-PD)

glucosylceramide

glucuronate
- trimetrexate g.

glucuronidation

glucuronide
- androstanediol g.

glucuronosyltransferase
- uridine 5′-diphosphate g.

GLUT
- glucose transporter protein

GLUT1–13
- glucose transporter protein 1 through 13

glutamic
- g. acid
- g. acid decarboxylase

glutamine-supplemented total parenteral nutrition

glutamyl
- gamma g.

glutamylcysteine synthetase

glutaraldehyde

glutaric
- g. acid
- g. aciduria type I

glutathione
- g. disulfide

g. ethylester
g. modification
g. monoethyl ester
g. S-transferase
g. S-transferase A1-1
g. transferase
glutathione-depleting agent
glutathione-S-transferase gene
gluten enteropathy-associated T-cell lymphoma
Glutose
glyceraldehyde phosphate dehydrogenase (GAPDH)
glycerin
glycerol
glyceryl
g. dinitrate (GDN)
g. trinitrate (GTN)
glycinate
glycine
N-myristoyl g.
N-terminal g.
glycocalyx
glycogen
g. acanthosis
g. storage disease
glycogenosis
hepatic g.
glycogen-rich cystadenoma
glycohistochemical marker
glycohistochemistry
glycol
interferon alfa-2b conjugated polyethylene g.
polyethylene g. (PEG)
glycolysis
glycolytic pathway
glycophorin
g. A
g. C
glycoprotein (gp)
g. A-80
EGP-2 g.
env g.
Ep-CAM g.
GA733-2 g.
gp100 g.
gp48 g.
gp75 g.
novel g.
SPARC g.
tumor-associated g. (TAG)

glycoprotein-72
tumor-associated g.-72 (TAG-72)
glycosaminoglycan
glycosidase
glycosylate
glycosylated
g. hemoglobin
g. protein
g. protein spanning viral envelope (gp41)
glycosylation
glycosyltransferase
glycyrrhetinic acid
glycyrrhizin
glyminox oral rinse
Glysennid
Gm antigen
GM-CFU
granulocyte-macrophage colony-forming unit
GM-CSF
granulocyte-macrophage colony-stimulating factor
rMu GM-CSF
GMK
green monkey kidney
GMK molecule
GMK vaccine
GMP
guanosine monophosphate
GMP-K
guanylate kinase
GNG
growing neural gas
GNG phase imaging
GnRH
gonadotropin-releasing hormone
GnRH analog
GO
gemtuzumab ozogamicin
goblet
g. cell
g. cell carcinoid (GCC)
g. cell-type adenocarcinoma
g. sign
GOG
Gynecologic Oncology Group
GOG staging system for ovarian cancer
goiter
adenomatous g.
colloid g.
diffuse toxic g.

NOTES

goiter *(continued)*
 dyshormonogenetic g.
 substernal g.
goitrous cretinism
gold (Au)
 radioactive g.
gold-198 (^{198}Au)
Goldblatt kidney
Goldenberg Snarecoil bone marrow biopsy needle
Goldie-Coldman
 G.-C. hypothesis
 G.-C. model
Goldman classification
Goldstein hematemesis
Golgi
 G. apparatus
 G. complex
 G. stack
Golgi-specific protein
Goltz syndrome
Gomori
 G. methenamine silver
 G. trichrome stain
gompertzian
 g. growth
 g. growth curve
 g. model
gonad
 maternal g.
gonadal irradiation
gonadoblastoma
 ovarian g.
gonadorelin
gonadotrope
gonadotropin
 chorionic g.
 human chorionic g. (hCG)
 human menopausal g.
 iodine ^{131}I murine MAb to human chorionic g.
 g. producing
gonadotropin-releasing
 g.-r. hormone (GnRH, GRH)
 g.-r. hormone agonist
 g.-r. hormone vaccine
gondii
 Toxoplasma g.
Gongylonema neoplasticum
goniometry
gonorrhea
gonorrhoeae
 Neisseria g.
Gonzales blood group
Gonzalez regimen
Goodpasture syndrome
Good syndrome
gooseneck deformity

gordonae
 Mycobacterium g.
Gorlin-Pindborg syndrome
Gorlin syndrome
GOS
 galactose oxidase-Schiff
 GOS reaction
goserelin acetate
gossypol
Gothenburg Breast Screening Trial
Gottron papule
gotu kola
Gower
 hemoglobin G.
gp
 gene product
 glycoprotein
gp41
 glycosylated protein spanning viral envelope
 gp41 epitope
 TM gp41
 gp41 transmembrane
gp100
 gp100 glycoprotein
 gp100 melanoma antigen
 gp100 peptide
gp120
 canarypox-HIV gp120
 V3 loop of gp120
gp160
 gp160 envelope
 recombinant gp160 (rgp160)
 gp160 recombinant vaccinia virus
gp100:209-217 peptide
gp209-2M immunodominant peptide
gp48 glycoprotein
gp75 glycoprotein
G6PD, G-6-PD
 glucose-6-phosphate dehydrogenase deficiency
 G6PD cell marker
 G6PD deficiency
grade
 Bartl g.
 Broders g.
 Edmondson g.
 Fuhrman nuclear g.
 Gleason g. 1-5
 histologic g.
 g. III oligoastrocytoma
 g. III oligodendroglioma
 g. I–IV astrocytoma
 g. I–IV GVHD
 nuclear g.
 Scarf-Bloom-Richardson g.
 Simpson surgical g.
 tumor g.
 tumor regression g. (TRG)

WHO g. I-IV
Wolfe g.
Gradenigo syndrome
gradient
    g. echo sequence
    Ficoll-Paque g.
    field g.
    magnetic field g.
    serum-ascites albumin g.
    X g.
    Y g.
gradient-recalled echo (GRE)
grading
    Edmondson-Steiner histologic g.
    Jaffe g.
    g. parameter
    Scharff-Bloom-Richardson g.
    Visick gastric cancer g.
Graffi virus
graft
    aortic g.
    aorticorenal g.
    aortofemoral bypass g.
    aortoiliac bypass g.
    arterial bypass g.
    autologous bone g.
    axillobifemoral bypass g.
    bifemoral g.
    bilateral myocutaneous g.
    bone g.
    bone-tendon-bone g.
    cytokine-mobilized peripheral
      blood g.
    g. disease (GVHD)
    donor g.
    g. failure
    heterologous g.
    isogeneic g.
    jejunal g.
    polytetrafluoroethylene g.
    g. rejection
    Sauvage filamentous velour g.
    in situ vein g.
    Sparks mandrel g.
    g. versus host disease (GVHD)
    g. versus host reaction (GVHR)
    g. versus immunocompetent cell
      effect
    g. versus leukemia (GVL)
    g. versus leukemia effect
    g. versus lymphoma effect
    g. versus myeloma effect
    g. versus tumor effect

Gram-negative
    G.-n. bacteria
    G.-n. enteric bacteria
    G.-n. pneumonia
    G.-n. rod
Gram-positive
    G.-p. bacteria
    G.-p. organism
Gram stain
granisetron hydrochloride
Granocyte
granular
    g. acute lymphoblastic leukemia
    g. calcification
    g. cell myoblastoma
    g. cell tumor
    g. leukocyte
    g. lymphocyte-proliferative disorder
      (GLPD)
granularis
    ependymitis g.
granularity
granulation
    toxic g.
granule
    alpha g.
    azurophilic g.
    basophilic g.
    delta g.
    dense g.
    E.E.S. G.'s
    effervescent citrocarbonate g.
    fine azurophilic g.
    Fordyce g.
    Neisser g.
    neurosecretory g.
    specific cytoplasmic g.
    sulfur g.
Granulex
granulin-epithelin precursor (GEP)
granulocyte
    g. colony-forming unit (G-CFU)
    g. colony-stimulating factor (G-
      CSF)
    g. count
    g., erythrocyte, monocyte,
      megakaryocyte colony-forming cell
      (GEMM-CFC)
    g. phagocytosis
    g. priming effect
    g. recombinant G-CSF
    g. transfusion

G

NOTES

granulocyte-macrophage
  g.-m. colony-forming unit (GM-CFU)
  g.-m. colony stimulating
  g.-m. colony-stimulating factor (GM-CSF)
  stimulating factor g.-m.
granulocytic
  g. kinetics
  g. leukemia
  g. marker
  g. sarcoma
granulocytopenia
granulocytopenic fever
granulocytosis
  paraneoplastic g.
granuloma, pl. **granulomata**
  actinic g.
  amebic g.
  g. annulare
  apical g.
  beryllium g.
  bilharzial g.
  coccidioidal g.
  dental g.
  g. endemicum
  eosinophilic g.
  g. faciale
  g. gangrenescens
  giant cell reparative g.
  g. gravidarum
  infectious g.
  g. inguinale
  laryngeal g.
  lethal midline g.
  lipoid g.
  lipophagic g.
  Majocchi g.
  malignant g.
  midline g.
  g. multiforme
  oily g.
  paracoccidioidal g.
  periapical g.
  g. pudendi
  g. pyogenicum
  reparative giant cell g.
  sarcoid g.
  g. telangiectaticum
  g. tropicum
  g. venereum
granulomatis
  Cephalosporium g.
granulomatosa
  cheilitis g.
granulomatosis
  allergic g.
  bronchocentric g. (BCG)
  g. disciformis

lipid g.
lipoid g.
lipophagia g.
lymphocytic angiitis and g.
lymphomatoid g.
g. siderotica
Wegener g.
granulomatous
  g. abscess
  g. angiitis
  g. arteritis
  g. calcification
  g. colitis
  g. cystitis
  g. disease
  g. endophthalmitis
  g. enteritis
  g. gastritis
  g. infection
  g. inflammation
  g. mastitis
  g. meningitis
  g. nocardiosis
  g. process
  g. prostatitis
  g. slack skin
  g. slack skin disorder
  g. slack skin syndrome
granulopoiesis
granulosa-stromal cell tumor
granulosus
  Echinococcus g.
granzyme
grape cell
grapeseed oil
grape-skin thin-walled lung cavity
Graseby pump
Graves disease
gravidarum
  granuloma g.
  hyperemesis g.
gravis
  myasthenia g.
gravity drainage
Gravol
Grawitz tumor
gray (Gy)
  g. matter fold
  g. platelet syndrome
  g. scale
  g. scale examination
gray/white matter interface
GRE
  gradient-recalled echo
great vessel
green
  g. cancer
  g. monkey kidney (GMK)
green-fluorescent protein (GFP)

Greenwald and Lewman method
Greenwood formula
Greig syndrome
grenz ray
grepafloxacin
Grey Turner sign
GRFoma
    growth hormone-releasing factor
      neuroendocrine tumor
GRH
    gonadotropin-releasing hormone
    growth hormone-releasing hormone
GRID
    gay-related immune deficiency
Grifulvin V
Grimelius stain
griseofulvin
Grisovin-FP
Gris-PEG
Groninger Intelligence Test, short form
  (GIT-V)
groove
    bicipital g.
    olfactory g.
    testiculoepididymal g.
Groshong catheter
gross
    G. cell surface antigen
    G. leukemia
    G. leukemia virus
    g. specimen
    g. total resection (GTR)
    g. tumor volume (GTV)
ground itch anemia
group
    ABO blood g.
    AIDS Clinical Treatment G.
      (ACTG)
    AIDS Clinical Treatment G. 214
      (ACTG 214)
    AIDS Clinical Treatment G. 325
      (ACTG 325)
    AIDS Clinical Treatment G. 334
      (ACTG 334)
    AIDS Clinical Treatment G. 349
      (ACTG 349)
    AIDS Vaccine Evaluation G.
      (AVEG)
    Auberger blood g.
    Austrian Breast Cancer Study G.
    blood g.
    Brown University Oncology G.
      (BrUOG)

    g. B streptococcal infection
    cancer and leukemia g. B
      (CALGB)
    Cartwright blood g.
    Children's Cancer G. (CCG)
    Children's Cancer Study G.
      (CCSG)
    Cooperative Oncology G.
    Cuneo Lung Cancer Study G.
      (CuLCaSG)
    determinant g.
    diagnostic-related g. (DRG)
    Diego blood g.
    Dombrock blood g.
    Duffy blood g.
    Early Breast Cancer Trialists'
      Collaborative G. (EBCTCG)
    Eastern Cooperative Oncology G.
      (ECOG)
    Gastrointestinal Tumor Study G.
      (GITSG, GTSG)
    Gonzales blood g.
    Gynecologic Oncology G. (GOG)
    high-frequency blood g.
    I blood g.
    Intergroup Rhabdomyosarcoma
      Study G. (IRSG)
    International Breast Cancer
      Study G. (IBCSG)
    International Germ Cell Cancer
      Collaborative G. (IGCCCG)
    International Mesothelioma
      Interest G. (IMIG)
    Kell blood g.
    Kell-Cellano blood g.
    Kidd blood g.
    labile methanesulfonate g.
    laser g.
    Lewis blood g.
    low-frequency blood g.
    Lutheran blood g.
    MN blood g.
    MNS blood g.
    National Cancer Institute
      Cooperative G.
    no-treatment control g.
    P blood g.
    Pediatric Oncology G. (POG)
    Philadelphia Bone Marrow
      Transplant G. (PBTG)
    Polycythemia Vera Study G.
      (PVSG)

G

NOTES

group *(continued)*
  Radiation Therapy Oncology G. (RTOG)
  reduced sulfhydryl g.
  Rh blood g.
  RSH g.
  self-help g.
  Southwest Oncology G. (SWOG)
  sulfhydryl g.
  support g.
  Taiwan Pediatric Oncology G. (TPOG)
  Veterans Administration Cooperative Urological Research G. (VACURG)
growing neural gas (GNG)
growth
  g. arrest lines
  g. factor dimerization
  g. factor mobilized autologous peripheral blood stem cell
  g. factor mobilized autologous peripheral blood stem cell transplantation
  g. factor receptor
  g. fraction
  g. fraction concept
  gompertzian g.
  horizontal g.
  g. hormone (GH)
  g. hormone deficiency (GHD)
  g. hormone-producing adenoma
  g. hormone release-inhibiting hormone (GH-RIH)
  g. hormone-releasing factor (GHRF, GH-RF)
  g. hormone-releasing factor neuroendocrine tumor (GRFoma)
  g. hormone-releasing hormone (GHRH, GH-RH, GRH)
  tumor g.
  uncoordinated cell g.
growth-related tumor marker ALP isoenzyme
GRP
  gastrin-releasing peptide
GRPR, GRP-R
  gastrin-releasing peptide receptor
Gruppo
  G. Interdisciplinare Valutazione Interventi in Oncologia (GIVIO)
  G. Italiano Malattie Ematologiche Maligne dell'Adulto (GIMEMA)
GSE
  genital self-examination
gsp protooncogene/oncogene
GSTM1 gene
GSTP1 gene
GSTT1 gene

GTD
  gestational trophoblastic disease
GTN
  glyceryl trinitrate
GTP
  deoxyguanosine triphosphate
GTP-binding protein
GTR
  gross total resection
GTSG *(var. of* GITSG)
GTV
  gross tumor volume
guaiac
  g. needle
  g. negative
  g. testing
Guama virus
guanidine thiocyanate method
guanidinium
guanine (G)
  methyl g.
guanosine
  arabinosyl g. (ara-G)
  dioxolane g.
  g. diphosphate (GDP)
  g. monophosphate (GMP)
  g. triphosphatase-activating protein
guanylate kinase (GMP-K)
guanylhydrazone
Guarnieri body
Guaroa virus
guidance
  angioscopic g.
  CryoGuide software-controlled ultrasound planning and g.
guide
  gutter g.
  guttering candle g.
  g. wire
guided imagery
guideline
  Mallinckrodt Institute g.'s
  MIR g.'s
guidewire
  angiographic g.
  extra-stiff g.
  open-ended g.
  Rosen g.
  spring-tipped g.
  Terumo g.
guilliermondii
  Candida g.
Gull renal epistaxis
gumma
  cerebral g.
  syphilitic g.
gummatous
  g. lesion
  g. syphilis

gun
> Biopty g.
> G. Hill hemoglobin

Gunderson-Sosin
> G.-S. modification
> G.-S. staging system

gustatory
> g. alteration
> g. sweating

Gustave-Roussy
> Institut G.-R.

gut
> g. mass
> g. replication

gut-associated lymphoid tissue (GALT)
Guthrie bacterial inhibition assay
gutter guide
guttering
> candle g.
> g. candle guide

GVAX pancreatic cancer vaccine
GVHD
> graft disease

> graft versus host disease
> > grade I–IV GVHD
> > hepatic chronic GVHD
> > steroid refractory acute GVHD

GVH disease
GVHR
> graft versus host reaction

GVL
> graft versus leukemia

Gy
> gray

gynandroblastoma
gynecologic
> g. cancer patient
> g. malignancy
> G. Oncology Group (GOG)
> G. Oncology Group staging system
> > for ovarian cancer
> g. tumor

gynecomastia
Gynkotek pump
gyrus
> cingulate g.

NOTES

G

H

heroin
Hounsfield unit
hydrogen
H antigen
H factor
H gene
H-2
H-2 antigen
H-2 complex
H9 cell
HA-1^A allele
HA-1^H allele
HAA
hepatitis-associated antigen
heterocyclic aromatic amine
Haagensen staging
haarscheibe tumor
HAART
highly active antiretroviral therapy
Haber toxicologic principle
habitus
body h.
HAD
hexamethylmelamine, Adriamycin, DDP
hadron therapy
HADS
Hospital Anxiety and Depression Scale
Haemate-P
Haemonetics Cell Saver
haemophilum
Mycobacterium h.
Haemophilus
H. *aegyptius*
H. *aphrophilus*
H. *ducreyi*
H. *gallinarum*
H. *influenzae*
H. *influenzae* meningitis
H. *influenzae* pneumonia
H. *influenzae* type b (Hib)
H. *pertussis*
Hafnia alvei
Hagedorn
H. and Jansen method
H. needle
Hageman factor
Haggitt classification
HA-HAase urine test
Hahnemann University Hospital technique
HAI
hepatic arterial infusion
hepatitis activity index

hair
h. loss
Schridde cancer h.
hairpin technique
hairy
h. cell
h. cell index
h. cell leukemia
h. epidermal nevus
h. gene
h. leukopenia
h. leukoplakia
Hakim
H. syndrome
H. valve and pump
halazepam
Halcion
Haldol
Ativan, Benadryl, H. (ABH)
Haley's M-O
Halfan
half-body radiation therapy
half-life
biologic h.-l.
effective h.-l.
elimination h.-l.
intracellular h.-l.
plasma h.-l.
Halfprin
half strength (HS)
half-value layer (HVL)
halichondrin B
Hall antidote
Hallervorden-Spatz disease
hallucis
adductor h.
halo
h. melanoma
perinuclear h.
Halodrin
halofantrine
halofuginone
halogenated pyrimidine
haloperidol
halopyrimidine
Halotestin
cyclophosphamide, Adriamycin, 5-fluorouracil, tamoxifen, H. (CAFTH)
cyclophosphamide, methotrexate, 5-fluorouracil, prednisone, tamoxifen, H. (CMFPTH)
dibromodulcitol, Adriamycin, vincristine, H. (DAVH)

H

Halotestin *(continued)*
  dibromodulcitol, Adriamycin,
    vincristine, tamoxifen, H.
    (DAVTH)
  etoposide, prednisone, Oncovin,
    cyclophosphamide, H. (EPOCH)
  etoposide, prednisone, Oncovin,
    Cytoxan, H. (EPOCH)
  vinblastine, Adriamycin,
    thiotepa, H. (VATH)
halothane anesthesia
halstedian
  h. concept
  h. concept of tumor spread
Halsted paradigm
Haltran
HAM
  hexamethylenamine, Adriamycin,
    melphalan
  hexamethylenamine, Adriamycin,
    methotrexate
  hexamethylmelamine, Adriamycin,
    melphalan
  hexamethylmelamine, Adriamycin,
    methotrexate
HAMA
  human antimouse antibody
Hamacher method
hamartoma
  angiomatous lymphoid h.
  astrocytic h.
  benign fetal h.
  chondroid h.
  fetal h.
  h. of iris
  lymphoid h.
  mesenchymal h.
  pulmonary chondroid h.
  retinal h.
  thymolipomatous h.
Hamazaki-Wesenberg body
Hamburger phenomenon
Hamilton Rating Scale for Depression
Hammarsten test
Hammerschlag method
Ham method
HAMP
  hexamethylenamine, Adriamycin,
    methotrexate, Platinol
hand
  h. antisepsis
  h. block
handicap
  physical h.
handle
  Amplatz radiolucent h.
handling
  drug h.

hand-mirror
  h.-m. cell leukemia
  h.-m. cell type
  h.-m. lymphocyte
Hand-Schüller-Christian disease
Hangar-Rose skin test antigen
hanging-block
  h.-b. culture
  h.-b. technique
hanging-drop culture
Hanks balanced salt solution
Hann filter
Hansel stain
Hansemann macrophage
Hansen disease
Hansenula anomala
Hantavirus
HAP
  hepatic arterial phase
  HAP image
haploidentical
haploidy
haplotype
  major histocompatibility complex h.
  MHC h.
happiness
  Atkinson Life H. (ATKLH)
hapten
  conjugated h.
  molecule h.
hapten-chelate construct
haptoglobin
hardening
  beam h.
Harding-Passey melanoma (HPM)
hard palate cancer
Hardy-Vezine classification system
Hardy-Zuckerman 2 feline sarcoma virus
harlequin appearance
Harris-Benedict equation
Harting body
Hartmann pouch
Hartnup disease
harvesting
  bone marrow h.
  cell h.
  stem cell marrow h.
Harvey sarcoma virus
Hashimoto
  H. disease
  H. thyroiditis
Hassall corpuscle
HAT
  hypoxanthine aminopterin thymidine
  HAT medium
Hautmann ileoneobladder
HAV
  hepatitis A virus

haversian
    h. canal
    h. canal of bone
Hawkeye SPECT application
Hayem solution
hazel
    witch h.
HB
  heart block
  hepatitis B
  hepatoblastoma
HBI
  hemibody irradiation
HBME-1 antibody
HBO
  hyperbaric oxygen
    HBO therapy
HBsAg
  hepatitis B surface antigen
HBV
  hepatitis B virus
    HBV DNA measurement
HC
  hydrocortisone
    Bancap HC
    Sustacal HC
HC2
  Hybrid Capture 2
    HC2 test
4-HC
  4-hydroperoxycyclophosphamide
h-caldesmon
    high molecular weight h-c.
H-CAP
  hexamethylenamine, cyclophosphamide,
    Adriamycin, Platinol
  hexamethylmelamine, cyclophosphamide,
    Adriamycin, Platinol
  hexamethylmelamine, Cytoxan,
    Adriamycin, Platinol
HCC
  hepatocellular carcinoma
HCCA
  hilar cholangiocarcinoma
HCFA
  Health Care Financing Administration
hCG
  human chorionic gonadotropin
hck protooncogene/oncogene
HCl
  hydrochloride
    aclarubicin HCl
    carubicin HCl

    chlormethine HCl
    doxorubicin HCl
    esorubicin HCl
    fadrozole HCl
    gemcitabine HCl
    hydromorphone HCl
    idarubicin HCl
    irinotecan HCl
    levamisole HCl
    liarozole HCl
    mycophenolate mofetil HCl
    pilocarpine HCl
    topotecan HCl
HCM
  hypercalcemia of malignancy
HCMV
  human cytomegalovirus
HCRC
  hereditary clear cell renal carcinoma
Hct
  hematocrit
HCTZ
  hydrochlorothiazide
HCV
  hepatitis C virus
HCV-RNA
  HCV-RNA HEAD
  HCV-RNA high-throughput
    extraction amplification and
    detection
  HCV-RNA NAT
H-D
  Hunter-Driffield
    H-D curve
HD
  heart disease
  hemodialysis
  Hirschsprung disease
  Hodgkin disease
  Huntington disease
  hydatid disease
HDARA-C
  high-dose ara-C
HDC
  high-dose chemotherapy
HDC/ASCR
  high-dose chemotherapy with autologous
    bone marrow or stem cell rescue
HDCh
  high-dose chemotherapy
HD-CNVp
  high-dose cyclophosphamide,
    mitoxantrone, VP-16

NOTES

H

HDC/SCR
   high-dose chemotherapy and stem cell
   rescue
HDCT, HD-CT
   high-dose chemotherapy
HDGF
   hepatoma-derived growth factor
HD-HIV
   Hodgkin disease and HIV infection
HDL
   high-density lipoprotein
HDM
   high-dose morphine
HDMTX
   high-dose methotrexate
HDMTX-CF
   high-dose methotrexate and citrovorum
   factor
HDMTX-LV
   high-dose methotrexate and leucovorin
HDPEB
   high-dose Platinol, etoposide, bleomycin
      HDPEB protocol
HDR
   high dose rate
      HDR brachytherapy
      HDR intracavitary radiation therapy
HDRA
   histoculture drug response assay
HDRIB
   high dose rate intracavitary
   brachytherapy
HDRV
   human diploid cell strain rabies vaccine
HDT
   high-dose therapy
HDV
   hepatitis delta virus
   hepatitis D virus
HD-VAC
   high-dose methotrexate, vinblastine,
   Adriamycin, cisplatin
HE
   hereditary elliptocytosis
H&E
   hematoxylin and eosin
HEAD
   high-throughput extraction amplification
   and detection
      HCV-RNA HEAD
head
   h. of bed (HOB)
   h. computed axial tomographic
      scan
   h. and neck cancer
   h. and neck mucosal melanoma
      (HNMM)
   h. and neck squamous cell
      carcinoma (HNSCC)

HEADS FIRST
   home, education, abuse, drugs, safety,
   friends, image, recreation, sexuality,
   threats
healing
   delayed h.
   faith h.
   primary h.
   wound h.
health
   H. Care Financing Administration
      (HCFA)
   National Institutes of H. (NIH)
health-related quality of life (HRQL)
heart
   apex of h.
   h. block (HB)
   h. disease (HD)
   water-bottle h.
Heartscan heart attack prediction test
heat
   h. exchanger
   h. perfusion
   h. shock protein 70 (hsp70)
   h. transfer mechanism
heated
   antiinhibitor coagulant complex,
      vapor h.
   h. intraoperative intraperitoneal
      chemotherapy (HIIC)
heater
   h. probe unit (HPU)
   resistance wire h.
heat-induced epitope retrieval (HIER)
heating
   hot source h.
   interstitial conductive h.
heat-mediated antigen retrieval
heat-stable alkaline phosphatase
heavy-chain
   h.-c. disease
   h.-c. immunoglobulin
**heavy membrane mitochondrial
   subcellular fraction**
HEC
   highly emetogenic chemotherapy
Hectorol
Hedinger syndrome
186-HEDP
heel-stick hematocrit
Heerfordt syndrome
Heidenhain iron hematoxylin stain
heilmannii
   Helicobacter h.
Heinz
   H. body
   H. body hemolytic anemia
Heinz-Ehrlich body
HEK293-p53-EGFP cellular testing

Hektoen, Kretschmer, and Welker
  protein
Hektoen phenomenon
HeLa cell
helical
  h. blood flow
  h. tomotherapy
Helicase mutation
helicis
  chondrodermatitis nodularis h.
Helicobacter
  H. heilmanii
  H. pylori
heliotrope erythema
Helistat
helium
  h. ion beam
  h. ion therapy
helium-neon (HeNe)
  h.-n. laser
Helixate FS
helix-loop-helix (HLH)
  h.-l.-h. structure
helix pomatia agglutinin (HPA)
helix-turn-helix (HTH)
HELLP
  hemolysis, elevated liver enzymes, low
    platelets
    HELLP syndrome
Helmes 3 antigen
helmet
  h. cell
  h. field
helminthiasis
helminthic infection
helminth infection
helminthoma
help
  B-cell h.
helper
  h. cell
  h. factor
  h. genome
  h. T lymphocyte
Hemabate
hemachrome
hemacytometer
hemadynamometer
hemafacient
Hemagard collection tube
hemagglutinating antibody
hemagglutination
  indirect h.

passive h.
reverse passive h.
h. titer
viral h.
hemagglutinin
  cold h.
hemangioblastoma
  capillary h.
  cerebellar h.
  cerebelloretinal h.
  cystic h.
  ventricular h.
hemangioblastomatosis
  cerebelloretinal h.
hemangioendothelial sarcoma
hemangioendothelioma
  epithelioid h. (EH)
  extranodal h.
  kaposiform h.
hemangioendotheliosis
hemangiofibroma
  juvenile h.
hemangioma
  arteriovenous h.
  capillary h.
  cavernous h.
  choroidal h.
  dumbbell-shaped spinal
    cavernous h.
  epidural cavernous h.
  epithelioid h.
  extraaxial cavernous h.
  extremity h.
  facial h.
  fatal h.
  giant h.
  hepatic h.
  infantile cutaneous h.
  pediatric h.
  spinal h.
  splenic h.
  subglottic h.
  vertebral h.
hemangiomatosis
hemangiopericytoma (HPC)
  meningeal h. (M-HPC)
hemangiopericytoma-like pattern
hemangiopericytomatous
hemangiosarcoma
hemapheresis
HemAssist
  H. blood substitute
  H. blood substitute for hemoglobin

NOTES

H

Hema-Strip HIV test
Hemasure r/LS red blood cell filtration
   system
hematemesis
   Goldstein h.
Hematinic
   Theragran H.
hematochezia
hematocrit (Hct)
   heel-stick h.
   h. phenomenon
hematocyte
hematogenous
   h. dissemination
   h. interstitial bacterial pneumonia
   h. metastasis
   h. osteomyelitis
hematogone
hematologic
   h. adverse effect
   h. complication
   h. disorder
   h. engraftment
   h. factor
   h. malignancy
   h. manifestation
   h. neoplasm
   h. reconstitution
   h. recovery time
   h. toxicity
hematology
   American Society of H. (ASH)
hematoma
   axillary h.
   basal ganglia h.
   bladder flap h.
   bowel wall h.
   epidural h.
   extradural h.
   mediastinal h.
   periaortic mediastinal h.
   perinephric h.
   umbilical cord h.
hematometra
hematometrocolpos
hematomyelia
hematophagia
hematopoiesis
   embryonal h.
   extramedullary h.
   Ogawa model for h.
   trilineage h.
hematopoietic
   h. cell surface antigen
   h. chimerism
   h. cobblestone area
   h. colony-stimulating factor
   h. CSF
   h. disorder

h. engraftment
h. function
h. growth factor
h. marrow
h. microenvironment
h. neoplasm
h. precursor
h. progenitor
h. progenitor cell
h. recovery
h. regulation
h. stem cell (HSC)
h. stem cell factor
h. stem cell support (HSCS)
h. stem cell transplantation (HSCT)
h. stem cell treatment
h. system
h. target cell
hematopoietic-inductive microenvironment
   model
hematopoietin-1
hematoporphyrin
   h. derivative (HPD)
   h. therapy
hematoxylin
   h. body
   Carazzi h.
   Clara h.
   h. and eosin (H&E)
   Lillie h.
hematoxylin-eosin stain
Hematrol
hematuria
HemeSelect test
heme synthesis
hemianopia, hemianopsia
   homonymous h.
hemibody
   h. irradiation (HBI)
   h. radiation
hemic calculus
hemicellulose
hemichorea-hemiballismus syndrome
hemidiaphragm
   accessory h.
hemihepatectomy
hemihypertrophy
Hemi-Kock neobladder
hemilaryngectomy
hemimandibulectomy
hemimelica
   dysplasia epiphysealis h.
hemin
hemipelvectomy
   internal h.
hemiscrotectomy
hemispheral astrocytoma
hemisphere
   cerebellar h.

cerebral h.
diffusely swollen h.
hemisyndrome
hemobilia
tropical h.
hemoblast
lymphoid h.
hemoblastic leukemia
Hemoccult
H. II SENSA
H. test
hemochromatosis
hereditary h.
Hemochron
H. Jr. Citrate PT assay
H. P214 glass-activated ACT tube
hemocyanin
keyhole limpet h. (KLH)
Hemocyte
hemocytoblastic leukemia
hemocytoblastoma
Hemo-Dial dialysate additive
hemodialysis (HD)
hemodilution
acute normovolemic h.
normovolemic h.
hemodynamically significant
hemodynamic catheterization
hemodynamics
Hemofil M
hemofiltration
continuous arteriovenous h.
(CAVH)
continuous venovenous h. (CVVH)
hemoglobin
h. A$_1$
h. A$_2$
h. A–Z
h. Chesapeake
h. electrophoresis
fast h.
fetal h.
h. glutamer-250 oxygen-based
therapeutic
glycosylated h.
h. Gower
Gun Hill h.
HemAssist blood substitute for h.
high-affinity h.
high molecular weight h.
h. Lepore
mean corpuscular h. (MCH,
MCHg)

muscle h.
nitric oxide h.
h. oxidation
oxidized h.
oxygenated h.
h. Portland
h. product
pyridoxylated stroma-free h.
h. Rainier
rHb1.1 recombinant h.
h. S-C disease
h. Seattle
slow h.
h. S-O-Arab disease
h. S-thalassemia disease
h. Yakima
hemoglobinemia
hemoglobinopathy
hemoglobinuria
marathon h.
paroxysmal cold h. (PCH)
paroxysmal nocturnal h. (PNH)
hemogram
hemojuvelin gene mutation
Hemolink
hemolysate
hemolysin
hot-cold h.
hemolysis
acute intravascular h.
cold antibody immune h.
h., elevated liver enzymes, low
platelets (HELLP)
extravascular h.
intravascular h.
hemolytic
h. anemia
h. anemia of newborn
h. complement assay
h. disease
h. disease of newborn
h. plaque assay
h. transfusion reaction
h. transfusion syndrome
h. uremic syndrome (HUS)
hemonectin
Hemonyne
hemopathology
hemopexin
hemophagocytic
h. histiocytic hyperplasia
h. lymphohistiocytosis
h. syndrome

NOTES

H

259

hemophagocytosis
hemophilia
  h. A, B, C
  acquired h.
  h. B, Leyden
  inherited h.
  h. neonatorum
hemophilia-associated AIDS
hemophiliac arthropathy
hemopoiesis
hemopoietic stem cell
hemoptysis
Hemopure solution
hemorrhage
  abdominal h.
  adrenal h.
  alveolar h.
  bladder h.
  catheter-induced pulmonary
    artery h.
  cerebellar h.
  cerebral h.
  colonic diverticular h.
  colorectal h.
  diffuse pulmonary alveolar h.
  diverticular h.
  Duret h.
  exsanguinating h.
  extraluminal h.
  germinal matrix h.
  germinal matrix-related h.
  intraperitoneal h.
  intratumoral h.
  labyrinthine h.
  petechial h.
  pulmonary artery h.
  related h.
  retinal h.
  vitreous h.
hemorrhagic
  h. conversion
  h. cystitis
  h. cystitis prophylaxis
  h. fever
  h. gastritis
  h. infarction
  h. necrosis
  h. neuroblastoma
  h. pancreatitis
  h. telangiectasia
  h. thrombocythemia
hemorrhoidal
  h. artery
  h. collateral
hemosiderin
  h. ring
  urine h.
hemosiderinuria

hemosiderosis
  idiopathic pulmonary h.
  pulmonary h.
  transfusion h.
  transfusion-related h.
hemostasis
hemostat
  D-Stat flowable h.
  microfibrillar collagen h.
hemostatic balance
Hemotene
Hendel
  H. correction
  H. correction of scalocephaly
HeNe
  helium-neon
  HeNe laser
Henle
  H. fibrin
  loop of H. (LH)
Henoch-Schönlein purpura
Henschke
  H. afterloader
  H. seed applicator
henselae
  Bartonella h.
Henson node
Hepanorm LMWH
hepaplastin test
heparin
  h. affinity chromatography
  calcium h.
  h. cofactor
  h. cofactor II
  h. lock
  low-dose h.
  low molecular weight h. (LMWH)
  Rotachrom H.
  sodium h.
  Stachrom h.
heparin-binding growth factor
heparin-fragment therapy
heparin-induced thrombocytopenia (HIT)
heparinization procedure
hepatic
  h. anaplastic sarcoma
  h. angiosarcoma
  h. arterial chemotherapy
  h. arterial dominant phase
  h. arterial embolization
  h. arterial infusion (HAI)
  h. arterial phase (HAP)
  h. chronic GVHD
  h. coagulation protein disorder
  h. cytochrome
  h. 2,6-dimethyl iminodiacetic acid
  h. flexure cancer
  h. glycogenosis
  h. hemangioma

h. infusion chemotherapy
h. iron content
h. iron index
h. lobe
h. metastasis
h. microsomal enzyme
h. neoplasm
h. nodule
h. non-Hodgkin lymphoma (HNHL)
h. parenchyma
h. P450 cytochrome system
h. portal perfusion
h. resection
h. schistosomiasis
h. segment
h. transaminase
h. tumor
h. venoocclusive disease (HVOD)
hepaticojejunostomy
hepatis
bacillary peliosis h.
hepatitis
h. activity index (HAI)
acute h.
h. A virus (HAV)
h. B (HB)
h. B immune globulin
h. B immune globulin human
h. B surface antigen (HBsAg)
h. B viral DNA load
h. B virus (HBV)
H. C check
chronic active h.
h. C virus (HCV)
h. D
h. delta virus (HDV)
h. D virus (HDV)
h. E virus (HEV)
h. F
fulminant h.
giant cell h.
h. G virus (HGV)
herpes simplex h.
infectious h. (IH)
non-A h.
non-B h.
radiation h.
serum h. (SH)
viral h. (VH)
hepatitis-associated antigen (HAA)
hepatobiliary cancer
hepatoblastoma (HB)
hepatocarcinogenesis

hepatocarcinoma
hepatocellular
h. cancer
h. carcinoma (HCC)
h. cholangiocarcinoma
hepatocyte
h. growth factor (HGF)
h. stimulating factor
hepatoerythropoietic porphyria
hepatoid adenocarcinoma
hepatolysin
hepatoma
malignant h.
hepatoma-derived growth factor (HDGF)
hepatomegaly
hepatopathy
paraneoplastic h.
hepatosplenic lymphoma
hepatosplenomegaly
hepatotoxicity
hepatotoxin
hepatotropic virus
HepCheck whole blood control
hepcidin gene mutation
Hep-Lock
hepsulfam
Heptalac
heptamer/nonamer sequence
heptic enlargement
heptic enlargment
heptoglobin
HER-2
HER-2 assay
HER-2 overexpressing breast tumor
HER-2 overexpressing ovarian tumor
HER-2 protein amplification
HER-2 protein overexpression
HER-2 protooncogene/oncogene
rhuMAb HER-2
HER-3
HER-3 assay
HER-3 coexpression
HER-4
HER-4 assay
HER-4 coexpression
HER-2-overexpressing breast carcinoma
herbal
h. medicine
h. remedy
h. tea
herbalism

NOTES

H

herbicide
    phenoxyacetic acid h.
Herbst registry
HercepTest immunohistochemical test
Herceptin
    H. antineoplasm therapy
    Evacet and H.
    Myocet and H.
herd immunity
hereditary
    h. acanthocytosis
    h. cancer
    h. chronic nephritis
    h. clear cell renal carcinoma
      (HCRC)
    h. coproporphyria
    h. disorder
    h. elliptocytosis (HE)
    h. familial cancer syndrome
    h. hemochromatosis
    h. hemorrhagic telangiectasia
    h. hyperphosphatasia
    h. leptocytosis
    h. methemoglobinemia
    h. motor-sensory neuropathy
    h. mucolipid storage cell
    h. multiple exostosis (HME)
    h. nephritis (HN)
    h. nonpolyposis colon cancer
      (HNPCC)
    h. nonpolyposis colorectal cancer
      (HNPCC)
    h. nonpolyposis colorectal
      carcinoma (HNPCC)
    h. pancreatitis
    h. papillary renal carcinoma
      (HPRC)
    h. papillary renal carcinoma
      syndrome
    h. persistence
    h. pyropoikilocytosis (HPP)
    h. retinoblastoma
    h. retinoblastoma-osteosarcoma
    h. spherocytosis (HS)
    h. stomatocytosis
    h. storage pool defect
    h. xerocytosis
heredity
Herendeen phenomenon
Heritage Panel
Hermansky-Pudlak syndrome
HER-2/neu
    HER-2/neu gene
    HER-2/neu oncoprotein
HER-2/*neu*-expressing cancer
HER-2/*neu* overexpression
hernia
    abdominal wall h.
    axial h.

    Bochdalek h.
    diaphragmatic h.
    duodenal h.
    hiatal h.
    h. metastasis
    h. neoplasm
herniation
    cervical disc h.
    disc h.
    subfalcine h.
    transdural h.
    transtentorial h.
heroin (H)
Herp-Check antibody test
herpes
    anal h.
    anorectal h.
    h. corneae
    h. digitalis
    h. facialis
    h. febrilis
    h. genitalis
    h. gestationis
    h. gladiatorum
    h. ICP47
    h. labialis
    h. menstrualis
    ocular h.
    h. progenitalis
    h. simplex (HS)
    h. simplex encephalitis
    h. simplex hepatitis
    h. simplex virus (HSV)
    h. simplex virus infection
    h. simplex virus-thymidine kinase
      (HSV-tk)
    h. simplex virus type 1 (HSV-1)
    h. simplex virus type 2 (HSV-2)
    h. simplex virus type 6 (HSV-6)
    h. simplex virus type 7 (HSV-7)
    h. viral therapy
    h. viral therapy of recurrent
      glioblastoma
    h. whitlow
    h. zoster
    h. zoster ophthalmicus
    h. zoster virus
herpesvirus
    human h. 1 (HHV-1)
    human h. 2 (HHV-2)
    human h. 3 (HHV-3)
    human h. 4 (HHV-4)
    human h. 5 (HHV-5)
    human h. 6 (HHV-6)
    human h. 7 (HHV-7)
    human h. 8 (HHV-8)
    Kaposi sarcoma-associated h.
      (KSHV)
    h. pneumonia

H. saimiri
    theta h.
    h. thymidine kinase cDNA
herpetic
    h. felon
    h. gingivostomatitis
    h. lesion
    h. neuritis
    h. proctitis
    h. ulcer
    h. whitlow
herpetiformis
    dermatitis h.
Herrick anemia
Hers disease
HERV
    human endogenous retrovirus
HERV-E
    human endogenous retrovirus E
HERV-K
    human endogenous retrovirus K
Heschl region
Hespan
heteroagglutination
heteroagglutinin
heteroantibody
heteroantigen
heteroaromatic replacement
heteroatom-substituted analog
heterochromatin
heterochromia iridis
heterocyclic
    h. amine carcinogen
    h. aromatic amine (HAA)
heterodimer
    karyopherin ab h.
heterodimerization
heteroduplex analysis
heterogeneic antigen
heterogeneity, heterogenicity
    allelic h.
    biologic h.
    genetic h.
    lineage h.
    subtype h.
    tissue h.
heterogeneous
heterogenetic antibody
heterogenic
heterogenicity (*var. of* heterogeneity)
heterogenous density
heterograft
heterohemagglutination

heterohybridoma
heteroimmune
heterokaryon
heterologous
    h. antigen
    h. graft
    h. tumor
heterolysin
heteronuclear decoupling
heterophil
    h. antibody
    h. antigen
heteroploid index
heteroserotherapy
heterotopia
    incomplete band h.
heterotopic ossification
heterotransplantation
heterozygosity
    loss of h. (LOH)
heterozygous
    h. achondroplasia
    h. familial hypercholesterolemia
HEV
    hepatitis E virus
Hewlett-Packard SONOS 1500 system
Hexa-CAF
    hexamethylmelamine, cyclophosphamide,
    methotrexate, 5-fluorouracil
hexachloride
    gamma-benzene h.
Hexadrol
hexamer
    palindromic h.
hexametazime (HMPAO)
hexamethylamine
hexamethylenamine
    h., Adriamycin, melphalan (HAM)
    h., Adriamycin, methotrexate
    (HAM)
    h., Adriamycin, methotrexate,
    Platinol (HAMP)
    h., cyclophosphamide, Adriamycin,
    Platinol (H-CAP)
hexamethylene bisacetamide (HMBA)
hexamethylmelamine (HMM, HXM)
    h., Adriamycin, DDP (HAD)
    h., Adriamycin, melphalan (HAM)
    h., Adriamycin, methotrexate
    (HAM)
    h., cyclophosphamide, Adriamycin,
    Platinol (H-CAP)

NOTES

H

hexamethylmelamine *(continued)*
  h., cyclophosphamide, methotrexate,
    5-fluorouracil (Hexa-CAF)
  h., Cytoxan, Adriamycin, Platinol
    (H-CAP)
hexamethylpropyleneamine oxime
  (HMPAO)
hexanoate
hexaphosphate
  inositol h.
Hexastat
hexose
  h. monophosphate
  h. monophosphate shunt
Hextend
Hexvix
Heymann nephritis
Heyman packing
Heyman-Simon
  H.-S. capsule
  H.-S. source
HFS
HGD
  high-grade dysplasia
HGF
  hepatocyte growth factor
HGF/C-Met autocrine loop
HGH
  human growth hormone
HGPIN
  high-grade prostatic intraepithelial
    neoplasia
HGSIL
  high-grade squamous intraepithelial
    lesion
HGV
  hepatitis G virus
HHM
  humoral hypercalcemia of malignancy
HHT
  homoharringtonine
HHV-1
  human herpesvirus 1
HHV-2
  human herpesvirus 2
HHV-3
  human herpesvirus 3
HHV-4
  human herpesvirus 4
HHV-5
  human herpesvirus 5
HHV-6
  human herpesvirus 6
HHV-7
  human herpesvirus 7
HHV-8
  human herpesvirus 8
5-HIAA
  5-hydroxyindoleacetic acid

6-HIAA
  6-hydroxyindoleacetic acid
  6-HIAA tumor marker
hiatal hernia
hiatus
  esophageal h.
Hib
  Haemophilus influenzae type b
hibernoma
hiccup, hiccough, pl. **hiccups**
Hicks-Pitney thromboplastin generation
  test
HID/AB
  high-iron diamine/Alcian blue
  HID/AB staining
HI-DAC, HiDAC
  high-dose cytosine arabinoside
hidden hyperdiploidy
hidradenitis
  eccrine h.
  neutrophilic eccrine h.
hidradenoma papilliferum
hidrocystoma
  apocrine h.
HIER
  heat-induced epitope retrieval
HIF
  HIV-inducing factor
HIF-1
  hypoxia-inducible factor-1
high
  h. dose rate (HDR)
  h. dose rate intracavitary
    brachytherapy (HDRIB)
  h. dose rate intracavitary therapy
  h. dose rate remote brachytherapy
  h. echogenicity
  h. index of suspicion
  h. linear energy transfer radiation
  h. molecular weight caldesmon
  h. molecular weight h-caldesmon
  h. molecular weight hemoglobin
  h. osmolar medium (HOM)
  H. Pure PCR template preparation
    kit
  h. signal intensity
  h. spatial resolution algorithm
high-affinity
  h.-a. antibody
  h.-a. hemoglobin
high-arched teeth
high-density
  h.-d. bile
  h.-d. lipoprotein (HDL)
high-dose
  h.-d. alkylating agent
  h.-d. arabinoside C (HiDAC)
  h.-d. ara-C (HDARA-C)
  h.-d. chemoradiotherapy

h.-d. chemotherapy (HDC, HDCh, HDCT, HD-CT)

h.-d. chemotherapy and autologous stem cell transplant

h.-d. chemotherapy and stem cell rescue (HDC/SCR)

h.-d. chemotherapy with autologous bone marrow or stem cell rescue (HDC/ASCR)

h.-d. chemotherapy with stem cell support

h.-d. cyclophosphamide, mitoxantrone, VP-16 (HD-CNVp)

h.-d. cytarabine

h.-d. cytosine arabinoside (HI-DAC, HiDAC)

h.-d. ECV consolidation chemotherapy

h.-d. etoposide, thiotepa, dose-adjusted carboplatin (TVCa)

h.-d. infusion

h.-d. ketoconazole

h.-d. ketoconazole plus alendronate

h.-d. methotrexate (HDMTX, HMTX)

h.-d. methotrexate, bleomycin, Adriamycin, cyclophosphamide, Oncovin, dexamethasone

h.-d. methotrexate and citrovorum factor (HDMTX-CF)

h.-d. methotrexate and leucovorin (HDMTX-LV)

h.-d. methotrexate, vinblastine, Adriamycin, cisplatin (HD-VAC)

h.-d. morphine (HDM)

h.-d. Platinol, etoposide, bleomycin (HDPEB)

h.-d. therapy (HDT)

high-energy

h.-e. phosphate reaction

h.-e. photon

higher seroincidence

high-fiber diet

high-frequency blood group

high-grade

h.-g. B-cell lymphoma

h.-g. cartilaginous tumor

h.-g. dysplasia (HGD)

h.-g. dysplastic adenoma

h.-g. immunoblastic histology

h.-g. malignant fibrous histiocytoma

h.-g. neutropenia

h.-g. prostatic intraepithelial neoplasia (HGPIN)

h.-g. squamous intraepithelial lesion (HGSIL, HSIL)

high-intensity

h.-i. zone (HIZ)

h.-i. zone lesion

high-iron diamine/Alcian blue (HID/AB)

highly

h. active antiretroviral therapy (HAART)

h. emetogenic chemotherapy (HEC)

high-performance

h.-p. liquid chromatography (HPLC)

h.-p. size-exclusion chromatography (HPSEC)

high-power field (hpf)

high-pressure liquid chromatography (HPLC)

high-resolution

h.-r. computed tomography (HRCT)

h.-r. CT

h.-r. CT scan

h.-r. multileaf collimator

h.-r. probe

high-risk

h.-r. breast cancer (HRBC)

h.-r. population

h.-r. primary breast cancer (HRPBC)

high-signal abnormality

high-throughput

h.-t. extraction amplification and detection (HEAD)

h.-t. screening (HTS)

h.-t. tissue microarray analysis

high-titer

h.-t. HHV-8 infection

h.-t. human herpesvirus 8 infection

h.-t. viremia

high-velocity flow pattern

Higoumenakia sign

HIIC

heated intraoperative intraperitoneal chemotherapy

hyperthermic intraperitoneal antiblastic perfusion

hyperthermic intraperitoneal intraoperative chemotherapy

HIK1083 antibody

hilar

h. adenopathy

h. biopsy

NOTES

H

hilar *(continued)*
 h. cell tumor
 h. cell tumor of ovary
 h. cholangiocarcinoma (HCCA)
 h. enlargement
 h. lymph node
 h. mass
 h. shadow
hilum, pl. **hila**
 renal h.
hilus
 splenic h.
HIMAC system
Himalayan yew
Hinton test
hippuric acid
Hirschsprung disease (HD)
hirsutism
hirudin
Hirudo medicinalis **leech**
histamine
 h. degranulation
 h. dihydrochloride
 h. H1 receptor
histaminemia
Histerone
 H. 100
 H. Injection
histidine decarboxylase
histioblast
histiocyte
 foamy h.
 sea-blue h.
histiocytic
 h. lymphoma
 h. medullary reticulosis
 h. necrotizing lymphadenitis
 h. neoplasm
 h. nodular Hodgkin disease
 h. proliferation
 h. sarcoma
 h. tissue
histiocytoma
 angiomatoid malignant fibrous h.
 benign fibrous h.
 high-grade malignant fibrous h.
 malignant fibrous h. (MFH)
 scrotal h.
histiocytosis
 diffuse cerebral h.
 Langerhans cell h. (LCH)
 malignant h.
 multicentric h.
 regressing atypical h.
 sea-blue h.
 systemic Langerhans cell h.
 h. X
histobath
histochemical method

histochemistry
 bone marrow h.
histocompatibility
 h. antigen
 h. complex
 h. gene
 h. testing
histocompatible donor
histoculture drug response assay (HDRA)
Histofine
 H. SAB-PO kit
 H. SAB-PO(M) detector kit
histofluorescence
histogram
 DNA h.
 dose-surface h.
 dose-volume h. (DVH)
 dose-wall h.
 erythrocyte h.
 leukocyte h.
 normalized dose-surface h.
 platelet h.
 z-dependent dose-volume h. (zDVH)
histograph
 Eppendorf pO_2 h.
histoid
 h. neoplasm
 h. tumor
histoincompatibility
histologic
 h. analysis
 h. architecture
 h. change
 h. coagulative tumor necrosis
 h. grade
 h. parameter
 h. subdivision
 h. subtype
histologically aggressive gastric non-Hodgkin lymphoma
histology
 cytology and h.
 h. and cytology
 favorable h.
 high-grade immunoblastic h.
 lymph node h.
 unfavorable h.
histolytica
 Entamoeba h.
histolyticum
 Clostridium h.
histone
 h. acetylation
 h. deacetylase inhibitor
 h. phosphorylation
histopathologic
 h. abnormality

h. analysis
h. examination
h. tumor classification
h. validation
Histoplasma capsulatum
histoplasmin
histoplasmosis
disseminated CNS h.
extrapulmonary h.
history
natural h.
pack-year smoking h.
histotope
histotoxic
histrelin implant
HIT
heparin-induced thrombocytopenia
Hitachi
H. H600 electron microscope
H. H7000 electron microscope
2-hit hypothesis
HIV
human immunodeficiency virus
HIV antibody
HIV antigenemia
clade B HIV
HIV concordance
HIV discordance
HIV encephalitis
HIV encephalopathy
E subtype of HIV
HIV immunoglobulin (HIVIG)
HIV latency
live-attenuated HIV
HIV necrotizing gingivitis
HIV necrotizing periodontitis
nonsyncytia-forming HIV
NSI variant of HIV
HIV nucleocapsid protein (p7)
HIV p25 antigen assay
HIV pathogenesis
HIV PCR assay
HIV protease inhibitor
HIV protein immunogen
HIV reverse transcriptase
HIV RNA
HIV RNA load
Salmonella-vectored HIV
HIV screening
HIV seronegative
HIV seropositive
HIV seropositivity

unintegrated HIV
HIV vaccine-induced humoral
immunity
HIV viral antigen
HIV visual analog scale
HIV-1
human immunodeficiency virus type 1
HIV-1 binding to CCR5
HIV-1 cytopathic effect
HIV-1 gp120 C4-V-3 peptide
HIV-1 replicative cycle
T-cell-tropic HIV-1
HIV-2
human immunodeficiency virus type 2
HIV/AIDS
Joint United Nations Programme
on HIV/AIDS (UNAIDS)
HIV-associated
HIV-a. lipodystrophy
HIV-a. minor motor deficit
HIV-a. nephropathy
HIV-a. non-Hodgkin lymphoma
(HIV-NHL)
HIV-a. PML
HIV-a. thrombocytopenia
HIV-1E
human immunodeficiency virus type 1E
Hivid
HIVIG
HIV immunoglobulin
HIVIG infusion
HIV-induced
HIV-i. apoptosis
HIV-i. disease
HIV-inducing factor (HIF)
HIVNET
human immunodeficiency virus project
network
HIV-NHL
HIV-associated non-Hodgkin lymphoma
HIV-PARSE
human immunodeficiency virus-patient-
reported status and experience
HIV-QAM
human immunodeficiency virus quality
audit marker
HIV-QOL
human immunodeficiency virus quality of
life
HIV-RNA PCR assay
HIV-specific CTL
HIV-TAT protein

NOTES

H

267

HIZ
  high-intensity zone
    HIZ lesion
HLA
  human leukocyte antigen
    HLA complex
    HLA disparity
    HLA sensitization
    HLA typing
HLA-A1
HLA-A2.1-positive colorectal cancer
HLA-B
HLA-B27
  human leukocyte antigen B27
HLA-B57
  human leukocyte antigen B57
HLA-C
HLA-D
HLA-DP
    class II gene product HLA-DP
HLA-DQ
    class II gene product HLA-DQ
HLA-DR
    class II gene product HLA-DR
HLA-DR 1, 5
HLA-identical
    HLA-i. donor
    HLA-i. sibling
    HLA-i. sibling transplant
HLA-L antigen
**HLA-matched peripheral blood
  mobilized hematopoietic progenitor
  cell transplantation**
HLA-nonidentical donor
HLH
    helix-loop-helix
    HLH domain
HLI
  human leukocyte interferon
HM
    hydatidiform mole
HMAF
    hydroxymethylacylfulvene
HMB45
    homatropine methylbromide
    HMB45 antibody
HMBA
    hexamethylene bisacetamide
hMCAF
    human macrophage-monocyte
      chemotactic and activating factor
HME
    hereditary multiple exostosis
HMFG
    human milk fat globule
hMLH1 gene
HMM
    hexamethylmelamine
    human malignant mesothelioma

HMPAO
    hexametazime
    hexamethylpropyleneamine oxime
hMSH2 gene
hMSH3 gene
HMTV
    human mammary tumor virus
HMTX
    high-dose methotrexate
HmX Hematology Flow Cytometer
HN
    hereditary nephritis
HN$_2$
    nitrogen mustard
HNHL
    hepatic non-Hodgkin lymphoma
HNMM
    head and neck mucosal melanoma
H-NMR study
HNPCC
    hereditary nonpolyposis colon cancer
    hereditary nonpolyposis colorectal cancer
    hereditary nonpolyposis colorectal
      carcinoma
      HNPCC carrier
HNSCC
    head and neck squamous cell carcinoma
HOA
    hypertrophic osteoarthropathy
HOAP-BLEO
    hydroxydaunomycin, Oncovin, ara-C,
      prednisone plus bleomycin
HOB
    head of bed
hobnail cell
Hodgkin
    H. cell
    H. disease (HD)
    H. disease and HIV infection
      (HD-HIV)
    H. disease staging
    H. lymphoma
    H. and Reed-Sternberg (HRS)
    H. sarcoma
Hoechst
    H. 33342 DNA staining
    H. dye
    H. dye method
Hofbauer cell
Hohn catheter
holandric gene
hold
    breath h.
holder
    Dale gastrostomy tube h.
    VBH head h.
    Vogele-Bale-Hohner head h.
holiday
    drug h.

holistic medicine
Holland classification
Hollenhorst plaque
Holliday junction
Hollister wound exudate absorber
hollow
    h. fiber assay
    h. needle
    h. organ
    h. ribbon
holmium:yttrium-argon-garnet (Ho:YAG)
    h.:y.-a.-g. laser
Holoxan
HOM
    high osmolar medium
homatropine methylbromide (HMB45)
home
    AIDS group h.
    h., education, abuse, drugs, safety,
      friends, image, recreation,
      sexuality, threats (HEADS FIRST)
    h. health care
    h. nutritional support
homeobox gene
homeodomain
homeopathy
homeostasis
    brain h.
    immunologic h.
homeostatic mechanism
Homer-Wright rosette
homing-induced apoptosis
hominis
    Blastocystis h.
    Dermatobia h.
    Pentatrichomonas h.
homocholic acid
homocystinemia
homocystinuria
homodimer
homogenate
homogeneity
homogeneously staining region (HSR)
homogenizer
    Wheaton tissue h.
homograft valve
homoharringtonine (HHT)
homolog, homologue
    cytokine h.
    human oncogene h.
homologous
    h. antigen

    h. disease
    h. tumor
homology
homonymous hemianopia
homopolymeric template
homotransplantation
homovanillic
    h. acid (HVA)
    h. acid level
homozygosity
homozygous
    h. achondroplasia
    h. familial hypercholesterolemia
Hong Kong disease
Honvol
hook
    skin h.
hookwire
    Kopans breast lesion localization h.
hookworm anemia
Hoover sign
HOPES
    human immunodeficiency virus overview
      of problems evaluation system
Hopkins
    H. Pain Rating Instrument (HPRI)
    H. rod
Hoppe-Seyler test
hordeolum
horizontal
    h. growth
    h. transmission
    h. transmission of virus
hormesis
hormonagogue
hormonal
    h. ablative therapy
    h. abnormality
    h. agent
    h. assay
    h. chemoprevention
    h. flare
    h. maneuver
    h. prevention
hormone
    adrenocorticotropic h. (ACTH)
    antidiuretic h. (ADH)
    Cancer and Steroid H. (CASH)
    corticotropin-releasing h. (CRH)
    endogenous h.
    exogenous h.
    follicle-stimulating h. (FSH)

NOTES

hormone *(continued)*
    follicle-stimulating hormone-releasing h. (FSH-RH)
    gonadotropin-releasing h. (GnRH, GRH)
    growth h. (GH)
    growth hormone release-inhibiting h. (GH-RIH)
    growth hormone-releasing h. (GHRH, GH-RH, GRH)
    human growth h. (HGH)
    immunoreactive parathyroid h. (iPTH)
    inappropriate secretion of antidiuretic h. (ISADH)
    intrauterine h.
    luteinizing h. (LH)
    luteinizing hormone-releasing h. (LHRH, LH-RH)
    lymphocyte-stimulating h.
    novel erythropoiesis-stimulating h.
    parathyroid h. (PTH)
    postmenopausal h. (PMH)
    prolactin-inhibiting h. (PIH)
    prolactin-releasing h. (PRH)
    h. receptor
    h. releasing
    h. replacement therapy (HRT)
    serum parathyroid h.
    sex h.
    steroid h.
    steroidal h.
    syndrome of inappropriate secretion of antidiuretic h. (SIADH)
    thyrocalcitonin h.
    thyroid h.
    thyroid-stimulating h. (TSH)
    thyrotropin-releasing h. (TRH)
hormone-dependent prostate cancer
hormone-naive disease
hormone-refractory
    h.-r. breast cancer
    h.-r. disease
    h.-r. prostate cancer (HRPC)
    h.-r. prostate carcinoma
hormonotherapy
horn
    h. cyst
    keratin h.
Horner syndrome
horse
    h. antihuman thymus globulin
    h. red blood cell
horseradish peroxidase
horseshoe kidney
hospice care
hospital
    H. Anxiety and Depression Scale (HADS)
    H. for Sick Children pain scale
    St. Jude Children's Research H. (SJCRH)
hospital-based registry
host
    h. cell
    h. defense
    h. defense mechanism
    h. factor
    h. immunity
    h. reaction
    h. rescue
    h. response
    h. response mechanism
    h. stroma
    tumor-bearing h.
    h. vector system
Ho staging classification
host-related factor
hot
    h. conization
    h. flash
    h. node
    h. source heating
hot-cold hemolysin
hot-water circulating suit
Hounsfield unit (H)
hourglass-shaped tumor
House-Brackmann grading scale
Howell-Jolly body
HOX11
    HOX11 oncogene
    HOX11 protooncogene/oncogene
Hoxsey treatment
Ho:YAG
    holmium:yttrium-argon-garnet
    Ho:YAG laser
    Ho:YAG LTK
Hp^{del}
    PCR detection of Hp^{del}
HPA
    helix pomatia agglutinin
    hypothalamic-pituitary-adrenal
    HPA suppression
H.P. Acthar Gel
HPC
    hemangiopericytoma
    soft tissue HPC
HPD
    hematoporphyrin derivative
HPETE
    hydroperoxyeicosatetraenoic acid
hpf
    high-power field
HPG
    hypothalamic-pituitary-gonadal
hPL
    human placental lactogen

HPLC
high-performance liquid chromatography
high-pressure liquid chromatography
HPM
Harding-Passey melanoma
HPMPC
3-hydroxy-2-phosphono-methoxypropyl
cytosine
hPMS1 gene
hPMS2 gene
HPP
hereditary pyropoikilocytosis
HPP-CFC bone marrow stem cell assay
4-HPR
N-(4-hydroxyphenyl)retinamide
hPR
human progesterone receptor
HPRC
hereditary papillary renal carcinoma
HPRC syndrome
HPRI
Hopkins Pain Rating Instrument
HPSEC
high-performance size-exclusion
chromatography
HPU
heater probe unit
HPU heat probe
HPV
human papillomavirus (type 16, 18)
human parvovirus
HPV 6, 11, 16, 18, 31, 45
HPV DNA status
HPV DNA testing
HPV E6 oncoprotein
HPV E7 oncoprotein
hRad9 protein
HRARE
hybrid rapid acquisition with relaxation
enhancement
H-ras
H-r. gene
H-r. oncogene
H-r. protooncogene/oncogene
HRBC
high-risk breast cancer
HRC
HRC gene
HRC region
HRCT
high-resolution computed tomography
HRCT scan

HRPBC
high-risk primary breast cancer
HRPC
hormone-refractory prostate cancer
HRQL
health-related quality of life
HRS
Hodgkin and Reed-Sternberg
HRS cell
HRT
hormone replacement therapy
HS
half strength
hereditary spherocytosis
herpes simplex
Hurler syndrome
Estratest HS
HS27
immortalized clones HS1 to HS27
HS27a
immortalized clone HS27a
HSAP tumor marker
HSC
hematopoietic stem cell
HSCS
hematopoietic stem cell support
HSCT
hematopoietic stem cell transplantation
HSIL
high-grade squamous intraepithelial
lesion
hsp70
heat shock protein 70
HSR
homogeneously staining region
hst (K-fgf) protooncogene/oncogene
HS-tk gene therapy
HSV
herpes simplex virus
HSV-1
herpes simplex virus type 1
HSV-2
herpes simplex virus type 2
HSV-6
herpes simplex virus type 6
HSV-7
herpes simplex virus type 7
HSV-tk
herpes simplex virus-thymidine kinase
HSV-tk with ganciclovir therapy
HSV-tk with ganciclovir therapy of
recurrent glioblastoma

NOTES

H

271

5-HT₃
> 5-hydroxytryptamine type 3

hTERC gene

hTERT
> human telomerase catalytic subunit

hTERT
> human telomerase reverse transcriptase
>> hTERT gene

HTH
> helix-turn-helix

HTLV
> human T-cell leukemia virus
> human T-lymphotrophic retrovirus

HTLV-I
> human T-cell leukemia virus type I
> human T-lymphotrophic virus type I
>> HTLV-I antibody-positive
>> HTLV-I retrovirus

HTLV-II
> human T-cell leukemia virus type II
> human T-lymphotrophic virus type II

HTLV-III
> human T-cell leukemia virus type III
> human T-lymphotrophic virus type III
>> virus HTLV-III

hTR
> human telomerase
>> hTR gene

HTS
> high-throughput screening

HU
> hydroxyurea
>> ara-C + HU

huan
> jin bu h.

huang
> ma h.

huC242 compound

HU-CSF
> human urinary colony-stimulating factor

Huët-Pelger nuclear anomaly

HuIFN
> human interferon

HuM195
> humanized monoclonal anti-CD33
>> antibody HuM195

hum
> venous h.

human
> albumin h. 5%, 25%
> h. alpha₁-protease inhibitor
> h. AML cell line
> h. androgen receptor
> h. androgen receptor gene
>> (HUMARA)
> antihemophilic factor h.
> h. antimouse antibody (HAMA)
> h. antiserum
> h. antithrombin III

h. antitoxin response
h. breast carcinoma virus
CD4 recombinant soluble h.
h. chorionic gonadotropin (hCG)
h. cytomegalovirus (HCMV)
h. dermal microvascular endothelial cell
h. diploid cell strain rabies vaccine (HDRV)
h. endogenous retrovirus (HERV)
h. endogenous retrovirus E (HERV-E)
h. endogenous retrovirus K (HERV-K)
h. endostatin protein
factor IX, purified h.
h. fibronectin fragment CH-296
h. gamma interferon
h. granulocyte-stimulating factor
h. growth factor
h. growth hormone (HGH)
h. hematopoietic progenitor cell antigen
h. hemopoietic tissue
hepatitis B immune globulin h.
h. herpesvirus 1 (HHV-1)
h. herpesvirus 2 (HHV-2)
h. herpesvirus 3 (HHV-3)
h. herpesvirus 4 (HHV-4)
h. herpesvirus 5 (HHV-5)
h. herpesvirus 6 (HHV-6)
h. herpesvirus 7 (HHV-7)
h. herpesvirus 8 (HHV-8)
Humate-P antihemophilic factor/von Willebrand factor complex h.
h. IFN-y quantikine ELISA kit
h. IgM monoclonal antibody to cytomegalovirus
immune globulin intravenous h.
h. immunodeficiency necrotizing gingivitis
h. immunodeficiency necrotizing periodontitis
h. immunodeficiency virus (HIV)
h. immunodeficiency virus antibody
h. immunodeficiency virus antigen
h. immunodeficiency virus assessment scale
h. immunodeficiency virus-associated minor motor deficit
h. immunodeficiency virus-associated nephropathy
h. immunodeficiency virus concordance
h. immunodeficiency virus 1 cytopathic effect
h. immunodeficiency virus discordance

h. immunodeficiency virus hyperimmune globulin infusion

h. immunodeficiency virus latency

h. immunodeficiency virus overview of problems evaluation system (HOPES)

h. immunodeficiency virus-patient-reported status and experience (HIV-PARSE)

h. immunodeficiency virus project network (HIVNET)

h. immunodeficiency virus quality audit marker (HIV-QAM)

h. immunodeficiency virus quality of life (HIV-QOL)

h. immunodeficiency virus 1 replicative cycle

h. immunodeficiency virus reverse transcriptase

h. immunodeficiency virus ribonucleic acid

h. immunodeficiency virus ribonucleic acid load

h. immunodeficiency virus ribonucleic acid polymerase chain reaction

h. immunodeficiency virus-specific cytotoxic T lymphocyte

h. immunodeficiency virus tat

h. immunodeficiency virus type 1 (HIV-1)

h. immunodeficiency virus type 2 (HIV-2)

h. immunodeficiency virus type 1E (HIV-1E)

h. immunodeficiency virus visual analog scale

h. interferon (HuIFN)

h. interleukin

h. interleukin for DA-cells

h. Jagged1 ligand

h. leukemia-associated antigen

h. leukocyte antigen (HLA)

h. leukocyte antigen B27 (HLA-B27)

h. leukocyte antigen B57 (HLA-B57)

h. leukocyte antigen restriction element

h. leukocyte Cw5 antigen

h. leukocyte interferon (HLI)

h. lymphoblastoid cell line

h. macrophage-monocyte chemotactic and activating factor (hMCAF)

h. malignant mesothelioma (HMM)

h. mammary tumor virus (HMTV)

h. menopausal gonadotropin

h. milk fat globule (HMFG)

h. oncogene homolog

h. papillomavirus-associated vulvovaginal lesion

h. papillomavirus DNA testing

h. papillomavirus (type 16, 18) (HPV)

h. parvovirus (HPV)

h. pathogenic retrovirus

h. placental lactogen (hPL)

plasma protein fraction h.

h. progenitor

h. progesterone receptor (hPR)

h. progesterone receptor gene polymorphism testing

rabies immune globulin h.

$Rh_o(D)$ immune globulin h.

h. serum albumin

h. T-cell leukemia/lymphoma virus

h. T-cell leukemia virus (HTLV)

h. T-cell leukemia virus (type 1-5)

h. T-cell leukemia virus type I (HTLV-I)

h. T-cell leukemia virus type II (HTLV-II)

h. T-cell leukemia virus type III (HTLV-III)

h. T-cell lymphotropic virus

h. telomerase (hTR)

h. telomerase catalytic subunit (hTERT)

h. telomerase reverse transcriptase (hTERT)

tetanus immune globulin h.

h. T-lymphotrophic retrovirus (HTLV)

h. T-lymphotrophic virus type I (HTLV-I)

h. T-lymphotrophic virus type II (HTLV-II)

h. T-lymphotrophic virus type III (HTLV-III)

h. tumor

h. umbilical vein endothelial cell (HUVEC)

NOTES

H

human *(continued)*
    h. urinary colony-stimulating factor (HU-CSF)
    h. urinary CSF
humanized
    h. anticancer bispecific antibody
    h. antihuman IL-2 receptor antibody (anti-Tac)
    h. anti-Tac
    h. monoclonal anti-CD33 antibody HuM195
human-leukocyte-antigen-identical transplant
human-murine xenograft
HUMARA
    human androgen receptor gene
HumaRAD compartmental radioimmunotherapy
HumaSPECT cancer imaging agent
Humate-P
    H.-P antihemophilic factor/von Willebrand factor complex
    H.-P antihemophilic factor/von Willebrand factor complex human
Humatin
HuMax-CD20
humeral diaphysis
humoral
    h. antibody
    h. factor
    h. hypercalcemia of malignancy (HHM)
    h. immunity
hump
    buffalo h.
hunter
    H. glossitis
    H. syndrome
Hunter-Driffield (H-D)
    H.-D. curve
Huntington
    H. chorea
    H. disease (HD)
Huntsman Cancer Institute
Hurler-Scheie compound
Hurler syndrome (HS)
Hurricaine
Hürthle
    H. cell carcinoma
    H. cell neoplasia
    H. cell tumor
HUS
    hemolytic uremic syndrome
HUTCH-1 antigen
Hutchinson
    H. lentigo
    H. melanotic freckle
    H. teeth
    H. triad

Hutchinson-Boeck
    H.-B. disease
    H.-B. syndrome
Hutchison-Gilford syndrome
HUVEC
    human umbilical vein endothelial cell
HVA
    homovanillic acid
HVL
    half-value layer
HVOD
    hepatic venoocclusive disease
HxGPRT
    hypoxanthine-guanine phosphoribosyl transferase
HXM
    hexamethylmelamine
hyal-1 testing
hyal-2 testing
hyaline
    h. cartilage matrix tumor
    h. leukocyte
    h. membrane disease
hyaline-vascular
    h.-v. Castleman disease
    h.-v. variant
hyaluronic
    h. acid
    h. acid testing
hyaluronidase
    h. overexpression
    h. testing
Hyams
    H. grading system
    H. grading system for esthesioneuroblastoma
H-Y antigen
Hyate:C
Hybolin
    H. Decanoate
    H. Improved Injection
hybrid
    A-form RNA-DNA h.
    H. Capture 2 (HC2)
    H. Capture 2 HPV DNA test
    H. Capture 2 test
    h. polyvalent synthetic peptide
    h. rapid acquisition with relaxation enhancement (HRARE)
    h. regimen
2-hybrid
    2-h. system
    2-h. yeast screen
hybridization
    comparative genomic h. (CGH)
    DNA in situ h.
    erbB2 blood fluorescent in situ h.
    erbB2 bone marrow fluorescent in situ h.

fluorescence in situ h. (FISH)
fluorescent in situ h. (FISH)
int-2 blood fluorescent in situ h.
int-2 bone marrow fluorescent in
  situ h.
in vitro h.
nucleic acid h.
h. protection assay
in situ h. (ISH)
Southern blot h.
subtraction h.

hybridoma
  h. antibody
  h. cell
  h. technique

Hybritech
  H. Free PSA test
  H. Tandem PSA ratio

hycamptamine

Hycamtin

hydatid
  h. cyst
  h. disease (HD)
  h. sand

hydatidiform mole (HM)

hydatidosis

Hydragran absorption dressing

hydralazine

hydration layer water

hydrazide analog

hydrazine sulfate

Hydrea

hydroacanthoma simplex

hydrocarbon
  h. inhalation
  polycyclic aromatic h. (PAH)
  polynuclear aromatic h. (PAH)

hydrocele
  idiopathic h.

hydrocephalus
  chronic communicating h.
  extraventricular obstructive h.

Hydrocet

hydrochloride (HCl)
  anagrelide h.
  bisantrene h.
  cefepime h.
  cimetidine h.
  cytarabine h.
  cytosine arabinosine h.
  daunomycin h.
  daunorubicin h.

h. dihydrate
diphenhydramine h.
doxorubicin h.
epirubicin h.
gemcitabine h.
granisetron h.
hydromorphone h.
hydroxydaunomycin h.
irinotecan h.
lidocaine h.
losoxantrone h.
mechlorethamine h.
melphalan h.
meperidine h.
metoclopramide h.
mitoxantrone h.
ondansetron h.
oxycodone h.
procarbazine h.
ranitidine h.
teloxantrone h.
topotecan h.
tripelennamine h.
zorubicin h.

hydrochlorothiazide (HCTZ)
  h. and spironolactone
  h. and triamterene

Hydrocil

hydrocodone
  h. and acetaminophen
  h. and aspirin
  h. and ibuprofen

hydrocolloid ulcer dressing

hydrocortisone (HC)
  dibucaine and h.
  intrathecal h.
  pramoxine and h.
  h. rectal
  h. sodium succinate

Hydrocortone
  H. Acetate injection
  H. Phosphate injection

hydroflumethiazide

hydrogen (H)
  h. ion concentration (pH)
  h. peroxide

Hydrogesic

hydrolase
  S-adenosylhomocysteine h.
    (AdoHcyase)

hydrolysis

hydrometer

NOTES

H

hydromorphone
  h. HCl
  h. hydrochloride
Hydro-Par
4-hydroperoxycyclophosphamide (4-HC)
  4-h. acid
**hydroperoxyeicosatetraenoic acid
  (HPETE)**
hydrophobic residue
hydrophone
hydrops
  h. fetalis
  immune h.
hydroquinone
hydrostatic reduction
hydrotherapy
hydroxamate peptidomimetic inhibitor
hydroxide
  aluminum h.
  magnesium h.
**3-hydroxy-2-phosphono-methoxypropyl
  cytosine (HPMPC)**
4-hydroxyandrostenedione
4-hydroxyanisole
3-hydroxy-benz[a]anthracene
3-hydroxy-benzo[a]pyrene
hydroxycarbamide
hydroxychloroquine
hydroxycobalamin
4-hydroxy-cyclophosphamide
hydroxydaunomycin
  h. hydrochloride
  h., Oncovin, ara-C, prednisone plus
    bleomycin (HOAP-BLEO)
  prednisone, Oncovin, ara-C,
    cyclophosphamide, h. (POACH)
hydroxyephedrine imaging agent
hydroxyethylamine moiety
hydroxyethyl starch
4-hydroxyifosfamide
5-hydroxyindoleacetic acid (5-HIAA)
6-hydroxyindoleacetic acid (6-HIAA)
4-hydroxy IPA
hydroxylase
  tyrosine h. (TH)
hydroxylation
  microsomal h.
  ring h.
hydroxymethotrexate
**hydroxymethylacylfulvene (HMAF, MGI-
  114)**
hydroxyprogesterone caproate
5-hydroxytryptamine
  5-h. type 3 (5-HT$_3$)
  5-h. type 3 receptor antagonist
5-hydroxytryptophan
hydroxyurea (HU)
  ara-C plus h. (ara-C/HU)
  L-asparaginase, BCNU, h.

cyclophosphamide, m-AMSA, h.
  (CMH)
cyclophosphamide, methotrexate, 5-
  fluorouracil, h. (CMFH)
Cytoxan, m-AMSA, hydroxyurea
  (CMH)
6-thioguanine, asparaginase,
  BCNU, h.
6-thioguanine, procarbazine,
  CCNU, h. (TPCH)
    6-thioguanine, procarbazine,
    dibromodulcitol, CCNU, 5-
    fluorouracil, h.
hydroxyzine
hyfrecation
Hy/Gestrone
hygiene
  oral h.
hygroma
  cystic h.
hylic tumor
Hylutin
Hymenolepis nana
hyoglossus muscle
hyoscyamine
  h., atropine, scopolamine, kaolin,
    pectin
  h., atropine, scopolamine, kaolin,
    pectin, opium
hyperactivity
hyperacute rejection
hyperalbuminemia
hyperaldosteronism
hyperalimentation
hyperammonemia
hyperamylasemia
  asymptomatic h.
hyperandrogenism
hyperargininemia
hyperbaric
  h. oxygen (HBO)
  h. oxygen therapy
hyperbetaalaninemia
hyperbetalipoproteinemia
hyperbilirubinemia
hyperbradykininemia
hypercalcemia
  h. of infancy
  h. of malignancy (HCM)
  paraneoplastic h.
  tumor-induced h.
hypercalciuria
hypercapnia
hypercarbia
hypercarotenemia
hypercellular cartilaginous neoplasm
hypercellularity
hypercementosis
hyperchlorhydria

hypercholesterolemia
  familial h.
  heterozygous familial h.
  homozygous familial h.
hyperchromatic
  h. nucleus
  h. spindle cell
hyperchromatism
hypercoagulability
  paraneoplastic h.
hypercoagulable state
hypercorticism
hypercortisolemia
hypercortisolism
hyper-CVAD
  hyperfractionated cyclophosphamide,
    vincristine, doxorubicin, dexamethasone
  hyper-CVAD regimen
hypercystinuria
hyperdense mass
hyperdiploid tumor
hyperdiploidy
  benzene-induced h.
  hidden h.
hyperemesis gravidarum
hyperemia
  reactive h.
hypereosinophilia
hypereosinophilic syndrome
hypererythrocythemia
hyperfibrinogenemia
hyperfractionated
  h. cyclophosphamide, vincristine,
    doxorubicin, dexamethasone
    (hyper-CVAD)
  h. radiation
  h. radiotherapy
hyperfractionation
  accelerated h. (AHF)
hypergammaglobulinemia
hypergastrinemia
hyperglycemia
hypergranular acute promyelocytic
  leukemia
hyperhemoglobinemia
HyperHep
hyperhomocysteinemia
hypericin
  oral h.
hypericum
hyperimmune
  h. cytomegalovirus globulin

  h. intravenous gamma globulin
  h. plasma
hyperimmunoglobulin M
hyperintense
  h. focus
  h. lesion
  h. signal
hyperintensity
  multifocal area of h.
  white matter h.
hyperkalemia
hyperkeratosis, pl. **hyperkeratoses**
  h. follicularis et parafollicularis in
    cutem penetrans
  uremic follicular h.
hyperkeratotic lesion
hyperlactemia
  asymptomatic h.
hyperleukocytosis
hyperlipasemia
hyperlipidemia
  familial combined h. (FCH)
hyperlipoproteinemia
hypermaturation
hypermetabolism
hypermethylation
  promoter h.
hypermutation
  somatic h.
hypernephroma
hyperorthokeratosis
hyperosmolality
hyperosmolar
hyperosmolarity
hyperostosis
  ankylosing h.
  bony h.
  diffuse idiopathic skeletal h.
  dysplastic cortical h.
  infantile cortical h.
hyperparakeratosis
hyperparathyroidism
  recurrent h.
hyperpathia
hyperpepsinogenemia
hyperphenylalaninemia
hyperphosphatasia
  hereditary h.
hyperphosphatemia
hyperpigmentation
  nail h.
  oral h.
hyperpigmented lesion

NOTES

H

hyperpituitarism
hyperplasia
    adenomatoid h.
    adenomatous h.
    adrenal h.
    adrenocortical h.
    alveolar epithelial h.
    angiofollicular lymph node h.
    angiofollicular lymphoid h.
    angiolymphoid h.
    atypical ductal h. (ADH)
    atypical lobular h.
    atypical regenerative h.
    benign prostatic h. (BPH)
    bone marrow lymphoid h.
    breast h.
    Brunner gland h.
    C-cell h.
    cutaneous lymphoid h.
    cystic glandular h.
    desquamated epithelial h.
    diet-induced coronary artery
      intimal h.
    ductal h.
    endometrial h. (EH)
    epithelial h.
    explosive follicular h.
    focal epithelial h.
    focal nodular h. (FNH)
    follicular h.
    follicular basal cell h.
    G-cell h.
    giant lymph node h.
    glandular h.
    glomerular mesangial h.
    hemophagocytic histiocytic h.
    idiopathic adrenal h. (IAH)
    idiopathic adrenocortical h. (IAH)
    immunoblastic h.
    intimal h.
    keratinizing h.
    lymph node h.
    lymphoid h.
    mantle zone h.
    micronodular h.
    mixed follicular h.
    mucous cell h. (MCH)
    multicentric angiofollicular
      lymphoid h.
    myointimal h.
    nodular regenerative h.
    papillary h.
    plasmacytic h.
    pneumocyte h.
    polymorphic B-cell h.
    pseudoangiomatous stromal h.
      (PASH)
    pulmonary lymphoid h.
    reactive lymphoid h.

    regenerative h.
    sebaceous gland h.
    tissue h.
    transient angiolymphoid h.
hyperplastic
    h. achondroplasia
    h. candidiasis
    h. cholecystosis
    h. gastropathy
    h. nodule
hyperpotassemia
hyperprolactinemia
hyperproliferative anemia
hyperproteinemia
hyperreflexia
    detrusor h.
hyperreninemic hypertension
hypersecretion
hypersensitivity
    alveolar h.
    delayed h.
    delayed-type h. (DTH)
    h. lymphadenopathy
    h. reaction
    sulfonamide h.
hypersplenic anemia
hypersplenism
hypertelorism
    ocular h.
hypertension
    arterial h.
    benign intracranial h.
    extrahepatic portal h.
    hyperreninemic h.
    IL-2 induced h.
    intracranial h.
    intrahepatic portal h.
    persistent pulmonary h.
    portal h.
    pregnancy-induced h. (PIH)
    pulmonary arterial h.
    renal allograft-mediated h.
    renovascular cause for h.
    thromboembolic pulmonary
      arterial h.
    venous h.
hypertensive intraarterial chemotherapy
hyperthermia
    anular phased-array h.
    external ultrasound h.
    interstitial ultrasound h.
    prostatic h.
    h. therapy
    h. treatment
    ultrasonic h.
    ultrasound h.
    whole body h.
hyperthermic
    h. antiblastic perfusion

h. intraperitoneal antiblastic
perfusion (HIIC)
h. intraperitoneal intraoperative
chemotherapy (HIIC)
h. limb perfusion
hyperthyroidism
hypertonic
h. glucose
h. saline
h. solution
hypertonica
polycythemia h.
hypertrichosis lanuginosa acquisita
hypertriglyceridemia
hypertrophic
h. osteoarthropathy (HOA)
h. pulmonary osteoarthropathy
hypertrophy
asymmetric septal h.
benign prostatic h. (BPH)
Brunner gland h.
compensatory h.
prostatic h.
segmental h.
septal h.
hyperuricemia
hypervascularized tumor
hyperviscosity syndrome
hypervitaminosis D
hypervolemia
hypesthesia (*var. of* hypoesthesia)
Hy-Phen
hypnoanalgesia
hypnoanesthesia
Hypnorm
hypoadrenalism
hypoalbuminemia
hypoaldosteronism
hypoaminoacidemia
hypobetalipoproteinemia
hypobilirubinemia
hypocalcemia
paraneoplastic h.
hypocapnia
hypocarbia
hypocellularity
bone marrow h.
hypocellular leukemia
hypochloremia
hypochlorhydria
hypocholesterolemia
hypochondroplasia
hypochromia

hypochromic
h. anemia
h. erythrocyte
hypocoagulable
hypocythemia
hypocytosis
hypodense lesion
hypodensity
nodal h.
white matter h.
hypodermoclysis
hypoeosinophilia
hypoesthesia, hypesthesia
facial h.
hypoferremia
hypofibrinogenemia
hypofibrinolytic state
hypofluorite
hypofractionated
h. radiation
h. radiation therapy
h. stereotactic radiotherapy
hypofractionation
hypogammaglobulinemia
acquired h.
primary h.
secondary h.
sex-linked h.
X-linked h.
hypogastric
h. node
h. plexus
hypogeusia
hypoglossal nerve palsy
hypoglycemia
non-islet cell tumor h. (NICTH)
hypogonadism
compensated h.
iatrogenic h.
hypogranular promyelocytic leukemia
hypogranulocytosis
hypointense
h. lesion
h. zone
hypokalemia
hypolipoproteinemia
hypolobulation
hypomagnesemia
hypometabolism
hypomethylating agent
hyponatremia
dilutional h.
volemic h.

NOTES

hypoparathyroidism
hypoperfusion
    cerebral h.
hypoperistalsis syndrome
hypophagia
hypopharyngeal
    h. cancer
    h. tumor
    h. wall
hypopharynx
hypophosphatasia
hypophosphatemic osteomalacia
hypophysectomy
hypophysis
hypophysitis
    lymphoid h.
hypopituitarism
hypoplasia
    bone marrow h.
    cartilage-hair h.
    cerebellar h.
    cerebral white matter h.
    lymphoid h.
    marrow h.
    renal h.
hypoplastic
    h. anemia
    h. myelodysplasia
hypopotassemia
hypoproliferative
    h. anemia
    h. thrombocytopenia
hypoproteinemia
hypopyon
hyporesponsiveness
hypotension
    arterial h.
    orthostatic h.
hypotestosteronemia
hypotetraploid region
hypothalamic
    h. amenorrhea
    h. blood flow
    h. glioma
    h. tumor
hypothalamic-pituitary-adrenal (HPA)
    h.-p.-a. axis
hypothalamic-pituitary-gonadal (HPG)
hypothermia treatment
hypothermic perfusion
hypothesis, pl. hypotheses
    Goldie-Coldman h.
    2-hit h.

incessant ovulation h.
Knudsen h.
Monro-Kellie h.
Norton-Simon h.
null h.
Starling h.
h. testing
hypothrombinemia
hypothyroidism
hypotonia
hypouricemia
hypovolemia
hypoxanthine aminopterin thymidine (HAT)
hypoxanthine-guanine phosphoribosyl transferase (HxGPRT)
hypoxemia
hypoxia
    anemic h.
    oxygen affinity h.
    tumor h.
hypoxia-inducible factor-1 (HIF-1)
hypoxia-mediated
    h.-m. malignant progression
    h.-m. tumor progression
hypoxic
    h. cell cytotoxic agent
    h. cell sensitizer
hypozincemia
Hyprogest 250
hysterectomy
    abdominal h.
    extrafascial h.
    laparoscopic-assisted radical vaginal h.
    laparoscopic supracervical h. (LSH)
    modified radical h.
    radical abdominal h.
    radical vaginal h.
    Rutledge classification of extended h.
    total abdominal h. (TAH)
    total vaginal h.
    vaginal h.
    Wertheim h.
    Wertheim-Okabayashi radical h.
hysterosalpingography
hystrix
    ichthyosis h.
Hytakerol
Hytinic
Hytrin

I
    iodine
    isoleucine
    I blood group
125I, I-125
    iodine-125
131I, I-131
    iodine-131
        Albumotope 131I
        antiferritin antibody linked to 131I
        131I antitenascin monoclonal
            antibody
        131I tositumomab
i(12p) marker chromosome
I-12t radioactive seed
IA
    intraarterial
    invasive aspergillosis
Ia antigen
IAB
    intermittent androgen blockade
IAC
    intraarterial chemotherapy
IAH
    idiopathic adrenal hyperplasia
    idiopathic adrenocortical hyperplasia
IAP
    immunosuppressive acidic protein
        IAP tumor marker
IAS
    intraarterial secretin
iatrogenic
    i. anemia
    i. arteriovenous fistula
    i. disease
    i. hypogonadism
    i. immunosuppression
    i. menopause
    i. TRD
iatropic symptom
IAVI
    International AIDS Vaccine Initiative
I-B1 radiolabeled antibody
ibandronate sodium
IBC
    inflammatory breast cancer
    iron-binding capacity
IBCA
    isobutyl cyanoacrylate
IBCSG
    International Breast Cancer Study Group
Iberet-Folic-500
Iberet-Liquid

IBMTR
    International Bone Marrow Transplant
        Registry
IBR
    immediate breast reconstruction
ibritumomab tiuxetan
IBT
    inflatable bone tamp
    intracavitary brachytherapy
IBTR
    ipsilateral breast tumor recurrence
ibudilast
ibuprofen
    hydrocodone and i.
ICA
    immunocytochemical assay
    internal carotid artery
    intracranial aneurysm
ICAM
    intercellular adhesion molecule
ICAM-1
    intercellular adhesion molecule-1
Icaps
ICBF
    intramyocardial coronary blood flow
ICC
    intraclass correlation coefficient
    intrahepatic cholangiocarcinoma
ICD
    International Classification of Diseases
ICD-O
    International Classification of Diseases
        for Oncology
ICE
    ifosfamide, carboplatin, etoposide
    immunoglobulin-complexed enzyme
        ICE disorder
ice
    carbon dioxide i.
    dry i.
iceberg
    i. phenomenon
    i. radiotherapy
ICED
    index of coexistent disease
ichthyosis
    acquired i.
    i. hystrix
ICIC
    International Cancer Information Center
ICL
    idiopathic CD4+ lymphocytopenia
ICM
    image cytometry
icosahedral coat protein

ICP47
>herpes ICP47
>viral gene ICP47

ICPO protein

ICR
>Institute for Cancer Research

ICRF
>bispiperazinedione

ICRU
>International Commission on Radiation
>Units and Measurements
>>ICRU reference point

ICS
>intracellular cytokine staining

ICSI
>intracytoplasmic sperm injection

ICS-PCR for MRD

icteric

icteroanemia

icterus
>i. neonatorum
>i. praecox

ICTP RIA kit

ICV
>intracerebroventricular
>>ICV reservoir

IDA
>idarubicin

Idamycin PFS

idarubicin (IDA)
>fluradabine, ara-C, G-CSF, i.
>(FLAG-ida)
>i. HCl

idarubicinol

IDC
>interdigitating dendritic cell
>intraductal carcinoma
>invasive ductal carcinoma

IDDM
>insulin-dependent diabetes mellitus

IDEC-Y2B8
>IDEC-Y2B8 radioimmunotherapy
>IDEC-Y2B8 radioimmunotherapy
>trial

identification
>cellular i.

idioagglutinin

idioheteroagglutinin

idiopathic
>i. adrenal hyperplasia (IAH)
>i. adrenocortical hyperplasia (IAH)
>i. CD4+ lymphocytopenia (ICL)
>i. follicular mucinosis
>i. growth hormone deficiency
>i. hydrocele
>i. hypertrophic subaortic stenosis
>i. hypochromic anemia
>i. megakaryocytic aplasia

>i. multiple pigmented hemorrhagic
>sarcoma
>i. myelofibrosis
>i. onychodysplasia
>i. plasmacytic lymphadenopathy
>i. pulmonary fibrosis (IPF)
>i. pulmonary hemosiderosis
>i. thrombocythemia
>i. thrombocytopenia
>i. thrombocytopenic purpura (ITP)
>i. venous thrombosis

idiotype
>i. antibody
>i. vaccination

idiotypic antigen

IDMTX
>intermediate-dose methotrexate

idoxifene

idoxuridine (IDU, IUDR, IUdR)

IDU
>idoxuridine
>injection drug user

IDX
>4′-iodo-4′-deoxydoxorubicin

IE
>immediate early
>>phosphorylation of IE
>>IE protein

IEF-PAGE
>isoelectric focusing polyacrylamide gel in
>electrophoresis

IEL
>intraepithelial lymphocyte

IEP
>immunoelectrophoresis

IFA
>immunofluorescence antibody
>incomplete Freund adjuvant
>silver stain

Ifex
>ifosfamide
>Ifex, mesna, Folex, 5-fluorouracil

iFind handheld device

IFLFA
>recombinant interferon alfa

IFM
>ifosfamide

IFN
>interferon
>>leukocyte-derived IFN

IFNa
>interferon alfa-2a
>>IFNa and CRA therapy

IFN-alfa-1

IFN-alfa-2

IFN-alfa-2b antibody

IFN-beta
>interferon beta
>>fibroblast-derived IFN-beta

IFN-G, IFN-g
  gamma interferon
  interferon gamma
IFN-psi
  immune cell-produced IFN-p.
IFOS
  ifosfamide
ifosfamide (Ifex, IFM, IFOS, IFX)
  i., carboplatin, etoposide (ICE)
  carboplatin, VePesid, i. (CVI)
  i. encephalopathy
  gemcitabine, cisplatin, i. (GIOP)
  i., mesna uroprotection,
    methotrexate, etoposide (IMVP-16)
  i., Platinol, Adriamycin (IPA)
  i., vincristine, actinomycin (IVA)
  vincristine, actinomycin D, i. (VAI)
IFP
  interstitial fluid pressure
IFS
  intrinsic fluorescence spectroscopy
IFSA
  individualized functional status
    assessment
IFX
  ifosfamide
Ig
  immunoglobulin
  anti-HDV Ig
  anti-HEV Ig
  Ig binding
  cytoplasmic Ig
  Ig gene
  platelet-associated Ig
  platelet-directed Ig
  variable region of Ig
  Ig V gene mutation
IgA
  immunoglobulin A
  IgA antibody
  mucosal IgA
  secretory IgA
  IgA synthesis
IGCCCG
  International Germ Cell Cancer
    Collaborative Group
IgD
  immunoglobulin D
IgE
  immunoglobulin E
IGF
  insulin-like growth factor

IGF-1
  insulin-like growth factor-1
IGF-2
  insulin-like growth factor-2
IGFBP
  insulin-like growth factor-binding protein
IgG
  immunoglobulin G
  anti-HAV IgG
  IgG kappa
IgG-ACA positive
IgM
  immunoglobulin M
  anti-HAV IgM
  anti-HBc IgM
igne
  erythema ab i.
IGRT
  image-guided radiotherapy
IgY antibody
IH
  infectious hepatitis
IHAC
  intrahepatic artery chemotherapy
IHC
  immunohistochemical
  immunohistochemistry
IHP
  isolated hepatic perfusion
IIEF
  International Index of Erectile function
IIIB-based gp120 antigen
IIRS
  Illness Intrusiveness Rating Scale
Ikaros isoform
IL
  interleukin
IL-1
  interleukin-1
    IL-1 receptor antagonist
IL-1–21
  interleukin-1 through interleukin-21
IL-1A
  interleukin-1A
IL-1alpha
  interleukin-1alpha
IL-1B
  interleukin-1B
  rMu IL-1B
IL-1beta
  interleukin-1beta
IL-2
  interleukin-2

NOTES

283

IL-2 *(continued)*
    IL-2 after allogeneic transplantation
    DAB389 IL-2
    IL-2 induced hypertension
    posttransplant IL-2
    recombinant human IL-2
    subcutaneous IL-2
    ultra-low dose IL-2

IL-3
    interleukin-3

IL-4
    interleukin-4
    recombinant human IL-4

IL-4R
    interleukin-4R

IL-6
    interleukin-6
    rMu IL-6

IL-7
    interleukin-7
    rMu IL-7

IL-10
    interleukin-10
    recombinant human IL-10

IL-11
    interleukin-11

IL-12
    interleukin-12

^{131}I-labeled
    ^{131}I-l. anti-CD20 antibody
    ^{131}I-l. anti-CD45 antibody
    ^{131}I-l. anti-CD45 antibody combined
      with CY and TBI
    ^{131}I-l. anti-CD45 antibody combined
      with CY and TBI regimen
    ^{131}I-l. B-cell-specific anti-CD20
      monoclonal antibody

ileitis
    backwash i.
    nonsclerosing i.

ileocolic intussusception
ileocolitis
ileocystoplasty
    LeDuc-Camey i.
ileoileal intussusception
ileoneobladder
    Hautmann i.
    W-shaped i.
ileus
    adynamic i.
    cecal i.
    colonic i.
    intestinal i.
ILGF
    insulin-like growth factor
Ilhéus virus

iliac
    i. lymph node
    i. wing
ilium, pl. **ilia**
ILL
    intermediate lymphocytic lymphoma
ill-defined mass
illness
    i. comorbidity
    dysenteric i.
    I. Intrusiveness Rating Scale (IIRS)
illuminator
    Mammo Mask i.
ilmofosine
Ilosone Pulvule
ILP
    isolated limb perfusion
IL-3Ra^{bright}
    interleukin-3Ra^{bright}
IM
    intramuscular
image
    i. analysis microscopy
    axial i.
    confocal i.
    i. cytometer
    i. cytometry (ICM)
    degradation of i.
    dynamic i.
    i. fusion
    HAP i.
    i. intensifier
    metabolite i.
    planar gamma camera i.
    quantitative PET i.
    T2-weighted i.
image-guided radiotherapy (IGRT)
imagery
    guided i.
    visual i.
imaging
    acoustic i.
    bone i.
    brain i.
    chemical shift i. (CSI)
    color Doppler i.
    color-flow Doppler i.
    continuous-wave Doppler i.
    cross-sectional i.
    CT-based volumetric i.
    diagnostic i.
    diffraction-enhanced i. (DEI)
    diffusion i.
    diffusion-weighted i. (DWI)
    diffusion-weighted MR i.
    3D proton MR spectroscopic i.
    dynamic contrast-enhanced magnetic
      resonance i. (DCE-MRI)
    dynamic magnetic resonance i.

Dynamic Optical Breast I. (DOBI)
dynamic volume i.
echo planar i. (EPI)
electronic portal i.
electrostatic i.
endocrine i.
endometrial chemical shift i.
endorectal coil magnetic
  resonance i.
endorectal MR i.
field-echo i.
functional magnetic resonance i.
  (fMRI)
generalized nephrographic phase i.
GNG phase i.
1H-nuclear magnetic resonance
  spectroscopic i.
isotope colloid i.
LAVA abdominal i.
LAVA liver i.
low-field magnetic resonance i.
lung perfusion i.
LymphoScan i.
magnetic resonance i. (MRI)
magnetic resonance spectroscopic i.
i. mass spectrometry
mediastinal cross-sectional i.
metaiodobenzylguanidine
  catecholamine i.
MIBG catecholamine i.
monoclonal antibody i.
multiplanar i.
myocardial perfusion i.
nuclear i.
PASTA i.
penile bulb i.
polarity-altered spectral selective
  acquisition i.
prediction of extracapsular prostate
  cancer extension with endorectal
  MR i.
radiolabeled antibody i.
radionuclide i.
spectroscopic i.
stereotactic CT i.
^{99m}Tc-HMPAO cerebral perfusion
  SPECT i.
^{99m}Tc-HMPAO SPECT i.
time-resolved i.
tumor viability i.
VIBRANT breast i.
imatinib mesylate

imbalance
  potassium i.
IMBC
  initially metastatic breast carcinoma
IMC
  internal mammary chain of lymph nodes
Imed
  I. Gemini PC-2 volumetric
    controller
  I. Gemini PC-2 volumetric pump
  I. infusion pump
Imerslünd-Graesbeck syndrome
Imerslünd syndrome
imexon injection
^{131}**I-mIB6**
  monoiodobenzylguanidine
I-MIBG
  iodine-131 metaiodobenzylguanidine
imidazole carboxamide
imidazotetrazine agent
imide
  immunomodulatory i.
IMIG
  International Mesothelioma Interest
    Group
    IMIG classification
5-iminodaunomycin
5-iminodaunorubicin
imipenem and cilastatin
imipramine
imiquimod
immature mediastinal teratoma
immediate
  i. breast reconstruction (IBR)
  i. early (IE)
immersion technique
immitis
  Coccidioides i.
immobilization
  sternooccipital-mandibular i. (SOMI)
immortal cell
immortalization
  spontaneous i.
immortalized
  i. clone
  i. clone HS27a
  i. clones HS1 to HS27
immotile cilia syndrome
ImmTher therapy
ImmuCyst
Immulite PSA assay
immune
  i. activation

NOTES

immune *(continued)*
  i. adherence
  i. agglutinin
  i. antibody
  i. anticancer effect
  i. cell
  i. cell-produced IFN-psi
  i. cell-produced interferon psi
  i. clearance
  i. complex
  i. complex disease
  i. complex disorder
  i. complex-dissociated p24 antigenemia
  i. deficiency
  i. enhancement
  i. flow cytometry
  i. function abnormality
  i. gamma globulin
  i. globulin intramuscular
  i. globulin intravenous
  i. globulin intravenous human
  i. hemolytic anemia
  i. hydrops
  i. interferon
  i. marker
  i. modulation
  i. modulator
  i. monitoring technique
  i. neutropenia
  i. pathogenesis
  i. reaction
  i. reconstitution
  i. response
  i. response gene
  i. serum
  i. state
  i. suppression
  i. suppressor
  i. suppressor gene
  i. surveillance
  i. system
  i. system anatomy
  i. thrombocytopenia
  i. thrombocytopenic purpura (ITP)
  i. tolerance
immune-enhancing drug
immune-mediated
  i.-m. anemia
  i.-m. antileukemia effect
  i.-m. destruction
  i.-m. therapy
  i.-m. thrombocytopenia
immune-stimulating agent
immunifacient
immunity
  acquired i.
  active i.
  adoptive i.

  antiviral i.
  cell-mediated i. (CMI)
  cellular i.
  community i.
  congenital i.
  familial i.
  genetic i.
  herd i.
  HIV vaccine-induced humoral i.
  host i.
  humoral i.
  inherent i.
  innate i.
  mucosal i.
  native i.
  radiation i.
  sterilizing i.
  i. transfer
  transplantation i.
immunization
  active i.
  allogeneic tumor cell i.
  autologous tumor cell i.
  CD34-derived dendritic cell i.
  nucleic acid i.
  passive i.
  peripheral monocyte-derived dendritic cell i.
  recombinant fowlpox and vaccinia viruses encoding the tyrosinase antigen i.
Immuno
  Feiba VH I.
Immuno1 Complexed PSA test
immunoadhesin
immunoadjuvant
immunoadsorption
  i. column
  i. technique
immunoarchitecture
immunoassay
  bacterial filtration-capture i.
  cyclosporine i.
  enzyme i. (EIA)
  ImmunoCard STAT rotavirus i.
  microlatex particle-mediated i.
  nephelometric i.
immunoaugmentative therapy
immunobead-binding assay test
immunobiology
immunoblast
immunoblastic
  i. hyperplasia
  i. lymphadenopathy
  i. lymphadenopathy-like T-cell lymphoma
  i. sarcoma
  i. sarcoma of B and T cells

immunoblot
    i. analysis
    carcinoma syndrome i.
    i. test
immunoblotting
ImmunoCard STAT rotavirus
  immunoassay
immunochemical marker
immunochemistry
immunochemotherapy
immunocompetent
    i. cell
    i. lymphocyte
immunocompromised
immunoconjugate
    chelate i.
    yttrium-90-labeled anti-B2 i.
immunocytochemical
    i. analysis
    i. assay (ICA)
    i. marker
    i. stain
immunocytochemistry
immunocytoma
    cutaneous i.
    lymphoplasmacytic i.
    lymphoplasmacytoid i.
    plasma cell i.
    polymorphic i.
immunocytometer
ImmunoCyt urine test
immunodeficiency
    cellular i.
    combined i.
    common variable i.
    phagocytic dysfunction disorder i.
    secondary i.
    severe combined i. (SCID)
    i. virus
immunodetection technique
immunodiagnosis
immunodiffusion
    Ouchterlony i.
    Oudin i.
immunodominance
immunodominant peptide
immunoelectrophoresis (IEP)
    countercurrent exchanger i.
    crossed i.
    2-dimensional i.
    Laurell i.
    rocket i.
immunofiltration

immunofixation
immunofluorescence
    i. analysis
    i. antibody (IFA)
    i. antibody assay
    indirect i.
    i. technique
immunofluorometric procedure
immunogen
    HIV protein i.
    protein i.
immunogenetic
immunogenic
    i. determinant
    i. tumor
immunogenicity
immunogenotypic analysis
immunogenotyping
immunoglobulin (Ig)
    i. A (IgA)
    i. alpha chain
    i. anticardiolipin antibody positive
    antihepatitis A virus i. G, M
    antihepatitis B core i. G
    antihepatitis delta virus i.
    antihepatitis E virus i.
    B-cell surface i.
    bovine i.
    chelated i.
    i. clonality determination
    cluster of differentiation 4 i. G
    (CD4-IgG)
    cytoplasmic i.
    cytotoxic lymphocyte activation
    antigen 4 i. (CTLA4Ig)
    i. D (IgD)
    i. delta chain
    i. E (IgE)
    i. epsilon chain
    i. G (IgG)
    i. G1
    i. gamma chain
    i. gene
    i. gene rearrangement
    heavy-chain i.
    i. heavy chain
    HIV i. (HIVIG)
    intracellular i.
    intravenous i. (IVIG)
    i. kappa chain
    i. lambda chain
    leukemia specific i.
    i. M (IgM)

NOTES

immunoglobulin *(continued)*
  i. mu chain
  platelet-associated i. (PAIg)
  platelet-directed i. (PDIg)
  i. preparation
  i. resilience
  secretory i.
  serum i.
  i. superfamily
  surface membrane i.
immunoglobulin-complexed enzyme (ICE)
immunohematology
immunohematopoietic stem cell
immunohistochemical (IHC)
  i. analysis
  i. diagnostic test
  i. localization
  i. marker
  i. staining
  i. technique
immunohistochemistry (IHC)
immunohistofluorescence
immunohistologic staining
immunohistology
  bone marrow i.
immunoliposome
immunologic
  i. characterization
  i. classification
  i. competence
  i. enhancement
  i. homeostasis
  i. memory
  i. method
  i. method of purging
  i. paralysis
  i. prophylaxis
  i. reconstitution
  i. recovery
  i. suppression
  i. surveillance
  i. tolerance
  i. unresponsiveness
immunologically sequestered site
immunology
  transplantation i.
  tumor i.
immunomodulating
  i. effect
  i. infection
immunomodulator (Imreg-1, Imreg-2)
immunomodulatory
  i. imide
  i. strategy
  i. therapy
immunopathogenesis
immunopathology
immunoperoxidase
  i. stain

  i. staining for cytokeratin
  i. tumor
immunophenotype
  altered i.
  biopsy i.
immunophenotypic
  i. analysis
  i. marker
immunophenotyping
immunophoresis
immunopotentiation
immunoprecipitation
immunoproliferative
  i. lesion
  i. small intestinal disease (IPSID)
immunoprophylaxis
immunoradioassay
immunoradiometric
  i. assay (IRMA)
  i. assay of antigen activity
immunoreaction
immunoreactive
  i. insulin
  i. parathyroid hormone (iPTH)
immunoreactivity
  p53 i.
immunoreceptor tyrosine-based activation motif (ITAM)
immunoregulation
immunoregulatory
  i. effector system
  i. factor expression
immunoresistance
immunorestorative
immunoscintigraphy
  anti-CEA antibody i.
immunoselection
immunosorbent
immunospot
  enzyme-linked i. (ELISPOT)
immunostain
immunostainer
  Ventana 320 automated i.
immunostaining
  Ki-67 i.
  vimentin i.
immunostimulation
immunostimulatory effect
immunosuppressant agent
immunosuppression
  iatrogenic i.
immunosuppressive
  i. acidic protein (IAP)
  i. drug
  i. modality
  i. therapy
immunosurveillance
immunotherapy
  active nonspecific i.

active specific i. (ASI)
adjuvant i.
adoptive i.
Calmette-Guérin i.
cellular i.
intralesional i.
intraperitoneal i.
nonspecific i.
Pacis BCG i.
passive humoral i.
specific i.
tumor i.
immunotolerance
immunotoxin
anti-TAP-72 i.
CD5-T lymphocyte i.
i. LMB-1
recombinant disulfide stabilized i.
recombinant single-chain i.
immunotoxin-mediated cytotoxicity
IMN
internal mammary lymph node chain
IMOxine
IMP
inosine monophosphate
impaction
fecal i.
impairment
memory i.
renal i.
impedance
acoustic i.
imperfecta
dentinogenesis i.
osteogenesis i.
Imperial Cancer Research Fund
implant
BrachySeed Pd-103 i.
Brånemark i.
carcinomatous i.
carmustine i.
cesium i.
Duros leuprolide i.
ear i.
i. geometry
histrelin i.
interstitial radium needle i.
intracavitary i.
^{192}Ir i.
$_{Ie}$Ir i.
iridium-192 i.
leuprolide acetate i.
planar I mesh i.

polifeprosan 20 with carmustine 3.85% i.
i. procedure
prostate seed i.
prosthetic i.
radioactive iodine-125 i.
radioactive palladium-103 seed i.
radioactive 103Pd seed i.
retropubic I-125 i.
seed i.
subpectoral i.
transperineal i.
transvaginal i.
tumor i.
Viadur i.
Vitrasert i.
Zoladex i.
implantable
i. drug delivery system
i. drug pump
i. infusion port
i. infusion pump
i. osmotic pump
i. vascular access device
implantation
palladium-103 i.
radon seed i.
seed i.
implanted pump
implanter
Wallner interstitial prostate i.
impotence
arteriogenic i.
impression
basilar i.
extrinsic i.
extrinsic esophageal i.
imprint cytology
imprinting
genomic i.
Imreg-1, Imreg-2
immunomodulator
IMRT
intensity-modulated radiation therapy
Imubind uPAR ELISA test kit
Imuran
Imuthiol
Imuvert
IMVP-16
ifosfamide, mesna uroprotection, methotrexate, etoposide
^{111}In, In-111
indium-111

NOTES

289

in
    i. situ
    i. situ assay
    i. situ carcinoma of vagina
    i. situ DNA nick end-labeling
    i. situ hybridization (ISH)
    i. situ vein graft
    i. toto
    i. vitro
    i. vitro antibody production (IVAP)
    i. vitro antibody production assay
    i. vitro antigen production
    i. vitro antiviral activity
    i. vitro fertilization
    i. vitro flow cytometric assay
    i. vitro hybridization
    i. vitro induction-remission
    chemotherapy
    i. vitro transcription assay
    i. vivo
    i. vivo binding
    i. vivo clonal expansion
    i. vivo gene transfer
    i. vivo labeling
    i. vivo optical spectroscopy 2000
    (INVOS 2000)
Inactine Pathogen Inactivation
inactivation
    Inactine Pathogen I.
    Knudsen hypothesis of tumor
    suppressor gene i.
    tumor suppressor gene i.
inactivator
    C1 i.
inanition
inappropriate
    i. secretion
    i. secretion of antidiuretic hormone
    (ISADH)
incentive
    suboptimal i.
incessant ovulation hypothesis
incidence rate
incidentaloma
    adrenal i.
incident pain
incision
    transurethral i.
    Weber-Fergusson i.
incisional biopsy
incisor
    fascial i.
inclusion
    Alder-Reilly i.
    i. cell
    i. cyst
    erythrocytic i.
    leukocytic i.
    mesothelial cell i.

incognitus
    Mycoplasma i.
incompatibility
    ABO i.
    Rh i.
incomplete
    i. band heterotopia
    i. Freund adjuvant (IFA)
    i. reconstitution
inconsequential symptom
incontinence
    bladder i.
    bowel i.
incontinentia pigmenti
increased
    i. M/E ratio
    i. signal
increment
    interscan i.
incrementi
    stadium i.
incubation period
incubative stage
IND
    investigational new drug
indanocine
indapamide
indazole
    isomer i.
independent jaws
Inderal LA
indeterminate cell
indeterminatus
    situs i.
index, pl. **indices, indexes**
    ankle-arm i. (AAI)
    ankle-brachial i. (ABI)
    apoptotic i. (AI)
    bifrontal i.
    biopsy volume i.
    body mass i. (BMI)
    Broca i.
    Broders i.
    chemotherapeutic i.
    i. of coexistent disease (ICED)
    congestion i.
    DNA i.
    end-diastolic sphericity i.
    EORTC i.
    European Organization for Research
    and Treatment of Cancer i.
    fluorescence i. (FI)
    free thyroxine i.
    free/total PSA i.
    fucosylation i.
    hairy cell i.
    hepatic iron i.
    hepatitis activity i. (HAI)
    heteroploid i.

International Prognostic I. (IPI)
karyopyknotic i.
Ki-67 i.
Krebs leukocyte i.
metastatic efficiency i. (MEI)
mitosis-karyorrhexis i. (MKI)
mitotic i.
mitotic-karyorrhectic i.
Nottingham prognostic i.
nuclear contour i.
Oral Mucositis I.
palliation i.
plasma cell labeling i. (PCLI)
proliferation i.
Quetelet i.
red blood cell distribution width i.
Sokal i.
Spitzer quality of life i.
Stuart i.
thymidine labeling i. (TLI)
tritiated thymidine labeling i. (TLI)
tumor gene i. (TGI)
Wintrobe i.
Index-Cancer
Functional Living I.-C. (FLIC)
Indiana pouch
Indian club needle
indication
indicator
prognostic i.
indices (*pl. of* index)
indicis
extensor i.
Indiclor
indigenous neoplasm
indigotica
indinavir trough concentration
indirect
i. bilirubin
i. detection
i. fluorescent antibody test
i. hemagglutination
i. immunofluorescence
indirubin
indium-111 (^{111}In, In-111)
i.-111 capromab pendetide dye
individual
seronegative i.
TMP-SMX-intolerant i.
trimethoprim-sulfamethoxazole
intolerant i.
virus-positive antibody-negative i.

individualized
i. functional status assessment
(IFSA)
i. mutant p53 peptide-pulsed
cultured autologous dendritic cell
therapy
indocyanine
i. green-enhanced phototherapy
i. green retention test
indole
indolent
i. disease
i. disseminated leukemia
i. disseminated lymphoma
i. extranodal lymphoma
i. lymphoid malignancy
i. lymphoid neoplasm
i. nodal lymphoma
indomethacin treatment
Indotec
induced
i. phagocytosis
i. sputum
i. sputum test
inducible protein 10 (IP-10)
InDuct
I. breast aspirator
I. breast microcatheter
induction
antimetabolite i.
i. and consolidation chemotherapy
decitabine-mediated i.
dorsal i.
double i. (DI)
i. failure
gene i.
remission i.
i. therapy
induction/maintenance
induction-remission chemotherapy
inductive interaction
indwelling vascular access catheter
ineligibility
AZT i.
infancy
desmoplastic cerebral astrocytoma
of i. (DCAI)
giant cell hepatitis of i.
hypercalcemia of i.
melanotic neuroectodermal tumor
of i. (MNTI)
transient hypogammaglobulinemia
of i.

NOTES

infantile
- i. astrocytoma
- i. choriocarcinoma syndrome
- i. cortical hyperostosis
- i. cutaneous hemangioma
- i. fibrosarcoma
- i. ganglioglioma
- i. monosomy 7 syndrome
- i. Refsum disease

infantisepticum
- *Corynebacterium i.*

Infantol

infarct
- basal ganglia i.
- bone i.
- Zahn i.

infarction
- acute myocardial i.
- bilateral i.
- bone i.
- bowel i.
- brainstem i.
- cerebral i.
- dural sinus thrombosis i.
- embolic i.
- hemorrhagic i.
- myocardial i. (MI)
- renal i.
- splenic i.
- transcatheter therapeutic i.

infection
- adenovirus i.
- amebic i.
- anaerobic i.
- bacterial i.
- *Bordetella pertussis* i.
- brain i.
- buccal space i.
- catheter i.
- congenital i.
- cutaneous viral i.
- cytomegalovirus i.
- deep-seated i.
- dermatophyte tinea i.
- disc space i.
- disseminated fungal i.
- disseminated *Penicillium marneffei* i.
- ectoparasitic i.
- Epstein-Barr i.
- genital human papillomavirus i.
- genitourinary i.
- granulomatous i.
- group B streptococcal i.
- helminth i.
- helminthic i.
- herpes simplex virus i.
- high-titer HHV-8 i.
- high-titer human herpesvirus 8 i.

- Hodgkin disease and HIV i. (HD-HIV)
- immunomodulating i.
- kala-azar i.
- multiplicities of i. (MOI)
- musculoskeletal i.
- *Mycoplasma* i.
- neurologic i.
- neutropenia-related bacterial i.
- nonopportunistic i.
- nosocomial i.
- odontogenic i.
- opportunistic i. (OI)
- paronychial i.
- per-event occupational i.
- pyogenic i.
- renal fungal i.
- respiratory i.
- salivary gland i.
- shunt i.
- skin i.
- Theiler virus i.
- transient i.
- i. tropism
- upper respiratory i.
- urinary tract i. (UTI)
- wound i.

infection-control practices

infectious
- i. granuloma
- i. hepatitis (IH)
- i. mononucleosis
- i. papillomavirus
- i. process
- i. virion

INFeD

Infergen

inferior pubic ramus

infertility
- secondary i.

infield recurrence

infiltrate
- alveolar i.
- benign i.
- consolidating i.
- fluffy i.
- Jessner lymphocytic i.
- localized i.
- lymphoplasmacytic i.
- nodular i.

infiltrating
- i. ductal carcinoma
- i. gland
- i. glioma
- i. lesion
- i. lobular carcinoma
- i. pneumonitis
- i. salivary duct carcinoma
- i. tumor

infiltration
- bone marrow i.
- brachial plexus i.
- diffuse fatty i.
- focal fatty i.
- leukemic i.
- pulmonary i.
- tumor i.

infiltrative
- i. astrocytoma
- i. disorder
- i. plaque

Infinia Hawkeye nuclear medicine system

inflammation
- bronchial i.
- esophageal i.
- granulomatous i.
- perirectal i.
- suppurative i.

inflammation/reactive atypia

inflammatory
- i. bowel disease
- i. breast cancer (IBC)
- i. breast carcinoma
- i. cholesteatoma
- i. cytokine
- i. demyelinating polyneuropathy
- i. fibrosarcoma
- i. fracture
- i. linear epidermal nevus
- i. lymph
- i. myofibroblastic tumor
- i. neuropathy
- i. polyp
- i. pseudotumor
- i. response
- i. T lymphocyte

inflatable bone tamp (IBT)

influenzae
- Haemophilus i.

influenza virus

informed consent

Inform HER-2/neu breast cancer test

infraclavicular lymph node

infradiaphragmatic Hodgkin disease

infratemporal fossa

infratentorial tumor

Infumed pump

Infumorph

infundibulum
- ductus i.
- follicular i.

Infusaid pump

infusate

Infuse-A-Port
- I.-A-P. catheter
- I.-A-P. infusion pump

infuser
- Paragon i.
- single-day i.

infusion
- allodonor lymphocyte i.
- balloon-occluded arterial i.
- cell i.
- i. chemotherapy
- continuous 3-day flavopiridol i.
- cyclophosphamide, Adriamycin, 5-fluorouracil by continuous i. (CAFFI)
- donor lymphocyte i.
- epidural i.
- flavopiridol i.
- hepatic arterial i. (HAI)
- high-dose i.
- HIVIG i.
- human immunodeficiency virus hyperimmune globulin i.
- intermittent high-dose i.
- intraarterial i.
- intramaxillary arterial i.
- intraportal i.
- intravenous i.
- isolated hepatic i.
- isolated limb i.
- limb i.
- locoregional i.
- low-dose i.
- multivitamin i.-12 (MVI-12)
- neuraxial opioid i.
- pediatric multivitamin i.
- i. port
- portal i.
- i. pump
- stem cell i.
- streptokinase i.
- systemic i.
- vasopressin i.
- viable donor lymphocyte i.
- i. wire

infusion-related
- i.-r. cytokine release syndrome (IRCRS)
- i.-r. fever

Infusor
- Baxter I.

NOTES

inguinal
    i. lymphadenectomy
    i. lymph node metastasis
    i. orchiectomy
inguinale
    granuloma i.
    lymphogranuloma i.
inhalant
    butyl nitrate i.
inhalation
    end i.
    hydrocarbon i.
    NebuPent I.
inherent
    i. drug resistance
    i. filter
    i. immunity
inheritance
    autosomal recessive i.
    genetic i.
inherited
    i. class II HLA deficiency
      syndrome
    i. hemolytic anemia
    i. hemophilia
inhibin
inhibiting gene
inhibition
    chemokine i.
    leukocyte adherence i.
    leukocyte migration i.
inhibitor
    absent radius thrombocytopenia i.
    ACE i.
    acrylic nucleotide reverse
      transcriptase i.
    allosteric i.
    5-alpha-reductase i.
    AMN107 aminopyrimidine i.
    angiogenesis i.
    anti-HIV protease i.
    anti-human immunodeficiency virus
      protease i.
    aromatase i. (AI)
    arresten angiogenesis i.
    bcr/abl tyrosine kinase i.
    calcium influx i.
    calmodulin i.
    chain-terminating i.
    c-kit i.
    cyclic urea-based i.
    cyclin-dependent kinase i.
    dioxopiperazine i.
    endogenous GAD i.
    endothelial cell growth i.
    eniluracil i.
    epidermal growth factor-tyrosine
      kinase i. (EGFR-TKI)
    factor II i.

    factor V i.
    factor VII i.
    factor IX i.
    factor X i.
    factor XI i.
    factor XII i.
    farnesyl protein transferase i.
    farnesyl transferase i. (FTI)
    fibrin i.
    fibrinogen i.
    i. of 5-FU metabolism
    histone deacetylase i.
    HIV protease i.
    human alpha$_1$-protease i.
    hydroxamate peptidomimetic i.
    integrase i.
    lipophilic topoisomerase I i.
    liposomal topoisomerase I i.
    matrix metalloproteinase i.
    Merrill-Dow polyamine i.
    microtubule i.
    mitotic i.
    monoamine oxidase i. (MAOI)
    nonnucleoside reverse
      transcriptase i. (NNRTI)
    nonpeptic i.
    nonspermicidal i.
    nonsteroidal aromatase i.
    nucleoside reverse transcriptase i.
      (NRTI)
    peptidic MMP i.
    phosphodiesterase i.
    plasminogen activator i. (PAI)
    plasminogen activator i. type I
    prostaglandin i.
    protease i. (PI)
    proteasome i.
    protein kinase i.
    proton pump i.
    ras pathway i.
    reverse transcriptase i. (RTI)
    secretory leukocyte protease i.
      (SLPI)
    selective serotonin reuptake i.
      (SSRI)
    separation phase i.
    signal transduction i. (STI)
    sodium-hydrogen exchanger i.
    specific *abl* tyrosine kinase i.
    spindle i.
    structure-based HIV protease i.
    structure-based human
      immunodeficiency virus protease i.
    substrate-based i.
    symmetry-based i.
    i. synthesis
    synthetic i.
    TAR i.
    tissue i.

topoisomerase (I-II) i.
tyrosine kinase i.
viral protease i.

inhomogeneity

initially metastatic breast carcinoma (IMBC)

initiative

International AIDS Vaccine I. (IAVI)

initio

ab i.

injectable

Innohep i.
tinzaparin sodium i.

injection

Adlone I.
Adrucil I.
A-HydroCort I.
alcohol i.
Amcort I.
A-methaPred I.
Andro-L.A. I.
Andropository I.
AquaMEPHYTON I.
Aranesp subcutaneous i.
argatroban i.
Aristocort Forte I.
Aristocort Intralesional I.
Aristospan Intraarticular I.
Aristospan Intralesional I.
Arranon i.
Astramorph PF I.
bolus i.
Camptosar i.
Celestone Phosphate I.
Cel-U-Jec I.
Cleocin Phosphate I.
DC i.
Decadron I.
Delatest I.
Delatestryl I.
dendritic cell i.
depGynogen I.
depMedalone I.
DepoCyt cytarabine liposomal i.
Depo-Estradiol I.
Depogen I.
Depo-Medrol I.
Depopred I.
Depo-Provera I.
Depo-Testosterone I.
Dilaudid I.
Dilaudid-HP I.

Dioval I.
D-Med I.
i. drug user (IDU)
Duralone i.
Duramorph I.
Duratest I.
epidural i.
epirubicin i.
Estra-L I.
Estro-Cyp I.
Everone I.
extraarachnoid i.
Faslodex i.
Ferrlecit sodium ferric gluconate complex in sucrose i.
fulvestrant i.
Histerone I.
Hybolin Improved I.
Hydrocortone Acetate i.
Hydrocortone Phosphate i.
imexon i.
intracytoplasmic sperm i. (ICSI)
intramuscular i.
intrathecal i.
intratumoral i.
iron sucrose i.
Kefurox I.
Kenaject I.
Kenalog I.
Key-Pred I.
Key-Pred-SP I.
Lincorex I.
Lyphocin I.
Medralone I.
Minocin IV I.
Miraluma I.
Monistat I.V. I.
M-Prednisol I.
Nebcin I.
Nydrazid I.
Ornidyl I.
Osmitrol I.
pegfilgrastim i.
Pentacarinat I.
Pentam-300 I.
pentostatin i.
percutaneous alcohol i.
percutaneous ethanol i. (PEI)
peripheral i.
Prednisol TBA I.
Rifadin I.
samarium-153 EDTMP i.
Solu-Cortef I.

NOTES

injection *(continued)*
    Solu-Medrol i.
    steroid i.
    Sublimaze I.
    Tac-3 I.
    Tac-40 I.
    Terramycin I.M. I.
    Tesamone I.
    tinzaparin sodium i.
    Toposar I.
    Triam-A I.
    Triam Forte I.
    Triamonide I.
    Tridil I.
    trigger point i. (TPI)
    Tri-Kort I.
    Trilog I.
    Trilone I.
    Triostat I.
    Vancocin I.
    Vancoled I.
    Zinacef I.
    zoledronic acid for i.

injury
    acute traumatic aortic i.
    aortic i.
    apophysial i.
    brachial plexus birth i.
    burn i.
    cervical i.
    drug-induced oxidant i.
    endothelial i.
    epiphysial plate i.
    mechanism of i.
    radiation i.
    tracheobronchial i. (TBI)
    traumatic i.
    unintentional i.

[111]In-labeled capromab pendetide
inlet
    thoracic i.
innate immunity
innocent tumor
Innohep injectable
INNO-LIA syphilis test
Innova
    I. 4100 flat-panel detector
    I. 4100 flat-panel x-ray system
Innovar
innovative therapy
inoculum, pl. **inocula**
    stem cell i.
inopexia
inorganic phosphorus
inosine
    i. monophosphate (IMP)
    i. pranobex
inositol hexaphosphate

inositus
    diabetes i.
Inoue balloon method
InPath cervical cancer screening device
INPC
    International Neuroblastoma Pathology
      Classification
INR
    international normalized ratio
insertion
    catheter i.
    double codon i.
    subclavian central venous
      catheter i.
insertional mutagenesis
inside-out technique
inside-the-needle infusion catheter
insipidus
    diabetes i. (DI)
Insomnia Formula Sleep Aide
inspiration
    degree of i.
    suspended i.
INSS
    International Neuroblastoma Staging
      System
    INSS stage
    INSS stage 1 tumor
instability
    atraumatic, multidirectional,
      bilateral i.
    dorsal intercalated segment i.
    microsatellite i. (MIN, MSI)
    vasomotor i.
instant glucose
instillation
    intrapleural i.
    intravesical i.
instillational therapy
institute
    I. for Cancer Research (ICR)
    Dana-Farber Cancer I. (DFCI)
    Huntsman Cancer I.
    Milan Cancer I.
    National Cancer I.
Institut Gustave-Roussy
institutional review board (IRB)
instrument
    Cell-Dyn Sapphire hematology i.
    Ceprate SC I. II
    Fatigue Assessment I. (FAI)
    Hopkins Pain Rating I. (HPRI)
    Kevorkian-Younge cervical
      biopsy i.
    LightCycler polymerase chain
      reaction analysis i.
    medical outcomes study-human
      immunodeficiency virus i.
    Rotex biopsy i.

insufficiency
  adrenal i.
  aortic i.
  renal i.
insufflation
  sterile talc i.
insular
  i. carcinoma
  i. carcinoma of thyroid
  i. pattern
insulin
  i. antagonist
  i. clearance
  immunoreactive i.
insulin-dependent diabetes mellitus (IDDM)
insulin-like
  i.-l. growth factor (IGF, ILGF)
  i.-l. growth factor-1 (IGF-1)
  i.-l. growth factor-2 (IGF-2)
  i.-l. growth factor-binding protein (IGFBP)
  i.-l. growth factor binding protein-3 assay
  i.-l. peptide
insulinoma
InSure assay
int-2
  int-2 blood fluorescent in situ hybridization
  int-2 bone marrow fluorescent in situ hybridization
  int-2 protooncogene/oncogene
intake
  caloric i.
Intal
integral
  i. dose
  i. uniformity
Integra PBS Pageblot test
integrase
  full-length i.
  i. inhibitor
  i. protein
integrated
  i. reference air-kerma (IRAK)
  i. trimodality approach
integration
  Blocked-Beam-Generator i.
  Clarkson i.
  monoclonal i.
  Rolfing structural i.
Integrilin

integrin
  i. antagonist
  i. subunit
integrin-matrix combination
integumentary barrier
Intelliject pump
intensification
  i. chemotherapy
  dose i.
  i. regimen
Intensified Radiographic Imaging System (IRIS)
intensifier
  image i.
intensity
  absolute dose i. (ADI)
  dose i. (DI)
  drug dose i. (DDI)
  fluorescent signal i.
  high signal i.
  radiation i.
  relative dose i. (RDI)
  signal i.
  summation dose i.
intensity-modulated
  i.-m. arc therapy
  i.-m. radiation therapy (IMRT)
intensive
  i. consolidation chemotherapy
  i. ductal carcinoma
intent
  curative i.
  palliative i.
intention-to-treat principle
interaction
  CD4-gp120 i.
  cell-cell cytoskeletal i.
  cell-matrix cytoskeletal i.
  cell-to-cell i.
  effector/target cell i.
  extracellular matrix/basement membrane i.
  inductive i.
  mind-body i.
  van der Waal i.
  viral host cell i.
interaortocaval lymph node
intercalator
  DNA i.
intercellular
  i. adhesion molecule (ICAM)
  i. adhesion molecule-1 (ICAM-1)
  i. bridge

NOTES

intercellular *(continued)*
  i. junction
  i. lymph
intercostal
  i. muscle
  i. nerve
  i. nerve sheath
intercourse
  active anal i.
  anal i.
  anal-digital i.
  anal-manual i.
  receptive anal i.
interdigitating
  i. dendritic cell (IDC)
  i. dendritic cell sarcoma
interdisciplinary team
interface
  bone-air i.
  gray/white matter i.
  loss of distinction at gray/white
    matter i.
interferon (IFN)
  alfa i.
  i. alfa
  i. alfa-2a (IFNa)
  i. alfa-2a, recombinant
  i. alfa-2b
  i. alfa-2b conjugated polyethylene
    glycol
  i. alfa-2b, recombinant
  i. alfa-2b and ribavirin combination
    pack
  i. alfa-n1
  i. alfa-n3
  all-*trans*-retinoic acid in
    combination with i.
  i. alpha therapy
  i. beta (IFN-beta)
  i. beta-1a
  consensus i.
  gamma i. (IFN-G, IFN-g)
  i. gamma (IFN-G, IFN-g)
  i. gamma-1b
  human i. (HuIFN)
  human gamma i.
  human leukocyte i. (HLI)
  immune i.
  intralesional i.
  leukocyte i.
  leukocyte-derived i.
  low-dose oral i.
  lymphoblastoid i.
  pegylated i.
  r-beta-ser i.
  recombinant alfa i.
  recombinant alfa-2b i.
  i. regulatory factor (IRF)

  i. regulatory factor 1 (IRF-1)
  i. regulatory factor 2 (IRF-2)
interferon-gamma-1b
interferon-n1
  alfa i.-n1
interferon-n3
  alfa i.-n3
**interferon-refractory chronic
  myelogenous leukemia**
interfollicular
  i. Hodgkin disease
  i. mitotic count
  i. pattern
  i. region
intergroup
  I. Osteosarcoma Protocol
  I. Rhabdomyosarcoma Study Group
    (IRSG)
  I. Rhabdomyosarcoma Study Group
    Presurgical Staging Classification
interindividual variability
interlesional therapy
interleukin (IL)
  cytokine i.
  endocervical i.
  human i.
  murine i.
  recombinant human i. (rhIL)
interleukin-1A (IL-1A)
interleukin-1 (IL-1)
interleukin-1B (IL-1B)
  murine i.-1B
interleukin-2 (IL-2)
  p55 component of high-affinity i.-2
  PEG i.-2
  polyethylene glycol-modified i.-2
    (PEG-IL-2)
  recombinant i.-2 (rIL-2)
interleukin-3 (IL-3)
  murine i.-3
  recombinant human i.-3 (rhIL-3)
interleukin-4 (IL-4)
  i.-4 fusion toxin
interleukin-4R (IL-4R)
interleukin-6 (IL-6)
  murine i.-6
interleukin-7 (IL-7)
  murine i.-7
interleukin-10 (IL-10)
interleukin-11 (IL-11)
  recombinant human i.-11 (rhIL-11)
interleukin-12 (IL-12)
  i.-12 and EPOCH chemotherapy
  recombinant human i.-12 (rhIL-12)
interleukin-3Ra^{bright} (IL-3Ra^{bright})
interleukin-1alpha (IL-1alpha)
interleukin-1beta (IL-1beta)
**interleukin-1 through interleukin-21 (IL-
  1–21)**

Interlink
 I. cannula
 I. injection cap
intermedia
 thalassemia i.
intermediate
 i. carcinoma
 i. lymphocytic lymphoma (ILL)
 malignant teratoma, i. (MTI)
 i. remodeling
intermediate-dose
 i.-d. methotrexate (IDMTX)
 i.-d. salvage regimen
intermediate-grade CD20-positive lymphoma
intermediate-sized trial
intermedius
 bronchus i.
intermittent
 i. androgen blockade (IAB)
 i. claudication
 i. high-dose infusion
 i. high-dose vitamin C
 i. pneumatic compression (IPC)
internal
 i. carotid artery (ICA)
 i. hemipelvectomy
 i. iliac arterial infusion chemotherapy
 i. inguinal ring
 i. mammary chain
 i. mammary chain of lymph nodes (IMC)
 i. mammary lymph node chain (IMN)
 i. mammary lymphoscintigraphy
 i. radiation
 i. radiation therapy
international
 I. AIDS Vaccine Initiative (IAVI)
 I. Bone Marrow Transplant Registry (IBMTR)
 I. Breast Cancer Study Group (IBCSG)
 I. Cancer Alliance
 i. cancer care
 I. Cancer Information Center (ICIC)
 i. classification of cancer of cervix
 I. Classification of Diseases (ICD)
 I. Classification of Diseases for Oncology (ICD-O)

 I. Commission on Radiation Units and Measurements (ICRU)
 I. Federation of Gynecology and Obstetrics (FIGO)
 I. Federation of Gynecology and Obstetrics nomenclature
 I. Germ Cell Cancer Collaborative Group (IGCCCG)
 I. Index of Erectile function (IIEF)
 I. Mesothelioma Interest Group (IMIG)
 I. Myeloma Foundation
 I. Neuroblastoma Pathology Classification (INPC)
 I. Neuroblastoma Staging System (INSS)
 i. normalized ratio (INR)
 I. Prognostic Index (IPI)
 I. Society of Pediatric Oncology (SIOP)
 I. Staging System
 I. System of Units (SI)
 I. Union Against Cancer (UICC)
 I. Union Against Cancer-RO resection
 I. Workshop and Conference on Human Leukocyte Differentiation Antigens
internodal tract
internuclear bridging
internucleosomal DNA fragmentation
interossei
 dorsal i.
interpersonal
 i. psychotherapist
 i. psychotherapy
interphase cytogenetics
interposition
 jejunal graft i.
interscan
 i. increment
 i. spacing
interstitial
 i. antigen-antibody complex
 i. bacterial pneumonia
 i. BCNU
 i. BCNU administered via wafer
 i. brachytherapy
 i. cell tumor
 i. cell tumor of testis
 i. conductive heating
 i. dendritic cell
 i. fluid pressure (IFP)

NOTES

interstitial *(continued)*
    i. irradiation
    i. keratitis
    i. nephritis
    i. photon-radiosurgical therapy
    i. radiation
    i. radiation therapy
    i. radiotherapy
    i. radium needle implant
    i. ultrasound hyperthermia
intersubunit
interuncal distance
interval
    basion-axial i.
    basion-dens i.
    i. cancer
    confidence i. (CI)
    disease-free i. (DFI)
    narrow interscan i.
    progression-free i.
intervention
    biliary i.
    coronary i.
    dietary i.
    new approaches to coronary i.
    i. study
interventional procedure
intervertebral foramen
intervillous thrombosis
intestinal
    i. carcinoid tumor
    i. crypt
    i. ileus
    lipophagic i.
    i. metaplasia
    i. mucin
    i. obstruction
    i. parasympathetic ganglion
intestinalis
    Giardia i.
    Septata i.
intestine
    large i.
    small i.
intima
    pulmonary artery i.
    tunica i.
intimal hyperplasia
intolerance
    AZT i.
intoplicine
intoxication
    psychogenic water i.
intraaabdominal desmoplastic small round cell tumor
intraabdominal
    i. mass
    i. relapse
intraarterial (IA)

    i. chemotherapy (IAC)
    i. cisplatin chemotherapy
    i. floxuridine
    i. infusion
    i. secretin (IAS)
    i. therapy
intraaxial
    i. lesion
    i. neoplasm
    i. schwannoma
    i. tumor
intrabronchial lesion
intracanalicular sarcoma
intracapsular
    i. metastasis
    i. tumor
intracavernous injection therapy
intracavitary
    i. balloon applicator
    i. brachytherapy (IBT)
    i. chemotherapy
    i. delivery
    i. implant
    i. irradiation
    i. particle radiation
    i. radium
    i. therapy
intracellular
    i. activation
    i. antigen
    i. compartment
    i. cytokine staining (ICS)
    i. cytokine staining assay
    i. glutathione level
    i. half-life
    i. immunoglobulin
    i. proteolysis
    i. target
    i. tripeptide
intracellulare
    Mycobacterium i.
intracerebral
    i. amyloidoma
    i. distribution
    i. ganglioglioma
    i. ganglioma
    i. nerve sheath tumor
    i. schwannoma
    i. spinal fluid chemotherapy
    i. stimulation
intracerebroventricular (ICV)
intraclass correlation coefficient (ICC)
intracranial
    i. aneurysm (ICA)
    i. bleeding
    i. ependymoma
    i. focal process
    i. hypertension
    i. mass

i. mass lesion
i. neoplasm
i. neuroblastoma
i. tumor
intra-CSF chemotherapy
intractable
   i. nausea
   i. pain
intracystic
   i. papillary carcinoma
   i. papilloma
intracytoplasmic sperm injection (ICSI)
intradecidual sign
intradermal administration
IntraDose injectable gel
intraductal
   i. brachytherapy
   i. breast carcinoma
   i. calcification
   i. carcinoma (IDC)
   i. component
   i. mucin-hypersecreting neoplasm
   i. oncocytic papillary carcinoma
     (IPOC)
   i. papillary carcinoma
   i. papillary mucinous neoplasm
     (IPMN)
   i. papillary mucinous tumor
     (IPMT)
   i. papillary neoplasm of pancreas
     (IPNP)
   i. papilloma
   i. papillomatosis
   i. ultrasonography
intradural
   i. epidermoidoma
   i. extramedullary lesion
   i. extramedullary mass
intraepidermal carcinoma
intraepithelial
   i. carcinoma
   i. cell
   i. lesion
   i. lymphocyte (IEL)
   i. neoplasia
   i. neoplasia of vagina
   i. neoplasia of vulva
   i. neoplasm
intrafamilial transmission
intragenomic localization
intraglandular
intrahepatic
   i. arterial chemoembolization

i. arterioportal fistula
i. artery chemotherapy (IHAC)
i. bile duct
i. biliary cancer
i. biliary neoplasm
i. biloma
i. cholangiocarcinoma (ICC)
i. cholestasis
i. delivery
i. portal hypertension
intralesional
   i. administration
   i. bleomycin
   i. curettage
   i. curettage of tumor
   i. 5-FU
   i. immunotherapy
   i. interferon
   i. therapy
   i. triamcinolone
intraligamentous myoma
intralobar fissure
intraluminal
   i. adenocarcinoma
   i. brachytherapy
   i. crystalloid
   i. filling defect
   i. irradiation
   i. pH
   i. pressure profile
   i. probe
intralymphatic
   i. emboli
   i. radioactivity administration
intramammary lymph node (intraMLN)
intramaxillary arterial infusion
intramedullary
   i. compartment neoplasm
   i. lesion
   i. radiodensity
   i. spinal cord metastasis (ISCM)
   i. tumor biopsy
intraMLN
   intramammary lymph node
intramucosal carcinoma
intramural
   i. invasion
   i. tumor
intramuscular (IM)
   i. chemotherapy
   immune globulin i.

NOTES

intramuscular *(continued)*
    i. injection
    i. juvenile xanthogranuloma
**intramyocardial coronary blood flow
(ICBF)**
intraneural perineurioma
intranodal
    i. hemorrhagic spindle cell tumor
    i. myofibroblastoma
in-transit metastasis
intraobserver error
intraocular
    i. lesion
    i. melanoma
    i. retinoblastoma
    i. spread
intraoperative
    i. electron beam radiotherapy
    i. endoscopy (IOE)
    i. functional mapping
    i. radiation
    i. radiation therapy (IORT)
    i. radiotherapy (IORT)
    i. ultrasonography (IOUS)
intraoral
    i. cone irradiation
    i. roentgentherapy
    i. swage technique
intraorbital
    i. granular cell tumor
    i. lesion
intraosseous
    i. bone lesion
    i. ganglion
    i. keratin cyst
    i. meningioma
intraparenchymal
    i. meningioma
    i. metastasis
    i. nerve sheath tumor
intrapartum
intraperitoneal
    i. drug administration
    i. hemorrhage
    i. hyperthermic chemotherapy
    (IPHC)
    i. immunotherapy
    i. paclitaxel
    i. perfusion
    i. thermochemotherapy
intrapleural
    i. chemotherapy
    i. delivery
    i. instillation
    i. talc
    i. tetracycline
intraportal infusion
intraprostatic androgen
intrapulmonary bronchogenic cyst

intrasellar
    i. lesion
    i. mass
intraspinal administration
intrasurgical rupture
intratesticular leiomyosarcoma
intrathecal (IT)
    i. block
    i. chemotherapy
    i. hydrocortisone
    i. injection
    i. methotrexate
    i. neurolysis
    i. route
    i. therapy
intrathoracic
    i. esophagogastrostomy
    i. lymphoproliferative disorder
    i. organ involvement
intratumoral
    i. fat
    i. hemorrhage
    i. injection
    i. metastasis
intrauterine
    i. hormonal exposure
    i. hormone
    i. hormone exposure
intravagal paraganglioma
intravaginal
    i. brachytherapy (IVBT)
    i. roentgentherapy
intravascular
    i. agent
    i. brachytherapy
    i. brachytherapy dosimetry
    i. coil
    i. consumption coagulopathy
    i. filling defect
    i. hemolysis
    i. lymph
    i. lymphoma
    i. lymphomatosis (IVL)
    i. radiation therapy
    i. radiotherapy
    i. stent
    i. tumor
    i. ultrasound
intravenous (I.V.)
    i. alimentation
    i. contrast media
    i. cytotoxic drug
    i. drug abuse (IVDA)
    i. drug user (IVDU)
    i. fluid
    immune globulin i.
    i. immunoglobulin (IVIG)
    i. infusion
    i. infusion chemotherapy

i. methylprednisolone
i. ozone therapy
i. pyelogram (IVP)
i. pyelography (IVP)
intravenous-enhanced MRI
intraventricular
i. chemotherapy
i. mass
i. therapy
i. tumor
intravesical
i. chemotherapy
i. instillation
i. therapy (IVT)
intravital lymphatic staining
intravitreal ganciclovir
intrinsic
i. coagulation pathway
i. fluorescence spectroscopy (IFS)
i. hemolytic anemia
i. radiosensitivity
i. tyrosine kinase activity
introducer
Cardak i.
Razi cannula i.
Intron A
intubation
endotracheal i.
intussusception
ileocolic i.
ileoileal i.
rectal i.
Invader assay
invagination
basilar i.
invariant antigenetic match
invasion
blood vessel i. (BVI)
Clark level of i.
deep i.
early stromal i.
extrathyroidal i.
intramural i.
level of i.
local i.
lymphatic vessel i. (LVI)
perineural i. (PNI)
Sarisol i.
seminal vesicle i. (SVI)
stage of i.
transmural i.
invasionis
stadium i.

invasive
i. adenocarcinoma
i. aspergillosis (IA)
i. biopsy
i. comedocarcinoma
i. ductal carcinoma (IDC)
i. lobular carcinoma
i. mole
i. papillotubular carcinoma
i. penile cancer
i. pulmonary aspergillosis (IPA)
i. solid tubular carcinoma
i. squamous cell carcinoma
i. therapy
i. thermometry
i. thymoma
inventory
Brief Fatigue I. (BFI)
brief pain i. (BPI)
Fatigue Symptom I. (FSI)
Multidimensional Fatigue I. (MFI, MFI-20)
Multidimensional Fatigue Symptom I.
State-Trait Anxiety I.
Wisconsin Brief Pain I.
Zung Depression I.
inverse
i. polymerase chain
i. segmental multileaf collimator
inverse-square law
inverted
i. follicular keratosis
i. papilloma (IP)
i. schneiderian papilloma
investigational
i. high-dose chemotherapy quartet
i. new drug (IND)
Invirase capsule
involucrin
involucrum, pl. **involucra**
involuting phase
involution
thymic i.
involved-field radiation
involvement
axillary node i.
bone marrow i.
capsular i.
celiac nodal i.
contiguous organ i.
extramedullary i.
extranodal i.

NOTES

303

involvement *(continued)*
    intrathoracic organ i.
    lymphomatous bone marrow i.
    lymphovascular i. (LVSI)
    nipple i.
    organ i.
    pagetoid epidermal i.
    supraclavicular node i.
INVOS 2000
    in vivo optical spectroscopy 2000
IOCM
    isosmolar contrast medium
iodide
    potassium i.
    saturated solution of potassium i. (SSKI)
    sodium i.
iodine (I)
    i. ^{131}I Lym-1 MAb
    i. ^{131}I murine MAb to alpha fetoprotein
    i. ^{131}I murine MAb to human chorionic gonadotropin
    i. ^{131}I murine MAb IgG2a to B cell
    I-Plant radioactive i.
    i. ^{131}I radiolabeled B1 MAb
    radioactive i.
iodine-125 (^{125}I, I-125)
    i.-125 brachytherapy seed
iodine-131 (^{131}I, I-131)
    i.-131 antiferritin treatment for hepatocellular cancer
    i.-131 metaiodobenzylguanidine (I-MIBG)
iodine-131-labeled B-lymphocyte stimulator
iodine-131-metaiodobenzylguanidine
iodoazomycin arabinoside
iodocholesterol scan
4′-iodo-4′-deoxydoxorubicin (IDX)
iododeoxyuridine (IUDR, IUdR)
iododoxorubicin
Iodopen
iodoquinol
Iodotope
IOE
    intraoperative endoscopy
ion
    reactive carbonium i.
ionafarnib
ionization
    surface-enhanced laser desorption and i. (SELDI)
ionizing radiation
IORT
    intraoperative radiation therapy
    intraoperative radiotherapy
iothalamate meglumine

Iotrex
IOUS
    intraoperative ultrasonography
IP
    inverted papilloma
IP-10
    inducible protein 10
IPA
    ifosfamide, Platinol, Adriamycin
    invasive pulmonary aspergillosis
    4-hydroxy IPA
IPC
    intermittent pneumatic compression
IPF
    idiopathic pulmonary fibrosis
IPHC
    intraperitoneal hyperthermic chemotherapy
IPI
    International Prognostic Index
I-Plant radioactive iodine
IPMN
    intraductal papillary mucinous neoplasm
IPMT
    intraductal papillary mucinous tumor
IPNP
    intraductal papillary neoplasm of pancreas
IPOC
    intraductal oncocytic papillary carcinoma
IPP
    isopropyl pyrrolizine
IPSID
    immunoproliferative small intestinal disease
ipsilateral
    i. breast tumor recurrence (IBTR)
    i. electron beam
    i. synchronous adrenalectomy
    i. tumor
iPTH
    immunoreactive parathyroid hormone
^{192}Ir
    iridium-192
        ^{192}Ir implant
        ^{192}Ir ribbon
        ^{192}Ir wire
^{194}Ir
    iridium-194
IRAK
    integrated reference air-kerma
IRB
    institutional review board
Ircon
IRCRS
    infusion-related cytokine release syndrome
Iressa

IRF
  interferon regulatory factor
  IRF staining pattern
IRF-1
  interferon regulatory factor 1
IRF-2
  interferon regulatory factor 2
iridis
  heterochromia i.
  rubeosis i.
iridium-192 (^{192}Ir)
  i.-192 implant
iridium-194 (^{194}Ir)
iridocyclectomy
iridotrabeculectomy
$_{Ie}$**Ir implant**
irinotecan
  i., folinic acid, 5-fluorouracil
    (FOLFIRI)
  i. HCl
  i. hydrochloride
  i. and oxaliplatin (IROX)
irinotecan-induced diarrhea
IRIS
  Intensified Radiographic Imaging System
iris
  i. fluorescein photography
  hamartoma of i.
  i. melanocytic tumor
  i. melanoma
Irish node
IRMA
  immunoradiometric assay
  prolifigen TPA IRMA
irofulven
iron (Fe)
  i. binding
  i. deficiency
  i. deposition
  i. dextran complex
  ferrous i.
  i. overload
  i. oxide
  i. oxide dextran colloid
  serum i.
  i. stain
  i. sucrose injection
  tissue i.
  i. transport
iron-binding
  i.-b. capacity (IBC)
  i.-b. capacity test
iron-deficiency anemia

iron-dextran particle
IROX
  irinotecan and oxaliplatin
  IROX regimen
irradiated
  i. blood
  i. field
  i. glioblastoma
irradiation
  abdominal i.
  accelerated partial breast i. (APBI)
  adjuvant i.
  axillary i.
  breast i.
  central lymphatic i.
  charged-particle i.
  craniospinal i. (CSI)
  endocavitary i.
  external beam photon i.
  external orthovoltage i.
  extracorporeal i.
  fractionated external beam i.
  fractionated total body i. (FTBI)
  gamma i.
  gated i.
  gonadal i.
  hemibody i. (HBI)
  interstitial i.
  intracavitary i.
  intraluminal i.
  intraoral cone i.
  local i.
  low LET external beam i.
  mantle i.
  mediastinal i.
  pelvic i.
  prophylactic cranial i. (PCI)
  rapid-fractionation i.
  regional i.
  single-fraction total body i.
  split-course i.
  stereotactic external beam i. (SEBI)
  subtotal lymphoid i. (STLI)
  subtotal nodal i. (STNI)
  surface i.
  total body i. (TBI)
  total lymphoid i. (TLI)
  total nodal i.
  UV i.
  whole abdominal i.
  whole abdominopelvic i. (WAP)
  whole lung i.

NOTES

irradiation *(continued)*
>   whole pelvic i.
>   whole pelvis i.

irradiation-produced sarcoma
irradiator
>   portable blood i.

irregularity
>   avulsive cortical i.

irreversible
>   i. monoclonal lymphoma
>   i. sickled cell (ISC)

irrigant
>   Neosporin G.U. I.

IRSG
>   Intergroup Rhabdomyosarcoma Study
>   Group
>   IRSG Presurgical Staging
>   Classification

**IS1000 gel documentation imaging
system**
ISADH
>   inappropriate secretion of antidiuretic
>   hormone

ISC
>   irreversible sickled cell

Iscador
ischemia
>   cerebral i.
>   chemotherapy-induced i.
>   myocardial i.
>   radiation-induced i.
>   radiation-related i.

ischial tuberosity
ischium
ISCM
>   intramedullary spinal cord metastasis

iseganan HCl oral solution
ISET
>   isolation by size of epithelial tumor cells
>   ISET assay

isethionate
>   pentamidine i.
>   piritrexim i.

ISH
>   in situ hybridization
>   ISH EBER technique

island
>   bone i.
>   cell i.
>   endometrial i.

islet
>   i. cell adenoma
>   i. cell neoplasm
>   i. cell tumor

isoallotypic determinant
isoantibody
isoantigen
isobologram analysis
isobutyl cyanoacrylate (IBCA)

isocarboxazid
isocenter dose
isocentral
isocentric 4-field box
isochromat
isochromatic
isochromosome 17q
isocyanate
isocytosis
isodose
>   i. curve
>   i. envelope
>   i. line
>   i. shift method

**isoelectric focusing polyacrylamide gel
in electrophoresis (IEF-PAGE)**
isoelectrofocusing
isoenzyme
>   creatine kinase-BB i. (CK-BB)
>   growth-related tumor marker
>   ALP i.
>   Regan i.
>   i. RNase

isoerythrolysis
isoflurane
isoform
>   CD44v6 i.
>   galectin-3 i.
>   Ikaros i.
>   oncogenic Ikaros i.

isogeneic
>   i. antigen
>   i. graft

isograft
isohemagglutinin
isoimmune neonatal thrombocytopenia
isoimmunity
isointense lesion
isolate
>   nonsyncytia-forming i.
>   primary i.
>   i. specific
>   T-cell line-adapted i.

isolated
>   i. heat perfusion
>   i. hepatic infusion
>   i. hepatic perfusion (IHP)
>   i. hepatic portal and arterial
>   perfusion
>   i. limb infusion
>   i. limb perfusion (ILP)
>   i. tumor cell (ITC)

isolation
>   i. perfusion therapy
>   i. by size of epithelial tumor cells
>   (ISET)

isoleucine (I)
**Isolex 300i magnetic stem cell selection
system**

isologous neoplasm
IsoMed
    I. Constant-Flow Infusion System
    I. implantable drug pump
isomer indazole
isometric
isomorphic gliosis
isoniazid
    i. resistant
    i. sensitive
    i. toxicity
isopentane
isophil
    i. antibody
    i. antigen
isoprenoid plant compound
Isoprinosine
isopropyl
    i. alcohol
    i. pyrrolizine (IPP)
Isordil
isosmolar contrast medium (IOCM)
isosorbide dinitrate
Isospora belli
isosporiasis
    chronic intestinal i.
isosulfan blue dye
isothiocyanate
    fluorescein i.
isotope
    beta-emitting i.
    i. colloid imaging
    i. dilution principle
    i. effect
    low LET i.
    poorly concentrated i.
    radioactive i.
isotretinoin
isotype
    M-component i.
isotypic determinant
isovaleric acidemia
Isovorin
issue
    end-of-life i.'s
    existential i.
    psychosocial i.
isthmus, pl. **isthmi**
    aortic i.
isthmusectomy
IT
    intrathecal
    IT MTX

ITAM
    immunoreceptor tyrosine-based activation motif
Itaqui virus
ITC
    isolated tumor cell
Itch-X
ITP
    idiopathic thrombocytopenic purpura
    immune thrombocytopenic purpura
      steroid-refractory ITP
itraconazole toxicity
IUDR, IUdR
    idoxuridine
    iododeoxyuridine
I.V.
    intravenous
      Aranesp I.V.
      Fucidin I.V.
      Gammar-P I.V.
      KVO-type I.V.
      Merrem I.V.
      Nystatin-LF I.V.
IVA
    ifosfamide, vincristine, actinomycin
      IVA seal
Ivalon particle
IVAP
    in vitro antibody production
IVBT
    intravaginal brachytherapy
IVDA
    intravenous drug abuse
IVDU
    intravenous drug user
Ivemark syndrome
IV-enhanced MRI
IVIG
    intravenous immunoglobulin
IVL
    intravascular lymphomatosis
Ivor-Lewis esophagectomy
IVP
    intravenous pyelogram
    intravenous pyelography
IVT
    intravesical therapy
Ivy bleeding time
ixabepilone
IX:Ag
    factor IX antigen
Ixodes
    I. dammini

NOTES

Ixodes (continued)
    I. scapularis

Jaa Amp
Jaccoud arthropathy
Jackson
    J. dilator
    J. staging system
    J. staging system for penile cancer
Jackson-Parker classification
Jacobson nerve
Jacobsson criteria
Jaffe grading
Jaksch anemia
Jamestown Canyon (JC)
Jamshidi
    J. adult needle
    J. liver biopsy needle
    J. muscle biopsy needle
Jamshidi-Kormed bone marrow biopsy
    needle
Jansen-type metaphysial
    chondrodysplasia
Jansky classification
Japanese
    J. B encephalitis virus
    J. variant
    J. V3 loop sequence
Jarisch-Herxheimer reaction
Jass grading system
jaundice
    obstructive j.
jaw
    asymmetric j.'s
    collimator j.
    independent j.'s
    keratocyst of j.
Jaworski body
JC
    Jamestown Canyon
    JC papovavirus
    JC virus
J chain
jejunal
    j. graft
    j. graft interposition
jejuni
    Campylobacter j.
jejunostomy
    percutaneous endoscopic j. (PEJ)
    j. tube
    Witzel j.
jelly
    Royal J.
jennerian
jennerization
Jensen sarcoma

Jerne
    J. plaque assay
    J. theory
    J. theory of antibody formation
Jeryl Lynn mumps virus
Jessner lymphocytic infiltrate
jet
    j. lavage
    j. nebulizer
    pressurized fluid j.
Jew
    Ashkenazi J.
Jewett
    J. classification of bladder
        carcinoma
    J. nail
Jewett-Marshall staging system
Jewett-Strong
    J.-S. staging
    J.-S. staging of bladder cancer
Jewett-Strong-Marshall
    J.-S.-M. staging
    J.-S.-M. staging of bladder cancer
Jewett-Whitmore classification
jin bu huan
jiroveci
    Pneumocystis j.
jitteriness
JNPA
    juvenile nasopharyngeal angiofibroma
Job syndrome
Joel scanning electron microscope
Johnsen score
Johns Hopkins Oncology Center
Johnson & Johnson waterproof tape
joining
    j. chain
    j. segment
joint
    AC j.
    acromioclavicular j.
    ankle j.
    atlantoaxial j.
    ball-and-socket j.
    calcaneocuboid j.
    Clutton j.
    diarthrodial j.
    j. effusion
    elbow j.
    flail j.
    j. pain
    J. United Nations Programme on
        HIV/AIDS (UNAIDS)
Jolly body

J

JON95
> oncoprotein JON95

Josephs-Diamond-Blackfan anemia

JPA
> juvenile pilocytic astrocytoma

jugular
> j. bulb
> j. catheter
> j. chain
> j. venous pressure
> j. venous pulse (JVP)

jugulare
> glomus j.
> tympanicum j.

jugulocarotid

jugulodigastric
> j. basin
> j. node

jugulotympanic paraganglioma

juice
> cancer j.

junction
> anomalous j.
> atrioventricular j.
> EG j.
> esophagogastric j.
> Holliday j.
> intercellular j.
> mucocutaneous j.
> rectosigmoid j.
> stromoepithelial j.

junctional zone

Junin virus

Junior Strength Motrin

jun protooncogene/oncogene

Jurkat
> J. cell
> J. cell line
> J. T-cell line

juvenile
> j. aponeurotic fibroma
> j. carcinoma
> j. chronic myelogenous leukemia
> j. fibroadenoma
> j. hemangiofibroma
> j. hyalin fibromatosis
> j. melanoma
> j. nasopharyngeal angiofibroma (JNPA)
> j. palmoplantar fibromatosis
> j. pilocytic astrocytoma (JPA)
> j. polyposis
> j. polyposis syndrome
> j. xanthogranuloma

juxtaarticular

juxtacortical
> j. osteogenic
> j. osteosarcoma
> j. sarcoma

juxtaepiphysial

juxtaglomerular tumor

juxtaposition

JVP
> jugular venous pulse

κ (*var. of* kappa)

K

  potassium

    K + 10

    K antigen

    K + Care

    K + Care Effervescent

    K meson

^{39}**K**

  potassium-39

Kabikinase

Kadesky staging system

Kadian Oral

Kadish

    K. staging

    K. staging of esthesioneuroblastoma

    K. staging system

Kagan staging system

Kahler disease

KAI1/CD82 gene

Kaiser ninhydrin test

kala-azar infection

kallikrein-2 protease level

kallikrein-inhibiting unit

Kallmann syndrome

Kampo medicine

kanamycin

kangri

    k. burn carcinoma

    k. cancer

kansasii

    Mycobacterium k.

Kantrex

Kaochlor SF

Kaodene

kaolin

    k. and pectin

    k. and pectin with opium

Kaon

Kaon-Cl

Kaon-Cl-10

Kaopectate

    K. Advanced Formula

    K. Maximum Strength Caplets

Kao-Spen

Kaplan-Meier survival curve

Kaposi

    K. sarcoma (KS)

    K. sarcoma-associated herpesvirus
    (KSHV)

    K. sarcoma-associated virus

    K. varicelliform eruption

kaposiform hemangioendothelioma

kappa, κ

    IgG k.

    k. light chain

kappa-beta

    receptor activator of nuclear
    factor k.-b. (RANK)

Karapandzic advancement flap

karenitecin

Karnofsky performance status (KPS)

Karr method

Karroo syndrome

Karst

    Ganoderma Lucidum K.

karyokinesis

karyolytic

karyometric analysis

karyometry

karyopherin

    k. ab heterodimer

    recombinant k.

karyopyknotic index

karyorrhectic cell

karyorrhexis

karyotype

    complex k.

karyotypic analysis

karyotyping

Kasabach-Merritt syndrome

Kasof

Kast syndrome

Katayama fever

Kauffmann-White scheme

kava

Kaybovite-1000

Kay Ciel

Kayexalate

Kaznelson syndrome

KC1 Delta coagulation analyzer

kD

    kilodalton

K-Dur 10, 20

Keasby tumor

keep vein open (KVO)

Keflex

Keflin, gentamicin, carbenicillin (KGC)

Keftab

Kefurox Injection

Kefzol

Kegel exercise

K-Electrolyte Effervescent

Kell

    K. antibody

    K. blood group

Kell-Cellano blood group

Kellgren disease

Kemadrin
Kemerovo virus
Kemron
Kenacort Oral
Kenaject Injection
Kenalog Injection
Kennedy disease
Kepivance
keratectomy
  photorefractive k.
keratin
  k. 34 E-12
  k. horn
  k. pearl
  k. staining
keratinization focus
keratinizing
  k. hyperplasia
  k. squamous cell carcinoma
keratinocyte
  dyskeratotic k.
  factor receptor k.
  k. growth factor (KGF)
  k. growth factor 2 (KGF-2)
  k. growth factor receptor (KGFR)
keratitis
  bacterial k.
  interstitial k.
  necrogranulomatous k.
keratoacanthoma
  giant aggressive k.
keratoconjunctivitis
  microsporidial k.
  k. sicca
keratocyst of jaw
keratocyte
keratoderma blennorrhagicum
keratopathy
  vortex k.
keratoplasty
  laser thermal k. (LTK)
  noncontact holmium:yttrium-argon-
    garnet laser thermal k.
keratosis, pl. keratoses
  acral palmoplantar k.
  actinic k.
  follicular k.
  frictional k.
  inverted follicular k.
  k. palmaris et plantaris
  palmoplantar k.
  smokeless tobacco k.
  snuff-dippers' k.
  solar k.
  stucco k.
  tobacco pouch k.
  vocal cord k.
kerma
  kinetic energy released in material

kerma-to-dose conversion factor
kernicterus
Kern marker
Kernohan
  K. grading system I-IV
  K. histologic grading system
  K. notch
Kestrone-5
ketamine
ketene
  propyl k.
ketoconazole
  high-dose k.
ketone body
ketoprofen (KT)
ketorolac tromethamine
ketosis
Ketron-Goodman
  K.-G. syndrome
  K.-G. variant
Kety-Schmidt method
keV, kev
  kiloelectron volt
Kevorkian-Younge cervical biopsy
  instrument
Keyes dermatologic punch
keyhole
  k. configuration
  k. limpet hemocyanin (KLH)
keyhole-shaped craniectomy
Key-Pred Injection
Key-Pred-SP Injection
key terminal enzyme
KG-1 cell
KGC
  Keflin, gentamicin, carbenicillin
K-Gen Effervescent
KGF
  keratinocyte growth factor
KGF-2
  keratinocyte growth factor 2
KGFR
  keratinocyte growth factor receptor
Khan scatter analysis
Ki-1
  Ki-1 antigen
  Ki-1 positive lymphoma
Ki-67
  Ki-67 immunostaining
  Ki-67 index
  Ki-67 monoclonal antibody
  Ki-67 nuclear antigen
Kidd
  K. antibody
  K. blood group
K-Ide
kidney
  absent k.
  k. adenocarcinoma

atypical angiomyolipoma of k.
k. cancer
canine k.
k. and cord block
duplex k.
ectopic k.
Goldblatt k.
green monkey k. (GMK)
horseshoe k.
Madin-Darby canine k.
myeloma k.
rhabdoid tumor of k.
k. transplant
kidney-fixing antibody
Kiel
K. classification of non-Hodgkin lymphoma
K. Pediatric Tumor Registry
K. tumor cell classification
Kienböck disease
Kikuchi lymphadenitis
kill
cell k.
fractional cell k.
log k.
logs of cell k.
killed
k. virus
k. virus vaccine
killer
k. cell
lymphokine-activated k. (LAK)
natural k. (NK)
kilodalton (kD)
128 k. neuronal protein
kiloelectron volt (keV, kev)
kilogram
coulombs per k. (c/kg)
kilovoltage (kV)
Kim-Ray Greenfield caval filter
KinAir bed
kinase
bcr/abl k.
creatine k. (CK)
Csk homologous k. (CHK)
cyclin-dependent k. (CDK)
cyclin-dependent k. 4
cytidylate/2′-deoxycytidylate k. (CMP/dCMP-K)
cytosolic thymidine k.
2′-deoxycytidine k. (dCK)
2′-deoxythymidine k. (dTK)

double-stranded RNA-activated protein k.
focal adhesion k. (FAK)
guanylate k. (GMP-K)
herpes simplex virus-thymidine k. (HSV-tk)
mitogen-activated protein k.
nucleoside 5′-diphosphate k. (NDK-K)
protein k.
pyruvate k.
receptor tyrosine k. (RTK)
RNA-dependent protein k. (PKR)
serine-threonine k.
serum thymidine k.
stress-activated protein k. (SAPK)
thymidine k. (TK)
thymidylate k.
transmembrane receptor tyrosine k.
tumor M2-pyruvate k.
tyrosine k.
kin-cohort design
Kinesis reagent kit
kinetic
k. energy released in material (kerma)
k. resistance
kinetic-based sequencing
kinetics
cell-cycle k.
exponential k.
granulocytic k.
kinetocyte
King-Armstrong unit
kink
cervicomedullary k.
kinking
aortic k.
kinoid
TNF-alpha k.
Kinyoun stain
Kionex
Ki-ras gene
kirilowii
Trichosanthes k.
Kirsten sarcoma virus
kit
cake mix k.
Cellfree Interleukin-2 Receptor k.
chemiluminescent substrate k.
cold k.
Confide HIV test k.
Corzyme k.

NOTES

kit *(continued)*
deoxyribonucleic acid probe k.
DNA polymerase assay k.
DNA probe k.
DNAzol k.
dye terminator cycle sequencing
core k.
Endogen Human VEGF ELISA k.
EZ::TN insertion k.
FastPrep DNA k.
Gen-Probe hybridization k.
High Pure PCR template
preparation k.
Histofine SAB-PO k.
Histofine SAB-PO(M) detector k.
human IFN-y quantikine ELISA k.
ICTP RIA k.
Imubind uPAR ELISA test k.
Kinesis reagent k.
Lectin-Link K.
k. ligand (KL)
Matritech NMP22 test k.
Melastatin test k.
Miraluma k.
Myelo-Nate k.
NMP22 test k.
PathVysion HER-2 DNA probe k.
PAXgene Blood RNA k.
PicoGreen dsDNA Quantitation K.
PICP RIA k.
Predicta Human TNF-alpha
ELISA k.
ProteinChip antibody capture k.
Puregene DNA Purification K.
QIAmp tissue k.
Quanta Lite ELISA autoimmune k.
radioimmunoassay k.
Reversecell Ag k.
RNA PCR core k.
SCC RIABEAD
radioimmunoassay k.
SC-HSV test k.
SureCell herpes test k.
UroVysion bladder cancer k.
UroVysion test k.
Vectastain Elite ABC k.
Vysis PathVysion HER-2 DNA
Probe K.
You-Bend hemodialysis
catheterization k.
kit protooncogene/oncogene
Kitzmiller test
KL
kit ligand
Klatskin
K. biliary adenocarcinoma
K. cholangiocarcinoma
K. needle

K. tumor
K. tumor classification
K-Lease
Klebsiella
K. oxytoca
K. pneumoniae
Kleihauer-Betke
K.-B. method
K.-B. stain
Kleihauer test
KLH
keyhole limpet hemocyanin
KLH molecule
Klinefelter syndrome (KS)
Klippel-Trenaunay-Weber syndrome
K-Lor
Klor-Con
Klor-Con/EF
Klorvess Effervescent
Klotrix
K-Lyte/Cl
K-Lyte Effervescent
Km antigen
K1myc
K1myc protein
K1myc transfectant
knee effusion
knife, pl. **knives**
Leksell gamma k.
knob
aortic k.
Knobloch syndrome
knockout
genetic k.
K-Norm
Knudsen
K. hypothesis
K. hypothesis of tumor suppressor
gene inactivation
Koate-HP
Kobak needle
Kobert test
Koch
K. phenomenon
K. postulate
K. pouch
Kocher-Cushing reflex
Kocher maneuver
Kodak Ektachem autoanalyzer
Koenen tumor
Kogenate
Kohn pore
koilocyte
koilocytotic cell
koilonychia
kola
gotu k.
Kolmer test
Kombucha tea

Konsyl
Konsyl-D
Konyne 80
Kopans
    K. breast lesion localization
    hookwire
    K. needle
Kostmann syndrome
Kowarsky test
Kozlowski-Tsuruta syndrome
K-Phos Neutral
KPS
    Karnofsky performance status
Krabbe disease
K-ras
    K-ras analysis
    K-ras gene
    K-ras oncogene
    K-ras protooncogene/oncogene
    K-ras mutation
Kraske procedure
Krebs
    K. cycle
    K. leukocyte index
Krigel staging system
Krishan
    K. procedure
    K. procedure for DNA analysis by
    flow cytometry
Kristalose
Krompecher carcinoma
Krukenberg tumor
krusei
    Candida k.
KS
    Kaposi sarcoma
    Klinefelter syndrome

    AIDS-associated KS
    salivary gland KS
KS-associated virus
KSHV
    Kaposi sarcoma-associated herpesvirus
KT
    ketoprofen
    Orudis KT
K-Tab
KTP
    potassium, titanyl, phosphate
    KTP laser
Kulchitsky cell
Kuopio Ischemia Heart Disease Risk
    Factor Study
Kupffer
    K. cell
    K. cell sarcoma
Ku protein
Kuru disease
Kuske breast template
Kussmaul sign
kV
    kilovoltage
Kveim
    K. antigen
    K. test
K-Vescent
KVO
    keep vein open
KVO-type I.V.
Kwik Board IV and arterial line
    stabilizer
kyphoplasty
Kyrle disease
Kytril tablet

NOTES

L1210
  L1210 leukemia
  murine leukemia L1210
L^d
  alloantigen L^d
L26 antigen
LA
  leuprolide acetate
  long-acting
    Dexone LA
    Inderal LA
    Trelstar LA
L-A
  long-acting
    Bicillin L-A
L.A.
  long-acting
    Dexasone L.A.
    Solurex L.A.
Labbé vein
LABC
  locally advanced breast cancer
labeling
  antibody l.
  pulse l.
  terminal deoxynucleotide transferase
    UTP nick-end l.
  terminal deoxynucleotidyl
    transferase-mediated digoxigenin-
    dUTP nick-end l. (TUNEL)
  terminal transferase-mediated dUTP-
    biotin nick-end l.
  triple-color fluorochrome l.
  in vivo l.
labial
  l. artery
  l. lentigo
labialis
  herpes l.
labile methanesulfonate group
lability
  genetic l.
labium majus
laboratory
  l. assay
  l. findings
  l. marker
  l. protocol
  l. study
  Venereal Disease Research L.
    (VDRL)
La Bross spot test
labrum-ligament complex (LLC)

labyrinth
  bony l.
  l. walking
labyrinthine hemorrhage
LAC
  laparoscopy-assisted colectomy
LACC
  Life After Cancer Care
laceration
  bladder l.
lac operon
Lactaid drops
lactamase
lactate
  calcium l.
  l. dehydrogenase
  plasma l.
  Ringer l.
lactated Ringer solution
lactating adenoma
lactescent blood
lactic
  l. acidemia
  l. acidosis
  l. dehydrogenase (LD, LDH)
Lactinex
Lactobacillus
  L. casei
  L. casei factor
  L. crispatus
  L. lactis Dorner factor
lactogen
  human placental l. (hPL)
Lactulax
lacunar cell
Ladd band
ladder effect
Ladendorff test
LAD-NSCLC
  locally advanced nonsmall-cell lung
    cancer
L.A.E. 20
Laënnec cirrhosis
Laetrile
LAF
  lymphocyte-activating factor
LAG
  lymphangiogram
LAHNC
  locally advanced head and neck cancer
LAK
  lymphokine-activated killer
    LAK cell
lake
  blood l.

L

laked blood
Laki-Lorand factor
Lallemand body
Lallemand-Trousseau body
LAM
    L-asparaginase and methotrexate
LAM-1
    leukocyte adhesion molecule-1
Lambert
    canal of L.
Lambert-Eaton myasthenic syndrome
lambertosis
lamblia
    Giardia l.
lambliasis
lamella, pl. lamellae
    basal l.
    coronoid l.
lamellated bone
lamellipodia
lamina, pl. laminae
    basal l.
    external elastic l.
    l. propria
laminar
    l. air flow
    l. fracture
laminated calcified concretion
laminin-5 y2 chain protein
laminin-8
laminin-9
laminin receptor
lamivudine
    l. triphosphate and azidothymidine (3TC/AZT)
    zidovudine and l.
lamp
    xenon flash l.
Lamprene
LANA
    lytic-associated nuclear antigen
Lanacane
Lanacaps
    Ferralyn L.
Lancefield classification
lancet
    Laser L.
landing zone
Landschutz tumor
Langat virus
Langer-Giedion syndrome (LGS)
Langerhans
    L. cell histiocytosis (LCH)
    L. dendritic cell (L-DC)
Langhans giant cell
lanreotide
Lansky score
lansoprazole
lanthanic

lanuginosa
LAP
    leucine aminopeptidase
    leukocyte alkaline phosphatase
    LAP test
laparoscope
    Combilight PDD 5133 l.
laparoscopic
    l. abdominal tumor diagnosis
    l. adrenalectomy
    l. colectomy
    l. lymphadenectomy
    l. microwave coagulation
    l. ovarian transposition
    l. supracervical hysterectomy (LSH)
    l. ultrasonography (LUS)
laparoscopic-assisted radical vaginal hysterectomy
laparoscopy
    robot-assisted l.
laparoscopy-assisted colectomy (LAC)
laparotomy
    staging l.
Laplace law
LAPOCA
    L-asparaginase, prednisone, Oncovin, cytarabine, Adriamycin
LAR
    low anterior resection
    Sandostatin LAR
Largactil
large
    l. agranular lymphocyte
    l. bowel
    l. cell calcifying Sertoli cell tumor (LCCSCT)
    l. cell carcinoma with neuroendocrine differentiation (LCCND)
    l. cell carcinoma with neuroendocrine features (LCNF)
    l. cell carcinoma with neuroendocrine morphology (LCCNM)
    l. cell immunoblastic lymphoma
    l. cell lung cancer
    l. cell neuroendocrine carcinoma (LCNEC)
    l. granular lymphocyte (LGL)
    l. granular lymphocyte antigen
    l. granular lymphocytic leukemia
    l. granular lymphocytosis
    l. intestine
    l. intestine neoplasm
    l. loop excision
    l. loop excision of transformation zone (LLETZ)
    l. noncleaved cell lymphoma
    l. noncleaved follicular center cell

l. operable breast cancer (LOBC)
l. plaque parapsoriasis
large-bore catheter
large-field radiotherapy
large-joint polyarthropathy
Lariam
Larmor
L. equation
L. frequency
Larrea tridentata
laryngeal
l. cancer
l. chondrosarcoma
l. granuloma
l. neoplasm
l. nerve
l. ventricle
laryngectomee
laryngectomy
salvage total l.
supraglottic l.
vertical partial l.
larynges (*pl. of* larynx)
laryngoesophagectomy
laryngofissure
laryngopharyngeal reflux (LPR)
laryngopharyngectomy
laryngopharyngoesophagectomy
laryngopharynx
laryngoscope
Dedo l.
laryngostroboscopy
larynx, pl. **larynges**
l. cancer
supraglottic l.
LAS
lymphadenopathy syndrome
LASA
linear analog self-assessment
laser
l. ablation
argon l.
argon-pumped dye l.
l. capture microdissection (LCM)
l. coagulation
l. conization
l. correlational spectroscopy (LCS)
l. destruction
endoscopic l.
l. group
helium-neon l.
HeNe l.
holmium:yttrium-argon-garnet l.

Ho:YAG l.
KTP l.
L. Lancet
l. microscopy
Nd:YAG l.
pulsed metal vapor l.
l. radiation
l. scanning
smart l.
l. surgery
l. therapy
l. thermal keratoplasty (LTK)
l. vaporization
laser-desorption ionization time-of-flight mass spectrometry
laser-induced fluorescence emission bronchoscopy
Lasix Special
Lassa fever virus
LAT
linker for activation of T cells
lata
condylomata lata
late
l. antigen
l. central nervous system toxicity (LCNST)
L. Effects of Normal Tissue (LENT)
l. fatal events
l. intensive therapy
l. radiation myelitis
latency
clinical l.
HIV l.
human immunodeficiency virus l.
molecular l.
latent
l. carcinoma
l. iron-binding capacity (LIBC)
l. membrane protein-1 (LMP-1)
l. stage
l. syphilis
lateral
l. aberrant thyroid carcinoma
l. field
l. pharyngeal wall
l. rhinotomy
latex
l. agglutination
l. condom
l. dam
Latino virus

NOTES

L

LATS
    long-acting thyroid stimulator
lattice theory
laudanum
Laue x-ray crystallography
laulimalide
Launois-Cléret syndrome
Laurell
    L. immunoelectrophoresis
    L. technique
Laurén
    L. classification
    L. classification of stomach cancer
laurocapram
    methotrexate and l.
LAV
    lymphadenopathy-associated virus
LAVA
    liver acquisitions with volume
        acceleration
    LAVA abdominal imaging
    LAVA liver imaging
lavage
    antral l.
    bronchoalveolar l. (BAL)
    ductal l. (DL)
    jet l.
    nipple duct l.
    peritoneal l.
LaVeen shunt
law
    Behring l.
    inverse-square l.
    Laplace l.
    least-square l.
lawn plate
laxative
    Fleet L.
Laxilose
layer
    boundary l.
    half-value l. (HVL)
lazaroid
lazy leukocyte syndrome (LLS)
LBC
    locoregional breast cancer
LBL
    lymphoblastic lymphoma
LBP
    liquid-based Papanicolaou
    LBP cytology
LCCND
    large cell carcinoma with neuroendocrine
        differentiation
LCCNM
    large cell carcinoma with neuroendocrine
        morphology
LCCSCT
    large cell calcifying Sertoli cell tumor

LCDD
    light chain deposition disease
L-CF
    leucovorin-citrovorum factor
LCH
    Langerhans cell histiocytosis
        systemic LCH
L-chain myeloma
LCIS
    lobular carcinoma in situ
lck
    lck oncogene
    lck protooncogene/oncogene
LCL
    lymphocytic lymphosarcoma
LCM
    laser capture microdissection
        LCM virus
LCNEC
    large cell neuroendocrine carcinoma
LCNF
    large cell carcinoma with neuroendocrine
        features
LCNST
    late central nervous system toxicity
LCR
    leurocristine
LCS
    laser correlational spectroscopy
LCSS
    Lung Cancer Symptom Score
LCT
    Leydig cell tumor
LD
    lactic dehydrogenase
    lethal dose
    lymphocyte defined
        LD antigen
L-DC
    Langerhans dendritic cell
LDH
    lactic dehydrogenase
        LDH agent
LDL
    low-density lipoprotein
LDO
    low dose oral
        Alferon LDO
LD-PCR
    long-distance polymerase chain reaction
LDR
    low dose rate
        LDR intracavitary radiation therapy
LE
    lupus erythematosus
        LE factor
        LE preparation

Le
Lewis
Le blood group antigen
lead time bias
leaf, pl. **leaves**
l. motion pattern
plantain l.
League of Nations staging
leak
anastomotic l.
calibrated l.
urine l.
leakage
bile l.
leaky gene
least-square law
leather-bottle stomach
leaves (*pl. of* leaf)
lecithin
lectin
l. agglutination
l. cell adhesion molecule
Ulex europaeus I l.
lectin-binding site
Lectin-Link Kit
LED
liposome-encapsulated doxorubicin
Ledderhose disease
Lederer anemia
Lederplex
LeDer stain
LeDuc-Camey ileocystoplasty
leech
Hirudo medicinalis l.
leeching
Leede-Rumpel phenomenon
LEEP
loop electrosurgical excision procedure
LEEP conization
Lee-White clotting time
left
l. ventricle (LV)
l. ventricle failure
leg
Barbados l.
l. swelling
l. ulcer
Legionella
L. pneumonia
L. pneumophila
legionellosis
Legionnaires disease
legume

Leiden
factor V L. (FVL)
LeIF
Leishmania elongation initiation factor
Leiner disease
leiomyofibroma
leiomyoma, pl. **leiomyomata**
atypical l.
bizarre l.
cellular l. (CL)
l. cutis
epithelioid l.
parasitic l.
symplastic l.
leiomyomatosis
benign metastasizing l. (BML)
l. peritonealis disseminata
leiomyomatous tumor
leiomyosarcoma
esophageal l.
gastric l.
intratesticular l.
retroperitoneal l.
uterine l.
Leishman
L. chrome cell
L. stain
Leishman-Donovan body
Leishmania
L. donovani
L. elongation initiation factor (LeIF)
L. tropica
leishmaniasis
Leksell
L. gamma knife
L. stereotactic system
LELC
lymphoepithelioma-like carcinoma
Lemierre syndrome
Lennert
L. classification
L. classification for follicular lymphoma
L. pattern
lenograstim support
Lenoltec No. 1–4
lens, pl. **lenses**
acoustic l.
lens-sparing external beam radiation therapy (LSRT)
LENT
Late Effects of Normal Tissue

NOTES

LENT *(continued)*
 LENT Consensus Conference
 LENT paradigm
lentigo
 Hutchinson l.
 labial l.
 l. maligna
 l. maligna melanoma (LMM)
lentil
 l. agglutination binding
 l. lectin affinity chromatography
lentinan
lentiviral
 l. vector
lentivirus
lepirudin
Lepore
 hemoglobin L.
 L. trait
 L. virus
lepra
 l. cell
 l. reaction
leprae
 Mycobacterium l.
lepromin
leprosy
leptin
 plasma l.
leptocytosis
 hereditary l.
leptomeningeal
 l. cancer
 l. carcinoma
 l. carcinomatosis
 l. cyst
 l. disease (LMD)
 l. enhancement
 l. failure
 l. lymphoma
 l. metastasis (LM)
 l. space
 l. tumor
leptospirosis
leridistim
Lesch-Nyhan syndrome
Leser-Trélat sign
lesion
 aberrant crypt focus l.
 acanthotic l.
 adenoidal l.
 admixture l.
 adnexal l.
 anal squamous intraepithelial l.
 angiocentric immunoproliferative l.
  (AIL)
 angiocentric lymphoproliferative l.
 angiomyoid l.
 anular constricting l.

aortic valve l.
atherosclerotic l.
l. attenuation
axillary skin l.
barrel-shaped l.
benign bone l.
benign lymphoepithelial l. (BLL)
benign lymphoproliferative l.
benign vascular l.
blastic l.
bone marrow l.
brain l.
breast l.
bubbly bone l.
cartilaginous l.
cavitary lung l.
cavitary small bowel l.
centrilobular l.
cherry red endobronchial l.
clonal l.
cochlear l.
comring-enhancing l.
constricting l.
cortical l.
cystic l.
destructive bone l.
diffuse ulcerative l.
discrete l.
dorsal root entry zone l.
dysplastic leukoplakia l.
endobronchial l.
endophytic l.
enhancing brain l.
eosinophilic fibrohistiocytic l.
epididymis l.
epidural extramedullary l.
exophytic l.
expansile unilocular well-demarcated
 bone l.
extraaxial l.
extracranial mass l.
extrahepatic l.
extramedullary l.
extratesticular l.
fibrohistiocytic nodular l.
focal hypoechoic l. (FHL)
genetic l.
gummatous l.
herpetic l.
high-grade squamous
 intraepithelial l. (HGSIL, HSIL)
high-intensity zone l.
HIZ l.
human papillomavirus-associated
 vulvovaginal l.
hyperintense l.
hyperkeratotic l.
hyperpigmented l.
hypodense l.

hypointense l.
immunoproliferative l.
infiltrating l.
intraaxial l.
intrabronchial l.
intracranial mass l.
intradural extramedullary l.
intraepithelial l.
intramedullary l.
intraocular l.
intraorbital l.
intraosseous bone l.
intrasellar l.
isointense l.
low-grade malignant cartilaginous l.
low-grade squamous
    intraepithelial l. (LGSIL, LSIL)
lung l.
lymphoepithelial l.
lymphoproliferative l.
lytic l.
lytic bone l.
melanocytic l.
mesenchymal l.
metachronous l.
metastatic l.
mucocutaneous l.
multilocular cystic l.
napkin-ring l.
neoplastic l.
nodular l.
nodule-in-nodule l.
nonneoplastic l.
nonperforative l.
ocular adnexal l.
optic nerve l.
orbital l.
osteolytic l.
papulovesicular l.
paucicellular l.
photon-deficient bone l.
pigmented l.
prechiasmal optic nerve l.
precursor l.
preneoplastic l.
radioresistant l.
reticulated l.
satellite l.
severe ulcerative l.
sinonasal l.
skin l.
skip l.
small bowel l.

solitary l.
space-occupying l.
squamous intraepithelial l. (SIL)
l. success
target l.
trabeculated bone l.
ulcerating l.
ulcerative l.
unilocular l.
vascular l.
vulvovaginal l.
Waldeyer ring l.
well-circumscribed l.
well-demarcated l.
LET
    linear energy transfer
lethal
    l. dose (LD)
    l. gene
    l. midline granuloma
lethality
lethargy
letrazuril
letrozole
Letterer-Siwe disease
Leu-8 antigen
leucine
    l. aminopeptidase (LAP)
    l. zipper
Leucomax
Leucotropin
leucovorin (LV)
    ara-C, hydrocortisone, mesna,
        prednisone, VP-16, l.
    l. calcium
    cisplatin, 5-fluorouracil, l. (CFL)
    l. and 5-fluorouracil (LV5FU2)
    5-fluorouracil given with eniluracil
        and low-dose l.
    high-dose methotrexate and l.
        (HDMTX-LV)
    MACOB with l.
    methotrexate, Adriamycin,
        cyclophosphamide, Oncovin,
        prednisone, bleomycin with l.
    mitoxantrone, 5-fluorouracil, l.
        (MFL)
    Novantrone, 5-fluorouracil, l. (NFL)
    l., Oncovin, methotrexate,
        Adriamycin, cyclophosphamide
        (LOMAC)
    oxaliplatin, 5-fluorouracil, l.
    Platinol, 5-fluorouracil, l. (PFL)

NOTES

L

leucovorin *(continued)*
>   Platinol, 5-fluorouracil plus
>   etoposide, methotrexate, l.
>   l., prednisone
>   l. rescue
>   l. rescue factor

L-leucovorin
leucovorin-citrovorum factor (L-CF)
leucovorin-modulated 5-FU
Leu-Dox
>   Nl-leucyldoxorubicin

leukapheresis
leukemia
>   acute basophilic l. (ABL)
>   acute biphenotypic l.
>   acute eosinophilic l.
>   acute erythroblastic l.
>   acute granulocytic l. (AGL)
>   acute hypocellular l.
>   acute hypogranular promyelocytic l.
>   acute lymphoblastic l. (ALL)
>   acute lymphoblastic myelogenous l.
>   acute lymphocytic l. (ALL)
>   acute lymphoid l.
>   acute megakaryoblastic l. (AMegL)
>   acute megakaryocytic l.
>   acute mixed lineage l.
>   acute monoblastic l. (AML, AMOL)
>   acute monocytic l. (AML, AMOL)
>   acute myeloblastic l. (AMBL)
>   acute myeloblastic myelogenous l.
>   acute myelocytic l. (AML)
>   acute myelogenous l. (AML)
>   acute myeloid l. (AML)
>   acute myelomonoblastic l. (AMMOL)
>   acute myelomonocytic l.
>   acute nonlymphoblastic l. (ANLL)
>   acute nonlymphocytic l. (ANLL)
>   acute nonlymphoid l.
>   acute progranulocytic l.
>   acute promyelocytic l. (APL, APML)
>   acute undifferentiated l. (AUL)
>   adult T-cell l. (ATL)
>   aggressive blastic natural killer l.
>   aggressive blastic NK l.
>   aleukemic l.
>   aleukocythemic l.
>   basophilic l.
>   basophilocytic l.
>   B-cell acute lymphoblastic l.
>   B-cell acute lymphocytic l.
>   B-cell chronic lymphocytic l.
>   Binet classification of chronic lymphocytic l. (stage A–C)
>   Binet staging system for chronic lymphocytic l.

>   biphenotypic l.
>   blast cell l.
>   blastic natural killer cell l.
>   BN acute myelocytic l.
>   brown Norwegian rat acute myelocytic l. (BNML)
>   Burkitt l.
>   CD22+ l.
>   CD33-positive acute myeloid l.
>   child lymphoblastic l.
>   chronic granulocytic l. (CGL)
>   chronic lymphocytic l. (stage A-C) (CLL)
>   chronic lymphoid l. (stage A-C)
>   chronic monocytic l.
>   chronic myelocytic l. (CML)
>   chronic myelogenous l. (CML)
>   chronic myeloid l. (CML)
>   chronic myelomonocytic l. (CMML)
>   chronic neutrophilic l.
>   chronic phase chronic myelogenous l. (CP-CML)
>   l. cutis
>   de novo acute myeloid l.
>   embryonal l.
>   eosinophilic l.
>   l. eradication
>   erythroblastic l.
>   feline l.
>   graft versus l. (GVL)
>   granular acute lymphoblastic l.
>   granulocytic l.
>   Gross l.
>   hairy cell l.
>   hand-mirror cell l.
>   hemoblastic l.
>   hemocytoblastic l.
>   hypergranular acute promyelocytic l.
>   hypocellular l.
>   hypogranular promyelocytic l.
>   indolent disseminated l.
>   l. inhibitory factor (LIF)
>   interferon-refractory chronic myelogenous l.
>   juvenile chronic myelogenous l.
>   L1210 l.
>   large granular lymphocytic l.
>   leukemic l.
>   leukopenic l.
>   LGL l.
>   lineage switch l.
>   lymphatic l.
>   lymphoblastic l.
>   lymphocytic l.
>   lymphoid l.
>   M3 acute myeloid l.
>   mast cell l.
>   mature cell l.
>   megakaryoblastic l.

megakaryocytic l.
meningeal l.
metachronous l.
microgranular acute
  promyelocytic l.
micromyeloblastic l.
mixed cell l.
mixed lineage l.
monoblastic l.
monocytic l.
myeloblastic l.
myelocytic l.
myelogenic l.
myelogenous l.
myeloid l.
myelomonoblastic l.
myelomonocytic l.
myelomonocytic l., chronic
  (CMML, MLC)
myelomonocytic l., subacute (MLS)
Naegeli type of monocytic l.
natural killer cell l.
neutrophilic l.
non-B-cell l.
nonlymphoblastic l.
nonlymphocytic l.
nonlymphoid l.
non-T-cell l.
null cell acute lymphocytic l.
null cell lymphoblastic l.
oral hairy l.
P-gp-negative l.
Philadelphia chromosome-negative
  chronic myelogenous l. (Ph-CML)
Philadelphia chromosome-positive
  chronic myelogenous l.
Philadelphia-positive l.
plasma cell l.
polymerase chain reaction-based
  method for acute promyelocytic l.
polymorphocytic l.
postthymic T-cell l.
pre-B acute lymphoblastic l.
precursor B acute lymphoblastic l.
precursor T acute lymphocytic l.
preplasmacytic l.
pre-T acute lymphocytic l.
progranulocytic l.
prolymphocytic l. (PLL)
promyelocytic l. (PML)
pure erythroid l.
Rai classification of chronic
  lymphocytic l. (stage 0–IV)

Rauscher l.
Rieder cell l.
Schilling type of monocytic l.
l. screen
smoldering l.
L. Society of America
l. specific immunoglobulin
splenic l.
stem cell l.
subleukemic l.
Taiwan Pediatric Oncology Group
  acute myeloid l. 901
T-cell acute lymphoblastic l.
T-cell prolymphocytic l.
t(15;17) cytogenic subtypes of
  acute myeloid l.
testicular l.
thrombocytic l.
thymic l.
l. transcript
leukemia/lymphoma
  adult T-cell l./l. (ATLL)
leukemic
  l. arthritis
  l. blast
  l. blast progenitor
  l. burden
  l. cell
  l. clone
  l. infiltration
  l. leukemia
  l. marker 43/43
  l. myelosis
  l. reticuloendotheliosis
leukemogenesis
leukemogenicity
leukemogenic potential
leukemoid reaction
Leukeran
  L., methotrexate, 5-fluorouracil
    (LMF)
  L., vinblastine, vincristine,
    prednisone (LVVP)
Leukine
leukoblast
leukoblastosis
leukocidin
  Neisser-Wechsberg l.
  Panton-Valentine l.
leukocoria
leukocytal
leukocyte
  acidophilic l.

NOTES

L

leukocyte *(continued)*
    l. acid phosphatase stain
    l. adherence
    l. adherence inhibition
    l. adhesion deficiency
    l. adhesion molecule-1 (LAM-1)
    agranular l.
    l. alkaline phosphatase (LAP)
    basophilic l.
    l. common antigen
    cystinotic l.
    l. diapedesis
    l. differential count
    endothelial l.
    eosinophilic l.
    filament polymorphonuclear l.
    globular l.
    granular l.
    l. histogram
    hyaline l.
    l. interferon
    mast l.
    l. migration
    l. migration inhibition
    motile l.
    multinuclear l.
    neutrophilic l.
    nonfilament polymorphonuclear l.
    nongranular l.
    nonmotile l.
    oxyphilic l.
    polymorphonuclear l.
    l. removal filter
    segmented l.
    l. transfusion
    transitional l.
    Türk l.
leukocyte-derived
    l.-d. IFN
    l.-d. interferon
leukocyte-poor red blood cell
leukocythemia
leukocytic
    l. crystal
    l. inclusion
    l. sarcoma
leukocytoblast
leukocytoclastic vasculitis
leukocytogenesis
leukocytoid
leukocytoma
leukocytopenia
leukocytoplania
leukocytopoiesis
leukocytosis
    lymphocytic l.
    monocytic l.
    neutrophilic l.
    terminal l.

leukodepletion filter
leukodystrophy
    globoid cell l.
leukoencephalitis
leukoencephalopathy
    disseminated necrotizing l.
    multifocal l.
    progressive multifocal l.
    radiation-induced l.
    spongiform l.
leukoerythroblastic
    l. anemia
    l. reaction
leukoerythroblastosis
leukofiltration
leukoglobulin
leukokinetics
leukokinin
leukokoria
leukolymphosarcoma
LeukoNet Filter
leukoneutropenia
leukopenia
    autoimmune l.
    hairy l.
    lymphocytic l.
leukopenic
    l. leukemia
    l. myelosis
leukoplakia
    hairy l.
    oral hairy l.
leukopoiesis
leukopoor
    l. blood component
    l. red blood cell
leukoreduction filter (LRF)
leukosarcoma
leukosarcomatosis
LeukoScan
leukosialin
leukostasis
Leukotrap
    L. RC system
    L. red cell storage system
leukotriene
Leu monoclonal antibody
leupeptin
Leuprogel
leuprolide
    l. acetate (LA)
    l. acetate implant
    l. acetate, vinblastine, Adriamycin,
       mitomycin (L-VAM)
leuprorelin acetate
leurocristine (LCR)
Leustatin
Leuvectin
levamisole

levamisole HCl
Levaquin
levator
    l. ani muscle
    l. veli palatini muscle
LeVeen radiofrequency ablation needle
  electrode
level
    air-fluid l.
    amylase l.
    attenuation l.
    bax expression l.
    $beta_2$-microglobulin l.
    Clark l.
    complement 3 l.
    complement 4 l.
    elevated bilirubin l.
    energy l.
    genetic l.
    homovanillic acid l.
    intracellular glutathione l.
    l. of invasion
    kallikrein-2 protease l.
    peak-dose l.
    phenotypic l.
    placental alkaline phosphatase l.
    plasma AT-III l.
    plasma proinsulin l.
    plasma uric acid l.
    prodrug l.
    prostaglandin E_2 l.
    serum creatinine phosphokinase l.
    serum neopterin l.
    serum phenytoin l.
    significance l.
    vanillylmandelic acid l.
level-dependent
    blood oxygenation l.-d. (BOLD)
Levi scale
levo-alpha-acetyl methadol
Levo-Dromoran
levoleucovorin
levonantradol
levorphanol
levosulpiride
Levo-T
Levothroid
levothyroxine
Levoxyl
Levy-Jennings chart
Levy, Rowntree, and Marriott method
Lewis (Le)

L. antibody
L. A, Y antigen
L. and Benedict method
L. blood group
L. blood group antigen
L. procedure
Lewisohn method
LexA DNA binding domain
lexidronam
Leyden
    hemophilia B, L.
Leydig
    L. cell
    L. cell adenoma
    L. cell tumor (LCT)
LFA
    lymphocyte function-associated antigen
LFA-1
    lymphocyte function-associated antigen 1
LFA-2
    lymphocyte function-associated antigen 2
LFA-3
    lymphocyte function-associated antigen 3
LFS
    Li-Fraumeni syndrome
LFT
    liver function test
Lf unit
LGD
    low-grade dysplasia
LGE
    linear gingival erythema
LGG
    low-grade glioma
LGL
    large granular lymphocyte
    LGL leukemia
LGM filter
lg-NHL
    low-grade non-Hodgkin lymphoma
LGS
    Langer-Giedion syndrome
LGSIL
    low-grade squamous intraepithelial lesion
LH
    loop of Henle
    luteinizing hormone
L/H
    lymphocytic/histiocytic
    L/H cell
    L/H nodular pattern
    L/H type

L

NOTES

Lhermitte
  L. sign
  L. syndrome
Lhermitte-Duclos disease
LHMT
  low-range heparin management test
LHRF
  luteinizing hormone-releasing factor
  LHRF agonist
LHRH, LH-RH
  luteinizing hormone-releasing hormone
  LHRH agonist
  LHRH analog
  LHRH antagonist
LHS
  lymphatic and hematopoietic system
Liacopoulos phenomenon
Liang and Pardee method
liarozole
  l. fumarate
  l. HCl
Liatest AT-III
LIBC
  latent iron-binding capacity
libido
liblomycin
Libman-Sacks endocarditis
library
  cDNA l.
  DNA l.
  gene l.
  phage combinatorial l.
  serological analysis of recombinant
    cDNA expression l.
lichen
  l. myxedematosus
  l. planus
  l. striatus
lichenoid
  l. drug eruption
  l. graft-versus-host disease
  l. reaction
Lichtheim plaque
lidamidine
lidocaine hydrochloride
LIF
  leukemia inhibitory factor
LIFE
  lung imaging fluorescence endoscope
  lung imaging fluorescent endoscopy
  LIFE Imaging System and White
    Light bronchoscopy
life
  L. After Cancer Care (LACC)
  European Organization for Research
    and Treatment of Cancer Core
    Quality of L.
  l. event

health-related quality of l. (HRQL)
human immunodeficiency virus
  quality of l. (HIV-QOL)
quality of l. (QOL)
  l. satisfaction
  l. table survival
LifePort infusion set
LifeSpex device
lifestyle modification
life-threatening disease
Li-Fraumeni
  L.-F. familial cancer syndrome
  L.-F. syndrome (LFS)
ligament
  anterior commissure l.
  anterior cruciate l.
  anterior spinal l.
  arcuate l.
  broad l.
  calcaneofibular l.
  gastrohepatic l.
  posterior longitudinal l. (PLL)
  l. of Treitz
ligand
  l. blotting
  CD40 l.
  c-kit l.
  Fas l. (FasL)
  FLT3 l.
  human Jagged1 l.
  kit l. (KL)
  Notch l.
  osteoprotegerin l. (OPGL)
  l. pathway
  receptor activator of nuclear factor
    kappa-B l. (RANKL)
  TNF-related apoptosis-inducing l.
  tumor necrosis factor-related
    apoptosis-inducing l. (TRAIL)
ligase
ligation of Fas
light
  l. chain deposition disease (LCDD)
  l. chain isotype suppression
  l. collection system
  L. criteria
  l. electrodesiccation
  l. microscopy
  Questran L.
  Wood l.
**LightCycler polymerase chain reaction
  analysis instrument**
light-induced
  l.-i. fluorescence endoscope
  l.-i. fluorescence endoscopic
    bronchoscopy
  l.-i. fluorescence endoscopy

l.-i. fluorescence endoscopy in combination with pharmacoendoscopy
light-scattering spectroscopy (LSS)
ligneous
Likert-type response pattern
Lillie hematoxylin
LIM
Lin-11, Isl-1, Mec-3 genes
LIM domain
limb
l. infusion
l. perfusion
l. salvage
Limberg flap
limbic encephalitis
limb-sparing surgery
limit
eye exposure l.
permissible exposure l.
limitation
beam l.
limited resection
limited-stage
l.-s. disease
l.-s. small cell lung cancer (LSSCLC)
limulus
l. amoebocyte lysate assay
l. anti-DPS factor
Lin-11
L.-11, Isl-1, Mec-3 gene domain
L.-11, Isl-1, Mec-3 genes (LIM)
LINAC
linear accelerator
LINAC gantry
LINAC radiosurgery
LINAC RS
LINAC-based stereotactic radiosurgery
LINAC-RS
linear accelerator-based radiosurgery
linamarin
Lincocin
lincomycin
Lincorex Injection
Linctus
L. Codeine Blac
L. With Codeine Phosphate
Lindau tumor
line
air-fluid l.
anterior junction l.
azygoesophageal l.

Beau l.
Cantlie l.
CEM/HIV-1 cell l.
central venous pressure l.
Chamberlain l.
Chaussier l.
epiphysial l.
FAMPAC cell l.
glomic cell l.
growth arrest l.'s
human AML cell l.
human lymphoblastoid cell l.
isodose l.
Jurkat cell l.
Jurkat T-cell l.
Muehrcke l.
MZ2-MEL clonal cell l.
pectinate l.
PICC l.
Sappey l.
l. sepsis
subclavian l.
suture l.
T-cell l.
tumor cell l.
lineage
B l.
chromaffin l.
l. fidelity
l. heterogeneity
macrophage l.
mixed l.
l. promiscuity
l. restriction
schwannian l.
l. switch
l. switch leukemia
lineage-associated
l.-a. antigen
l.-a. gene
linear
l. accelerator (LINAC)
l. accelerator-based radiosurgery (LINAC-RS)
l. accelerator-based SRS
l. accelerator radiosurgery
l. analog self-assessment (LASA)
l. density
l. energy transfer (LET)
l. epidermal nevus
l. epitope
l. gingival erythema (LGE)
l. lichen planus

NOTES

linear *(continued)*
  l. porokeratosis
  l. regression analysis
linearity
  absolute l.
  differential l.
Linell-Ljungberg classification
linezolid
linguagram
  morsicatio l.
lingual
  l. artery
  l. nerve
lingua plicata
linguine sign
ling zhi
linitis
  l. plastica
  l. plastica carcinoma
link
  Waldmar l.
linkage
  l. analysis
  chemical l.
  l. dysequilibrium
  l. effector
linked to dipalmitoyl phosphatidylethanolamine
linker for activation of T cells (LAT)
Linomide
Linson electronic cell counter
Lioresal
liothyronine
liotrix
lip
  l. cancer
  l. shave
lipasemia
lipemia retinalis
lipemic
lipid
  l. cell neoplasm
  l. conjugate
  l. cyst
  l. granulomatosis
  l. moiety
  monophosphoryl l. A
  l. peroxidation
  l. pheresis
  l. profile
  l. sphingomyelin
  l. tail
lipid-associated sialic acid
lipid-coated virus
lipid-containing vesicle
lipid-independent anti-atherosclerotic property
Lipidox
Lipiodol

lipiodol CT scan
Lipisorb dressing
Lipitor
lipoatrophic phenotype
lipoatrophy
lipoblastomatosis
lipodystrophy
  HIV-associated l.
  l. syndrome
lipofibroma
lipofuscin deposit
lipogranuloma
lipogranulomatosis
  disseminated l.
Lipo-Hepin
lipoid
  l. granuloma
  l. granulomatosis
lipoma, pl. **lipomata**
  mediastinal l.
  pericallosal l.
  l. sarcomatosum
lipomatosis
  central sinus l.
  epidural l.
lipopeptide
  MALP-2 l.
lipophage
  foamy l.
lipophagia granulomatosis
lipophagic
  l. granuloma
  l. intestinal
lipophilic
  l. cationic complex
  l. prodrug
  l. topoisomerase I inhibitor
lipopolysaccharide
lipoprotein (LP)
  high-density l. (HDL)
  low-density l. (LDL)
lipoproteinemia
liposarcoma
  myxoid l.
  pleomorphic l.
  retroperitoneal l.
  l. of uterus
liposomal
  l. annamycin
  l. anthracycline
  l. cytarabine
  l. daunorubicin
  l. daunorubicin citrate
  l. doxorubicin
  l. MTP-PE
  l. nystatin
  l. preparation
  l. topoisomerase I inhibitor

l. tretinoin
l. vincristine
liposomally encapsulated daunorubicin
liposome
dactinomycin-loaded l.
MPL-containing l.
polycation l. (PCL)
vincristine sulfate l.
liposome-encapsulated
l.-e. doxorubicin (LED)
l.-e. recombinant
lipothymoma
Lipovite
Lipowitz metal
Lipschütz body
liquefaciens
Enterobacter l.
Moraxella l.
liquefaction
Liquichek Hematology-16 Control
liquid
l. crystal thermography
l. extraction
l. nitrogen
radiation l.
Sustacal L.
Theragran L.
Titralac Plus L.
Tums Extra Strength L.
X-Prep L.
liquid-based
l.-b. Papanicolaou (LBP)
l.-b. Papanicolaou cytology
Lisch nodule
lissencephaly-pachygyria spectrum
Listeria monocytogenes
listeriosis
lithium carbonate
lithotripsy
biliary l.
electrohydraulic l. (EHL)
littoral cell
live
l. vector vaccine
l. viral vector
live-attenuated
l.-a. HIV
l.-a. human immunodeficiency virus
l.-a. lentiviral vaccine
l.-a. recombinant *Salmonella typhi*
liver
l. abscess

l. acquisitions with volume acceleration (LAVA)
l. biopsy
l. cancer
l. capsule
l. cell carcinoma
l. failure
l. function test (LFT)
l. metastasis
l. transaminase
l. tumor
undifferentiated embryonal sarcoma of l. (UESL)
venoocclusive disease of l.
VOD of l.
liver-directed therapy
liver-kidney
l.-k. microsomal type 1 antibody target assay
l.-k. microsome 1
living
activities of daily l. (ADL)
Livingstone-Wheeler regimen
LKB Wallac 1277 automatic gamma counter
LKM1
LKM1 antibody
LKM1 assay
LKV-Drops
LLC
labrum-ligament complex
LLETZ
large loop excision of transformation zone
LLLT
low-level laser therapy
Lloyd syndrome
LLS
lazy leukocyte syndrome
LM
leptomeningeal metastasis
LMB-1
immunotoxin LMB-1
LMB-2
anti-Tac(Fv)-PE38 LMB-2
LMD
leptomeningeal disease
LMF
Leukeran, methotrexate, 5-fluorouracil
LMM
lentigo maligna melanoma
L-MNA
N-monomethyl-L-arginine

NOTES

L

331

LMP
low malignant potential
LMP-1
latent membrane protein-1
LMWH
low molecular weight heparin
Hepanorm LMWH
L-myc oncogene
LNPF
lymph node permeability factor
LNRS
lymph node revealing solution
load
hepatitis B viral DNA l.
HIV RNA l.
human immunodeficiency virus
ribonucleic acid l.
plasma viral l.
viral l.
loading
l. dose
front l.
lobaplatin
lobar bronchus
LOBC
large operable breast cancer
lobe
accessory l.
azygos l.
hepatic l.
lobectomy
sleeve l.
thoracoscopic l.
loboisthmusectomy
lobradimil and carboplatin
Lobstein disease
lobular
l. carcinoma
l. carcinoma in situ (LCIS)
l. neoplasia
lobularity
lobulated submucosal mass
local
l. anesthesia
l. anesthetic
l. boost
l. control
l. excision
l. invasion
l. irradiation
l. radiation
l. radiation therapy
l. recurrence (LR)
l. recurrence-free survival (LRFS)
l. surgery
local-acting radioisotope
localization
immunohistochemical l.
intragenomic l.

percutaneous l.
l. of prostate cancer
radiotherapy l.
localized
l. fibrous mesothelioma
l. infiltrate
l. mastocytoma
l. prostate carcinoma (LPC)
l. tumor
localizing sign
locally
l. advanced breast cancer (LABC)
l. advanced head and neck cancer
(LAHNC)
l. advanced melanoma
l. advanced nonsmall-cell lung
cancer (LAD-NSCLC)
loci (*pl. of* locus)
lock
field l.
heparin l.
locoregional
l. breast cancer (LBC)
l. control
l. disease (LR)
l. failure (LRF)
l. failure-free survival (LRFFS)
l. field radiotherapy
l. infusion
l. recurrence
l. relapse
l. spread
l. transfection
loculated pleural fluid
loculus, pl. **loculi**
locus, pl. **loci**
ATPase l.
chromosome 19q l.
l. material
microsatellite l.
quantitative trait l. (QTL)
Snell H l.
lodoxamide tromethamine
Loevit cell
Lofstrand crutch
log
l.'s of cell kill
l. effect
l. infectious virus titer
l. kill
log-kill model
log-rank test
LOH
loss of heterozygosity
LOH at 16q
lollipop follicle
LOMAC
leucovorin, Oncovin, methotrexate,
Adriamycin, cyclophosphamide

lomefloxacin
lometrexol
Lomotil
lomustine
> doxorubicin and l. (DL)
> procarbazine, Oncovin, l. (POC)

lonafarnib
Lone Star fever
long
> l. arm of chromosome (q)
> l. terminal repeat (LTR)

long-acting (L-A, LA, L.A.)
> l.-a. thyroid stimulator (LATS)
> l.-a. thyroid stimulator protector

long-bone radiograph
long-distance polymerase chain reaction (LD-PCR)
longevity quotient (LQ)
longitudinal relaxation
long-term
> l.-t. nonprogressor (LTNP)
> l.-t. storage
> l.-t. survivor

longus
> adductor l.
> extensor carpi radialis l. (ECRL)
> extensor digitorum l. (EDL)
> extensor hallucis l. (EHL)
> extensor pollicis l. (EPL)

lonidamine
Lonox
loop
> conductive l.
> l. diathermy
> duodenal l.
> efferent l.
> l. electrosurgical excision procedure (LEEP)
> l. of Henle (LH)
> HGF/C-Met autocrine l.
> paracrine l.

loose-leaf tobacco
loperamide
lophosphamide
Lopid
lopinavir
LOPP
> chlorambucil, vincristine, procarbazine, prednisone
> LOPP chemotherapy

Loprox
lorazepam

Lorcet
> L. 10/650
> L. Plus

Lorcet-HD
lordosis quotient (LQ)
Lorenzo oil
Lortab ASA
losartan
Losec
losoxantrone hydrochloride
loss
> CD4+ T-cell l.
> chromosome 1p and 19q l.
> l. of distinction
> l. of distinction at gray/white matter interface
> hair l.
> l. of heterozygosity (LOH)
> weight l.

Lossen rule
Lostorfer corpuscle
lotion
> Vitec l.

lovastatin
low
> l. anterior resection (LAR)
> l. columnar cell
> l. dose oral (LDO)
> l. dose rate (LDR)
> l. dose rate intracavity therapy
> l. LET external beam irradiation
> l. LET isotope
> l. linear energy transfer radiation
> l. malignant potential (LMP)
> l. malignant potential epithelial ovarian tumor
> l. molecular weight heparin (LMWH)
> l. molecular weight oxidizing agent
> l. volume disease

low-density lipoprotein (LDL)
low-dose
> l.-d. chemotherapy
> l.-d. helical scanning technique
> l.-d. heparin
> l.-d. infusion
> l.-d. oral interferon

low-energy linear accelerator
lower
> l. brachial plexopathy
> l. clivus

lowered tumor antigenicity
low-field magnetic resonance imaging

NOTES

low-frequency blood group
low-grade
    l.-g. astrocytoma
    l.-g. B-cell lymphoma
    l.-g. carcinoma
    l.-g. CD20-positive lymphoma
    l.-g. dysplasia (LGD)
    l.-g. fibromyxoid sarcoma
    l.-g. glioma (LGG)
    l.-g. malignant cartilaginous lesion
    l.-g. non-Hodgkin lymphoma (lg-NHL)
    l.-g. oligodendroglioma
    l.-g. squamous intraepithelial lesion (LGSIL, LSIL)
low-intensity preparative regimen
low-level
    l.-l. laser therapy (LLLT)
    l.-l. viral replication
low-molecular keratin stain
low-power field (lpf)
low-range heparin management test (LHMT)
low-residue diet
lox/Cre system of site-specific recombination
Lozol
LP
    lipoprotein
    lumbar puncture
    lymphomatoid papulosis
    lymphomatous polyposis
LPC
    localized prostate carcinoma
lpf
    low-power field
L-phase variant
LPHD
    lymphocyte-predominant Hodgkin disease
L-phenylalanine mustard (L-PAM)
LPL
    lymphoplasmacytoid lymphoma
LPR
    laryngopharyngeal reflux
LQ
    longevity quotient
    lordosis quotient
    LQ ratio
LR
    local recurrence
    locoregional disease
LRF
    leukoreduction filter
    locoregional failure
LRFFS
    locoregional failure-free survival
LRFS
    local recurrence-free survival

LRP
    lung resistance-related protein
LSA2L2 chemotherapy protocol
LSH
    laparoscopic supracervical hysterectomy
LSIL
    low-grade squamous intraepithelial lesion
LSRT
    lens-sparing external beam radiation therapy
LSS
    light-scattering spectroscopy
LSSCLC
    limited-stage small cell lung cancer
LT
    Beta LT
LT-alpha
    lymphotoxin-alpha
LT-beta
    lymphotoxin-beta
LTC-IC bone marrow stem cell assay
LTK
    laser thermal keratoplasty
    Ho:YAG LTK
LTNP
    long-term nonprogressor
LTR
    long terminal repeat
L-tryptophan
^{177}Lu
    lutetium-177
lucanthone
lucent band
Lucey-Driscoll syndrome
luciferase assay reagent
Lucké
    L. adenocarcinoma
    L. virus
Ludwig Trial
Luebering-Rapaport pathway
Lugano
    L. classification
    L. classification for testicular tumor
Lugol
    L. dye esophagoscopy
    L. solution
Lukatret
Lukes-Butler classification
Lukes-Collins
    L.-C. classification
    L.-C. classification of non-Hodgkin lymphoma
lumbar puncture (LP)
lumbosacral plexopathy
lumen, pl. **lumina, lumens**
luminal
    l. pH
    l. stent
luminometer

lump
    dominant l.
lung
    air-filled l.
    1-l. anesthesia
    l. block
    l. cancer
    l. cancer screening
    L. Cancer Symptom Scale
    L. Cancer Symptom Score (LCSS)
    compressed l.
    consolidated l.
    l. cyst
    l. function testing
    l. imaging fluorescence endoscope (LIFE)
    l. imaging fluorescent endoscopy (LIFE)
    l. lesion
    nonexpansile l.
    l. perfusion imaging
    l. resistance-related protein (LRP)
    respirator l.
    l. shielding
    trapped l.
Lunyo virus
Lupron
    L. Depot
    L. Depot-3 Month
    L. Depot-4 Month
    L. Depot-Ped
    L. Pediatric
    L., Velban, Adriamycin, Mutamycin (L-VAM)
lupus
    l. erythematosus (LE)
    l. vasculopathy
lupus-like anticoagulant
Luria-Delbruck
    L.-D. fluctuation test
    L.-D. model
lurtotecan
LUS
    laparoscopic ultrasonography
Luse body
lusitaniae
    Candida l.
luteinized
    l. thecoma
    l. thecoma of ovary
luteinizing
    l. hormone (LH)
    l. hormone-releasing factor (LHRF)

    l. hormone-releasing factor agonist
    l. hormone-releasing hormone (LHRH, LH-RH)
    l. hormone-releasing hormone agonist
lutetium-177 (^{177}Lu)
lutetium texaphyrin
Lu-Tex
Lutheran
    L. antibody
    L. blood group
Lutrepulse
Lutrin
Luxol fast blue stain
LV
    left ventricle
    leucovorin
    LV plus 5-FU
L-VAM
    leuprolide acetate, vinblastine, Adriamycin, mitomycin
    Lupron, Velban, Adriamycin, Mutamycin
L-Vax vaccine
LV5FU2
    leucovorin and 5-fluorouracil
LVI
    lymphatic vessel invasion
LVSI
    lymphovascular involvement
LVVP
    Leukeran, vinblastine, vincristine, prednisone
lwoffii
    Acinetobacter l.
Ly antigen
Lyb antigen
lycopene
lye stricture
lyl B cell
lyl-1 oncogene activation
Lym-1 monoclonal antibody
Lyman model
Lyme
    L. borreliosis
    L. disease
    L. disease vaccine
lymph
    aplastic l.
    l. channel
    euplastic l.
    inflammatory l.
    intercellular l.
    intravascular l.

NOTES

lymph *(continued)*
l. node
l. node basin
l. node biopsy
l. node drainage
l. node fibrosis
l. node histology
l. node hyperplasia
l. node metastasis
l. node permeability factor (LNPF)
l. node revealing solution (LNRS)
l. node staging
l. node station
plastic l.
tissue l.

lymphadenectomy
bilateral l.
complete l.
elective l.
3-field l.
inguinal l.
laparoscopic l.
Meigs pelvic l.
paraaortic l.
pelvic l.
perihilar l.
retroperitoneal l.
sentinel l.
staging l.

lymphadenitis
dermatopathic l.
histiocytic necrotizing l.
Kikuchi l.
mesenteric l.
postvaccinial l.
subacute necrotizing l.

lymphadenoma
l. cell
sebaceous l.

lymphadenopathy
angioblastic l.
angioimmunoblastic l. (AIL)
axillary l.
benign l.
bulky l.
dermatopathic l.
hypersensitivity l.
idiopathic plasmacytic l.
immunoblastic l.
massive l.
mediastinal l.
paraaortic l.
paratracheal l.
pelvic l.
peripancreatic l.
persistent generalized l. (PGL)
plasmacytic l.
retroperitoneal l.
secondary axillary l.

l. syndrome (LAS)
toxoplasmosis l.
lymphadenopathy-associated virus (LAV)
lymphadenosis
benign l.
lymphangioendothelial sarcoma
lymphangiogram (LAG)
lymphangiography
bipedal l.
l. effect
lymphangiohemangioma
lymphangioleiomyomatosis
lymphangioma
cystic l.
pancreatic cystic l.
retroperitoneal l.
simple capillary l.
lymphangiomyomatosis
lymphangiosarcoma
lymphangitic carcinomatosis
lymphangitis carcinomatosa
lymphapheresis
lymphatic
l. drainage
l. drainage of genitalia
l. drainage pattern
l. and hematopoietic system (LHS)
l. leukemia
l. mapping
l. metastasis
parapharyngeal l.
l. permeation
l. sarcoma
l. shunt
l. spread
l. system
l. tracking
l. trunk
l. vessel invasion (LVI)
lymphatica
pseudopolyposis l.
lymphaticovenous shunt
lymphaticum
angioma l.
Lymphazurin
lymphedema
l. alert bracelet
postmastectomy l.
lymphoblast
lymphoblastic
l. leukemia
l. lymphoma (LBL)
l. lymphoma-leukemia
l. transformation
lymphoblastoid interferon
lymphoblastoma
lymphochip technology
LymphoCide
lymphocyst

lymphocytapheresis
lymphocyte
    l. activator
    amplifier T l.
    anti-CD3 stimulated peripheral
        blood l.
    antitumor cytotoxic l.
    autologous T l.
    B l.
    binucleated l.
    clonal B l.
    cloned peripheral blood l.
    l. count
    cytotoxic T l. (CTL)
    l. defined (LD)
    l. depleted
    l. depletion
    l. enzyme stain
    l. function antigen
    l. function-associated antigen (LFA)
    l. function-associated antigen 1
        (LFA-1)
    l. function-associated antigen 2
        (LFA-2)
    l. function-associated antigen 3
        (LFA-3)
    l. gene rearrangement
    hand-mirror l.
    helper T l.
    human immunodeficiency virus-
        specific cytotoxic T l.
    l. immune globulin
    immunocompetent l.
    inflammatory T l.
    intraepithelial l. (IEL)
    large agranular l.
    large granular l. (LGL)
    l. migration
    l. mitogenic factor
    monocytoid B l.
    natural killer l.
    neoplastic l.
    null l.
    peptide activated l.
    peripheral blood l. (PBL)
    plasmacytoid l.
    polymorphonuclear l.
    l. proliferation
    l. proliferation assay
    l. recirculation
    l. recombinase
    small l.

splenic marginal zone lymphoma
    without villous l.'s
splenic marginal zone lymphoma
    with villous l.'s
stem cell l.
l. subset
T l.
thymic l.
l. transformation
tumor-associated l. (TAL)
tumor-infiltrating l. (TIL)
unfractionated l.
villous l.
lymphocyte-activating factor (LAF)
lymphocyte-depletion Hodgkin disease
lymphocyte-mediated cytolysis
**lymphocyte-predominant Hodgkin disease
    (LPHD)**
lymphocyte-stimulating hormone
lymphocytic
    l. angiitis
    l. angiitis and granulomatosis
    l. bronchitis
    l. choriomeningitis
    l. interstitial pneumonia
    l. leukemia
    l. leukemoid reaction
    l. leukocytosis
    l. leukopenia
    l. lymphoma
    l. lymphosarcoma (LCL)
    l. nodular Hodgkin disease
    poorly differentiated l.
    l. thyroiditis
    well-differentiated l.
lymphocytic/histiocytic (L/H)
lymphocytoma
lymphocytopenia
    idiopathic CD4+ l. (ICL)
lymphocytopoiesis
lymphocytosis
    large granular l.
lymphoepithelial
    l. cyst
    l. lesion
    l. tumor
lymphoepithelioid cell lymphoma
lymphoepithelioma
    salivary gland l.
lymphoepithelioma-like
    l.-l. carcinoma (LELC)
    l.-l. carcinoma of skin
lymphogenous metastasis

NOTES

L

337

lymphogranuloma
    l. benignum
    l. inguinale
    l. malignum
    Schaumann l.
    venereal l.
    l. venereum
    l. venereum antigen
    l. venereum virus
lymphogranulomatosis
lymphography
lymphohistiocytic variant
lymphohistiocytosis
    erythrophagocytic l.
    familial erythrophagocytic l.
    familial hemophagocytic l.
    hemophagocytic l.
lymphoid
    l. gland
    l. hamartoma
    l. hemoblast
    l. hemoblast of Pappenheim
    l. hyperplasia
    l. hypophysitis
    l. hypoplasia
    l. inflammatory pseudotumor
    l. interstitial pneumonia
    l. leukemia
    l. marker
    l. neoplasm
    l. organ
    l. proliferation
    l. stem cell
    l. tissue
    l. tumor
lymphokine
    cellular l.
    l. production
lymphokine-activated
    l.-a. killer (LAK)
    l.-a. killer cell
lympholeukocyte
lympholytic agent
lymphoma
    acute lymphoblastic l.
    adult T-cell l. (ATL)
    African Burkitt l.
    aggressive good-prognosis non-Hodgkin l. (AGPNHL)
    aggressive histology l. (AHL)
    AIDS-related primary central nervous system l.
    anaplastic large cell l. (ALCL)
    anaplastic large cell Ki-1-positive l.
    angiocentric NK-cell l.
    angiocentric T-cell l.
    angioimmunoblastic lymphadenopathy-like T-cell l.

angioimmunoblastic lymphadenopathy with dysproteinemia-like T-cell l.
angioimmunoblastic T-cell l. (ATCL)
angiotropic large cell l.
anorectal l.
B-cell l.
B-cell non-Hodgkin l. (B-NHL)
benign l.
Bennett classification of l.
Berard classification for follicular l.
biclonal follicular l.
body cavity non-Hodgkin l.
Burkitt l.
Burkitt-like l.
B-zone small lymphocytic l.
CD22+ l.
CD20-positive l.
central nervous system l.
centroblastic follicular l.
centrocytic follicular l.
centrocytoid centroblastic l.
cerebral l.
chronic lymphocytic l.
CNS l.
colorectal l.
cutaneous angiocentric T-cell l.
cutaneous T-cell l. (CTCL)
diffuse aggressive l.
diffuse histiocytic l. (DHL)
diffuse intermediate lymphocytic l.
diffuse large B-cell l. (DLBCL)
diffuse large cell l. (DLCL)
diffuse mixed small and large cell l.
diffuse poorly differentiated l. (DPDL)
diffuse small cell lymphocytic l.
dural arachnoid l.
effusion l.
endemic Burkitt l.
enteropathy-associated T-cell l. (EATL)
Epstein-Barr virus-positive sinonasal l.
erythrophagocytic T-gamma l.
extranodal follicular l.
extranodal Ki-1 anaplastic large cell l.
extranodal natural killer T-cell l.
follicle center l.
follicular non-Hodgkin l.
gastric MALT l.
gastrointestinal l.
gluten enteropathy-associated T-cell l.
hepatic non-Hodgkin l. (HNHL)
hepatosplenic l.

high-grade B-cell l.
histiocytic l.
histologically aggressive gastric
  non-Hodgkin l.
HIV-associated non-Hodgkin l.
  (HIV-NHL)
Hodgkin l.
immunoblastic lymphadenopathy-like
  T-cell l.
indolent disseminated l.
indolent extranodal l.
indolent nodal l.
intermediate-grade CD20-positive l.
intermediate lymphocytic l. (ILL)
intravascular l.
irreversible monoclonal l.
Kiel classification of non-
  Hodgkin l.
Ki-1 positive l.
large cell immunoblastic l.
large noncleaved cell l.
Lennert classification for
  follicular l.
leptomeningeal l.
low-grade B-cell l.
low-grade CD20-positive l.
low-grade non-Hodgkin l. (lg-NHL)
Lukes-Collins classification of non-
  Hodgkin l.
lymphoblastic l. (LBL)
lymphocytic l.
lymphoepithelioid cell l.
lymphoma-depleted Hodgkin l.
lymphoplasmacytic l.
lymphoplasmacytoid l. (LPL)
malignant l.
MALT l.
MALT/marginal zone l.
mantle cell l. (MCL)
mantle zone l.
marginal zone B-cell l. (MZBCL)
mediastinal large B-cell l.
Mediterranean abdominal l.
Memorial Sloan-Kettering staging
  of childhood l.
metastatic l.
mixed lymphocytic-histiocytic l.
mixed small cleaved and large
  cell l.
monocytoid B-cell l. (MBCL)
monomorphic l.
mucosa-associated lymphoid
  tissue l. (MALToma)

multiclonal follicular l.
multilobated T-cell l.
nasal T-cell/natural killer cell l.
natural killer-like T-cell l.
nodal marginal zone B-cell l.
nodular histiocytic l.
nodular poorly differentiated
  lymphocytic l. (NPDL)
noncleaved-cell l.
non-Hodgkin l. (NHL)
non-Hodgkin thyroid l. (NHTL)
nonimmunoblastic diffuse large B-
  cell l.
nonnasal CD56+T/NK cell l.
North American Burkitt l.
null cell anaplastic large cell l.
l. of ocular adnexa
ocular adnexal l.
ovarian l.
l. of ovary
panniculitis-like T-cell
  subcutaneous l.
pediatric l.
peripheral T-cell l.
perirenal l.
peritoneal l.
plasmablastic l.
plasmacytoid lymphocytic l.
pleomorphic T-cell l.
polymorphic B-cell l.
poorly differentiated lymphocytic l.
  (PDLL)
postthymic T-cell l.
precursor B-cell l.
pretarget lymphoma trial for non-
  Hodgkin l.
primary brain l. (PBL)
primary breast l. (PBL)
primary cardiac l.
primary central nervous system l.
  (PCNSL)
primary cerebral non-Hodgkin l.
  (PCNHL)
primary CNS l.
primary effusion l.
primary extranodal l. (PENL)
primary mediastinal B-cell l.
primary orbital l.
primary refractory Burkitt l.
pseudo-T-cell l.
pyothorax-associated pleural l.
Rappaport classification of l.
recurrent l.

NOTES

lymphoma *(continued)*
    refractory CD22+ B-cell l.
    renal l.
    L. Research Foundation of America
    retroperitoneal l.
    Revised European-American L.
     (REAL)
    l. screen
    secondary CD30+ anaplastic large
     cell l.
    sinonasal l.
    sinusoidal large cell l.
    skeletal l.
    small cleaved cell l.
    small lymphocytic l.
    small noncleaved cell l.
    spinal epidural l.
    splenic B-cell l.
    sporadic Burkitt l.
    subcutaneous panniculitic T-cell l.
    synchronous primary bilateral
     breast l.
    systemic l.
    T-cell lymphoblastic l.
    T-cell-rich B-cell l.
    testicular non-Hodgkin l.
    T-gamma l.
    thymic l.
    thyroid l.
    true histiocytic l.
    T-zone l.
    U-cell l.
    uterine corpus l.
    Waldeyer ring l.
    well-differentiated lymphocytic l.
     (WDLL)
    Working Formulation of non-
     Hodgkin l.
lymphoma-depleted Hodgkin lymphoma
lymphomagenesis
lymphoma-leukemia
    lymphoblastic l.-l.
• **lymphomatoid**
    l. granulomatosis
    l. panniculitis
    l. papulosis (LP)
lymphomatosis
    intravascular l. (IVL)
lymphomatosum
    cystadenoma l.
    papillary cystadenoma l.
lymphomatous
    l. bone marrow involvement
    l. mass
    l. meningitis
    l. polyposis (LP)
    l. type
lymphomyeloma

lymphopenia
    CD4 l.
lymphophagocytosis
lymphoplasmacytic
    l. immunocytoma
    l. infiltrate
    l. lymphoma
lymphoplasmacytoid
    l. cell
    l. immunocytoma
    l. lymphoma (LPL)
    l. morphology
lymphopoiesis
    thymus-dependent l.
lymphoproliferation
    posttransplantation l.
lymphoproliferative
    l. activity
    l. disorder
    l. lesion
    l. syndrome
    X-linked l. (XLP)
lymphoprotease
LymphoRad
lymphoreticular
    l. cell
    l. malignancy
    l. tumor
lymphosarcoma
    follicular l. (FLSA)
    lymphocytic l. (LCL)
lymphosarcomatosis
LymphoScan
    L. imaging
    L. Tc99m-labeled murine antibody
     fragment
lymphoscintigraphy
    cutaneous l.
    internal mammary l.
lymphotoxic antibody
lymphotoxin-alpha (LT-alpha)
lymphotoxin antitumor activity
lymphotoxin-beta (LT-beta)
lymphovascular involvement (LVSI)
Lynbya majuscula
Lynch cancer family syndrome (I, II)
Lyon phenomenon
lyophilization
lyophilized
    l. acemannan
    l. Cytoxan
    l. human AT-III
    l. recombinant interferon
     formulation
Lyphocin Injection
lysate
    cell l.
lysin

lysine
> contiguous l.

lysis
> acute tumor l. (ATL)
> clot l.
> complement l.
> complement-mediated l.
> euglobulin clot l.
> tumor l.

Lysodren
lysosomal storage disease
lysosome

lysozyme
lyssa body
lyt-10
> lyt-10 oncogene activation
> lyt-10 protooncogene/oncogene

Lyt antigen
lytic
> l. bone lesion
> l. lesion
> l. viral replication

lytic-associated nuclear antigen (LANA)
lyt-1 protooncogene/oncogene

NOTES

L

μ (*var. of* mu)

M
  mitoxantrone
  M antigen
  immunoglobulin M (IgM)
  M phase
  M protein

M2
  vincristine, carmustine,
    cyclophosphamide, melphalan,
    prednisone

M195 monoclonal antibody anti-CD33

M344
    M344 antibody
    M344 antigen

M3 acute myeloid leukemia

MA
  matrix
  megestrol acetate

MAA
  macroaggregated albumin

MAB
  maximal androgen blockade

MAb
  monoclonal antibody
    iodine ^{131}I Lym-1 MAb
    iodine ^{131}I radiolabeled B1 MAb
    ovarian rhenium-186 MAb
    PM-81 MAb

MAb-170

MAb-B43.13
    OvaRex MAb-B43.13

MAb-L6

MABOP
  Mustargen, Adriamycin, bleomycin,
    Oncovin, prednisone

MabThera

MAC
  methotrexate, actinomycin D,
    chlorambucil
  methotrexate, actinomycin D,
    cyclophosphamide
  methotrexate, Adriamycin,
    cyclophosphamide
  mitomycin C, Adriamycin,
    cyclophosphamide
  Mycobacterium avium complex
    MAC III

Mac-1 antigen

Mac-2 binding protein (Mac-2BP)

Macaca nemestrina

M2A Capsule

Mac-2BP
  Mac-2 binding protein

MACC
  methotrexate, Adriamycin,
    cyclophosphamide, CCNU
  methotrexate, ara-C, cyclophosphamide,
    CCNU

MacConkey agar

MacFarlane serum method

Machado-Guerreiro test

Machado test

machine
    Brown-Bovari m.
    cobalt megavoltage m.
    megavoltage m.
    neutron therapy m.
    Ventana Immuno-automated m.

MACHO
  methotrexate, asparaginase,
    cyclophosphamide,
    hydroxydaunomycin, Oncovin
  methotrexate, asparaginase, Cytoxan,
    hydroxydaunomycin, Oncovin

Machupo virus

MACOB
  methotrexate, Adriamycin,
    cyclophosphamide, Oncovin, bleomycin
    MACOB with leucovorin

MACOP-B
  methotrexate, Adriamycin,
    cyclophosphamide, Oncovin,
    prednisone, bleomycin

macroadenoma
    pituitary m.
    prolactin-secreting m.

macroaggregated albumin (MAA)

Macrobid

macrobiotic diet

macrocalcification

macrocephaly

macrocephaly-cutis
    m.-c. marmorata telangiectatica
      congenita (M-CMTC)
    m.-c. marmorata telangiectatica
      congenita syndrome

macrocyclic polyamine

macrocyst
    adrenocortical m.

macrocythemia

macrocytic anemia

macrocytosis

Macrodantin

macrofollicular
    m. adenoma
    m. thyroid papillary carcinoma

macrogammaglobulinemia
    Waldenström m.

M

343

macroglobulinemia
  Waldenström m.
macroglossia
macrolide
macromolecular
  m. nonlipid compound
  m. polar compound
macromolecule
macronodular cirrhosis
macronutrient
macrophage
  alveolar m.
  armed m.
  m. chemotactic factor
  colony-forming unit–granulocyte, erythrocyte, megakaryocyte, m. (CFU-GEMM)
  m. colony-stimulating factor (M-CSF)
  fixed m.
  free m.
  m. growth factor
  Hansemann m.
  m. inflammatory protein (MIP)
  m. inflammatory protein-1 alpha (MIP-1a, MIP-1 alpha)
  m. inflammatory protein I (MIP-I)
  m. inflammatory protein II (MIP-II)
  m. lineage
  m. lineage antigen
  monocyte-derived m.
  murine m.
  m. oxidative burst
  peritoneal m.
  m. phagocytic activity
  pulmonary alveolar m.
  tumor-associated m. (TAM)
  m. tumoricidal activity
  m. variant
macrophage-activating factor (MAF)
macrophage-derived chemokine (CXCR4)
macrophage-tropic
  m.-t. HIV strain
  m.-t. human immunodeficiency virus strain
macrophagocyte
macroscopic
  m. magnetic moment
  m. residual disease
macular edema
macule
  pigmented m.
maculopathy
MAD
  MeCCNU and Adriamycin

MADDOC
  mechlorethamine, Adriamycin, dacarbazine, DDP, Oncovin, cyclophosphamide
  MADDOC chemotherapy
Madin-Darby canine kidney
MAF
  macrophage-activating factor
Maffucci
  M. disease
  M. syndrome
mafosfamide
MAG
  multifocal atrophic gastritis
magaldrate and simethicone
Magano classification
magic mouthwash
Maglucate
Magnacal
magnesemia
magnesia
  Phillips' Milk of M.
magnesium
  m. chloride
  m. citrate
  m. gluconate
  m. hydroxide
  m. hydroxide and mineral oil emulsion
  m. oxide
  m. salicylate
  m. sulfate
magnetic
  m. bead
  m. field gradient
  m. induction device
  m. microsphere
  m. resonance (MR)
  m. resonance arthrography
  m. resonance elastography (MRE)
  m. resonance imaging (MRI)
  m. resonance imaging thermometry
  m. resonance spectroscopic imaging
  m. resonance spectroscopic imaging-guided brachytherapy
  m. resonance spectroscopy (MRS)
  m. therapy
magnetically responsive microsphere
magnetite in tumor targeting
magnetization
  equilibrium m.
  m. transfer (MT)
magnetotherapy
magnification (X)
  electronic m.
  m. mammography

magnitude

m. preparation-rapid acquisition gradient echo

vector m. (VM)

magnus

adductor m.

Magonate

Magrath-modified regimen

MAGS

microscopic angiogenesis grading system

ma huang

MAI

Mycobacterium avium-intracellulare

MAID

mesna, Adriamycin, ifosfamide, dacarbazine

mesna, Adriamycin, interleukin-3, dacarbazine

Mesnex, Adriamycin, Ifex, dacarbazine

MAIDS

murine-acquired immunodeficiency syndrome

main

m. biliary duct (MBD)

m. pancreatic duct (MPD)

m. papillary duct

m. pulmonary artery (MPA)

maintenance chemotherapy

Mainz pouch

maitake mushroom

maitansine (*var. of* maytansine)

Majocchi granuloma

major

m. aphthae

m. gene

m. histocompatibility complex (MHC)

m. histocompatibility complex antigen

m. histocompatibility complex haplotype

m. histocompatibility type

thalassemia m.

majus

labium m.

majuscula

Lynbya m.

MAK-6

monoclonal anticytokeratin MAK-6 cocktail

Makonde virus

malabsorption

paraneoplastic m.

malabsorptive diarrhea

malariae

Plasmodium m.

malarial rosette

Malassezia furfur

malate

sunitinib m.

maldescended testis

MALDI-TOF-MS

matrix-assisted laser desorption/ionization time-of-flight mass spectrometry

male

m. breast carcinoma (MBC)

m. germ line tumor

m. pseudohermaphroditism

Ray staging system of urethral cancer in m.'s

m. sexual dysfunction

maleate

diethyl m. (DEM)

rosiglitazone m.

thiethylperazine m.

male-to-female transmission

malformation

anorectal m.

arteriovenous m.

capillary m.

central nervous system m.

cerebral arteriovenous m.

cerebrovascular m.

cystic adenomatoid m.

extremity m.

split hand/split foot m. (SHFM)

Malherbe

calcifying epithelioma of M.

maligna

lentigo m.

malignancy

B-cell m.

enteropancreatic m.

eradication of m.

extrapelvic m.

gastrointestinal m.

gynecologic m.

hematologic m.

humoral hypercalcemia of m. (HHM)

hypercalcemia of m. (HCM)

indolent lymphoid m.

lymphoreticular m.

meningeal m.

metachronous m.

mimicker of m.

M

NOTES

malignancy *(continued)*
 occult primary m. (OPM)
 pelvic m.
 secondary m.
 solid tumor m.
 synchronous m.
 Tac-expressing m.
 T-cell m.
 tumor m.
 uroepithelial m.
 urogenital m.
 vulvar m.
malignant
 m. acini prostate gland
 m. angioendotheliomatosis
 m. astrocytoma
 m. carcinoid syndrome
 m. cell
 m. degeneration
 m. down
 m. effusion
 m. epithelial neoplasm
 m. epithelioid mesothelioma (MEM)
 m. fibrous histiocytoma (MFH)
 m. fibrous histiocytoma of bone
 m. fibrous histiocytoma of soft tissue
 m. giant cell tumor (MGCT)
 m. glioma
 m. granuloma
 m. hepatoma
 m. histiocytosis
 m. lentigo melanoma
 m. lymphoma
 m. lymphoproliferative disorder
 m. mastocytosis
 m. melanoma in situ
 m. mixed mesodermal tumor (MMMT)
 m. mixed müllerian tumor
 m. mixed oligoastrocytoma
 m. myeloma (MM)
 m. myoepithelioma (MME)
 m. nephrosclerosis
 m. ovarian teratoma
 m. ovarian tumor
 m. peripheral nerve sheath tumor (MPNST)
 m. pheochromocytoma
 m. pleural mesothelioma (MPM)
 m. progression
 m. reticulosis
 m. salivary gland tumor (MST)
 m. schwannoma
 m. small round cell tumor
 m. teratoma (MT)
 m. teratoma, intermediate (MTI)
 m. teratoma, trophoblastic (MTT)
 m. thrombocytopenia

 m. trichilemma tumor
 m. tumor of cervix
malignum
 adenoma m.
 lymphogranuloma m.
Malin syndrome
Mallamint
Mallinckrodt
 M. Institute guidelines
 M. Institute of Radiology Afterloading Vaginal Applicator (MIRALVA)
malmoense
 Mycobacterium m.
malnutrition
malondialdehyde
malpighian corpuscle
MALP-2 lipopeptide
malposition of branch pulmonary artery
MALT
 mucosa-associated lymphoid tissue
  MALT function
  MALT lymphoma
Maltlevol
MALT/marginal zone lymphoma
MALToma
 mucosa-associated lymphoid tissue lymphoma
maltophilia
 Stenotrophomonas m.
 Xanthomonas m.
malt soup extract
Maltsupex
mammaglobin breast cancer protein
mammalian cell
mammary
 m. aspiration specimen (MAS)
 m. aspiration specimen cytology test (MASCT)
 m. gland mass
 m. parenchymal stimulation
 m. serum antigen (MSA)
 m. tumorigenesis
mammastatin
Mammex TR computer-aided mammography diagnosis system
mammogram
 craniocaudal m.
 x-ray m. (XMG)
mammography
 computed tomography laser m. (CTLM)
 CT laser m.
 digital m.
 magnification m.
 optical m.
 screening m.
 1-view m.

2-view m.
x-ray m.
Mammo Mask illuminator
mammoplasty
augmentation m.
**MammoReader computer-aided detection
system**
MammoSite
M. brachytherapy (MSB)
M. Radiation Therapy System
M. RTS
M. RTS balloon interstitial device
Mammotest Plus breast biopsy system
mammotome
Biopsys m.
M. core biopsy device
Mammoviewer
mAMSA, m-AMSA
amsacrine
mAMSA, azacitidine, etoposide
(MAZE)
man
eugonadal m.
management
disease m.
energy conservation and activity m.
(ECAM)
genomic disease m.
pain m.
Manchester
M. LDR implant system
M. system for brachytherapy
M. system for radium therapy
Mancini plate
mandible
pipestem m.
protruding m.
mandibulectomy
coronal m.
marginal m.
mandibulotomy
Mandol
mandrillaris
Balamuthia m.
MANE
Morrow Assessment of Nausea and
Emesis
maneuver
hormonal m.
Kocher m.
Mendelsohn m.
Queckenstedt m.
manic-depressive

manifestation
cardiopulmonary m.
hematologic m.
ocular m.
oral m.
manifesto
alternative treatment activist m.
manipulation
bile duct m.
manner
paracrine m.
mannitol
mannose monooleate
mannosyl
manometric testing
mansoni
Schistosoma m.
mantle
m. cell
m. cell lymphoma (MCL)
cerebral m.
m. irradiation
m. radiotherapy
m. zone
m. zone hyperplasia
m. zone lymphoma
m. zone nodule
m. zone pattern
Mantoux method
manual
m. differential
m. lymph drainage (MLD)
m. lymphedema treatment
MAO
monoamine oxidase
MAOI
monoamine oxidase inhibitor
Maox
MAP
melphalan, Adriamycin, prednisone
mitomycin C, Adriamycin, Platinol
map
bladder m.
cancer m.
cerebral blood volume m.
genetic linkage m.
Mapap
mapping
activation m.
brain m.
functional m.
gene m.
intraoperative functional m.

M

NOTES

mapping *(continued)*
    lymphatic m.
    qualitative m.
    sentinel node m.
maprotiline
Maranox
marantic endocarditis
marathon hemoglobinuria
Marburg virus
marcellomycin
march
    m. anemia
    M. disease
marchalko cell
Marchand cell
Marchiafava-Micheli disease
Marcillin
Marek herpesvirus disease
Marfan syndrome
Margesic H
margin
    anal m.
    close m.'s
    disc m.
    epidermoid carcinoma of anal m.
    periarticular m.
    m. of resection
    tumor m.
marginal
    m. mandibulectomy
    m. zone
    m. zone B-cell lymphoma
      (MZBCL)
    m. zone cell
    m. zone pattern
marginalized
marijuana, marihuana
    m. patch
marimastat
    matrix metalloproteinase
      inhibitor, m. (MRM)
Marinol
marinum
    Mycobacterium m.
Marituba virus
marker
    AFP tumor m.
    alkaline phosphatase isoenzyme
     tumor m.
    allotypic m.
    alpha fetoprotein tumor m.
    m. ALZ-50
    B-cell m.
    B-hCG tumor m.
    biochemical m.
    biologic m.
    bone resorption m.
    CA1-18 tumor m.
    CA15-3 breast cancer tumor m.

CA15-3 RIA serum tumor m.
CA19-9 tumor m.
CA27.29 tumor m.
CA50 tumor m.
CA72-4 tumor m.
CA125 ovarian tumor m.
CA125-11 tumor m.
CA195 tumor m.
CA549 breast cancer tumor m.
CA M26 tumor m.
CA M29 tumor m.
CASA tumor m.
cathepsin B, L m.
CD5 m.
CEA tumor m.
cell-lineage m.
cell surface m.
cellular m.
chromosomal sex m.
chromosome 14q tumor m.
CK-BB tumor m.
clonal m.
CYFRA 21-1 tumor m.
epithelial m.
FT tumor m.
genetic m.
glycohistochemical m.
G6PD cell m.
granulocytic m.
6-HIAA tumor m.
HSAP tumor m.
human immunodeficiency virus
  quality audit m. (HIV-QAM)
IAP tumor m.
immune m.
immunochemical m.
immunocytochemical m.
immunohistochemical m.
immunophenotypic m.
Kern m.
laboratory m.
leukemic m. 43/43
lymphoid m.
MCA tumor m.
M-CSF serum m.
megakaryocytic m.
membrane m.
MicroMark tissue m.
monocytic m.
MSA tumor m.
myeloid m.
neuron-specific enolase tumor m.
NSE lung cancer tumor m.
oncofetal m.
OVX1 serum m.
PAP tumor m.
prognostic serum m.
proliferation m.
PSA prostate cancer tumor m.

RNAse tumor m.
SCC tumor m.
serum tumor m.
sialic acid tumor m.
sigmaS tumor m.
sitz m.
SLX tumor m.
specific reverse transcriptase-
polymerase chain reaction m.
surrogate m.
T-cell m.
TPA tumor m.
tumor activity m.
marking
genetic m.
m. technique
Markov
M. model
M. process
marneffei
Penicillium m.
Maroteaux-Lamy syndrome
marrow
m. ablation
bone m. (BM)
calvarial m.
m. cell
donor bone m.
m. edema
facial m.
m. failure syndrome
m. fibrosis
m. graft rejection
hematopoietic m.
m. hypoplasia
myelophthisis m.
nonpurged m.
pediatric fatty m.
m. progenitor
purged m.
purging of m.
m. recovery
red m.
m. toxic drug
m. transplant
unmodified m.
marrow-ablative chemoradiation
MARS
Mevacor Atherosclerosis Regression
Study
Marschalko-type plasma cell
Marshall-Jewett-Strong classification
MARstem

MART-1
melanoma antigen recognized by T cell
MART-1 peptide
Martinez
M. technique
M. Universal Perineal Interstitial
Template (MUPIT)
MAS
mammary aspiration specimen
MAS cytology test
Masaoka
M. staging system
M. staging system for thymoma
MASCC/ISOO
Multinational Association of Supportive
Care in Cancer/International Society for
Oral Oncology
MASCT
mammary aspiration specimen cytology
test
masculinization
masked virus
Mason-Pfizer monkey virus
masoprocol
maspin protein
mas protooncogene/oncogene
mass
abdominal m.
abdominopelvic m.
adnexal m.
adrenal cystic m.
anterior mediastinal m.
articular m.
atomic m.
benign m.
bleeder in tumor m.
brain m.
bulky m.
calcified renal m.
cardiophrenic angle m.
cauliflower-like m.
cerebellopontine angle m.
chest m.
m. collision stopping power
complex chest m.
cystic adrenal m.
cystic chest m.
cystic pelvic m.
dense brain m.
dominant m.
dumbbell m.
dysplasia-associated lesion or m.
(DALM)

NOTES

mass *(continued)*
    exophytic gut m.
    extracardiac m.
    extramedullary m.
    extrauterine pelvic m.
    extravascular m.
    fallopian tube m.
    gut m.
    hilar m.
    hyperdense m.
    ill-defined m.
    intraabdominal m.
    intracranial m.
    intradural extramedullary m.
    intrasellar m.
    intraventricular m.
    lobulated submucosal m.
    lymphomatous m.
    mammary gland m.
    mediastinal m.
    mesenteric m.
    ovarian m.
    pediatric m.
    pelvic m.
    pineal m.
    posterior mediastinal m.
    pulsatile m.
    m. radiative stopping power
    renal m.
    residual tumor m.
    retroperitoneal residual tumor m.
     (RRTM)
    m. spectrophotometer (MS)
    m. spectrophotometric detector
    subinsular m.
    submucosal m.
    thalamic-hypothalamic m.
    tumor m.
Massachusetts Medical Society
massage
    shiatsu m.
massive lymphadenopathy
Masson
    M. pseudoangiosarcoma
    M. trichrome stain
mast
    m. cell
    m. cell disease
    m. cell growth factor
    m. cell leukemia
    m. cell nevus
    m. cell sarcoma
    m. leukocyte
Mastadenovirus
mastectomy
    extended radical m.
    modified radical m. (MRM)
    non-skin-sparing m. (non-SSM)
    prophylactic contralateral m. (PCM)

    radical m.
    segmental m.
    skin-sparing m. (SSM)
    subcutaneous m.
    total simple prophylactic m.
    m. with immediate reconstruction
     (MIR)
mastitis
    cystic m.
    granulomatous m.
    plasma cell m.
mastocytoma
    localized m.
mastocytosis
    malignant m.
    systemic m.
Masugi nephritis
MAT
    multiple agent therapy
match
    invariant antigenetic m.
matched
    m. lymphocyte transfusion
    m. peripheral dose (MPD)
    m. related donor
    m. sibling donor (MSD)
    m. unrelated donor (MUD)
matchline technique
mater
    dura m.
material
    anthracotic m.
    ballistic m.
    bolus m.
    kinetic energy released in m.
     (kerma)
    locus m.
    orthotic m.
    ShearBan orthotic m.
    Superflab bolus m.
maternal
    m. gonad
    m. humoral immune response
    m. serum alpha fetoprotein
     (MSAFP)
maternal-fetal transmission
mathematical modeling technique
MAT-LyLu variant
matrices (*pl. of* matrix)
Matrigel
matriptase
Matritech NMP22 test kit
matrix, pl. **matrices (MA)**
    acquisition m.
    m. antigen
    m. breakdown
    cisplatin/collagen m.
    extracellular m. (ECM)
    m. metalloproteinase (MMP)

m. metalloproteinase-2
m. metalloproteinase-2 assay
m. metalloproteinase inhibitor
m. metalloproteinase inhibitor,
  marimastat (MRM)
p17 m.
protein m.
m. protein
**matrix-assisted laser desorption/ionization
time-of-flight mass spectrometry
(MALDI-TOF-MS)**
mats gene
matter
normal-appearing white m.
  (NAWM)
perilesional white m.
supratentorial gray m.
supratentorial white m.
Mattis Dementia Rating Scale
Matuhasi-Ogata phenomenon
Matulane
cyclophosphamide, Oncovin,
  prednisone, bleomycin,
  Adriamycin, M. (COP-BLAM)
maturation
m. arrest
disharmonic delayed osseous m.
mature
m. cell leukemia
m. cystic teratoma
m. fibrosis
m. mediastinal teratoma
m. ovarian teratoma
Maurer dot
Maxamine
Maxaquin
maxilla, pl. **maxillae, maxillas**
short m.
maxillary
m. sinus
m. sinus carcinoma
maxillectomy
maximal
m. androgen blockade (MAB)
m. drug concentration (C_{max})
m. flow rate
maximum
m. cytoreductive benefit
m. depth (D_{max})
m. permissible dose (MPD)
M. Strength Anbesol
m. tolerated dose (MTD)

Maxipime
Max protein
Maxzide
Mayaro virus
**Mayfield/ACCISS stereotactic
workstation**
May-Grunwald stain
May-Hegglin
M.-H. anomaly
M.-H. syndrome
Mayneord F factor
Mayo Lung Project (MLP)
maytansine, maitansine
MAZE
mAMSA, azacitidine, etoposide
mazepine
Mazicon
M-BACOD
methotrexate, bleomycin, Adriamycin,
  cyclophosphamide, Oncovin,
  dexamethasone
m-BACOD
moderate-dose methotrexate, bleomycin,
  Adriamycin, cyclophosphamide,
  Oncovin, dexamethasone
M-BACOS
methotrexate, bleomycin, Adriamycin,
  cyclophosphamide, Oncovin, Solu-
  Medrol
MBC
male breast carcinoma
metastatic breast cancer
metastatic breast carcinoma
methotrexate, bleomycin, cisplatin
  cutaneous MBC
MBCL
monocytoid B-cell lymphoma
MBD
main biliary duct
MBP
modified Bagshawe protocol
myelin base protein
MC
mitomycin C
MC-540
merocyanine 540
  MC-540 photoirradiation
Mc1 antibody
Mc5 antibody
MCAF
recombinant human MCAF
MCA tumor marker

NOTES

MCBP
melphalan, cyclophosphamide, BCNU, prednisone

MCC
Merkel cell carcinoma
mutated in colon cancer
MCC gene

McCabe-Fletcher classification

McCoy culture medium

MCD
mean central dose
multicentric Castleman disease

McDonough sarcoma virus

MCE
minimal cytotoxic epitope

McFarlane skin flap

McGill-Melzack pain score

McGill Pain Questionnaire (MPQ)

MCH
mean corpuscular hemoglobin
mucous cell hyperplasia

MCHC
mean corpuscular hemoglobin concentration

MCHg
mean corpuscular hemoglobin

mCi
millicurie

McIndoe-Hayes construction

McKrae herpes simplex virus

MCL
mantle cell lymphoma

McLeod
M. phenotype
M. syndrome

M-CMTC
macrocephaly-cutis marmorata telangiectatica congenita
M-CMTC syndrome

McNemar test

M-component isotype

MCP
melphalan, cyclophosphamide, prednisone
metacarpophalangeal
monocyte chemotactic protein

MCPT
Monte Carlo photon transport
MCPT simulation

MCR
morphine-controlled release

M-CSF
macrophage colony-stimulating factor
M-CSF serum marker

MCT
medullary carcinoma of thyroid

MCV
mean corpuscular volume
methotrexate, cisplatin, vinblastine

McWhirter technique

M.D.
M.D. Anderson Cancer Center
M.D. Anderson cancer staging
M.D. Anderson grading system
M.D. Anderson Hospital classification
M.D. Anderson tumor score system

mda-7
melanoma differentiation-associated gene

MDAS
Memorial Delirium Assessment Scale

MDLO
metoclopramide, dexamethasone, lorazepam, ondansetron

MDM2
MDM2 gene
MDM2 oncogene

MDMS
methylene dimethane sulfonate

MDR
multidrug resistance
multiple drug resistance

mdr1
mdr1 gene
mdr1 oncogene

MDR-TB
multidrug-resistant tuberculosis

MDS
myelodysplastic syndrome
MDS system

2-ME
2-methoxyestradiol

M/E
myeloid/erythroid
M/E ratio

meal
barium m.

mean
m. central dose (MCD)
m. corpuscular hemoglobin (MCH, MCHg)
m. corpuscular hemoglobin concentration (MCHC)
m. corpuscular volume (MCV)
m. optical density (MOD)
m. perfusate temperature
m. plasma volume (MPV)
m. platelet volume (MPV)

measles-mumps-rubella (MMR)

measles vaccine

measure
anthropometric m.

measured beam data

measurement
ankle-brachial pressure m.
automated cardiac flow m. (ACFM)
bidimensional tumor m.

end-diastolic velocity m.
HBV DNA m.
International Commission on
 Radiation Units and M.'s (ICRU)
multicolor immunofluorescence m.
peripheral blood mononuclear cell
 hepatitis B virus m.
meatus
 acoustic m.
 external auditory m.
Mebaral
mebendazole
MEC
 moderately emetogenic chemotherapy
MECC
 micellar electrokinetic capillary
  chromatography
MeCCNU
 methyl-CCNU
 semustine
  MeCCNU and Adriamycin (MAD)
  cyclophosphamide, Oncovin,
   MeCCNU (COM)
  cyclophosphamide, Oncovin,
   bleomycin, methotrexate,
   Adriamycin, MeCCNU
  5-fluorouracil, Adriamycin,
   MeCCNU (FAMe, FAME)
  5-fluorouracil, Adriamycin,
   mitomycin C, MeCCNU
   (FAMMe)
  MeCCNU, Oncovin, 5-fluorouracil
   (MOF)
  MeCCNU, Oncovin, 5-fluorouracil
   plus streptozocin (MOF-STREP)
mechanism
 autocrine m.
 effector m.
 epigenetic m.
 heat transfer m.
 homeostatic m.
 host defense m.
 host response m.
 m. of injury
 tumorigenic m.
mechlorethamine
 m., Adriamycin, dacarbazine, DDP
 m., Adriamycin, dacarbazine, DDP,
  Oncovin, cyclophosphamide
  (MADDOC)
 m., Adriamycin, dacarbazine, DDP,
  Oncovin, cyclophosphamide
  chemotherapy

cytarabine, bleomycin, Oncovin, m.
 (CytaBOM)
m. hydrochloride
melphalan, Oncovin, m.
m., Oncovin, bleomycin (MOB)
m., Oncovin, methotrexate,
 prednisone (MOMP)
m., Oncovin, prednisone (MOP)
m., Oncovin, prednisone,
 bleomycin, Adriamycin,
 procarbazine (MOP-BAP)
m., Oncovin, procarbazine (MOPr)
m., Oncovin, procarbazine,
 prednisone (MOPP)
m., Oncovin, procarbazine,
 prednisone, bleomycin (MOPP-
 BLEO)
m., Oncovin, procarbazine,
 prednisone, high-dose bleomycin
m., Oncovin, procarbazine,
 prednisone, low-dose bleomycin
m., Oncovin, procarbazine,
 prednisone plus Adriamycin,
 bleomycin, vinblastine
 (MOPP/ABV)
m., Oncovin, procarbazine,
 prednisone plus Adriamycin,
 bleomycin, vinblastine, dacarbazine
 (MOPP/ABVD)
m., vinblastine, procarbazine,
 prednisone (MVPP)
m., vincristine, vinblastine,
 procarbazine, prednisone (MVVPP)
meclofenamate sodium
MeCy
 methotrexate and cyclophosphamide
MED
 minimum effective dose
 multiple epiphysial dysplasia
Meda-Cap
media (*pl. of* medium)
medial lethal dose
median survival time (MST)
mediastinal
 m. cross-sectional imaging
 m. germ cell tumor
 m. hematoma
 m. irradiation
 m. large B-cell lymphoma
 m. lipoma
 m. lymphadenopathy
 m. lymph node
 m. mass

M

NOTES

mediastinal *(continued)*
    m. mesenchymal tumor
    m. neoplasm
    m. nodal station
    m. pathology
    m. pleura
    m. seminoma
    m. teratoma
mediastinitis
mediastinoscopy
mediastinum testis
mediated cell death
mediator
    m. cell
    chemical m.
    redox m.
mediator-related symptom
medical
    m. alert bracelet
    m. castration
    m. internal radiation dose (MIRD)
    m. internal radiation dosimetry
      (MIRD)
    m. oncology
    m. outcomes study (MOS)
    m. outcomes study-human
      immunodeficiency virus (MOS-
      HIV)
    m. outcomes study-human
      immunodeficiency virus instrument
    M. Research Council (MRC)
    m. therapy
medicamentosa
    dermatitis m.
medicated
    Zilactin-B M.
medication
    concomitant m.
    m. event monitoring system
      (MEMS)
    exogenous immunosuppressant m.
medicine
    African traditional m.
    allopathic m.
    alternative m.
    Ayurvedic m.
    complementary and alternative m.
      (CAM)
    complementary and alternative
      cancer m.
    diagnostic contrast m.
    herbal m.
    holistic m.
    Kampo m.
    mind-body m.
    National Center for Complementary
      and Alternative M. (NCCAM)
    nuclear m. (NM)
    Society of Nuclear M. (SNM)

Systemized Nomenclature of M.
    (SNOMED)
mediorenal tumor
Mediterranean
    M. abdominal lymphoma
    M. fever
    M. Kaposi sarcoma (MEKS)
medium, pl. **media**
    bolus administration of intravenous
      contrast m.
    m. chain triglycerides
    diatrizoate meglumine
      radiopaque m.
    Dulbecco Modified Eagle M.
      (DMEM)
    Eagle basal m.
    Eagle minimum essential m.
    HAT m.
    high osmolar m. (HOM)
    intravenous contrast media
    isosmolar contrast m. (IOCM)
    McCoy culture m.
    otitis media
    Thorotrast contrast m.
Medralone Injection
Medrol Dosepak
medroxyprogesterone acetate (MPA)
Medtronic infusion pump
medullary
    m. bone
    m. carcinoma of thyroid (MCT)
    m. cyst
    m. cystic disease
    m. duct epithelium
    m. sarcoma
    m. thymoma
    m. thyroid cancer
    m. thyroid carcinoma (MTC)
medulloblastoma
    recurrent m.
medulloepithelioma
MeFA
    methyl-CCNU, 5-fluorouracil,
      Adriamycin
mefenamic acid
mefloquine
Mefoxin
MegaBac
Mega B Complex
megacaryoblast *(var. of* megakaryoblast)
megacaryocyte *(var. of* megakaryocyte)
Megace oral suspension
megacolon
    aganglionic m.
megaelectron volt (MeV)
megakaryoblast, megacaryoblast
megakaryoblastic leukemia
megakaryocyte, megacaryocyte
    m. colony-forming unit

m. colony-stimulating factor (MEG-CSF)

m. growth and development factor (MGDF)

m. progenitor

vacuolated m.

megakaryocytic

m. blastic phase

m. leukemia

m. marker

megakaryocytopoiesis

megaloblast

megaloblastic anemia

megalocytosis

megaprosthesis

Megaton

megavitamin therapy

megavolt (MeV)

megavoltage

m. computed tomography

m. computed tomography-assisted stereotactic radiosurgery

m. computed tomography scanner

m. CT

m. CT-assisted stereotactic radiosurgery

m. CT scanner

m. external radiotherapy

m. machine

m. radiation

m. radiography

Megazinc Pink adhesive tape

MEG-CSF

megakaryocyte colony-stimulating factor

megestrol acetate (MA)

meglumine

diatrizoate m.

iothalamate m.

MEI

metastatic efficiency index

meibomian gland carcinoma

Meige disease

Meigs

M. pelvic lymphadenectomy

M. syndrome

Meigs-Okabayashi procedure

meiosis

MEKS

Mediterranean Kaposi sarcoma

MEL

melphalan

Melacine regimen

melanin

tumoral m.

melanoacanthoma

melanocarcinoma

melanocyte

uveal m.

melanocytic

m. lesion

m. nevus

melanocytoma

melanocytosis

meningeal m.

ocular m.

melanoma

acral-lentiginous m.

acral lentiginous m.

amelanotic m.

anorectal m.

m. antigen recognized by T cell (MART-1)

balloon-cell m.

benign juvenile m.

Bombriski m.

Breslow classification for malignant m.

Breslow thickness in malignant m.

m. cell lysate vaccine

choroidal m.

ciliary body m.

Clark staging system for malignant m.

Cloudman m.

conjunctival m.

cutaneous m. (CM)

cutaneous malignant m. (CMM)

desmoplastic neurotropic m. (DNM)

m. differentiation-associated gene (*mda*-7)

disseminated m.

familial atypical multiple mole m. (FAMMM)

halo m.

Harding-Passey m. (HPM)

head and neck mucosal m. (HNMM)

intraocular m.

iris m.

juvenile m.

lentigo maligna m. (LMM)

locally advanced m.

malignant lentigo m.

melanotic m.

m. metastasis

M

NOTES

melanoma *(continued)*
    metastatic malignant m.
    minimal deviation m.
    mucosal m.
    multiple primary m. (MPM)
    murine m.
    node-negative m.
    nodular m.
    nondesmoplastic m.
    nonmetastatic m.
    ocular m.
    posterior uveal m.
    primary m.
    regional m.
    satellite focus of m.
    Spitz-like m.
    spitzoid malignant m.
    subungual m.
    superficial spreading m.
    tapioca m.
    m. theraccine
    thin m.
    ulcerated m.
    uveal m.
    vulvar m.
    m. whole cell vaccine
melanoma-associated antigen
melanoma/astrocytoma syndrome
melanoma-inhibitory activity (MIA)
melanoma-specific antigen
melanomatosis
melanosis
    Becker m.
    Dubreuilh precancerous m.
    premalignant m.
melanosome
melanotic
    m. carcinoma
    m. melanoma
    m. neuroectodermal tumor
    m. neuroectodermal tumor of
      infancy (MNTI)
    m. sarcoma
Melastatin
    M. gene
    M. test kit
melatonin
melena
melengestrol acetate
melenic stool
Melimmune-1
Melimmune-2
Mellaril
mellitus
    diabetes m. (type 1-3)
    insulin-dependent diabetes m.
      (IDDM)
    non-insulin-dependent diabetes m.
      (NIDDM)

meloxicam
melphalan (MEL, MPL)
    m., Adriamycin, prednisone (MAP)
    BCNU, etoposide, ara-C, m.
      (BEAM, mini-BEAM)
    m., cyclophosphamide, BCNU,
      prednisone (MCBP)
    m., cyclophosphamide, prednisone
      (MCP)
    m., 5-fluorouracil,
      medroxyprogesterone acetate
      (MFP)
    m., 5-fluorouracil, Provera (MFP)
    hexamethylenamine, Adriamycin, m.
      (HAM)
    hexamethylmelamine,
      Adriamycin, m. (HAM)
    m. hydrochloride
    m., Oncovin, mechlorethamine
    m., Oncovin, methylprednisolone
    m. plus prednisone (MPL+PRED)
    m., prednisolone (MP)
    m. and thiotepa
melphalan/etoposide
    paclitaxel/cyclophosphamide and
      high-dose m./e.
melphalan/prednisone
MelVax
MEM
    malignant epithelioid mesothelioma
membrane
    basement m.
    m. bleb formation
    Bruch m.
    glomerular basement m. (GBM)
    m. marker
    mucous m.
    Nytran m.
    plasma m.
    prostate-specific m. (PSM)
    thyrohyoid m.
membranoproliferative glomerulonephritis (MPGN)
membranous
    m. glomerulopathy
    m. pattern
    m. stenosis
memorial
    M. Delirium Assessment Scale
      (MDAS)
    M. dimension averaging method
    M. Pain Assessment Card (MPAC)
    M. Sloan-Kettering Cancer Center
    M. Sloan-Kettering protocol
    M. Sloan-Kettering staging
    M. Sloan-Kettering staging of
      childhood lymphoma
    M. Symptom Assessment Scale
      (MSAS)

M. Symptom Assessment Scale (MSAS)

M. Symptom Assessment Scale-Psychological (MSAS-Psych)

memory
immunologic m.
m. impairment
m. phenomenon
m. T cell

MEMS
medication event monitoring system

MEN
multiple endocrine neoplasia

MEN1
multiple endocrine neoplasia type 1
MEN1 gene

menadione
Menadol
Mendelsohn maneuver
Menest
Mengo virus
meningeal
m. carcinoma
m. carcinomatosis
m. fibrosis
m. hemangiopericytoma (M-HPC)
m. leukemia
m. malignancy
m. melanocytosis
m. sarcoma

meningioma
atypical m.
cerebellopontine angle m.
clivus m.
cystic intraparenchymal m.
ectopic m.
fibrous m.
globular m.
intraosseous m.
intraparenchymal m.
olfactory groove m.
oncocytic m.
parasagittal m.
periauricular m.
perioptic m.
secretory m.
sphenoid ridge m.
spinal m.
suprasellar m.
syncytial m.
temporal m.
tentorial m.

transitional m.
tuberculum sellae m.

meningismus
meningitis, pl. **meningitides**
AIDS-related lymphomatous m.
aseptic m.
bacterial m.
carcinomatous m.
cryptococcal m.
Cryptococcus neoformans m.
epidural m.
granulomatous m.
Haemophilus influenzae m.
lymphomatous m.
neoplastic m.
Salmonella m.
tuberculous m.

meningocele
cervical m.

meningococcal
meniscus, pl. **menisci**
menogaril
menometrorrhagia
menopausal symptom
menopause
iatrogenic m.

menorrhagia
menotropin
menstrual function
menstrualis
herpes m.

mensuration
mental retardation
MEP
mitomycin C, etoposide, Platinol

Mepergan
meperidine
m. hydrochloride
m. and promethazine

mephenytoin
mephobarbital
Mepilex foam dressing
MePr
methylprednisolone

Mepron
merbarone
mercaptopurine
ara-C, daunorubicin, prednisolone, m.
cytarabine, daunorubicin, prednisolone, m.

NOTES

M

mercaptopurine *(continued)*
daunorubicin, cytarabine,
prednisone, m. (DCPM)
methotrexate plus m. (MTX+MP)
6-mercaptopurine (6-MP)
prednisone, Oncovin,
methotrexate, 6-m. (POMP)
Mercedes-Benz sign
MERFS
Multicenter European Radiofrequency
Survey
Meritene
Merkel
M. cell
M. cell carcinoma (MCC)
M. cell tumor
merocyanine 540 (MC-540)
meropenem
merozoite
Merrem I.V.
Merrill-Dow polyamine inhibitor
mertiatide
mesenchymal
m. bone tumor
m. chondrosarcoma
m. hamartoma
m. lesion
m. neoplasm
m. sex cord stromal tumor
m. stromal cell
mesenchyme
nonspecific m.
mesenchymoma
atrial m.
mesenteric
m. cyst
m. lymphadenitis
m. lymph node
m. mass
m. panniculitis (MP)
m. phlegmon
mesenteritis
retractile m.
mesentery
mesh
Dexon m.
Prolene m.
meshwork
trabecular m.
M-Eslon
mesna
m., Adriamycin, ifosfamide,
dacarbazine (MAID)
Adriamycin, ifosfamide,
dacarbazine, m.
m., Adriamycin, interleukin-3,
dacarbazine (MAID)
m., ifosfamide, mitoxantrone,
etoposide (MIME)

m., ifosfamide, Novantrone,
etoposide (MINE)
m., ifosfamide, Novantrone,
etoposide plus etoposide,
methylprednisolone, high-dose ara-
C, *cis*-platinum (MINE/ESHAP)
m., ifosfamide, Novantrone,
etoposide plus etoposide, Solu-
Medrol, ara-C, Platinol
m., ifosfamide, Novantrone, Taxol
(MINT)
m. rescue, ifosfamide, carboplatin,
etoposide (MICE)
m. uroprotection
m. uroprotection and etoposide
vincristine, doxorubicin,
cyclophosphamide, dactinomycin
plus ifosfamide with m. (VAdCA
+ I/E)
Mesnex, Adriamycin, Ifex, dacarbazine
(MAID)
mesoblastic nephroma
mesoderm
mesodermal sarcoma
mesometanephric carcinoma
meson
K m.
mu m.
negative pi m.
pi m.
mesonephric
m. adenocarcinoma
m. carcinoma
m. duct
mesonephroid tumor
mesonephroma
mesopharynx
mesorectal lymph node
mesorectum
mesothelial
m. cell
m. cell inclusion
m. tissue
mesothelioma
asbestos-related m.
atrioventricular node m.
biphasic malignant m.
Butchart classification of
malignant m.
m. cancer
cystic m.
diffuse malignant peritoneal m.
diffuse pleural m.
epididymal m.
epithelioid m.
human malignant m. (HMM)
localized fibrous m.
malignant epithelioid m. (MEM)
malignant pleural m. (MPM)

papillary m.
pericardial m.
peritoneal m.
pleural m.
sarcomatoid malignant m.
messenger
m. ribonucleic acid
m. RNA (mRNA)
Mestinon
mestranol
mesylate
crisnatol m.
Desferal M.
dezaguanine m.
dolasetron m.
exatecan m.
imatinib m.
nafamostat m.
nelfinavir m.
m. salt
saquinavir m.
MET
MET PET
MET PET scan
metaanalysis
metabolic
m. aberration
m. acidosis
m. alkalosis
m. complication
m. emergency
metabolism
glucose m.
inhibitor of 5-FU m.
m. in intraperitoneal chemotherapy
prostaglandin endoperoxide m.
pyrimidine m.
redox m.
metabolite
catecholamine m.
m. image
metacarpophalangeal (MCP)
metachronous
m. adenoma
m. carcinoma
m. disease
m. lesion
m. leukemia
m. malignancy
m. metastasis
m. presentation
m. testicular germ cell tumor

metagenesis
deletion m.
metaiodobenzylguanidine (MIBG)
m. catecholamine imaging
iodine-131 m. (I-MIBG)
m. scintigraphy
metal
Lipowitz m.
trace m.'s
metalloproteinase
matrix m. (MMP)
tissue inhibitor of m. (TIMP)
metalloproteinase-1
tissue inhibitor of matrix m.-1
(TIMP-1)
metalloproteinase-2
matrix m.-2
metalloproteinase-like, disintegrin-like, cysteine-rich protein
metalloproteinase-proteolytic enzyme
metallothionein (MT)
metamyelocyte
metanephric blastema
metaperiodate
sodium m.
metaphysial, metaphyseal
m. chondrodysplasia
m. lucent band
metaplasia
agnogenic myeloid m. (AMM)
Barrett m.
epithelial m.
focal squamous m.
gallbladder florid pyloric gland m.
intestinal m.
myelofibrosis with myeloid m.
(MMM)
myeloid m.
nephrogenic m.
osteocartilaginous m.
polycythemia vera with myeloid m.
postpolycythemic myeloid m.
primary myeloid m.
pseudopyloric m.
pyloric gland m.
secondary myeloid m.
squamous m.
symptomatic myeloid m.
viral-induced atypical squamous m.
metaplastic
m. carcinoma
m. epithelium
m. pyloric gland

NOTES

M

metarubricyte
metastagenicity
metastasectomy
    adrenal m.
metastasis, pl. **metastases**
    adnexal m.
    adrenal m.
    aortic node m.
    axillary node m.
    biochemical m.
    blastic m.
    bone m.
    bony m.
    brain m.
    breast m.
    calcified liver m.
    calcifying m.
    calvarial m.
    cavitating m.
    celiac lymph node m.
    cerebral m.
    clivus m.
    cutaneous m.
    cystic m.
    distant m. (DM)
    drop m.
    echopenic liver m.
    extracapsular m.
    extrapulmonary m.
    extraregional m.
    extrathoracic m.
    floxuridine in hepatic m.
    free from distant m. (FFDM)
    hematogenous m.
    hepatic m.
    hernia m.
    inguinal lymph node m.
    intracapsular m.
    intramedullary spinal cord m.
    (ISCM)
    in-transit m.
    intraparenchymal m.
    intratumoral m.
    leptomeningeal m. (LM)
    liver m.
    lymphatic m.
    lymph node m.
    lymphogenous m.
    melanoma m.
    metachronous m.
    microscopic m.
    multiple synchronous metastases
    nodal m.
    nonhemorrhagic melanoma m.
    occult m.
    orbital m.
    ovarian cancer m.
    paracardiac m.
    parasellar m.

    parenchymal brain m.
    peritoneal implant m.
    placental m.
    port site m.
    pulmonary m.
    punctate m.
    sarcoma m.
    site-specific m.
    skeletal m.
    skip m.
    solitary splenic m.
    sphenoid sinus m.
    stomach cancer m.
    testicular m.
    transarticular skip m.
    tumor, node, m. (TNM)
    uterine sarcoma m.
    Virchow m.
metastasize
Metastat
metastatic
    m. adenocarcinoma
    m. breast cancer (MBC)
    m. breast carcinoma (MBC)
    m. carcinoid syndrome
    m. cascade
    m. contamination
    m. deposit
    m. efficiency index (MEI)
    m. lesion
    m. lung cancer
    m. lymph node tumor
    m. lymphoma
    m. lymphoma of CNS
    m. malignant melanoma
    m. renal cell carcinoma (mRCC)
    m. squamous carcinoma of head
      and neck (MSCHN)
Metastron
metatypical carcinoma
Metchnikoff cellular immunity theory
meter
    AvocetPT rapid prothrombin
      time m.
met gene
methacrylate
    methyl m.
methadol
    levo-alpha-acetyl m.
methadone
Methadose
methanol
    m. extraction residue
    m. extraction residue of bacillus
      Calmette-Guérin vaccine
    m. freezing method
methemalbumin
methemoglobin (MHB)

methemoglobinemia
    acquired m.
    congenital m.
    hereditary m.
    toxic m.
methemoglobinemic
methemoglobinuria
Methergine
methimazole
methionine
Methitest tablet
method
    affinity-based m.
    antibody linkage m.
    antihemophilic factor m. M
    automated m.
    avidin-biotin-peroxidase complex m.
    Berger point kernel m.
    Berkson-Gage m.
    m. of Bernie Siegel
    biplane m.
    Brecher-Cronkite m.
    Breen and Tullis m.
    Breslow microstaging m.
    Brochner-Mortensen m.
    Brookmeyer-Crowley m.
    cancer-detection m.
    Clark microstaging m.
    m. clotting assay
    colorimetric m.
    coverslip m.
    cyanmethemoglobin quantitative m.
    cytocentrifuge m.
    cytochemical staining m.
    Dacie m.
    double balloon m.
    epitope retrieval m.
    Fahraeus m.
    Feldenkrais m.
    fibrin plate m.
    Fiske and Subbarow m.
    Folin and Wu m.
    George and Desu m.
    Greenwald and Lewman m.
    guanidine thiocyanate m.
    Hagedorn and Jansen m.
    Ham m.
    Hamacher m.
    Hammerschlag m.
    histochemical m.
    Hoechst dye m.
    immunologic m.
    Inoue balloon m.

    isodose shift m.
    Karr m.
    Kety-Schmidt m.
    Kleihauer-Betke m.
    Levy, Rowntree, and Marriott m.
    Lewis and Benedict m.
    Lewisohn m.
    Liang and Pardee m.
    MacFarlane serum m.
    Mantoux m.
    Memorial dimension averaging m.
    methanol freezing m.
    modified Powell m.
    neck region-lifting m.
    neutralization index m.
    Nikiforoff m.
    Oliver-Rosalki m.
    Paris m.
    Pembrey m.
    pharmacologic m.
    polymerase chain reaction-based m.
    power law TAR m.
    push-wedge m.
    restriction fragment length
      polymorphism m.
    Sahli m.
    Sanger m.
    score m.
    Seldinger m.
    Simonton m.
    Simplate m.
    single balloon m.
    single-stick m.
    single-tube m.
    Spearman rank correlation m.
    step-and-shoot m.
    Stockholm m.
    Student-Newman-Keuls m.
    trocar drainage m.
    TUNEL m.
    Westergren m.
    Wintrobe and Landsberg m.
methodology
    assay m.
Methosarb
methotrexate (MTX)
    m., actinomycin D, chlorambucil
      (MAC)
    m., actinomycin D,
      cyclophosphamide (MAC)
    m., Adriamycin, cyclophosphamide
      (MAC)

NOTES

M

methotrexate *(continued)*

Adriamycin, cyclophosphamide, m. (ACM)

m., Adriamycin, cyclophosphamide, CCNU (MACC)

m., Adriamycin, cyclophosphamide, Oncovin, bleomycin (MACOB)

m., Adriamycin, cyclophosphamide, Oncovin, prednisone, bleomycin (MACOP-B)

m., Adriamycin, cyclophosphamide, Oncovin, prednisone, bleomycin with leucovorin

Adriamycin, 5-fluorouracil, m. (AFM)

Adriamycin, vinblastine, m. (AVM)

m. and arabinoside C (MTX/ara-C)

m., ara-C, cyclophosphamide, CCNU (MACC)

L-asparaginase and m. (LAM)

m., asparaginase, cyclophosphamide, hydroxydaunomycin, Oncovin (MACHO)

m., asparaginase, Cytoxan, hydroxydaunomycin, Oncovin (MACHO)

L-asparaginase, ifosfamide, m. (AIM)

BCNU, bleomycin, VePesid, prednisone, m. (BBVP-M)

m., bleomycin, Adriamycin, cyclophosphamide, Oncovin, dexamethasone (M-BACOD)

m., bleomycin, Adriamycin, cyclophosphamide, Oncovin, Solu-Medrol (M-BACOS)

m., bleomycin, cisplatin (MBC)

m., bleomycin, DDP

bleomycin, Oncovin, m.

bleomycin, Oncovin, prednisone, Adriamycin, mechlorethamine, m. (BOPAM)

m., calcium leucovorin rescue, Adriamycin, cisplatin, bleomycin, cyclophosphamide, dactinomycin

CCNU, procarbazine, m. (CPM)

m., cisplatin, vinblastine (MCV)

m. and cyclophosphamide (MeCy)

cyclophosphamide, Adriamycin, m. (CAM)

cyclophosphamide, Adriamycin, VP-16, prednisone, m. (CAVPM)

cyclophosphamide, CCNU, m. (CCM)

cyclophosphamide, Oncovin, m. (COM, COMe)

cyclophosphamide, Oncovin, 5-fluorouracil/cyclophosphamide, Oncovin, m.

cyclophosphamide, vincristine, m. (CVM)

cytarabine, bleomycin, Oncovin, m.

cytosine arabinoside, etoposide, m. (CEM)

Cytoxan, Oncovin, 5-fluorouracil plus Cytoxan, Oncovin, m.

m., doxorubicin, cyclophosphamide, etoposide, mecloretamine, vincristine, procarbazine

m. and 5-fluorouracil (MF)

5-fluorouracil and m. (FUM)

5-fluorouracil, Adriamycin, m. (FAMTX)

5-fluorouracil, Adriamycin, cyclophosphamide, m. (FAC-M)

5-fluorouracil, Adriamycin, Cytoxan, m. (FAC-M)

5-fluorouracil, doxorubicin, m.

m., 5-fluorouracil, epirubicin, vincristine (MFEV)

5-fluorouracil, Novantrone, m. (FNM)

hexamethylenamine, Adriamycin, m. (HAM)

hexamethylmelamine, Adriamycin, m. (HAM)

high-dose m. (HDMTX, HMTX)

intermediate-dose m. (IDMTX)

intrathecal m.

m. and laurocapram

m., leucovorin, Adriamycin, cyclophosphamide, Oncovin, prednisone, bleomycin

m., leucovorin, bleomycin, Adriamycin, cyclophosphamide, Oncovin, dexamethasone

m. LFP solution

M. LPF Sodium

m., mechlorethamine, Oncovin, procarbazine, prednisone (MMOPP)

Oncovin and m.

m., Oncovin, L-asparaginase, dexamethasone (MOAD)

m., Oncovin, cyclophosphamide, Adriamycin (MOCA)

m., Oncovin, 5-fluorouracil (MOF)

m., Oncovin, PEG-asparaginase, prednisone (MOAP)

Platinol, 5-fluorouracil, m. (PFM)

m., Platinol, 5-fluorouracil, leucovorin, calcium (MPFL)

m. plus mercaptopurine (MTX+MP)

prednisone, L-asparaginase, daunomycin, VM-26, m.

prednisone, m.-leucovorin, Adriamycin, cyclophosphamide, etoposide plus cytarabine, bleomycin, Oncovin, methotrexate (ProMACE-CytaBOM)

prednisone, methotrexate-leucovorin, Adriamycin, cyclophosphamide, etoposide plus cytarabine, bleomycin, Oncovin, m. (ProMACE-CytaBOM)

procarbazine, ifosfamide, m. (PRIME)

pulse m.

m. sodium

m., vinblastine, Adriamycin, cisplatin (MVAC)

vincristine, bleomycin, m. (VBM)

vincristine, doxorubicin, prednisone, asparaginase, 6-mercaptopurine, m.

vincristine, etoposide, prednisone, Adriamycin, m. (VEPA-M)

VP-16-213, Adriamycin, m. (VAM)

m. with rescue

methotrexate/arabinoside C regimen

methotrimeprazine

methoxsalen sterile solution

2-methoxyestradiol (2-ME)

methoxyisobutylisonitrile (MIBI)

technetium-99m m. (^{99m}Tc MIBI)

methsuximide

methyclothiazide

methydiphosphonate bone scan

methyl

m. benzoate

m. guanine

m. methacrylate

m. nitrosourea

methylacetylenic putrescine

methylation

DNA m.

methylation-specific polymerase chain reaction

methylbromide

homatropine m. (HMB45)

methyl-CCNU (MeCCNU)

m.-CCNU, 5-fluorouracil, Adriamycin (MeFA)

5-fluorouracil, Adriamycin, m.-CCNU (FAM-C)

streptozocin, Adriamycin, m.-CCNU (SAM)

methylcellulose

methyldopa

methylene

m. blue

m. dimethane sulfonate (MDMS)

methylenetetrahydrofolate reductase (MTHFR)

methylergonovine

methylglyoxal-*bis*-guanylhydrazone (MGBG)

methylhydrazine

procarbazine m.

methylmercaptopurine riboside (MMPR)

methylnaltrexone (MNTX)

methylphenidate

methylprednisolone (MePr, MP)

m. acetate

Adriamycin, bleomycin, vinblastine, dacarbazine, m. (ABVD-MP)

doxorubicin, methylprednisolone, cytosine arabinoside, and cisplatin alternating with methotrexate, bleomycin, cyclophosphamide, doxorubicin, vincristine, and m.

intravenous m.

melphalan, Oncovin, m.

m., Oncovin, procarbazine (MOP)

m. pulse therapy (MPPT)

m. sodium succinate

vincristine, Adriamycin, m. (VAMP)

methylsergide

methyl-*tert*-butyl ether

methyltestosterone

estrogen and m.

methyltyrosine

alpha m.

methylxanthine

Meticorten

metoclopramide

m., dexamethasone, lorazepam, ondansetron (MDLO)

m. hydrochloride

metolazone

metoprine

met protooncogene/oncogene

metrizoate

metrofibroma

metronidazole

metronomic chemotherapy

metrorrhagia

Metvix PDT

MetXia

MetXia-P450

metyrapone

M

NOTES

metyrosine
MeV
    megaelectron volt
    megavolt
Mevacor Atherosclerosis Regression
    Study (MARS)
Mexate
Mexican
    M. hat cell
    M. hat erythrocyte
    M. hat sign
mexiletine
Meyer-Betz disease
Meyer dysplasia
Mezlin
mezlocillin
MF
    methotrexate and 5-fluorouracil
    mitomycin and 5-fluorouracil
    mycosis fungoides
MFEV
    methotrexate, 5-fluorouracil, epirubicin,
      vincristine
MFH
    malignant fibrous histiocytoma
MFI, MFI-20
    Multidimensional Fatigue Inventory
MFL
    mitoxantrone, 5-fluorouracil, leucovorin
MFP
    melphalan, 5-fluorouracil,
      medroxyprogesterone acetate
    melphalan, 5-fluorouracil, Provera
M1G8
      monoclonal antibody M1G8
MGBG
    methylglyoxal-*bis*-guanylhydrazone
MGCT
    malignant giant cell tumor
MGDF
    megakaryocyte growth and development
      factor
MGI-114
    hydroxymethylacylfulvene
MGUS
    monoclonal gammopathy of
      undetermined significance
MHA-TPA
    microhemagglutination assay-*Treponema*
      pallidum assay
MHB
    methemoglobin
MHC
    major histocompatibility complex
      MHC class II antigen
      MHC class I-restricted cytolytic
        activity
      MHC haplotype
      MHC receptor expression

MHC-restricted cytotoxic T cell
M-HPC
    meningeal hemangiopericytoma
MI
    myocardial infarction
MIA
    melanoma-inhibitory activity
Miacalcin Nasal Spray
MIB-1 expression
MIBB breast biopsy system
MIBG
    metaiodobenzylguanidine
      MIBG bone scan
      MIBG catecholamine imaging
MIBI
    methoxyisobutylisonitrile
      ^{99m}Tc MIBI
MIC
    minimum inhibitory concentration
      MIC tube
MICA
    microinvasive cervical cancer
      MICA gene
micafungin
Micatin Topical
MICB gene
MICE
    mesna rescue, ifosfamide, carboplatin,
      etoposide
micellar electrokinetic capillary
    chromatography (MECC)
Michaelis
    M. buffer
    M. complex
    M. constant
Michaelis-Menten pharmacokinetic
    behavior
michellamine B
Mick
    M. afterloading needle
    M. seed applicator
miconazole
MICRhoGAM
microabscess
    Pautrier m.
microadenoma
    adrenocorticotropin m.
    pituitary m.
    prolactin-secreting m.
microangiopathic hemolytic anemia
microangiopathy
    mineralizing m.
    thrombotic m. (TMA)
microarray
microassay for amino levulinate acid
    dehydratase
microbial flora

microbicide
    topical m.
    vaginal m.
microbiology
microbody
microcalcification
    ductal m.
    tumoral m.
microcarcinoma
    papillary m. (PMC)
microcarrier
    CultiSpher-G m.
    permeable collagen m.
MicroCatheter
    FirstCyte M.
microcatheter
    Cordis coaxial m.
    InDuct breast m.
microcentrifuge
microcephaly
    cytomegalovirus with m.
microchimerism
    persistent fetal m.
microchip DNA array
microculture tetrazolium dye assay
microcystic
    m. adenoma
    m. eccrine carcinoma
    m. formation
microcytosis
microcytotoxicity assay
microdeletion
    chromosome 22q11 m. (CATCH
    22)
microdissected
microdissection
    laser capture m. (LCM)
    Piezo Power M.
microdissector
microdosimetry
microelectrode
    Eppendorf pO$_2$ m.
microelectrophoresis
microencapsulation assay
microenvironment
    bone marrow m.
    hematopoietic m.
microexcision
microextension
microfibrillar collagen hemostat
microfluorometry
microfollicular adenoma
microgametocyte

microgastria-limb reduction anomaly
microglial cell
microglioma
microgranular acute promyelocytic
    leukemia
microhemagglutination assay-*Treponema*
    ***pallidum* assay (MHA-TPA)**
microhomology
microinvasive
    m. carcinoma
    m. carcinoma classification
    m. cervical cancer (MICA)
Micro-K 10 Extencaps
microlatex particle-mediated
    immunoassay
microlesion
micro liquid extraction
microlithiasis
    alveolar m.
micromanipulation
MicroMark tissue marker
micromegakaryocyte
micrometastasis, pl. **micrometastases**
    systemic m.
micrometastatic
micromultileaf
    m. collimator
    m. collimator system
micromyeloblastic leukemia
micronest
    endocrine cell m.
micronodular hyperplasia
Micronor
micronucleus, pl. **micronuclei**
micronutrient
microorganism
micropapillary
    m. serous carcinoma (MPSC)
    m. serous ovarian carcinoma
microphage
microplate
    m. plasma methotrexate assay
    m. plasma MTX assay
Micropore tape
MicroPrep 2 centrifuge
microsatellite
    m. instability (MIN, MSI)
    m. instability testing
    m. locus
microscope
    Hitachi H600 electron m.
    Hitachi H7000 electron m.

M

NOTES

microscope *(continued)*
    Joel scanning electron m.
    Zeiss Axioskop m.
microscopic
    m. angiogenesis grading system
      (MAGS)
    m. metastasis
    m. residuum
    m. seeding
microscopically normal tissue
microscopy
    confocal m.
    electron m.
    epiluminescence m.
    image analysis m.
    laser m.
    light m.
    transmission electron m. (TEM)
microSelectron-HDR afterloader
microsomal hydroxylation
microsome
    liver-kidney m. 1
microspectrofluorometry
microsphere
    acrylic m.
    Bead Block polyvinyl alcohol
      embolic m.
    degradable starch m.
    Embosphere m.
    gelatin-encapsulated nitrogen m.
    magnetic m.
    magnetically responsive m.
    paramagnetic m.
    silastic m.
    SIR-Spheres m.
    starch m.
    therapeutic m.
Microspora
Microsporida
microsporidial keratoconjunctivitis
microsporidiosis
Microsporum canis
microstaging
microti
    Babesia m.
microtiter blood typing system
microtrabecular hepatocellular carcinoma
microtron
    racetrack m.
microtubule
    m. assembly
    depolymerization of m.
    m. inhibitor
    polymerization of m.
microvacuolation
microvacuolization
microvascular anastomosis

microvesicular hepatic steatosis
microvessel density (MVD)
microvillus, pl. microvilli
microwave
    m. coagulation therapy
    m. epitope retrieval technique
    m. fixation
    transurethral m. (TURM)
Microzide
Midamor
Midas II automated stainer
midazolam
Middeldorpf tumor
middle
    m. ear
    m. upper arm circumference
      (MUAC)
Middlebrook
    M. agar
    M. broth
Middlebrook-Dubos hemagglutination
    test
midline
    m. catheter
    m. granuloma
    m. malignant reticulosis
midplane
    m. depth
    m. dose
MIFA
    mitomycin, 5-fluorouracil, Adriamycin
mifepristone
migrans
    visceral larva m.
migrant pattern
migrated
    m. monocyte
    m. tumor
migration
    cell m.
    embolus m.
    leukocyte m.
    lymphocyte m.
    neutrophil m.
    phagocyte m.
migrational abnormality
migratory tumor
Mikulicz
    M. disease
    M. syndrome
Mikulicz-Radecki syndrome
Mikulicz-Sjögren syndrome
Milan Cancer Institute
9-mile fever
milk
    m. factor
    m. fat globule protein
    m. thistle

Miller Behavioral Style Scale
millicurie (mCi)
milligram
>femtomoles per m. (fmol/mg)

million
>parts per m. (ppm)
>M. Women Study

Millipore ultrafree-CL centrifugal filter
millisievert (mSv)
mil/raf protooncogene/oncogene
miltefosine
milzbrand
MIME
>mesna, ifosfamide, mitoxantrone,
>etoposide

MIMIC
>Multivane Intensity Modulation
>Compensator

mimicker of malignancy
MIN
>microsatellite instability
>multiple intestinal neoplasia

Min
>modifier of M. (MOM)

mind-body
>m.-b. interaction
>m.-b. medicine

MINE
>mesna, ifosfamide, Novantrone, etoposide

MINE/ESHAP
>mesna, ifosfamide, Novantrone, etoposide
>plus etoposide, methylprednisolone,
>high-dose ara-C, *cis*-platinum

mineral
>m. fiber
>m. oil

mineralizing microangiopathy
mineralocorticoid
miner's anemia
Ming criteria
mini-BEAM
>BCNU, etoposide, ara-C, melphalan

mini-COAP
>Cytoxan, Oncovin, ara-C, prednisone

Mini-Gamulin Rh
minimal
>m. cytotoxic epitope (MCE)
>m. deviation adenocarcinoma
>m. deviation melanoma
>m. differentiation
>m. peripheral dose (MPD)
>m. residual disease (MRD)

minimi
>opponens digiti m. (ODM)

minimum
>m. effective dose (MED)
>m. flow rate
>m. inhibitory concentration (MIC)
>m. tolerance dose

minimyelogram
mining
>uranium m.

miniprobe
Mini Quant D-dimer test system
minisatellite
>m. allele
>m. DNA

Minitran Patch
Minocin IV Injection
minocycline
minor histocompatibility antigen
Minot-Murphy diet
minoxidil
MINT
>mesna, ifosfamide, Novantrone, Taxol

minute
>double m.

miosis
miotic
MIP
>macrophage inflammatory protein

MIP-1a, MIP-1 alpha
>macrophage inflammatory protein-1 alpha

MIP-I
>macrophage inflammatory protein I

MIP-II
>macrophage inflammatory protein II

MIR
>mastectomy with immediate
>reconstruction
>>MIR guidelines
>>MIR intrauterine tandem
>>MIR system

MiraLax
Miraluma
>M. injection
>M. kit

MIRALVA
>Mallinckrodt Institute of Radiology
>Afterloading Vaginal Applicator

MIRD
>medical internal radiation dose
>medical internal radiation dosimetry

Mirels scoring system
mirostipen

NOTES

mirror
    beam-splitting m.
mirtazapine
MIS
    müllerian-inhibiting substance
misery perfusion syndrome
mismatch
    m. repair (MMR)
    m. repair gene
mismatched related donor
misonidazole
misoprostol
mispair
missense mutation
missing block
mistletoe extract
MIT-C, MITO-C
    mitomycin C
Mithracin
mithramycin
mitindomide
MITO-C (*var. of* MIT-C)
mitocarcin
mitochondrial
    m. antibody
    m. deoxyribonucleic acid
      polymerase gamma
    m. DNA
    m. DNA mutation
    m. DNA polymerase gamma
    m. dysfunction
    m. encephalomyopathy
    m. hydroxylase enzyme
    m. oxidative phosphorylation
    m. respiratory chain enzyme
    m. respiratory chain enzyme
      complex
mitochondrium, pl. **mitochondria**
mitocromin
mitogen
    pokeweed m.
mitogen-activated protein kinase
mitogenic factor
mitogillin
mitoguazone
mitolactol
mitomalcin
mitomycin
    Adriamycin, bleomycin,
      cyclophosphamide, m. C (ABCM)
    m., Adriamycin, Platinol
    Adriamycin, vincristine, m. C
      (AVM)
    m. C (MC, MIT-C, MITO-C,
      MMC, MTC)
    m. C, Adriamycin,
      cyclophosphamide (MAC)
    m. C, Adriamycin, Platinol (MAP)
    m. cardiotoxicity

    m. C, etoposide, Platinol (MEP)
    m. C and 5-FU (Nigro protocol)
    cisplatin, doxorubicin, m. C
    m. C, Oncovin, bleomycin,
      cisplatin (MOB-III)
    m. and 5-fluorouracil (MF)
    m., 5-fluorouracil, Adriamycin
      (MIFA)
    5-fluorouracil, Adriamycin, m.
      (FAM)
    5-fluorouracil, Oncovin, m. C
      (FOM, FOMi)
    ftorafur, Adriamycin, m. C
      (FURAM)
    leuprolide acetate, vinblastine,
      Adriamycin, m. (L-VAM)
    streptonigrin, 6-thioguanine,
      cyclophosphamide, actinomycin, m.
      (STEAM)
    m. and vinblastine (MV)
    vinblastine and m. (VM)
    vinblastine, Adriamycin, m.
    vinblastine, Adriamycin, m. C
      (VAM)
    m., vinblastine, Platinol (MVP)
mitonafide
mitoquidone
mitosis, pl. **mitoses**
    quantal m.
mitosis-karyorrhexis index (MKI)
mitosper
mitotane
mitotic
    m. figure
    m. index
    m. inhibitor
    m. spindle agent
mitotic-karyorrhectic index
mitotoxicity
mitoxantrone (DHAD, M, MTZ)
    m. and cytarabine
    fludarabine, ara-C, m. (FAM)
    fludarabine, cytarabine, m. (FLAM)
    m., 5-fluorouracil, leucovorin
      (MFL)
    m. hydrochloride
    m., ifosfamide, VePesid (MIV)
    m., VePesid, thiotepa (MVT)
    m., vinblastine, cyclophosphamide
      (MVC)
    m., vinblastine, 5-fluorouracil
    m., vincristine, 5-fluorouracil
      (MVF)
    m., vincristine, procarbazine,
      prednisone
    m. and VP-16 (MV)
    m., VP-16, thiotepa (MVT)
mitozolomide

mitral
    m. regurgitation
    m. stenosis (MS)
    m. valve prolapse (MVP)
Mitrolan Chewable Tablet
Mitsuda antigen
Mitsuyasu staging system
MIV
    mitoxantrone, ifosfamide, VePesid
mixed
    m. cell leukemia
    m. cell sarcoma
    m. cryoglobulinemia
    m. donor-host hematopoietic chimerism
    m. follicular hyperplasia
    m. germ cell tumor
    m. histology tumor
    m. leukocyte culture (MLC)
    m. lineage
    m. lineage leukemia
    m. lymphocyte culture
    m. lymphocyte reaction
    m. lymphocytic-histiocytic lymphoma
    m. mesodermal tumor
    m. müllerian sarcoma
    m. müllerian tumor (MMT)
    m. oligoastrocytoma
    m. opioid agonist-antagonist
    m. ovarian mesodermal sarcoma
    m. pattern
    m. photon-electron technique
    m. sex cord-stromal tumor
    m. small cleaved and large cell lymphoma
    m. thymoma
    m. tumor of salivary gland
    m. tumor of skin
mixed-cellularity
    m.-c. Hodgkin disease
    m.-c. type
mixed-type carcinoma
mixture
    barium m.
    racemic m.
MKI
    mitosis-karyorrhexis index
M/L
    monocyte/lymphocyte
    M/L ratio
MLC
    mixed leukocyte culture

multileaf collimator
myelomonocytic leukemia, chronic
MLD
    manual lymph drainage
MLH1 gene
MLL gene
MLM gene
MLNS
    mucocutaneous lymph node syndrome
MLP
    Mayo Lung Project
MLS
    myelomonocytic leukemia, subacute
MM
    malignant myeloma
    multiple myeloma
MMC
    mitomycin C
    multicentric mammary carcinoma
MME
    malignant myoepithelioma
MMF
    mycophenolate mofetil
MMM
    myelofibrosis with myeloid metaplasia
MMMT
    malignant mixed mesodermal tumor
M-mode tracing
M195 monoclonal antibody anti-CD33
MMOPP
    methotrexate, mechlorethamine, Oncovin, procarbazine, prednisone
MMP
    matrix metalloproteinase
MMPR
    methylmercaptopurine riboside
MMR
    measles-mumps-rubella
    mismatch repair
      MMR gene
MMT
    mixed müllerian tumor
MN blood group
MNS blood group
MNTI
    melanotic neuroectodermal tumor of infancy
MNTX
    methylnaltrexone
M-O
      Haley's M-O
MO1 antigen

M

NOTES

MoAb
    monoclonal antibody
        MoAb 425 antibody
MOAD
    methotrexate, Oncovin, L-asparaginase,
      dexamethasone
MOAP
    methotrexate, Oncovin, PEG-
      asparaginase, prednisone
MOB
    mechlorethamine, Oncovin, bleomycin
    Mustargen, Oncovin, bleomycin
Mobetron
    M. intraoperative radiation therapy
      treatment system
    M. mobile, self-shielded electron
      accelerator
MOB-III
    mitomycin C, Oncovin, bleomycin,
      cisplatin
mobile
    cecum m.
mobility shift assay
mobilization
    stem cell m.
mobilizing agent
Mobin-Uddin filter
Mobist
MOCA
    methotrexate, Oncovin,
      cyclophosphamide, Adriamycin
moccasin appearance
MOCHA
    Multicenter Oral Carvedilol Heart Failure
    Assessment
MOD
    mean optical density
modafinil
modality
    immunosuppressive m.
Modane
    M. Bulk
    M. Soft
mode
    amplitude m.
    m. I, II additivity
    stimulated echo acquisition m.
      (STEAM)
model
    AIDS risk-reduction m.
    Couch m.
    fluid mosaic m.
    Gail breast cancer risk m.
    Goldie-Coldman m.
    gompertzian m.
    hematopoietic-inductive
      microenvironment m.
    log-kill m.
    Luria-Delbruck m.

    Lyman m.
    Markov m.
    multistage Markov m.
    Ogawa m.
    Preventive Health M. (PHM)
    primate m.
    risk-assessment m.
    Skipper-Schabel m.
    stillbirth and death m.
    m. system
    systemic m.
    Trentin hematopoietic-inductive
      microenvironment m.
modeling
    accurate beam m.
    m. derivation
    electromagnetic m.
    thermal m.
    ultrasonographic m.
moderate-dose methotrexate, bleomycin,
    Adriamycin, cyclophosphamide,
    Oncovin, dexamethasone (m-BACOD)
moderately
    m. differentiated adenocarcinoma
    m. emetogenic chemotherapy
      (MEC)
ModFit DNA analysis
modification
    beam m.
    Gehan-Gilbert m.
    glutathione m.
    Gunderson-Sosin m.
    lifestyle m.
    Musshoff m.
    neuroanatomic m.
    posttranslation m.
    posttranslational m.
    Rosch m.
modified
    m. Bagshawe protocol (MBP)
    m. citrus pectin
    m. Powell method
    m. radical hysterectomy
    m. radical mastectomy (MRM)
    m. Simpson rule
    m. systemic Berlin-Frankfurt-
      Munster therapy
modifier
    effect m.'s
    m. of Min (MOM)
    multidimensional analysis beam m.
    response m.
modifying gene
Modrastane
Modrefen
Modrenal
Moducal
modulation
    amplitude m.

antigenic m.
biochemical m.
immune m.
m. potential

modulator
combined m.'s
estrogen receptor m.
immune m.
multidrug resistance m.
selective estrogen receptor m.
(SERM)

MOF
MeCCNU, Oncovin, 5-fluorouracil
methotrexate, Oncovin, 5-fluorouracil

mofetil
mycophenolate m. (MMF)

MOF-STREP
MeCCNU, Oncovin, 5-fluorouracil plus
streptozocin

Mohs micrographic surgery
MOI
multiplicities of infection

moiety, pl. moieties
glucopyranoside m.
hydroxyethylamine m.
lipid m.
purine m.

Moiré photography
moist
m. desquamation
m. snuff

Moi-Stir
M.-S. oral spray
M.-S. Swabsticks

molar
mulberry m.
m. pregnancy

mold
dematiaceous m.
filter m.
m. therapy

mole
Breus m.
complete hydatidiform m. (CHM)
hydatidiform m. (HM)
invasive m.
partial hydatidiform m. (PHM)

molecular
m. approach
m. cell biology
m. chaperone
m. cloning

M. Dynamics Personal Densitometer
SI
m. epidemiology
m. genetic analysis
m. genetics
m. genetic technique
m. hybridization study
m. latency
m. target-based screen
m. weight

molecule
accessory adhesion m.
adhesion m.
antiangiogenic m.
BiTE m.
cell adhesion m.
cleaved polyprotein precursor m.
(p55)
costimulatory m.
dasatinib m.
desmoglein adhesion m.
E-cadherin adhesion m.
fibronectin adhesion m.
GMK m.
m. hapten
intercellular adhesion m. (ICAM)
KLH m.
lectin cell adhesion m.
negative angiogenic m.
neural cell adhesion m.
nitroxide tempo m.
polyprotein precursor m.
positive angiogenic m.
proangiogenic m.
retinoid-related m.
signaling lymphocytic activation m.
(SLAM)
signal transducing m. STAT 5
stress-induced MHC class I-
related m.

molecule-1
intercellular adhesion m.-1 (ICAM-
1)
leukocyte adhesion m.-1 (LAM-1)
platelet endothelial cell
adhesion m.-1 (PECAM-1)
vascular cell adhesion m.-1
(VCAM-1)

molgramostim
Moll
adenocarcinoma of M.

NOTES

M

molluscum
    m. contagiosum
    m. corpuscle
Moloney test
Molony murine leukemia virus
Molulsky dye reduction test
molybdenum
Molypen
MOM
    modifier of Min
moment
      macroscopic magnetic m.
MOMP
    mechlorethamine, Oncovin, methotrexate, prednisone
Mönckeberg sclerosis
Mondini dysplasia
Mondor disease
Moniliaceae
moniliasis
moniliid
Monistat-Derm Topical
Monistat I.V. Injection
monitor
    CoaguChek Pro/DM m.
    patient dose m.
    m. unit (MU)
monitoring
    Electrophysiologic Study Versus Electrocardiographic M. (ESVEM)
    p53 fluorescent m.
    physiologic m.
    m. technique
    therapeutic drug m. (TDM)
monoamine
    m. oxidase (MAO)
    m. oxidase inhibitor (MAOI)
monoblastic leukemia
monoblast predominance
monocellular suspension
monochemotherapy
monochromatic photography
Monocid
Monoclate-P
monoclonal
    m. antibodies against gastric mucins
    m. antibody (MAb, MoAb)
    m. antibody A103 fine-needle aspiration biopsy
    m. antibody anticancer vaccine
    m. antibody B43.13
    m. antibody B72.3
    m. antibody-defined antigen
    m. antibody imaging
    m. antibody M1G8
    m. antibody PC10
    m. antibody S5

    m. antibody therapy
    m. anticytokeratin (MAK-6)
    m. band
    m. gammopathy
    m. gammopathy of undetermined significance (MGUS)
    m. integration
    m. mouse anti-ELAM-1
    m. mouse anti-human TNF receptor p60
    m. mouse anti-ICAM-1
    m. mouse anti-VCAM-1
    m. origin
    m. rat anti-human TNF receptor p80
    m. spike
monoclonality
monocrotaline
monocyte
    m. chemoattractant protein 1
    m. chemotactic and activating factor
    m. chemotactic protein (MCP)
    m. colony-stimulating factor
    m. inflammatory protein
    m. lineage antigen
    migrated m.
    m. presenting
    m. tissue factor
monocyte-derived macrophage
monocyte/lymphocyte (M/L)
    m./l. ratio
monocyte-macrophage progenitor
monocyte-tropic strain
monocytic
    m. leukemia
    m. leukemoid reaction
    m. leukocytosis
    m. marker
    m. sarcoma
monocytogene
monocytogenes
    Listeria m.
monocytoid
    m. B cell
    m. B-cell lymphoma (MBCL)
    m. B lymphocyte
monocytopenia
monocytopoiesis
monocytosis
Monodox
monogamous
Mono-Gesic
monohistiocyte
monoiodobenzylguanidine (^{131}I-mIB6)
monoisocentric technique
monokine
monomeric precursor

monomorphic
> m. adenoma
> m. lymphoma

mononeuritis multiplex
mononeuropathy multiplex
Mononine
mononuclear
> m. cell
> m. phagocyte

mononucleosis
> Epstein-Barr m.
> infectious m.

mononucleosis-like symptom
monooctanoin
monooleate
> mannose m.
> polyethylene sorbitan m.

monophasic
monophosphate
> adenosine m. (AMP)
> cyclic guanosine m. (cGMP)
> deoxyadenosine m. (dAMP)
> fludarabine m. (FAMP)
> guanosine m. (GMP)
> hexose m.
> inosine m. (IMP)
> uradine m. (UMP)

5′-monophosphate
> 2′,3′-dideoxycytidine 5′-m. (ddCMP)

monophosphated acyclic adenine nucleoside analog
monophosphoryl lipid A
monophyletic cluster
monosomy
> m. 5q-syndrome
> m. 7 syndrome

Monospot test
monostotic fibrous dysplasia
monotherapy
> ddI m.
> nucleoside analog m.
> Proxinium m.

monoxide
> diffusing capacity of lung for carbon m. (DLCO)

Monro foramen colloid cyst
Monro-Kellie hypothesis
Monte
> M. Carlo photon transport (MCPT)
> M. Carlo photon transport simulation

Montgomery gland

month
> Lupron Depot-3 M.
> Lupron Depot-4 M.

Mooser cell
MOP
> mechlorethamine, Oncovin, prednisone
> methylprednisolone, Oncovin, procarbazine

MOP-BAP
> mechlorethamine, Oncovin, prednisone, bleomycin, Adriamycin, procarbazine

MOPP
> mechlorethamine, Oncovin, procarbazine, prednisone

MOPP/ABV
> mechlorethamine, Oncovin, procarbazine, prednisone plus Adriamycin, bleomycin, vinblastine

MOPP/ABVD
> mechlorethamine, Oncovin, procarbazine, prednisone plus Adriamycin, bleomycin, vinblastine, dacarbazine

MOPP-BLEO
> mechlorethamine, Oncovin, procarbazine, prednisone, bleomycin

MOPr
> mechlorethamine, Oncovin, procarbazine

Moraxella
> *M. bovis*
> *M. catarrhalis*
> *M. liquefaciens*

morbidity rate
morbilliform rash
Morbillivirus
MORE
> Multiple Outcomes for Raloxifene Evaluation
> MORE trial

More-Dophilus
moriendi
> ars m.

morpheaform basal cell carcinoma
morphea-type basal cell carcinoma
morphine
> high-dose m. (HDM)
> M. HP
> subcutaneous m.
> m. sulfate (MS)
> m. sulfate controlled release
> m. sulfate controlled-release suppository (MS-CRS)
> m. sulfate extended-release capsule

morphine-controlled release (MCR)

M

NOTES

morphine-potentiated
m.-p. HIV replication
m.-p. human immunodeficiency virus replication
morphogen
morphogenetic protein
morpholino anthracycline
morphologic
m. analysis
m. classification
m. pattern
morphology
large cell carcinoma with neuroendocrine m. (LCCNM)
lymphoplasmacytoid m.
spindle cell m.
m. system CAS-200
morphometry
nuclear m.
morphonuclear
Morquio syndrome
Morrow Assessment of Nausea and Emesis (MANE)
morsicatio
m. buccarum
m. linguagram
mortality
m. rate ratio
treatment-related m. (TRM)
Morton neuroma
morular cell
MOS
medical outcomes study
mosaic
m. genome
m. genome structure
m. pattern
Moschcowitz thrombotic thrombocytopenic purpura disease
MOS-HIV
medical outcomes study-human immunodeficiency virus
Mosler sign
mos protooncogene/oncogene
Mosse syndrome
Mossuril virus
Mostofi
M. classification
M. histologic typing
motexafin gadolinium
mother cell
mother-to-child transmission (MTCT)
motif
immunoreceptor tyrosine-based activation m. (ITAM)
protein m.
zinc finger m.
motile leukocyte

motility
antroduodenal m.
motion
perturbed water m.
Motofen
motor
m. cortex
m. neuronopathy
m. neuropathy
Motrin
Junior Strength M.
Mott
M. body
M. cell
mottling pattern
mountain anemia
mouth
floor of m.
Mouth-Aid
Orajel M.-A.
mouthwash
chamomile m.
chlorhexidine m.
magic m.
movement therapy
moving boundary electrophoresis
moving-strip technique
moxifloxacin
MP
melphalan, prednisolone
mesenteric panniculitis
methylprednisolone
ara-C + DNR + PRED + MP
6-MP
6-mercaptopurine
MPA
main pulmonary artery
medroxyprogesterone acetate
MPAC
Memorial Pain Assessment Card
MPD
main pancreatic duct
matched peripheral dose
maximum permissible dose
minimal peripheral dose
myeloproliferative disorder
MPFL
methotrexate, Platinol, 5-fluorouracil, leucovorin, calcium
MPGN
membranoproliferative glomerulonephritis
MPIF
myeloid progenitor inhibitory factor
MPIF-1
myeloid progenitor inhibitory factor-1
MPL
melphalan
MPL-containing liposome

MPL+PRED
melphalan plus prednisone
MPLV
myeloproliferative leukemia virus
MPM
malignant pleural mesothelioma
multiple primary melanoma
MPNST
malignant peripheral nerve sheath tumor
MPPT
methylprednisolone pulse therapy
MPQ
McGill Pain Questionnaire
M-Prednisol Injection
mps1-induced arrest
MPSC
micropapillary serous carcinoma
MPV
mean plasma volume
mean platelet volume
MPV nomogram
MQOL-HIV
Multidimensional Quality of Life
Questionnaire for Persons with Human
Immunodeficiency Virus
MR
magnetic resonance
MR arthrography
MR spectroscopy
1.5-T MR imaging system
MRC
Medical Research Council
mRCC
metastatic renal cell carcinoma
MRD
minimal residual disease
ICS-PCR for MRD
MRE
magnetic resonance elastography
MR-guided focused ultrasound
MRI
magnetic resonance imaging
dynamic contrast-enhanced MRI
echo planar MRI
fat-suppressed MRI
functional MRI
intravenous-enhanced MRI
IV-enhanced MRI
multiplanar MRI
proton-density-weighted MRI
RODEO MRI
spoiled gradient-recalled echo MRI
1.5 tesla MRI

MRI thermometry
ultrafast MRI
MRI-based stereotactic biopsy
MRM
matrix metalloproteinase inhibitor,
marimastat
modified radical mastectomy
mRNA
messenger RNA
rev mRNA
TNF-alpha mRNA
MRP
multidrug resistance protein
MRS
magnetic resonance spectroscopy
MS
mass spectrophotometer
mitral stenosis
morphine sulfate
multiple sclerosis
myasthenic syndrome
MS Contin
MS Contin Oral
MSA
mammary serum antigen
muscle-specific actin
MSA tumor marker
MSAFP
maternal serum alpha fetoprotein
MSAS
Memorial Symptom Assessment Scale
MSAS-Psych
Memorial Symptom Assessment Scale-
Psychological
MSB
MammoSite brachytherapy
MSCHN
metastatic squamous carcinoma of head
and neck
MS-CRS
morphine sulfate controlled-release
suppository
MSD
matched sibling donor
MSD Enteric-Coated ASA
MSH2 gene
MSH3 (hMSH3) gene
MSI
microsatellite instability
MSI testing
MST
malignant salivary gland tumor
median survival time

NOTES

M

MSTS
  American Musculoskeletal Tumor
    Society
mSv
  millisievert
MT
  magnetization transfer
  malignant teratoma
  metallothionein
MT-2 cell
MTA
  multitargeted antifolate
MTC
  medullary thyroid carcinoma
  mitomycin C
MTC-DOX
  doxorubicin adsorbed to magnetic
    targeted carrier
MTCT
  mother-to-child transmission
MTD
  maximum tolerated dose
M.T.E.-4
M.T.E.-5
M.T.E.-6
MTHFR
  methylenetetrahydrofolate reductase
MTI
  malignant teratoma, intermediate
MTN blot
MTP
  muramyl tripeptide
MTP-PE
  muramyl tripeptide
    phosphatidylethanolamine
    liposomal MTP-PE
M-tropic strain
MTS
  Muir-Torre syndrome
MTS1 gene
MTT
  malignant teratoma, trophoblastic
MTX
  methotrexate
    IT MTX
MTX/ara-C
  methotrexate and arabinoside C
    MTX/ara-C regimen
MTX, HiDAC, sequential CTX
MTX+MP
  methotrexate plus mercaptopurine
MTZ
  mitoxantrone
MU
  monitor unit
mu, μ
  mu meson
  mu receptor

MUAC
  middle upper arm circumference
MUC1 antigen
Mucha-Habermann disease
mucicarmine stain
mucin
  m. core protein
  m. core protein-1
  gastric m.
  intestinal m.
  monoclonal antibodies against
    gastric m.'s
mucinosa
  alopecia m.
mucinosis, pl. mucinoses
  alopecia mucinosa/follicular m.
    (AM/FM)
  follicular m.
  idiopathic follicular m.
  papular m.
mucinous
  m. adenocarcinoma
  m. adenocarcinoma of ovary
  m. cystadenocarcinoma
  m. cystadenoma
  m. cystadenoma of ovary
  m. duct ectasia
  m. eccrine carcinoma
  m. tumor
mucin-producing tumor
mucocele
  appendix m.
  breast m.
mucocutaneous
  m. candidiasis
  m. junction
  m. lesion
  m. lymph node syndrome (MLNS)
  m. reaction
mucoepidermoid
  m. carcinoma
  m. tumor
mucoid adenocarcinoma
Mucomyst
Mucoplex
mucopolypeptide
mucopolysaccharide
mucopolysaccharidosis,
  pl. **mucopolysaccharidoses**
mucoprotein
  Tamm-Horsfall m.
  TH m.
Mucor
mucormycosis
mucosa, pl. mucosae
  antral m.
  buccal m.
  deranged m.
  endocervical m.

gastric oxyntic m.
gingival m.
oral m.
oropharyngeal m.
rectal m.

mucosa-associated
m.-a. lymphoid tissue (MALT)
m.-a. lymphoid tissue function
m.-a. lymphoid tissue lymphoma
  (MALToma)

mucosal
m. barrier
m. biopsy
m. ecology
m. IgA
m. immune response
m. immunity
m. melanoma
m. neuroma
m. resection
m. thickening
m. toxicity
m. wave

mucositis
chemotherapy-related m.
oral m.
oropharyngeal m.
radiation m.

mucous
m. cell hyperplasia (MCH)
m. colitis
m. membrane
m. membrane exposure
m. patch

MUC1 antigen
MUC2 protein
MUD
matched unrelated donor
MUD transplant

Muehrcke line
Muenster protocol
MUGA
multiple gated acquisition
MUGA scan

mu-HCD
mu-heavy-chain disease

mu-heavy-chain disease (mu-HCD)
Muir-Torre
M.-T. syndrome (MTS)
M.-T. syndrome of hereditary
  nonpolyposis colon cancer

mulberry molar
mule-spinners' cancer

mullein
Müller
M. duct body
M. empyema
M. empyema catheter

müllerian
m. adenosarcoma
m. duct
m. duct formation and fusion
m. peritoneal tumor
m. sarcoma
m. sarcoma of uterus
m. structure
m. tumor

müllerian-inhibiting substance (MIS)
MulTE-PAK-4
MulTE-PAK-5
multiagent chemotherapy
multicenter
M. AIDS Cohort Study
M. European Radiofrequency
  Survey (MERFS)
M. Oral Carvedilol Heart Failure
  Assessment (MOCHA)
m. trial

multicentric
m. angiofollicular lymphoid
  hyperplasia
m. Castleman disease (MCD)
m. histiocytosis
m. malignant glioma
m. mammary carcinoma (MMC)

multicentricity
multiclonal follicular lymphoma
multiclonality
multicoil array technique
multicolony-stimulating factor
multicolor
m. data analysis
m. immunofluorescence
  measurement

multicopy suppressor screen
multidermatomal herpes zoster
multidimensional
m. analysis
m. analysis beam modifier
M. Fatigue Inventory (MFI, MFI-
  20)
M. Fatigue Symptom Inventory
m. flow cytometry
M. Quality of Life Questionnaire
  for Persons with Human

NOTES

M

multidimensional *(continued)*
> Immunodeficiency Virus (MQOL-HIV)

multidrug
> m. regimen
> m. resistance (MDR)
> m. resistance-associated mutation
> m. resistance detoxification
> m. resistance modulator
> m. resistance protein (MRP)

multidrug-resistant
> m.-r. phenotype
> m.-r. tuberculosis (MDR-TB)

multifactorial

multifocal
> m. area
> m. area of hyperintensity
> m. atrophic gastritis (MAG)
> m. encephalitis
> m. leukoencephalopathy
> m. myoclonus

multifocality
> tumor m.

multiforme
> erythema m.
> glioblastoma m. (GBM)
> granuloma m.
> supratentorial glioblastoma m.

multigene transcript

Multikine

multileaf collimator (MLC)

multilineage origin

multilobated
> m. nucleus
> m. T-cell lymphoma

multilocular
> m. cystic lesion
> m. peritoneal inclusion cyst

multilocularis
> *Echinococcus m.*

multilog effect

multimerization

multimodal
> m. physical therapy
> m. treatment

multimodality
> m. therapy
> m. treatment program

Multinational Association of Supportive Care in Cancer/International Society for Oral Oncology (MASCC/ISOO)

multinuclear leukocyte

multinucleated osteoclastic giant cell

multiparous

multipeptide

multiplanar
> m. gradient refocused
> m. imaging

> m. MRI
> m. reconstruction

multiple
> m. adjuvant
> m. agent therapy (MAT)
> m. basal cell neuroma syndrome
> m. core biopsies
> m. daily fraction
> m. drug resistance (MDR)
> m. endocrine neoplasia (MEN)
> m. endocrine neoplasia type 1 (MEN1)
> m. endocrine neoplasia type 2b
> m. endocrinoplasia
> m. endpoints
> m. epiphysial dysplasia (MED)
> m. gated acquisition (MUGA)
> m. gated acquisition scan
> m. hamartoma syndrome
> m. hereditary exostosis
> m. idiopathic hemorrhagic sarcoma
> m. intestinal neoplasia (MIN)
> m. lymphomatous polyposis
> m. marker reverse transcriptase-polymerase chain reaction assay
> m. myeloma (MM)
> m. myeloma staging
> m. myelomatosis
> m. noninguinal sites
> m. organ failure
> M. Outcomes for Raloxifene Evaluation (MORE)
> M. Outcomes of Raloxifene Evaluation trial
> m. primary melanoma (MPM)
> m. primary neoplasm
> m. sclerosis (MS)
> m. synchronous metastases

multiple-drug resistance gene

multiplex
> dysplasia epiphysealis m.
> mononeuritis m.
> mononeuropathy m.
> myeloma m.
> myelomatosis m.

multiplicities of infection (MOI)

multiploid tumor

multiploidy

multipotent hematopoietic progenitor

multipotential

Multi-Pro biopsy needle

multipuncture test

multistage Markov model

multisweep

multisystem organ failure

multitargeted
> m. antifolate (MTA)
> m. chemotherapy

multitherapy
 Di Bella m.
Multivane Intensity Modulation Compensator (MIMIC)
multivariate logistic regression analysis
multivitamin infusion-12 (MVI-12)
multivitamin-mineral formula
multivoxel spectroscopy
multocida
 Pasteurella m.
mummified cell
mumps
 m. skin test antigen
 m. virus
MUPIT
 Martinez Universal Perineal Interstitial Template
murabutide
mural thrombus
muramidase
muramyl
 m. dipeptide
 m. dipeptide derivative
 m. tripeptide (MTP)
 m. tripeptide phosphatidylethanolamine (MTP-PE)
murine
 m. colony-forming unit
 m. fibroblast transformation
 m. granulocyte-macrophage colony-stimulating growth factor
 m. interleukin
 m. interleukin-3
 m. interleukin-6
 m. interleukin-7
 m. interleukin-1B
 m. leukemia L1210
 m. leukemia P388
 m. L6 monoclonal antibody
 m. lymphocytic choriomeningitis virus
 m. macrophage
 m. melanoma
 m. monoclonal anticancer vaccine
 m. protein
 recombinant m. (rMu)
 m. sarcoma
 m. sarcoma virus
 m. tumor cell
murine-acquired immunodeficiency syndrome (MAIDS)

muris
 Cryptosporidium m.
muromonab-CD3
Murphy staging system
Murray Valley encephalitis virus
Murri disease
muscle
 abductor m.
 accessory m.
 m. actin
 anconeus m.
 ciliary m.
 constrictor m.
 detrusor m.
 digastric m.
 external oblique m.
 extraocular m.
 genioglossus m.
 geniohyoid m.
 m. hemoglobin
 hyoglossus m.
 intercostal m.
 levator ani m.
 levator veli palatini m.
 mylohyoid m.
 obturator internus m.
 omohyoid m.
 m. pain
 palatoglossus m.
 palatopharyngeus m.
 paralaryngeal m.
 pectineus m.
 pectoral m.
 pharyngeal constrictor m.
 piriformis m.
 m. relaxant
 m. sarcoma
 serratus anterior m.
 smooth m.
 sternocleidomastoid m.
 striated m.
 styloglossus m.
 tensor veli palatini m.
 transverse rectus abdominis m. (TRAM)
 vocalis m.
 m. weakness
muscle-specific actin (MSA)
muscular diaphragm
muscularis propria
musculoaponeurotic structure
musculocutaneous flap

NOTES

musculoskeletal
    m. infection
    m. system
musculus uvulae
mushroom
    maitake m.
music therapy
Musshoff modification
mustard
    Adriamycin plus L-phenylalanine m.
      (Adria + L-PAM, Adria + L-PAM)
    bleomycin, Adriamycin, CCNU,
      Oncovin, nitrogen m. (BACON)
    bleomycin, Adriamycin,
      methotrexate, Oncovin,
      nitrogen m. (BAMON)
    nitrogen m. (HN$_2$, NM)
    phenylalanine m. (PAM)
    L-phenylalanine m. (L-PAM)
    phosphoramide m.
    spirohydantoin m.
    uracil m. (UM)
Mustargen
    M., Adriamycin, bleomycin,
      Oncovin, prednisone (MABOP)
    M., Oncovin, bleomycin (MOB)
    M., Oncovin, procarbazine,
      prednisone
mutagen
mutagenesis
    m. assay
    insertional m.
mutagenicity
Mutamycin
    Lupron, Velban, Adriamycin, M.
      (L-VAM)
mutant
    m. cell
    m. gene
    m. Ras peptide-pulsed dendritic
      cell therapy
    site-directed m.
mutated in colon cancer (MCC)
mutation
    AT m. (ATM)
    BRCA1 m.
    BRCA1 gene m.
    BRCA gene m.
    cancerous m.
    cancer-related m.
    codon m.
    dominant lethal m.
    E-cadherin m.
    founder m.
    gain-of-function m.
    genetic m.
    germline m.
    Helicase m.
    m. in hematopoietic tissue

    hemojuvelin gene m.
    hepcidin gene m.
    Ig V gene m.
    K-ras m.
    missense m.
    mitochondrial DNA m.
    multidrug resistance-associated m.
    p53 gene m.
    Ras gene family point m.
    Rb m.
    resistance-associated m.
    resistance-conferring m.
    somatic m.
    threonine 215 tyrosine m.
    transcriptional m.
    wimp m.
mutational
    m. spectrum
    m. strategy
mutually monogamous relationship
MV
    mitomycin and vinblastine
    mitoxantrone and VP-16
MVAC
    methotrexate, vinblastine, Adriamycin,
      cisplatin
M-Vax vaccine
MVC
    mitoxantrone, vinblastine,
      cyclophosphamide
      MVC 9 + 3
MVD
    microvessel density
MVF
    mitoxantrone, vincristine, 5-fluorouracil
      MVF chemotherapy protocol
MVI-12
    multivitamin infusion-12
M.V.I.
    M.V.I. Concentrate
    M.V.I. Pediatric
MVP
    mitomycin, vinblastine, Platinol
    mitral valve prolapse
MVPP
    mechlorethamine, vinblastine,
      procarbazine, prednisone
MVT
    mitoxantrone, VePesid, thiotepa
    mitoxantrone, VP-16, thiotepa
      MVT chemotherapy protocol
MVVPP
    mechlorethamine, vincristine, vinblastine,
      procarbazine, prednisone
myalgia
Myambutol
myasthenia gravis
myasthenic syndrome (MS)

myb
    myb oncogene
    myb protein
    myb protooncogene/oncogene
myc
    myc epitope
    myc oncogene
    myc protein
    myc protooncogene/oncogene
Mycelex-G Topical
Mycelex Troche
mycetoma
Mycifradin Sulfate
Myciguent
Mycinettes
MYCN protooncogene
mycobacterial protein
mycobacteriosis
    atypical m.
    nontuberculous m.
Mycobacterium
    M. avium complex (MAC)
    M. avium-intracellulare (MAI)
    M. bovis
    M. chelonae
    M. fortuitum
    M. genavense
    M. gordonae
    M. haemophilum
    M. intracellulare
    M. kansasii
    M. leprae
    M. malmoense
    M. marinum
    M. scrofulaceum
    M. tuberculosis
    M. ulcerans
    M. xenopi
Mycobutin
Mycogen II Topical
Mycolog-II Topical
Myconel Topical
mycophenolate
    m. mofetil (MMF)
    m. mofetil HCl
Mycoplasma
    M. incognitus
    M. infection
    M. pneumoniae
mycoplasmal
Mycosel agar
mycosis, pl. **mycoses**

m. fungoides (MF)
m. fungoides/Sézary syndrome
Mycostatin
mycotic stomatitis
Mycotoruloides
Mycotoruloides
mycotoxin
Myco-Triacet II
myelin
    m. base protein (MBP)
    m. basic protein assay
    m. pallor
myelinolysis
    central pontine m. (CPM)
    extrapontine m.
myelitis
    late radiation m.
    radiation m.
    radiation-induced transverse m.
    transverse m.
myeloablation
myeloablative
    m. chemoradiotherapy
    m. chemotherapy
    m. conditioning
myeloblast
myeloblastic leukemia
myeloblastoma
myelocyte
    eosinophilic m.
myelocytic
    m. crisis
    m. leukemia
    m. leukemoid reaction
myelocytoma
myelocytomatosis
myelodysplasia
    de novo m.
    hypoplastic m.
    secondary m.
myelodysplastic
    m. cancer
    m. syndrome (MDS)
myelofibrosis
    acute m.
    idiopathic m.
    m. with myeloid metaplasia (MMM)
myelogenic
    m. leukemia
    m. sarcoma
myelogenous leukemia

NOTES

myelogram
    cervical m.
myelographic block
myelography
    extraarachnoid m.
    staging m.
myeloid
    m. blood element
    m. colony-forming capacity
    m. depletion
    m. disease
    m. engraftment
    m. growth factor
    m. leukemia
    m. lineage antigen
    m. marker
    m. metaplasia
    m. precursor cell
    m. progenitor
    m. progenitor factor 1
    m. progenitor inhibitory factor
      (MPIF)
    m. progenitor inhibitory factor-1
      (MPIF-1)
    m. sarcoma
myeloid-associated antigen
myeloid/erythroid (M/E)
    m./e. ratio
myelokathexis
myeloleukemia
myelolipoma
    adrenal m.
myelolymphocyte
myeloma
    amyloidosis of multiple m.
    Bence Jones m.
    CALLA-positive m.
    m. cell
    Durie-Salmon classification of
      multiple m.
    endothelial m.
    giant cell m.
    m. kidney
    L-chain m.
    malignant m. (MM)
    multiple m. (MM)
    m. multiplex
    nonsecreting m.
    nonsecretory m.
    osteosclerotic m.
    plasma cell m.
    m. protein
    smoldering multiple m.
    solitary m.
myeloma-induced amyloidosis
myelomalacia
    cystic m.

myelomatosis
    multiple m.
    m. multiplex
myelomonoblastic leukemia
myelomonocyte
myelomonocytic
    m. antigen
    m. leukemia
    m. leukemia, chronic (CMML,
      MLC)
    m. leukemia, subacute (MLS)
Myelo-Nate
    M.-N. kit
    M.-N. needle
    M.-N. set
myelopathic anemia
myelopathy
    carcinomatous m.
    cystic m.
    paracarcinomatous m.
    vacuolar m.
myeloperoxidase stain
myelophthisic anemia
myelophthisis marrow
myelopoiesis
myelopoietin growth factor
myeloproliferative
    m. disorder (MPD)
    m. leukemia virus (MPLV)
myelosarcoma
myelosarcomatosis
myelosclerosis
myelosis
    aleukemic m.
    chronic megakaryocytic m.
    chronic nonleukemic m.
    erythremic m.
    leukemic m.
    leukopenic m.
    nonleukemic m.
    subleukemic m.
myelosuppression
    m. chemotherapy
    dose-limiting m.
myelosuppressive chemotherapy
myelotomy
    commissural m.
myelotoxic drug
myelotoxicity
    chemotherapy-induced m.
myiasis
    furuncular m.
Mykrox
myl
    myl oncogene
    myl protooncogene/oncogene
Myleran
Mylocel tablet
mylohyoid muscle

Mylotarg
Mylovenge therapeutic vaccine
myoablative therapy
myoblast
myoblastoma
    granular cell m.
myocardia (*pl. of* myocardium)
myocardial
    m. cell
    m. fibrosis
    m. function
    m. infarction (MI)
    m. ischemia
    m. perfusion imaging
    m. toxicity
myocarditis
myocardium, pl. myocardia
Myocet and Herceptin
myoclonus
    multifocal m.
myocutaneous
    m. flap
    transverse rectus abdominis m.
    (TRAM)
myocytoma
myoD
    myoD gene
    myoD protein
myoepithelial
    m. differentiation
    m. sialadenitis
myoepithelioma
    malignant m. (MME)
myofibrillar dropout
myofibroblastic
    m. feature
    m. tumor
myofibroblastoma
    intranodal m.
myofibrohistiocytic proliferation
myofibroma
Myoflex
myogenesis
myoglobin
myoid cell
myointimal hyperplasia
myokymia
myokymic discharge
myoma, pl. myomata
    intraligamentous m.

myomalacia
myomatous polyp
myomectomy
myometrium
myopathy
    azidothymidine m.
    AZT m.
    carcinomatous m.
    steroid m.
myopharyngeal stricture
Myoplex
myosarcoma
myosis
    endolymphatic stromal m.
myositis
    necrotizing m.
myristate
myristic acid
myristoylation
myristoyl-coenzyme A
Mysoline
Mytrex F Topical
myxedematosus
    lichen m.
myxochondrofibrosarcoma
myxofibroma
myxofibrosarcoma
myxoid
    m. cell pattern
    extraskeletal m.
    m. liposarcoma
    m. stroma
myxoma, pl. myxomata, myxomas
    atrial m.
    reaction intramuscular m.
    m. sarcomatosum
myxomatodes
    carcinoma m.
myxopapillary ependymoma
myxosarcoma
myxovirus
MZ2-MEL clonal cell line
MZBCL
    marginal zone B-cell lymphoma
M-Zole 7 Dual Pack

M

NOTES

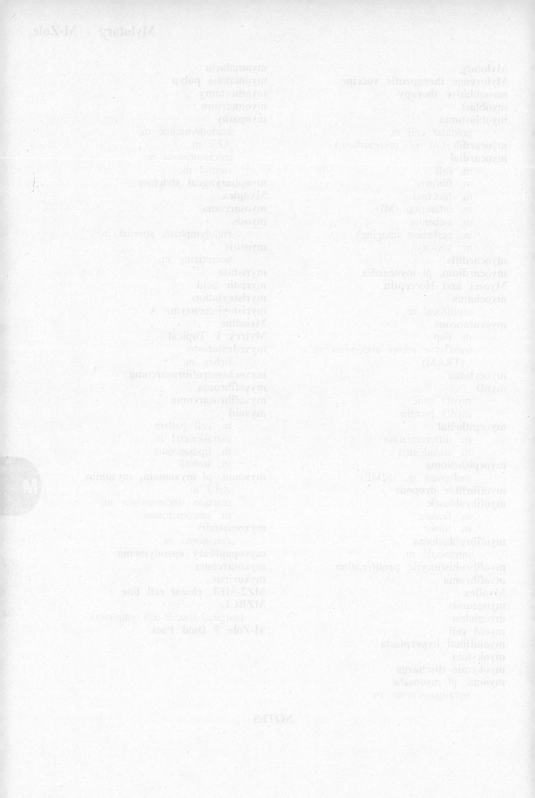

N
Alferon N
N-9
nonoxynol-9
N901 blocked ricin
Na
sodium
²³Na
sodium-23
²⁴Na
sodium-24
NAAD
neoadjuvant androgen deprivation
nabilone
NABTT
new approaches to brain tumor therapy
nabumetone
NAC
N-acetyl-L-cysteine
nitrogen mustard, Adriamycin, CCNU
N-acetylation polymorphism
N-acetyl-b-D-glucosaminidase
N-acetyl-L-cysteine (NAC)
N-acetyltransferase
NACT
neoadjuvant chemotherapy
NAD
no active disease
no appreciable disease
nadir blood count
Nadopen-V
Nadostine
NADPH, NADP
nicotinamide adenine dinucleotide
phosphate
NADPH enzyme
NADPH-dependent oxidase
Naegeli
N. type
N. type of monocytic leukemia
NAF
nipple aspirate fluid
nipple aspiration fluid
nafamostat mesylate
nafcillin
nafidimide
naftifine
Naftin
Nageotte cell
nail
n. hyperpigmentation
Jewett n.
Smith-Petersen n.
naive T cell

naked DNA vector vaccine
Na-K exchange pump
nalbuphine
Nalfon
nalidixic acid
Nallpen
naloxone (NX)
naltrexone
NA-MYCN gene
nana
Hymenolepis n.
nandrolone phenpropionate
nanocolloid
technetium-labeled n.
nanodosimetry
nanogram
NanoInvasive therapy
nanomolar concentration
nanoparticle
naphthalene sulfonate polymer
naphthyl
alpha n.
naphthylurea
polysulfonated n.
napkin-ring lesion
Naprosyn
naproxen
Naqua
Nardil
narrow
n. collimation
n. interscan interval
narrowing
arteriolar n.
colonic n.
degenerative n.
disc space n.
duodenal n.
esophageal n.
NARS
neuropsychiatric-acquired
immunodeficiency syndrome
NARS rating scale
NART
National Adult Reading Test
nasal
n. cavity cancer
n. fossa tumor
n. spray
n. T-cell/natural killer cell
lymphoma
n. thickening
n. vestibule
n. vestibule cancer

N

Nasalcrom
nasobiliary tube (NBT)
nasogastric (NG)
   n. feeding
nasopharyngeal
   n. cancer
   n. carcinoma (NPC)
   n. carcinoma in situ (NPCIS)
nasopharynx cancer
NAT
   nucleic acid testing
      HCV-RNA NAT
national
   N. Adult Reading Test (NART)
   N. Alliance of Breast Cancer
      Organizations
   N. Association of Tumor Registrars
      (NATR)
   N. Cancer Institute
   N. Cancer Institute Common
      Toxicity Criteria (NCI-CTC)
   N. Cancer Institute Cooperative
      Group
   N. Cancer Institute Protocol 89-C-
      41
   N. Center for Complementary and
      Alternative Medicine (NCCAM)
   N. Center for Health Statistics
      (NCHS)
   N. Childhood Cancer Foundation
   N. Coalition for Cancer
      Survivorship
   N. Collaborative Diethylstilbestrol
      Adenosis Project (DESAD)
   N. Colorectal Cancer Roundtable
      (NCCRT)
   N. Comprehensive Cancer Network
      (NCCN)
   N. Institute of Allergy and
      Infectious Disease (NIAID)
   N. Institutes of Health (NIH)
   N. Institute of Standards and
      Technology (NIST)
   N. Lung Transplant Patient
      Association
   N. Marrow Donor Program
      (NMDP)
   N. Prostatic Cancer Project criteria
   N. Surgical Adjuvant Breast and
      Bowel Project (NSABP)
   N. Surgical Adjuvant Breast
      Project (NSABP)
   N. Wilms Tumor Study (NWTS)
native
   n. L-asparaginase
   n. immunity
NATR
   National Association of Tumor Registrars

Natulan
natural
   n. antibody
   n. disease
   n. history
   n. killer (NK)
   n. killer activity
   n. killer cell
   n. killer cell antigen
   n. killer cell leukemia
   n. killer-like T-cell lymphoma
   n. killer lymphocyte
   n. selection theory
   n. variation
natural-end cancer
Naturetin
nausea
   intractable n.
Navelbine
Navigator gamma ray detector
NAWM
   normal-appearing white matter
Naxen
NBCC
   nevoid basal cell carcinoma
NBCCS
   nevoid basal cell carcinoma syndrome
NB-DNJ
   N-butyldeoxynojirimycin
NBS
   Nijmegen breakage syndrome
NBT
   nasobiliary tube
N-butyldeoxynojirimycin (NB-DNJ)
NC
   nucleocapsid
9-NC, 9NC
   9-nitrocamptothecin
NCCAM
   National Center for Complementary and
      Alternative Medicine
NCCN
   National Comprehensive Cancer Network
NCCRT
   National Colorectal Cancer Roundtable
NCHS
   National Center for Health Statistics
NCI-CTC
   National Cancer Institute Common
      Toxicity Criteria
NCT
   neoadjuvant chemotherapy
NDF
   neu differentiation factor
NDK-K
   nucleoside 5'-diphosphate kinase
NDMA
   N-nitrosodimethylamine

NDV
    Newcastle disease virus
    NDV therapy
Nd:YAG laser
NE
    neuroendocrine
    neutropenic enterocolitis
NEAD
    near-UV excited autofluorescence
      diagnosis
    NEAD system
Nearly Me breast form
near-total thyroidectomy
near-UV
    n.-UV excited autofluorescence
      diagnosis (NEAD)
    n.-UV excited autofluorescence
      diagnosis system
Nebcin Injection
nebulizer
    DeVilbiss n.
    Emerson-Segal Medimizer
      demand n.
    Fisons n.
    jet n.
    PulmoMate n.
    Schuco n.
    Selrodo n.
NebuPent Inhalation
NEC
    neuroendocrine carcinoma
neck
    metastatic squamous carcinoma of
      head and n. (MSCHN)
    osteosarcoma of head and n.
      (OSHN)
    n. region-lifting method
    squamous cell carcinoma of head
      and n. (SCCHN)
necrobiotic xanthogranuloma
necrogranulomatous keratitis
necrolysis
necrolytic migratory erythema
necropsy specimen
necrosis, pl. **necroses**
    acute tubular n.
    aortic wall n.
    aseptic n.
    avascular n. (AVN)
    coagulation n.
    coagulative tumor cell n.
    cortical n.
    cystic medial n.

    fast n.
    hemorrhagic n.
    histologic coagulative tumor n.
    radiation n.
    subcutaneous fat n.
    tumor cell n.
necrotic
    n. cell death
    n. core
    n. ulceration
necrotizing
    n. fasciitis
    n. myositis
    n. stomatitis
    n. superficial tracheobronchitis
    n. ulcerative gingivitis
NED
    no evidence of disease
NED-SD
    no evidence of disease-stationary disease
needle
    Abrams biopsy n.
    abscission n.
    Accucore II biopsy n.
    Ackermann n.
    Amersham CDCS A-type n.
    Amplatz angiography n.
    Amplatz TLA n.
    aspiration n.
    atraumatic n.
    Autovac n.
    Baltaxe-Mitty-Pollack n.
    Bauer Temno biopsy n.
    BD bone marrow biopsy n.
    beveled-tip n.
    Bierman n.
    biopsy n.
    n. biopsy
    Biopty-Cut biopsy n.
    Buerger prostatic n.
    butterfly n.
    cesium n.
    Chiba n.
    Conrad-Crosby bone marrow
      biopsy n.
    Cope biopsy n.
    dumbbell n.
    Eclipse blood collection n.
    Ferris bone marrow aspiration n.
    flexible biopsy n.
    Franklin-Silverman biopsy n.
    Franseen n.

N

NOTES

needle *(continued)*
    Goldenberg Snarecoil bone marrow
      biopsy n.
    guaiac n.
    Hagedorn n.
    hollow n.
    Indian club n.
    Jamshidi adult n.
    Jamshidi-Kormed bone marrow
      biopsy n.
    Jamshidi liver biopsy n.
    Jamshidi muscle biopsy n.
    Klatskin n.
    Kobak n.
    Kopans n.
    Mick afterloading n.
    Multi-Pro biopsy n.
    Myelo-Nate n.
    noncoring Huber n.
    percutaneous n.
    Pharmaseal n.
    pleural biopsy n.
    n. puncture
    ^{226}Ra n.
    Ring drainage catheter n.
    Rosenthal aspiration n.
    Rotex n.
    Rutner biopsy n.
    scalp vein n.
    sheathed n.
    skinny n.
    Sure-Cut n.
    2-n. technique
    Teflon-coated n.
    Temno biopsy n.
    Terry-Mayo n.
    tie-on n.
    Tocantins bone marrow biopsy n.
    n. track
    transaxillary n.
    Travenol biopsy n.
    trocar n.
    Tru-Cut liver biopsy n.
    Turkel n.
    Tworek bone marrow-aspirating n.
    Vacutainer n.
    Veenema-Gusberg prostatic
      biopsy n.
    Veress n.
    Vim-Silverman n.
    Waterfield n.
    Westcott n.
    Zavala lung biopsy n.
NEF
  negative factor
nef
    n. expression
    n. gene

    n. gene-deleted virus
    n. protein
nef-deleted virus
negative
    n. angiogenic molecule
    breakpoint cluster region-n. (BCR-
      negative)
    E rosette n.
    n. factor (NEF)
    fluorescent dye efflux n.
    guaiac n.
    Philadelphia chromosome n. (Ph-
      negative)
    n. pi meson
    replication error n. (RER−)
    Rh n.
    n. selection procedure
    tumor receptor protein n.
NegGram
Negri
    N. body
    N. corpuscle
Neill-Mooser body
Neisser granule
Neisseria gonorrhoeae
neisserial
Neisser-Wechsberg leukocidin
nelarabine
nelfinavir mesylate
Nelson
    N. syndrome
    N. tumor
nemestrina
    Macaca n.
neoadjuvant
    n. androgen deprivation (NAAD)
    n. chemotherapy (NACT, NCT)
    n. therapy
neoangiogenesis
    bone marrow n.
neoantigen
neoantigenic
neobladder
    Hemi-Kock n.
    orthotopic n.
Neo-Calglucon
neocarzinostatin
Neo-Codema
neocytosis
neodymium:yttrium-aluminum-garnet
Neo-Estrone
neoformans
    Cryptococcus n.
Neo-fradin
neoglycoprotein
neogullet
NeoLipid compound
Neoloid
Neomark

Neo-Minophagen
    Stronger N.-M. C
neomycin and polymyxin B
neonatal anemia
neonatorum
    anemia n.
    hemophilia n.
    icterus n.
neon particle
Neopap
neoplasia
    anal intraepithelial n. (AIN)
    anogenital squamous
      intraepithelial n.
    B-cell n.
    cervical intraepithelial n. (CIN)
    colon n.
    endocrine n.
    endometrial intraepithelial n. (EIN)
    esophagogastric n.
    gestational trophoblastic n.
    high-grade prostatic
      intraepithelial n. (HGPIN)
    Hürthle cell n.
    intraepithelial n.
    lobular n.
    multiple endocrine n. (MEN)
    multiple endocrine n. type 1
      (MEN1)
    multiple endocrine n. type 2b
    multiple intestinal n. (MIN)
    ovarian intraepithelial n.
    preinvasive urothelial n.
    prostatic intraepithelial n. (PIN)
    vulvar intraepithelial n. (VIN)
neoplasm
    actin-positive spindle cell n.
    adrenal n.
    adrenocortical n.
    alpha islet cell n.
    autochthonous n.
    B-cell n.
    biliary n.
    bone n.
    borderline malignant epithelial
      ovarian n.
    bronchopulmonary n.
    cavitating n.
    cervical intraepithelial n. (CIN)
    choroid plexus n.
    colonic n.
    connective tissue n.
    cranial nerve n.

    cutaneous n.
    cystic adrenal n.
    ductectatic mucinous cystic n.
    dysontogenetic n.
    epithelial n.
    esophageal n.
    external ear n.
    extrahepatic n.
    fibrillary astrocytic n.
    germ cell n.
    gestational trophoblastic n.
    glioneuronal n.
    hematologic n.
    hematopoietic n.
    hepatic n.
    hernia n.
    histiocytic n.
    histoid n.
    hypercellular cartilaginous n.
    indigenous n.
    indolent lymphoid n.
    intraaxial n.
    intracranial n.
    intraductal mucin-hypersecreting n.
    intraductal papillary mucinous n.
      (IPMN)
    intraepithelial n.
    intrahepatic biliary n.
    intramedullary compartment n.
    islet cell n.
    isologous n.
    large intestine n.
    laryngeal n.
    lipid cell n.
    lymphoid n.
    malignant epithelial n.
    mediastinal n.
    mesenchymal n.
    multiple primary n.
    neuroendocrine n.
    ovarian lipid cell n.
    ovarian malignant epithelial n.
    papillary cystic n.
    pearly n.
    pineal gland n.
    plasma cell n.
    primary n.
    prostate n.
    radiation-induced n. (RIN)
    second malignant n. (SMN)
    skeletal n.
    smooth muscle n.
    spindle cell n.

NOTES

N

neoplasm *(continued)*
    n. staging
    supratentorial extraventricular
      ependymal n.
    T-cell n.
    thoracic spinal n.
    thymic epithelial n.
    transitional cell n.
    trochlear nerve n.
    trophoblastic n.
    vaginal intraepithelial n. (VAIN)
    vulvar intraepithelial n. (VIN)
neoplastic
    n. acini
    n. angiogenesis
    n. arachnoiditis
    n. cell
    n. clone
    n. follicle
    n. lesion
    n. lymphocyte
    n. meningitis
    n. polyp
    n. proliferating
      angioendotheliomatosis
    n. state
    n. urothelium
neoplasticum
    Gongylonema n.
neopterin
Neoral
    Sandimmune N.
Neosar
NeoSpect diagnostic imaging agent
Neosporin G.U. Irrigant
Neo-Tabs
NeoTect imaging agent
Neotrace-4
Neotrofin
NeoVadrin B Complex
neovagina
neovasculature
    tumor n.
Neovastat
nephelometric immunoassay
nephrectomy
    radical n.
nephritis
    acute diffuse bacterial n.
    acute focal bacterial n.
    acute interstitial n. (AIN)
    bacterial n.
    chronic n.
    diffuse bacterial n.
    hereditary n. (HN)
    hereditary chronic n.
    Heymann n.
    interstitial n.
    Masugi n.

    radiation n.
    tubulointerstitial n.
nephroblastoma
    cystic partially differentiated n.
    polycystic n.
Nephro-Calci
nephrocalcinosis
Nephro-Fer
nephrogenic
    n. adenoma
    n. metaplasia
    n. rest
nephroma
    congenital mesoblastic n.
    cystic n.
    mesoblastic n.
nephromalacia
nephron-sparing surgery
nephropathic cystinosis
nephropathy
    analgesic n.
    Balkan n.
    biopsy-proven typical n.
    HIV-associated n.
    human immunodeficiency virus-
      associated n.
    radiation n.
    typical n.
    uric acid n.
nephrosclerosis
    malignant n.
nephroscope
    flexible n.
    percutaneous n.
    rigid n.
nephroscopy
    percutaneous n.
nephrostolithotomy
    caliceal n.
nephrostomy
    percutaneous n.
nephrotic syndrome
nephrotoxicity
    cisplatin n.
nephrotoxin
    concurrent n.
nephroureterectomy
Nephrox Suspension
neptamustine
NER
    no evidence of recurrence
NERD
    no evidence of recurrent disease
nerve
    accessory n.
    acoustic n.
    alveolar n.
    n. block
    n. cell tumor

facial n.
n. growth factor
intercostal n.
Jacobson n.
laryngeal n.
lingual n.
n. paralysis
peripheral n.
phrenic n.
recurrent laryngeal n.
sarcoma of peripheral n.
n. sheath malignant tumor
spinal accessory n.
trigeminal n.
trochlear n.
vagus n.

nerve-sparing
n.-s. cryosurgery
n.-s. radical retropubic
prostatectomy

nervosa
anorexia n.

nervous system

NESP
novel erythropoiesis-stimulating protein

nest
cancer n.
solid cell n.
squamoid n.
Walthard n.

nested primer

NET
neuroendocrine tumor

netilmicin

network
artificial neural n. (ANN)
cytokine n.
Early Detection Research N.
(EDRN)
human immunodeficiency virus
project n. (HIVNET)
National Comprehensive Cancer N.
(NCCN)
neural n.
n. theory

neu
neu differentiation factor (NDF)
neu oncogene

Neufeld reaction

Neulasta

Neumann cell

Neumega

Neumune

Neupogen

neural
n. cell adhesion molecule
n. network
n. tissue

neuraminidase

neuraxial
n. desmoplastic neuroepithelial
tumor
n. opioid infusion

neuraxis
n. radiation
n. radiotherapy
n. staging
n. tumor

neuregulin

neurilemoma
Antoni n.

neurinoma
acoustic n.

neuritis
ethambutol-induced optic n.
herpetic n.
optic n.

neuroablation

neuroablative technique

neuroadenolysis

neuroanatomic modification

neuroaugmentation

neuroblastoma
cerebral n.
connatal n.
Evans stages of n. (I–IV)
hemorrhagic n.
intracranial n.
occult n.
olfactory n. (ONB)

neurocutaneous syndrome

neurocytoma
central n.

neurodevelopment testing

neurodiagnostic evaluation

neuroectoderma
primitive n.

neuroectodermal tumor

neuroendocrine (NE)
n. cancer
n. carcinoma (NEC)
n. cell
n. differentiation
n. neoplasm
n. small cell carcinoma
n. tumor (NET)

N

NOTES

neuroepithelial tumor
neuroepithelioma
    primitive n.
neurofibroma
    aryepiglottic fold n.
    cutaneous n.
    facial n.
    plexiform n.
    skin n.
    storiform n.
neurofibromatosis (NF)
    abortive n.
    n. 2 gene
    segmental n.
    von Recklinghausen n.
neurofibromin
neurofibrosarcoma
neurogastrointestinal peptide
neurogenic
    n. sarcoma
    n. tumor
neuroimaging
neuroimmunology
neurokinin-1 (NK₁)
    n.-1 antagonist aprepitant
    n.-1 receptor antagonist
neuroleptic
    n. agent
    n. malignant syndrome
neuroleukin
neurologic
    n. abnormality
    n. adverse effect
    n. assessment
    n. examination
    n. infection
    n. paraneoplastic syndrome
neurolysis
    celiac plexus n.
    intrathecal n.
neurolytic nerve block
neuroma
    acoustic n.
    digital n.
    facial n.
    Morton n.
    mucosal n.
    postamputation n.
    trigeminal n.
neuromatosa
    elephantiasis n.
neuromedin B receptor (NMB-R)
neuromuscular
    n. function
    n. toxicity
neuromyopathy
    carcinomatous n.

neuronal
    n. apoptotic process
    n. tumor
neuronal-glial tumor
neuronopathy
    motor n.
    sensory n.
    subacute motor n.
    subacute sensory n.
neuron-restrictive silencing factor
neuron-specific
    n.-s. enolase (NSE)
    n.-s. enolase tumor marker
Neurontin
neurooncology
    tumor n.
neuropathic pain
neuropathicum
neuropathy
    acute n.
    carcinomatous n.
    chemotherapy-induced peripheral n.
    compression n.
    cranial n.
    cryptococcal optic n.
    dose-limiting n.
    hereditary motor-sensory n.
    inflammatory n.
    motor n.
    optic n.
    oxaliplatin-induced n.
    paraneoplastic sensorimotor
      peripheral n.
    paraneoplastic sensory n.
    peripheral n.
    postherpetic n.
    sensorimotor peripheral n.
    sensory n.
    trigeminal n.
    Vinca-related n.
neuropilin (NRP)
    n. 1 (NRP1)
    n. 2 (NRP2)
    n. 1, 2 assay
neuropraxia
neuropsychiatric-acquired
    n.-a. immunodeficiency syndrome
      (NARS)
    n.-a. immunodeficiency syndrome
      rating scale
neuropsychological test profile
neuroradiological findings
neuroradiology
    American Society of N. (ASN)
neurorehabilitation strategy
neurosarcoidosis
neurosarcoma
neurosecretory granule
neurosensory retina

Neurostat Mark II cryoanalgesia system
neurostimulating procedure
neurosurgery
    ablative n.
neurosurgical approach
neurosyphilis
    asymptomatic n.
    n. cryptomeningitis
    symptomatic n.
neurotensin
    n. receptor type 1 (NT-R-1)
    n. receptor type 2 (NT-R-2)
    n. receptor type 3 (NT-R-3)
neurotensinoma
neuroticum
neurotized melanocytic nevus (NMN)
neurotoxicity
    peripheral n.
neurovascular bundle (NVB)
Neu-Sensamide
neutral
    n. endopeptidase
    K-Phos N.
neutralization
    cisplatin n.
    n. epitope
    n. index method
neutralizing
    n. antibody
    n. antibody to vascular endothelial
      growth factor
Neutra-Phos-K
NeuTrexin
neutron
    n. beam
    n. beam radiation
    n. capture therapy
    fast n.
    n. technique
    n. therapy machine
neutropenia
    acquired n.
    autoimmune n.
    benign ethnic n.
    congenital n.
    drug-induced n.
    ethnic n.
    febrile n.
    high-grade n.
    immune n.
    severe congenital n.
neutropenia-related bacterial infection

neutropenic
    n. colitis
    n. enterocolitis (NE)
    n. fever
neutrophil
    n. alkaline phosphatase
    n. engraftment
    n. lobe count
    n. migration
    n. migration-inhibition factor
    Pelger-Huët n.
    polymorphonuclear n.
    n. pooling
    n. recovery
    n. reserve
neutrophil-activating peptide
neutrophilia
neutrophilic
    n. cell
    n. eccrine hidradenitis
    n. leukemia
    n. leukocyte
    n. leukocytosis
    n. xanthoma
neutrophilopenia
neutropoiesis
nevi (*pl. of* nevus)
Nevin staging
nevirapine
nevocellular nevus
nevoid
    n. basal cell cancer syndrome
    n. basal cell carcinoma (NBCC)
    n. basal cell carcinoma syndrome
      (NBCCS)
nevoxanthoendothelioma
nevus, pl. **nevi**
    atypical n.
    Becker pigmented hairy
      epidermal n.
    benign n.
    cellular blue n.
    choroidal n.
    common acquired n.
    dysplastic n.
    ectopic n.
    epidermal n.
    epithelial cell n.
    n. flammeus
    giant melanocytic n.
    hairy epidermal n.
    inflammatory linear epidermal n.
    linear epidermal n.

NOTES

nevus *(continued)*
    mast cell n.
    melanocytic n.
    neurotized melanocytic n. (NMN)
    nevocellular n.
    organoid n.
    sebaceous n.
    n. sebaceus
    spindle cell n.
    Spitz n.
    systematized epidermal n.
    n. verrucosis
    n. of vulva
    white sponge n.
new
    n. approaches to brain tumor therapy (NABTT)
    n. approaches to coronary intervention
    n. bone formation
    N. International Staging System
    n. methylene blue N stain
    n. tuberculin
newborn
    hemolytic anemia of n.
    hemolytic disease of n.
Newcastle
    N. disease
    N. disease virus (NDV)
    N. disease virus therapy
Newman-Keuls procedure
Newvicon camera tube
Nezelof
    N. syndrome
    N. type of thymic alymphoplasia
NF
    neurofibromatosis
NF-κB, NF-kB
    nuclear factor kappa beta
NF-1 gene
NF-2 gene
NFAT
    nuclear factor of activated T cell
NF-kB *(var. of NF-κB)*
    nuclear factor kappa beta
NFL
    Novantrone, 5-fluorouracil, leucovorin
N-2 fluorenylacetamide
NG
    nasogastric
Ng-monomethyl-L-arginine
NGR-endostatin
NHL
    non-Hodgkin lymphoma
NHS-activated HiTrap affinity column
NHTL
    non-Hodgkin thyroid lymphoma
N-(4-hydroxyphenyl)retinamide (4-HPR)
niacin

NIAID
    National Institute of Allergy and Infectious Disease
Niaspan
Nichols radioimmunoassay
nick translation
nicotinamide
    accelerated radiotherapy with carbogen and n. (ARCON)
    n. adenine dinucleotide
    n. adenine dinucleotide phosphate (NADPH, NADP)
nicotine
    n. dependence
    n. stomatitis
Nicotinex
NICTH
    non-islet cell tumor hypoglycemia
NIDDM
    non-insulin-dependent diabetes mellitus
Niemann-Pick disease
nifedipine
Niferex
Niferex-PN
niger
    Aspergillus n.
night sweats
nigra
    dermatosis papulosis n.
nigricans
    acanthosis n.
Nigro protocol
niguldipine
NIH
    National Institutes of Health
Nijmegen breakage syndrome (NBS)
Nikiforoff method
Nilandron
NI-leucyldoxorubicin (Leu-Dox)
Nilstat
nilutamide
nimodipine
nimorazole
Nimotop
nimustine (ACNU)
Nipent
Nippe test
nipple
    adenoma of n.
    aortic n.
    n. aspirate fluid (NAF)
    n. aspiration cytology
    n. aspiration fluid (NAF)
    deep to n.
    n. discharge
    n. duct lavage
    n. involvement
    Paget disease of n.
    supernumerary n.

nipple-areolar reconstruction
NIST
> National Institute of Standards and Technology

nitazoxanide (NTZ)
nitrate
> gallium n.
> vinblastine, ifosfamide, gallium n. (VIG)

nitric
> n. oxide (NO)
> n. oxide hemoglobin
> n. oxide synthase

nitrite
> amyl n.

nitroaromatic
nitrobenzylthioinosine
Nitro-Bid Ointment
nitroblue tetrazolium
9-nitrocamptothecin (9-NC, 9NC)
Nitro-Dur Patch
nitrofurantoin
Nitrogard Buccal
nitrogen
> blood urea n. (BUN)
> liquid n.
> n. mustard (HN$_2$, NM)
> n. mustard, Adriamycin, CCNU (NAC)
> n. mustard, vincristine, procarbazine, prednisone/doxorubicin, bleomycin, vinblastine

nitrogen-phosphorus detector
nitroglycerin
Nitroglyn Oral
nitroimidazole compound
Nitrolingual Translingual Spray
Nitrol Ointment
Nitrong
> N. Oral Tablet
> N. SR

nitrosamine
> tobacco-specific n. (TSNA)

nitrosomethylurea
nitrosourea
> methyl n.

Nitrostat Sublingual
nitrous oxide
nitroxide tempo molecule
NIVA
> noninvasive vascular assessment

> arterial NIVA
> venous NIVA

NIZ
> noninfarct zone

Nizoral
NK
> natural killer
> NK activity
> NK cell

NK$_1$
> neurokinin-1
> NK$_1$ antagonist aprepitant
> NK$_1$ CNS receptor

N-linked glycosylated site
NM
> nitrogen mustard
> nuclear medicine

nm23 gene
nm23-H1 protein
NMB-R
> neuromedin B receptor

NMDP
> National Marrow Donor Program

N-methyl-D-aspartate
N-methylhydrazine
NMN
> neurotized melanocytic nevus

N-monomethyl-L-arginine (L-MNA)
NMP
> nuclear matrix protein

NMP22 test kit
NMR
> nuclear magnetic resonance
> continuous-wave NMR
> NMR spectroscopy

NMSC
> nonmelanoma skin cancer

N-myc
> *N-myc* copy number
> N-myc oncogene

N-myristoyl
> N-m. glycine
> N-m. transferase

N,N-diethyl-2-[4-(phenylmethyl)phenoxy]ethanamine.HCl
NNI site
N-nitroso compound (NOC)
N-nitrosodimethylamine (NDMA)
NNRTI
> nonnucleoside reverse transcriptase inhibitor

NO
> nitric oxide

NOTES

N

no
- no active disease (NAD)
- no appreciable disease (NAD)
- no evidence of disease (NED)
- no evidence of disease-stationary disease (NED-SD)
- no evidence of recurrence (NER)
- no evidence of recurrent disease (NERD)
- no response (NR)

NOC
- N-nitroso compound

Nocardia
- *N. asteroides*
- *N. pneumonia*

nocardiosis
- granulomatous n.
- pulmonary n.

nociceptive pain
nocodazole
nodal
- n. basin
- n. enlargement
- n. hypodensity
- n. marginal zone B-cell lymphoma
- n. metastasis
- n. sampling
- n. staging procedure

nodal enlargement
node
- accessory lymph n.
- antetracheal n.
- aortic lymph n.
- atrioventricular n.
- A-V n.
- axillary lymph n. (ALN)
- axillary sentinel lymph n. (ASLN)
- azygos lymph n.
- cartilaginous n.
- celiac lymph n.
- cervical lymph n.
- Cloquet n.
- common iliac lymph n.
- diaphragmatic lymph n.
- facial lymph n.
- first-echelon lymph n.
- Henson n.
- hilar lymph n.
- hot n.
- hypogastric n.
- iliac lymph n.
- infraclavicular lymph n.
- interaortocaval lymph n.
- internal mammary chain of lymph n.'s (IMC)
- intramammary lymph n. (intraMLN)
- Irish n.
- jugulodigastric n.
- lymph n.

- mediastinal lymph n.
- mesenteric lymph n.
- mesorectal lymph n.
- nonsentinel lymph n. (NSN)
- obturator lymph n.
- paraaortic lymph n.
- paracaval lymph n.
- parotid lymph n.
- pelvic lymph n.
- periaortic lymph n.
- precaval lymph n.
- retrocrural lymph n.
- retropharyngeal lymph n.
- Rotter n.
- second-echelon lymph n.
- N. Seeker surgical radiation detection system
- sentinel lymph n. (SLN)
- Sister Mary Joseph n.
- solitary lymph n.
- spinal accessory lymph n.
- subcarinal lymph n.
- submandibular lymph n.
- submental lymph n.
- Troisier n.
- tumor-draining lymph n. (TDLN)
- Virchow n.
- Virchow-Trosier n.

node-negative
- n.-n. disease
- n.-n. melanoma
- n.-n. patient
- n.-n. primary tumor

node-positive disease
nodes of Rouviere
nodular
- n. disorder
- n. fasciitis
- n. histiocytic lymphoma
- n. hyperintense focus
- n. infiltrate
- n. lesion
- n. melanoma
- n. panencephalitis
- n. partial remission (nPR)
- n. pattern
- n. poorly differentiated lymphocytic lymphoma (NPDL)
- n. regenerative hyperplasia
- n. sclerosing Hodgkin disease (NSHD)
- n. sclerosis
- n. thickening

nodule
- adenomatoid n.
- cerebral n.
- cold n.
- echogenic n.

fatty dysplastic regenerative
  hepatic n.
hepatic n.
hyperplastic n.
Lisch n.
mantle zone n.
prostatic hyperplastic n.
pulmonary n.
red-blue n.
siderotic n.
Sister Mary Joseph n.
violaceous n.
nodule-in-nodule lesion
nogalamycin
Noguchi test
noise
  acoustic n.
nolatrexed dihydrochloride
Nolvadex tablet
nomenclature
  FIGO n.
  International Federation of
    Gynecology and Obstetrics n.
nominal standard dose (NSD)
nomogram
  MPV n.
non-A hepatitis
nonalkylating agent
nonangiogenic cell
nonapeptide
nonaxial beam technique
nonbacterial endocarditis
non-B-cell leukemia
nonbenzodiazepine anxiolytic
non-B hepatitis
non-Burkitt subtype
noncausal association
nonchromaffin paraganglioma
noncisplatinum
noncleaved-cell lymphoma
noncomplex PSA
**noncontact holmium:yttrium-argon-garnet
  laser thermal keratoplasty**
nonconvoluted type
noncoplanar
  n. beam
  n. beam technique
noncoring Huber needle
noncovalent
noncurative resection
nondesmoplastic melanoma
nondysgerminoma
nonencapsulated sclerosing tumor

nonepithelial tumor
nonexpansile lung
nonferromagnetic MR-compatible frame
**nonfilament polymorphonuclear
  leukocyte**
nongerminoma germ cell tumor
nongranular leukocyte
nonhematologic toxicity
nonhematopoietic
  n. element
  n. growth factor
  n. stem cell
nonhemorrhagic melanoma metastasis
nonhistone
non-Hodgkin
  n.-H. lymphoma (NHL)
  n.-H. thyroid lymphoma (NHTL)
nonhuman bile acid
nonicteric
nonimmune hydrops fetalis
**nonimmunoblastic diffuse large B-cell
  lymphoma**
nonimmunogenic
  n. murine tumor cell
  n. tumor
noninfarct zone (NIZ)
noninfiltrating lobular carcinoma
**non-insulin-dependent diabetes mellitus
  (NIDDM)**
noninvasive
  n. thermometry
  n. tubular carcinoma
  n. vascular assessment (NIVA)
noni plant
**non-islet cell tumor hypoglycemia
  (NICTH)**
nonleukemic myelosis
nonlinear
  n. least squares regression analysis
  n. sampling
nonlymphoblastic leukemia
nonlymphocytic leukemia
nonlymphoid leukemia
nonmaleficence
nonmelanoma skin cancer (NMSC)
nonmetastatic melanoma
**nonmitogenic humanized anti-CD3
  antibody**
nonmotile leukocyte
nonmucinous adenocarcinoma
nonmyeloablative
  n. allogeneic stem cell transplant
  n. conditioning

N

NOTES

nonmyelosuppressive
  n. agent
  n. toxicity
nonnasal CD56+T/NK cell lymphoma
nonneoplastic
  n. disease
  n. lesion
  n. T cell
nonnucleated
nonnucleoside
  n. reverse transcriptase inhibitor
    (NNRTI)
  n. reverse transcriptase inhibitor
    binding site
nonopioid analgesic
nonopportunistic infection
nonossifying fibroma
nonosteogenic fibroma
nonoverlapping toxicity concept
nonoxynol-9 (N-9)
nonparametric
nonpeptic inhibitor
nonperforative lesion
nonpharmacological approach
nonpharmacologic therapy
nonpilocytic astrocytoma
nonpolyposis colorectal cancer
nonprogressor
  long-term n. (LTNP)
  short-term n.
nonpurged marrow
nonreciprocal translocation
nonresponder
nonrhabdomyosarcoma soft tissue
  sarcoma
nonsaturable drug
nonsclerosing
  n. ileitis
  n. tumor
nonsealed radionuclide therapy
nonsecreting myeloma
nonsecretor
nonsecretory myeloma
nonseminomatous
  n. germ cell tumor (NSGCT)
  n. testicular germ cell tumor
    (NSTGCT)
nonsense codon
nonsentinel lymph node (NSN)
non-skin-sparing mastectomy (non-SSM)
nonskull base chordoma (NSBC)
nonsmall
  n. cell
  n. cell carcinoma (NSCC)
  n. cell lung cancer (NSCLC)
  n. cell lung carcinoma (NSCLC)
  n. cell lung carcinoma with
    neuroendocrine differentiation
    (NSCLC-ND)

nonspecific
  n. esterase
  n. esterase stain
  n. immunotherapy
  n. interstitial pneumonitis
  n. mesenchyme
  n. reaction
  n. staining
nonspermicidal inhibitor
nonsplit supraclavicular field
nonsquamous carcinoma
non-SSM
  non-skin-sparing mastectomy
nonsteroidal
  n. antiandrogen (NSAA)
  n. antiestrogen
  n. antiinflammatory drug (NSAID)
  n. aromatase inhibitor
nonstructural gene
nonsyncytia-forming
  n.-f. HIV
  n.-f. human immunodeficiency virus
  n.-f. isolate
nonsyncytium-inducing (NSI)
  n.-i. chemokine (CC-CKR-5)
nonsystemic
non-T-cell leukemia
non-T, non-B acute lymphocytic
  leukemia of childhood
nontreponemal antibody titer
nontuberculous mycobacteriosis
nonunion
  bony n.
  n. of fracture
nonviremic
Noonan syndrome
NOPHO
  Nordic Society for Pediatric Hematology
    and Oncology
NOPP
  Novantrone, Oncovin, procarbazine,
    prednisone
Norcet
Norco
Nordic Society for Pediatric
  Hematology and Oncology (NOPHO)
Norelin
norethindrone
norethynodrel
norfloxacin
Norgesic Forte
normal
  n. clonal CD4+ T cell
  n. hematopoietic cell
  n. tissue
  n. variant
normal-appearing white matter
  (NAWM)

normalization
  assay n.
normalized dose-surface histogram
normoblast
  basophilic n.
  orthochromic n.
  polychromatophilic n.
normocellularity
normochromic
  n. anemia
  n. erythrocyte
normocytic
  n. anemia
  n., normochromic anemia
normocytosis
normogram
  body surface n.
  dosing n.
normovolemia
normovolemic hemodilution
Norport pump
Norpramin
Norrie disease
Norris corpuscle
Nor-tet oral
North American Burkitt lymphoma
northern
  N. blot
  N. blot analysis
  N. blot test
Norton-Simon hypothesis
nortriptyline
Norvir
Norwalk agent
Norwegian
  brown N. (BN)
  N. scabies
NOS
  not otherwise specified
nose
  n. bolus
  saddle n.
nosocomial
  n. anemia
  n. infection
notch
  apical n.
  n. gene family
  Kernohan n.
  N. ligand
  thyroid n.
not otherwise specified (NOS)
no-touch technique

no-treatment control group
Nottingham prognostic index
Novamoxin
Novantrone
  N., 5-fluorouracil, leucovorin (NFL)
  Oncovin, prednisone, etoposide, N.
    (OPEN)
  N., Oncovin, procarbazine,
    prednisone (NOPP)
Novapren
Novasen
Novastan
novel
  n. erythropoiesis-stimulating
    hormone
  n. erythropoiesis-stimulating protein
    (NESP)
  n. form
  n. form of consolidation
    chemotherapy
  n. glycoprotein
  n. therapeutic strategy
novo
  de n.
Novo-Aloprazol
Novo-AZT
novobiocin
Novo-Carbamaz
Novo-Chlorpromazine
Novo-Clopate
Novo-Cloxin
Novo-Cromolyn
Novo-Cyproterone
Novo-Difenac-K
Novo-Difenac-SR
Novo-Diflunisal
Novo-Dipiradol
Novo-Doxepin
Novo-Doxylin
Novo-Famotidine
Novo-Fibrate
Novo-Flurprofen
Novo-Folacid
Novo-Furan
Novo-Gesic-C8
Novo-Gesic-C15
Novo-Gesic-C30
Novo-Hexidyl
Novo-Hydrazide
Novo-Keto-EC
Novo-Lexin
Novo-Methacin
Novo-Mucilax

N

NOTES

Novo-Naprox
Novo-Nifedin
Novo-Pen-VK
Novo-Piroxicam
Novo-Pramine
Novo-Prednisone
Novo-Profen
Novo-Propoxyn
Novo-Pyrazone
Novo-Ranidine
Novo-Rythro Encap
Novo-Semide
NovoSeven
    N. Coagulation Factor VIIa
    N. Coagulation Factor VIIa
    recombinant
Novo-Soxazole
Novo-Spiroton
Novoste Beta-Cath delivery system
Novo-Sundac
Novo-Tamoxifen
Novo-Tetra
Novo-Thalidone
Novo-Tolmetin
Novo-Triamzide
Novo-Trimel
Novo-Tripramine
Novo-Zolamide
NOX enzyme
N-oxide
NPC
    nasopharyngeal carcinoma
NPCIS
    nasopharyngeal carcinoma in situ
NPDL
    nodular poorly differentiated lymphocytic
    lymphoma
N-phosphonacetyl-L-aspartate (PALA)
nPR
    nodular partial remission
NR
    no response
      NR antigen
N-ras
    N-r. gene
    N-r. oncogene
    N-r. protooncogene/oncogene
NRC
    Nuclear Regulatory Commission
NR-LU-10 antibody
NRP
    neuropilin
NRP1
    neuropilin 1
NRP2
    neuropilin 2
NRTI
    nucleoside reverse transcriptase inhibitor

NSAA
    nonsteroidal antiandrogen
NSABP
    National Surgical Adjuvant Breast and
    Bowel Project
    National Surgical Adjuvant Breast
    Project
      NSABP protocol
      NSABP protocol B23
NSAID
    nonsteroidal antiinflammatory drug
NSBC
    nonskull base chordoma
NSCC
    nonsmall cell carcinoma
NSCLC
    nonsmall cell lung cancer
    nonsmall cell lung carcinoma
NSCLC-ND
    nonsmall cell lung carcinoma with
      neuroendocrine differentiation
NSD
    nominal standard dose
NSE
    neuron-specific enolase
      NSE lung cancer tumor marker
NSGCT
    nonseminomatous germ cell tumor
NSHD
    nodular sclerosing Hodgkin disease
NSI
    nonsyncytium-inducing
      NSI variant
      NSI variant of HIV
NSN
    nonsentinel lymph node
NST
    nutrition support team
NSTGCT
    nonseminomatous testicular germ cell
    tumor
Ntaya virus
N-telopeptide (NTX)
N-terminal glycine
NT-R-1
    neurotensin receptor type 1
NT-R-2
    neurotensin receptor type 2
NT-R-3
    neurotensin receptor type 3
NTX
    N-telopeptide
NTZ
    nitazoxanide
Nu-Alprax
Nu-Amoxi
Nu-Ampi
Nubain
Nu-Carbamazepine

Nu-Cephalex
Nu-Cimet
nuclear
- n. atypia
- n. bubbling artifact
- n. cell
- n. condensation
- n. contour index
- n. convolution
- n. DNA
- n. factor
- n. factor of activated T cell (NFAT)
- n. factor kappa beta (NF-κB, NF-kB)
- n. fragmentation
- n. grade
- 1H-n. magnetic resonance spectroscopic imaging
- n. hormone receptor
- n. imaging
- n. magnetic resonance (NMR)
- n. magnetic resonance spectroscopy
- n. matrix protein (NMP)
- n. medicine (NM)
- n. membrane abnormality
- n. morphometry
- n. organizing region
- n. proliferation antigen
- N. Regulatory Commission (NRC)
- n. spin density
- n. stratification
- n. unrest

nuclear-cytoplasmic ratio
nuclease-resistant phosphorothioate oligodeoxynucleotide
nucleated
- n. cell count
- n. erythrocyte
- n. red blood cell

nuclei (*pl. of* nucleus)
nucleic
- n. acid
- n. acid-binding protein
- n. acid construct
- n. acid hybridization
- n. acid immunization
- n. acid testing (NAT)
- n. acid vaccination
- n. acid vector

nucleocapsid (NC)
- n. protein

nucleolar organizing region

nucleoside
- n. analog
- n. analog monotherapy
- n. 5′-diphosphate kinase (NDK-K)
- n. phosphonate
- n. phosphotransferase
- physiologic n.
- pyrimidine n.
- n. reverse transcriptase inhibitor (NRTI)

5′-nucleotidase
nucleotide
- purine n.
- pyrimidine n.
- n. sequence analysis

Nucletron simulator
nucleus, pl. **nuclei**
- basal n.
- dentate n.
- hyperchromatic n.
- multilobated n.
- pleomorphic n.
- red n.
- vesicular n.

Nu-Cloxi
Nu-Cotrimox
Nu-Derm foam island dressing
Nu-Diclo
Nu-Diflunisal
Nu-Doxycycline
Nu-Famotidine
Nu-Flurprofen
Nu Gauze dressing
Nu-Gemfibrozil
Nu-Ibuprofen
Nu-Indo
Nu-Iron
Nu-Ketoprofen
Nu-Ketoprofen-E
null
- n. cell
- n. cell acute lymphocytic leukemia
- n. cell anaplastic large cell lymphoma
- n. cell lymphoblastic leukemia
- n. hypothesis
- n. lymphocyte

nulliparous patient
nullizygosity
numb chin syndrome
number
- average gradient n.
- *N-myc* copy n.

N

NOTES

Numorphan
Nu-Naprox
Nu-Nifedin
Nu-Pen-VK
Nupercainal
Nu-Pirox
Nuprin
Nu-Propranolol
Nu-Ranit
nurse
    n. cell
    n. cell environment
    oncology certified n. (OCN)
nurse-patient ratio
Nu-Sulfinpyrazone
nut
    areca n.
    betel n.
Nu-Tetra
NutraPrep LoSo prep
Nutren with fiber
Nu-Triazide
nutrient artery
Nu-Trimipramine
nutrition
    enteral n.
    glutamine-supplemented total
      parenteral n.
    parenteral n.
    n. support team (NST)
    total enteral n.
    total parenteral n. (TPN)

nutritional
    n. assessment
    n. deficiency
    n. disorder
    n. prevention
    n. status
    n. support
    n. therapy
Nutropin
Nuvance
Nuvion
NVB
    neurovascular bundle
NWTS
    National Wilms Tumor Study
NX
    naloxone
    regional lymph nodes cannot be
      addressed
    Talwin NX
Nyaderm
Nydrazid Injection
NY-ESO-1 protein
nystatin
    framycetin, colistin, n. (FRACON)
    liposomal n.
    n. and triamcinolone
Nystatin-LF I.V.
Nystat-Rx
Nystex
Nytran membrane
NYVAC

O

oxygen
O antigen
autotransplantation O

O-9

octoxynol-9

OA

ovarian ablation

OAF

off-axis factor

Oakley-Fulthorpe technique

OAP

Oncovin, ara-C, prednisone

OAP-BLEO

Oncovin, ara-C, prednisone, bleomycin

OAR

off-axis ratio
organs at risk
OAR value

OARS

Optimal Atherectomy Restenosis Study

oat

o. cell
o. cell carcinoma
o. cell lung cancer
o. cell tumor

OB

Chromagen OB

OBC

operable breast cancer

OBD

optimum biologic dose

O6-benzylguanine

obligate chain terminator

oblimersen sodium

obliterans

atherosclerosis o.
balanitis xerotica o.
endarteritis o.
radiation-associated endarteritis o.

obstetrics

International Federation of
Gynecology and O. (FIGO)

obstructing carcinoma

obstruction

airway o.
aqueductal o.
arachnoid villi o.
biliary tract o.
biliary tree o.
bladder outlet o.
bowel o.
bronchial o.
catheter o.
colonic o.

common bile duct o.
distal common bile duct o.
duodenal o.
duodenal-gastric outlet o.
extrahepatic binary o.
gastric outlet o.
intestinal o.
superior vena caval o. (SVCO)
ureteral o.
vascular o.
venous o.

obstructive

o. colorectal cancer
o. jaundice
o. lung disease
o. uropathy

obturator

o. fascia
o. internus muscle
o. lymph node

OC

oral contraceptive

occlusion

angiographic o.
arterial o.
balloon test o.
cerebral sinovenous o.
coronary o.
dural sinus o.
fresh thrombotic o.
percutaneous thermal o.
plastic stent o.
sinus o.
thrombotic o.
transcatheter o.

occult

o. bleeding
o. blood
o. blood in stool
o. blood testing
o. cancer
o. clonal B-cell population
o. metastasis
o. neuroblastoma
o. papillary carcinoma
o. primary malignancy (OPM)
o. tumor cell

occulta

spina bifida o.

occupational

O. Safety and Health
Administration bloodborne
pathogen standard
o. transmission

O

OCN
oncology certified nurse
OCR
off-center ratio
OCT
optical coherence tomography
Octagam
Octostim
octoxynol-9 (O-9)
OctreoScan 111 radioactive imaging agent
octreotide
o. acetate
o. pamoate
o. scan
$[^{90}Y]$-DOTA-D-Ph^{1}1-Tyr^3 o.
Ocufen Ophthalmic
ocular
o. adnexa
o. adnexal inflammatory pseudotumor
o. adnexal lesion
o. adnexal lymphoid proliferation
o. adnexal lymphoma
o. herpes
o. hypertelorism
o. manifestation
o. melanocytosis
o. melanoma
o. radiation therapy (ORT)
o. rhabdomyosarcoma
o. toxicity
o. toxoplasmosis
oculoectodermal syndrome
oculogyric crisis
oculoplethysmography (OPG)
Ocuvite
ODAC
Oncologic Drugs Advisory Committee
O-DAP
Oncovin, dianhydrogalactitol, Adriamycin, Platinol
ODM
opponens digiti minimi
odontoblastoma
odontogenic
o. epithelium
o. fibroma
o. infection
o. pain
o. tumor
odontoma
ODT
orally disintegrating tablet
Zofran ODT
odynophagia
OER
oxygen enhancement ratio
Oestrilin

off-axis
o.-a. factor (OAF)
o.-a. plane
o.-a. ratio (OAR)
off-center ratio (OCR)
off-core
office-based cryoablation
off-resonance
rotating delivery of excitation o.-r. (RODEO)
ofloxacin
Ogawa
O. model
O. model for hematopoiesis
Ogen Vaginal cream
O-glycanase enzyme
O-glycosylation
OI
opportunistic infection
oil
BAL in O.
brominated o.
castor o.
flaxseed o.
Fleet Flavored Castor O.
grapeseed o.
Lorenzo o.
mineral o.
pomegranate o.
progesterone in o.
rapeseed o.
o. tumor
oily granuloma
ointment
Anusol O.
Catrix O.
Chloresium o.
Elase O.
Ethezyme papain-urea debriding o.
Nitro-Bid O.
Nitrol O.
Panafil o.
Santyl o.
Terra-Cortril o.
OKB7 monoclonal antibody
OKT3
OKT3 anti-CD3 monoclonal antibody
Orthoclone OKT3
OKT4 cell
OKT8 cell
Okuda
O. stage I-III
O. staging
olanzapine
olecranon fracture
oleic acid
oleogranuloma

olfactory
- o. groove
- o. groove meningioma
- o. neuroblastoma (ONB)

oligemia
oligoadenylate synthetase
oligoastrocytoma
- anaplastic o.
- benign mixed o.
- grade III o.
- malignant mixed o.
- mixed o.
- recurrent vermian o.
- o. tumor
- vermian o.

oligoclonal
- o. band
- o. population

oligodendrocyte
oligodendrocytoma
oligodendroglial tumor
oligodendroglioma
- anaplastic o.
- bifrontal o.
- grade III o.
- low-grade o.
- subependymal o.

oligodeoxynucleotide
- nuclease-resistant phosphorothioate o.

oligohydramnios
oligolysine backbone
oligomer
oligomerization
oligomerize
oligonucleotide
- allele-specific o. (ASO)
- antisense o.
- antitelomerase antisense o.
- o. probe TC62

oligoribonucleotide
oligos
- antisense o.

oligosaccharide
oligospermia
olivacine
Oliver-Rosalki method
Ollier disease
olpadronate
oltipraz
Olympus
- O. GF-UM30P echoendoscope
- O. GIF-2T20 end-viewing endoscope
- O. SD-9L-1 snare

OMAD
- Oncovin, methotrexate, Adriamycin, dactinomycin

omalizumab
omega
- Pearl O.

omega-3 polyunsaturated fatty acid
Omenn syndrome
omentectomy
omentum, pl. **omenta**
omeprazole stimulation test
Ommaya spinal fluid reservoir
Omnicef
Omniferon
Omnifix tape
Omni-Flow 4000 Plus
omohyoid muscle
omphalocele
OMS Oral
onapristone
ONB
- olfactory neuroblastoma

Oncaspar
onchocerciasis
oncocytic
- o. adenocarcinoma
- o. cholangiocarcinoma
- o. hepatocellular tumor
- o. meningioma

oncocytoma
oncofetal
- o. antigen
- o. fibronectin
- o. marker
- o. protein

OncoGel
oncogene
- abl o.
- o. activation
- amplified o.
- bcl-1 o.
- bcl-2 o.
- bcl-3 o.
- B-lym o.
- B-RAF o.
- can o.
- CDK4 o.
- c-erbB2 o.
- c-ets o.
- c-fms o.

NOTES

O

oncogene *(continued)*
    c-fos o.
    CHOP/GADD153 o.
    c-myb o.
    c-myc o.
    dek o.
    E2A o.
    erb B o.
    o. expression
    fms o.
    gli o.
    HOX11 o.
    H-ras o.
    K-ras o.
    lck o.
    L-myc o.
    MDM2 o.
    mdr1 o.
    myb o.
    myc o.
    myl o.
    neu o.
    N-myc o.
    N-ras o.
    p53 o.
    PBX1 o.
    PDGF-a receptor o.
    RAR-alpha o.
    ras o.
    Rb1 o.
    rel o.
    rhombotin/Ttg-1 o.
    rhombotin/Ttg-2 o.
    R-ras o.
    tal o.
    tal-1 o.
    tan-1 o.
    tcl-1 o.
    tcl-2 o.
    tcl-3 o.
    tcl-4 o.
oncogenesis
    radiation o.
    viral o.
oncogenic
    o. agent
    o. Ikaros isoform
    o. virus
oncogenomics
oncogenous osteomalacia
oncologia
    Gruppo Interdisciplinare Valutazione Interventi in O. (GIVIO)
oncologic
    O. Drugs Advisory Committee (ODAC)
    o. emergency

oncologist
    radiation o.
    surgical o.
oncology
    American Society of Clinical O. (ASCO)
    American Society of Preventive O. (ASPO)
    American Society for Therapeutic Radiology and O. (ASTRO)
    o. certified nurse (OCN)
    International Classification of Diseases for O. (ICD-O)
    International Society of Pediatric O. (SIOP)
    medical o.
    Multinational Association of Supportive Care in Cancer/International Society for Oral O. (MASCC/ISOO)
    Nordic Society for Pediatric Hematology and O. (NOPHO)
    O. Nurses Association
    O. Nursing Society (ONS)
    psychosocial o.
    radiation o.
    Society of Gynecologic O. (SGO)
    Society of Surgical O. (SSO)
    surgical o.
    o. treatment
Oncolym radiolabeled monoclonal antibody
oncolysate
    vaccinia melanoma o. (VMO)
Oncolysin B
Onconase
Oncophage cancer vaccine
oncoplastic carcinoma
oncoprotein
    fusion o.
    HER-2/neu o.
    HPV E6 o.
    HPV E7 o.
    o. JON95
    P210 bcr/abl o.
OncoRad
    O. for bladder
    O. OV103
    O. PR
    O. Prostate
OncoScint
    O. CR103
    O. CR/OV
    O. OV103
    O. PR
    O. scan
oncostatin M (OSM)
oncosuppressor gene
oncotaxonomy

Onco-TCS
Oncotech assay
OncoTrac
OncoVax-CL
OncoVax-Pr
Oncovin
Adriamycin, prednisone, O. (APO)
O., ara-C, prednisone (OAP)
O., ara-C, prednisone, bleomycin
(OAP-BLEO)
O. and L-asparaginase
cyclophosphamide, Adriamycin, O.
(CAO)
cyclophosphamide, Adriamycin,
methotrexate, etoposide, O.
(CAMEO)
cyclophosphamide,
hydroxydaunomycin, O. (CHO)
cyclophosphamide, hydroxyurea,
actinomycin D, methotrexate, O.,
citrovorum factor, Adriamycin
(CHAM-OCA, CHAMOCA)
cyclophosphamide, methotrexate, 5-
fluorouracil, Adriamycin, O.
cytosine arabinoside, high-dose
methotrexate, leucovorin, O.
(CAMELEON)
cytosine arabinoside, methotrexate,
leucovorin, O. (CAMLO)
daunorubicin, azacitidine, ara-C,
prednisone, O. (DZAPO)
O., dianhydrogalactitol, Adriamycin,
Platinol (O-DAP)
etoposide, cyclophosphamide,
hydroxydaunomycin, O.
etoposide, methotrexate, actinomycin
D, cyclophosphamide, O. (EMA-
CO, EMACO)
etoposide, methotrexate, actinomycin
D, cyclophosphamide, O. (EMA-
CO, EMACO)
O. and methotrexate
O., methotrexate, Adriamycin,
dactinomycin (OMAD)
methotrexate, asparaginase,
cyclophosphamide,
hydroxydaunomycin, O. (MACHO)
methotrexate, asparaginase, Cytoxan,
hydroxydaunomycin, O. (MACHO)
prednisone, ara-C, 6-thioguanine,
cyclophosphamide, O. (PATCO)
O., prednisone, L-asparaginase
(OPAL)

O., prednisone, etoposide,
Novantrone (OPEN)
O., procarbazine, prednisone (OPP)
O., procarbazine, prednisone,
Adriamycin (OPPA)
O., procarbazine, prednisone,
Adriamycin, cyclophosphamide
O., procarbazine, prednisone,
Adriamycin plus
cyclophosphamide, Oncovin,
procarbazine, prednisone
(OPPA/COPP)
6-thioguanine, rubidomycin, ara-C,
methotrexate, prednisolone,
cyclophosphamide, O.
O., (vincristine), citrovorum factor,
Adriamycin
ondansetron
o. hydrochloride
metoclopramide, dexamethasone,
lorazepam, o. (MDLO)
Ondrox
One-Alpha
onion skin
onion-skinning pattern
Onkolox
ON-Q pain management infusion
system
ONS
Oncology Nursing Society
Ontak
ontogenic
POK erythroid myeloid o.
(Pokeman)
Onxol
onychodysplasia
idiopathic o.
onycholysis
periarticular thenar erythema and o.
(PATEO)
onychomycosis
onychoosteodysplasia
Ony-Clear Spray
ONYX-015 anticancer agent
oocytic ribonuclease
oogenesis
ookinete
oophorectomy
prophylactic o. (PO)
oophoritis
CMV o.
oophoropexy

O

NOTES

oophorus
  cumulus o.
oozing
  venous o.
opacity
  vitreous o.
OPAL
  Oncovin, prednisone, L-asparaginase
  OPAL knowledge-entry system
OPEN
  Oncovin, prednisone, etoposide,
  Novantrone
open
  keep vein o. (KVO)
  o. reading frame (ORF)
open-ended guidewire
opening
  aortic o.
  esophageal o.
open-tube rigid bronchoscope
operable breast cancer (OBC)
operation
  biliary-enteric anastomosis o.
  Finzi-Harmer o.
  second-look o.
  Whipple o.
operator gene
operon
  lac o.
OPG
  oculoplethysmography
  ophthalmoplethysmography
OPGL
  osteoprotegerin ligand
ophthalmic
  Ocufen O.
  o. plaque
  Tobrex O.
  Vira-A O.
  Viroptic O.
  Voltaren O.
ophthalmicus
  herpes zoster o.
  zoster o.
ophthalmologic abnormality
ophthalmoplethysmography (OPG)
opiate withdrawal
opioid
  o. agonist
  o. analgesic
  o. antagonist
  o. receptor
  rectal o.
  o. rotation
opioid-induced constipation
opium
  o. alkaloid
  belladonna and o.

  hyoscyamine, atropine, scopolamine,
    kaolin, pectin, o.
  kaolin and pectin with o.
  o. tincture
OPM
  occult primary malignancy
OPN
  osteopontin
OPP
  Oncovin, procarbazine, prednisone
OPPA
  Oncovin, procarbazine, prednisone,
    Adriamycin
OPPA/COPP
  Oncovin, procarbazine, prednisone,
    Adriamycin plus cyclophosphamide,
    Oncovin, procarbazine, prednisone
opponens digiti minimi (ODM)
opportunist
  seminated fungal o.
opportunistic
  o. infection (OI)
  o. pathogen
opportunity
  window of o.
oprelvekin
OpSite
  O. dressing
  O. TFD
opsoclonus
opsoclonus-myoclonus
  paraneoplastic o.-m.
opsomyoclonus syndrome
opsonin
opsonization
opsonizing antibody
optic
  o. atrophy
  o. chiasm disease
  o. nerve lesion
  o. neuritis
  o. neuropathy
  o. pathway glioma
optical
  O. Biopsy System
  o. coherence tomography (OCT)
  o. mammography
  o. signature
Opticrom
optimal
  O. Atherectomy Restenosis Study
    (OARS)
  o. cytoreduction
  o. therapeutic response
optimum biologic dose (OBD)
option
  adjuvant treatment o.
  treatment o.

Optrin
ora, pl. **orae**
Orabase-B
Orabase-O
Orabase with Benzocaine
orae (*pl. of* ora)
Orajel
    O. Brace-Aid oral anesthetic
    O. Maximum Strength
    O. Mouth-Aid
oral
    Ansaid O.
    Aristocort O.
    Atolone O.
    o. bioavailability
    o. bisphosphonate
    o. candidiasis
    Cataflam O.
    o. cavity
    o. cavity cancer
    Ceftin O.
    Celestone O.
    Cleocin HCl O.
    Cleocin Pediatric O.
    o. complication
    o. contraceptive (OC)
    o. copulation
    Cortef O.
    Curretab O.
    Cytomel O.
    Decadron Oral
    Delta-Cortef O.
    Dilaudid O.
    o. dose
    Dynacin O.
    o. epithelial cell genetic
      fingerprinting
    o. epithelial cell genotyping
    Estrace O.
    o. hairy leukemia
    o. hairy leukoplakia
    o. hygiene
    o. hypericin
    o. hyperpigmentation
    Indocin SR O.
    Kadian O.
    Kenacort O.
    Lamisil O.
    low dose o. (LDO)
    o. manifestation
    Medrol O.
    Mephyton O.
    MS Contin O.

    o. mucosa
    o. mucosal epithelium
    o. mucositis
    O. Mucositis Assessment Scale
    O. Mucositis Index
    Nitroglyn O.
    Noroxin O.
    Nor-tet O.
    OMS O.
    Oramorph SR O.
    Panmycin O.
    Pediapred O.
    o. perifosine
    Prelone O.
    o. premalignancy
    Proglycem O.
    Provera O.
    o. rehydration therapy
    Rifadin O.
    Rimactane O.
    Roxanol SR O.
    o. shark cartilage
    Sinequan O.
    o. spray
    o. squamous cell carcinoma
      (OSCC)
    Sumycin O.
    Terramycin O.
    Tetracap O.
    o. thrush
    o. ulcer
    Vancocin O.
    Voltaren-XR O.
    o. VP-16
    o. wound
    o. wound rinse
Oralet
    Fentanyl O.
orally disintegrating tablet (ODT)
Oral-Turinabol
Oramed
Oramorph SR Oral
orange
    acridine o.
OraQuick test
OraRinse
Orasept
Orasol
OraSure test
Ora-Swab
Ora-Testryl
Orathecin
Orbenin

NOTES

O

orbital
    o. exenteration
    o. lesion
    o. metastasis
    o. radiotherapy
    o. rhabdomyosarcoma
    o. sarcoidosis
orbitotomy
orchiectomy
    inguinal o.
    radical o.
    radical inguinal o.
    transscrotal o.
orchitis
Oretic
Orexin
ORF
    open reading frame
organ
    o.'s at risk (OAR)
    capillary beds of o.'s
    epithelioglandular o.
    o. failure
    hollow o.
    o. involvement
    lymphoid o.
    target o.
    o. tolerance dose (OTD)
    o. toxicity
    o. transplant
    o. volume
    o. of Zuckerkandl
organic erectile dysfunction
organism
    Gram-positive o.
    pleuropneumonia-like o.
organization
    AIDS service o. (ASO)
    National Alliance of Breast
      Cancer O.'s
    preferred provider o. (PPO)
    World Health O. (WHO)
organochlorine
organogenesis
organoid
    o. nevus
    o. tumor
organ-restricted lymphoid subset
organ-specific antigen
orgasmic problem
Orifer F
origin
    anomalous o.
    fever of unknown o. (FUO)
    monoclonal o.
    multilineage o.
    unknown o.
ormaplatin
Ormond disease

Ornidyl Injections
ornithine
    o. decarboxylase
    o. transcarbamylase (OTC)
    o. transcarbamylase deficiency
    o. transcarbamylase deficiency gene
orofacial carcinoma
oropharyngeal
    o. cancer
    o. mucosa
    o. mucositis
orphan
orphan
    enteric cytopathogenic bovine o.
      (ECBO)
    enteric cytopathogenic human o.
    enteric cytopathogenic monkey o.
      (ECMO)
    enterocytopathogenic human o.
      (ECHO)
orphenadrine, aspirin, caffeine
ORT
    ocular radiation therapy
orthochromatic erythroblast
orthochromic
    o. erythrocyte
    o. normoblast
Orthoclone
    O. OKT3
    O. OKT3 monoclonal antibody
orthogonal view
Ortho-mune antibody
ortho-para-DDD
orthophenyldiamine
orthophenylenediamine dihydrochloride
orthostatic hypotension
orthotic material
orthotopic
    o. diversion
    o. glioma
    o. neobladder
    o. xenograft
orthovoltage
    o. beam
    o. radiation
Orudis KT
Oruvail
Orzel UFT/leucovorin calcium
OS
    osteosarcoma
    overall survival
os, pl. ossa
    cervical o.
    external o.
Os-Cal 500
OSCC
    oral squamous cell carcinoma
oscillation therapy
oseltamivir

OSHA
> OSHA bloodborne pathogen standard

OSHN
> osteosarcoma of head and neck

Osler
> O. disease
> O. triad

OSM
> oncostatin M

Osmitrol Injection

Osmoglyn

osmotherapy

osmotic
> o. fragility test
> o. pump

ossa (*pl. of* os)

osseointegration

osseous sarcoma

ossicle
> accessory o.

ossification
> diaphysial o.
> ectopic o.
> enchondral o.
> endochondral o.
> heterotopic o.

osteoarthritis
> erosive o.

osteoarthropathy
> hypertrophic o. (HOA)
> hypertrophic pulmonary o.

osteoblast

osteoblastic sarcoma

osteoblastoma

osteocarcinoma

osteocartilaginous metaplasia

osteochondrodystrophy

osteochondroma
> solitary o.

osteochondromatosis
> bursal o.

osteochondrosarcoma

osteoclast-activating factor

osteoclastic

osteoclastoma giant cell tumor

osteocystoma

osteodysplastic slender-bone disorder

osteofibroma

osteogenesis imperfecta

osteogenic
> juxtacortical o.
> o. sarcoma

> o. sarcomatosis
> telangiectatic o.

osteoid
> o. osteoma
> o. sarcoma
> o. stroma
> tumor o.

osteolysis
> essential o.

osteolytic
> o. lesion
> o. sarcoma

osteoma, pl. **osteomas, osteomata**
> cancellous o.
> choroidal o.
> osteoid o.

osteomalacia
> hypophosphatemic o.
> oncogenous o.

osteomyelitis
> bacterial o.
> BCG o.
> hematogenous o.

osteomyocutaneous
> o. free flap
> o. free-tissue transfer

osteonecrosis
> bisphosphonate-associated o.
> dysbaric o.

osteopenia

osteophyte
> anterior o.

osteopontin (OPN)
> plasma o.

osteoporosis prevention drug

osteoprotegerin ligand (OPGL)

osteoradionecrosis

osteosarcoma (OS)
> o. antigen
> o. antigen-associated monoclonal antibody
> o. of bone
> chondroblastic o.
> epithelioid o.
> extraosseous o.
> extraskeletal o.
> extremity o.
> fibroblastic o.
> o. of head and neck (OSHN)
> juxtacortical o.
> parosteal o.
> periosteal o.

NOTES

osteosarcoma *(continued)*
    surface o.
    telangiectatic o.
osteosclerosis
    diffuse o.
osteosclerotic myeloma
Ostoforte
Ostofresh formula
ostomy
OTC
    ornithine transcarbamylase
        OTC deficiency
        OTC gene
OTD
    organ tolerance dose
otitis media
ototoxicity
    cisplatin-induced o.
OTR
    Ovarian Tumor Registry
Ouchterlony immunodiffusion
Oudin immunodiffusion
OutBound disposable syringe infusion system
OV103
    OncoRad OV103
    OncoScint OV103
ova (*pl. of* ovum)
ovale
    Plasmodium o.
OvaRex MAb-B43.13
ovarian
    o. ablation (OA)
    o. cancer (OVCA)
    o. cancer metastasis
    o. carcinoid tumor
    o. carcinoma (OVCA)
    o. choriocarcinoma
    o. cyst
    o. cystectomy
    o. cystic teratoma
    o. dysfunction
    o. dysgenesis
    o. dysgerminoma
    o. embryonal teratoma
    o. endometrioid carcinoma
    o. epithelial carcinoma
    o. epithelial tumor (OVET)
    o. epithelium
    o. failure
    o. follicle
    o. function
    o. gonadoblastoma
    o. granulosa-stromal cell tumor
    o. granulosa-theca cell tumor
    o. hilar cell tumor
    o. intraepithelial neoplasia
    o. lipid cell neoplasm
    o. lymphoma

    o. malignant epithelial neoplasm
    o. mass
    o. mesodermal sarcoma
    o. proliferative cystadenoma
    o. rhenium-186 MAb
    o. tubular adenoma
    O. Tumor Registry (OTR)
ovary
    Chinese hamster o. (CHO)
    coelomic epithelium of o.
    epithelial cancer of o.
    hilar cell tumor of o.
    luteinized thecoma of o.
    lymphoma of o.
    mucinous adenocarcinoma of o.
    mucinous cystadenoma of o.
    palpable postmenopausal o.
    stromal carcinoid of o.
    teratoblastoma of o.
    teratocarcinoma of o.
    thecoma of o.
    undifferentiated carcinoma of o.
Ovastat
O-Vax vaccine
OVCA
    ovarian cancer
    ovarian carcinoma
overall survival (OS)
overdevelopment
    bone o.
overexpressed receptor
overexpression
    c-erbB2 o.
    HER-2/*neu* o.
    HER-2 protein o.
    hyaluronidase o.
    p53 protein o.
overgrowth
    epiphysial o.
overirradiation
overlay
    Geo-Matt therapeutic foam o.
overload
    African iron o.
    circulatory o.
    iron o.
    volume o.
overmedication
over-the-needle infusion catheter
OVET
    ovarian epithelial tumor
ovoid
    afterloading tandem and o.
    tandem and o.
ovulation
ovum, pl. **ova**
    blighted o.
OVX1 serum marker

owl's
- o. eye appearance
- o. eye inclusion body

Owren disease

Owren-Koller buffer

oxacillin

oxaliplatin
- 5-fluorouracil, folinic acid, o. (FOLFOX)
- o., 5-fluorouracil, leucovorin folinic acid, leucovorin, 5-fluorouracil, gemcitabine, o. (FOLFUGEM-OX)
- gemcitabine plus o. (GEMOX)
- irinotecan and o. (IROX)
- o. with leucovorin and 5-fluorouracil (FOLFOX)

oxaliplatin/capecitabine combination

oxaliplatin-induced neuropathy

Oxandrin

oxandrolone

oxantrazole

oxaprozin

oxathiolane

oxazaphosphorine alkylating agent

oxazepam

oxiconazole

oxidase
- monoamine o. (MAO)
- NADPH-dependent o.

oxidase-Schiff
- galactose o.-S. (GOS)

oxidation
- o. of fatty acids
- hemoglobin o.

oxidative
- o. burst
- o. phosphorylation
- o. stress

oxide
- iron o.
- magnesium o.
- nitric o. (NO)
- nitrous o.
- ultrasmall superparamagnetic iron o.

oxidized
- o. cellulose
- o. hemoglobin
- o. lipoprotein(a) assay

oxidizing retroviral finger

oxidronate

Oxilan

oxime
- hexamethylpropyleneamine o. (HMPAO)
- technetium-99m hexamethylpropyleneamine o. (^{99m}Tc-HMPAO)

oximeter

oximetry
- pulse o.

Oxistat Topical

oxisuran

ox red blood cell

Oxsoralen-Ultra

Oxycel

Oxycocet

Oxycodan

oxycodone
- o. and acetaminophen
- o. and aspirin
- o. hydrochloride

OxyContin II

oxygen (O)
- o. affinity hypoxia
- o. delivery
- o. demand
- o. enhancement ratio (OER)
- hyperbaric o. (HBO)
- o. reduction product
- o. therapeutic
- o. therapy

oxygenated hemoglobin

oxygenation
- extracorporeal membrane o.
- tumor o.

oxygenator
- extracorporeal membrane o.

oxygen-based therapeutic system

oxygen-reactive radical

Oxygent

oxyhemoglobin

oxymetholone

oxymorphone

oxyphenbutazone

oxyphilic
- o. adenoma
- o. leukocyte

oxypurinol stone

oxytetracycline

oxytoca
- *Klebsiella o.*

oxytocin

Oyst-Cal 500

Oystercal 500

NOTES

O

Oz antigen
ozogamicin
    gemtuzumab o. (GO)

ozone treatment

π (*var. of* pi)
P
    P blood group
    P factor
P-170
    P-glycoprotein
^{32}P, P32
    phosphorus-32
        chromic phosphate ^{32}P
        ^{32}P intraperitoneal treatment
        Phosphocol ^{32}P
p
    short arm of chromosome
3p
    chromosome 3p
9p
    chromosome 9p
16p
    chromosome 16p
17p
    chromosome 17p
    p53 gene on chromosome 17p
P3C541b
    gag lipopeptide P3C541b
p7
    cleaved polyprotein precursor molecule
      product
    HIV nucleocapsid protein
p9
    cleaved polyprotein precursor molecule
      product
p16 protein
p17 matrix
p24
    cleaved polyprotein precursor molecule
      product
        p24 antigenemia
        p24 capsid
        p24 protein
p30 protein
P32 (*var. of* ^{32}P)
***p40* T-cell growth factor**
p53
        p53 adenoviral gene
        p53 analysis
        p53 fluorescent monitoring
        p53 gene
        p53 gene mutation
        p53 gene on chromosome 17p
        p53 immunoreactivity
        p53 oncogene
        p53 phosphoprotein
        p53 protein
        p53 protein overexpression
    wild-type p53

p53-dependent signal transduction
p55
    cleaved polyprotein precursor molecule
        p55 component of high-affinity
          interleukin-2
        p55 precursor
        p55 protein
p60
      monoclonal mouse anti-human TNF
        receptor p60
p66/51 polymerase
p80
      monoclonal rat anti-human TNF
        receptor p80
p150 protein
p170 protein
p185 protein
P210 bcr/abl oncoprotein
P388
      murine leukemia P388
P450
      retroviral cytochrome P450
PA
    pathology
    pernicious anemia
    pituitary adenoma
    posteroanterior
    pulmonary artery
        PA chest film
        PA portal
        PA projection
PAB
    peripheral androgen blockade
PABA
    paraaminobenzoic acid
PAB-Esc-C
    Platinol, Adriamycin, bleomycin,
      escalating doses of Cytoxan
PAC
    Platinol, Adriamycin, cyclophosphamide
    premature atrial contraction
PAC-1
    Platinol, Adriamycin, cyclophosphamide
PACE
    5-fluorouracil, cisplatin, cytarabine,
      caffeine
    Platinol, Adriamycin, cyclophosphamide,
      etoposide
        PACE chemotherapy protocol
pachydermatosis
pachydermia
pachydermoperiostosis
pachymeninx, pl. **pachymeninges**
pachyonychia congenita
Pacific yew

Pacis
P. BCG
P. BCG immunotherapy
pack
interferon alfa-2b and ribavirin combination p.
M-Zole 7 Dual P.
packed
p. cell volume (PCV)
p. erythrocytes
p. red blood cells
packing
p. for bleeding
Heyman p.
pack-year smoking history
paclitaxel (PTX)
p. and docetaxel
p. and doxorubicin
estramustine plus p.
intraperitoneal p.
polyglutamate p. (PG-TXL)
Tocosol P.
paclitaxel/cyclophosphamide and high-dose melphalan/etoposide
paclitaxel-resistant tumor
pad
gelatin sponge p.
padding
antral p.
PadKit sample collection system
PAGE
polyacrylamide gel electrophoresis
2D PAGE
Paget
P. carcinoma
P. disease
P. disease of nipple
pagetic
pagetoid
p. epidermal involvement
p. reticulosis
PAH
polycyclic aromatic hydrocarbon
polynuclear aromatic hydrocarbon
PAI
plasminogen activator inhibitor
PAIg
platelet-associated immunoglobulin
pain
abdominal p.
acute p.
bone p.
p. cascade
chronic p.
p. cocktail
dysesthetic p.
existential p.
flank p.

incident p.
intractable p.
joint p.
p. management
muscle p.
neuropathic p.
nociceptive p.
odontogenic p.
phantom limb p.
pleuritic p.
radicular p.
somatic p.
spiritual p.
visceral p.
PALA
N-phosphonacetyl-L-aspartate
Palafer
palate
palatine process
palatoglossus muscle
palatopharyngeus muscle
palifermin
palindrome
palindromic hexamer
palisade-like arrangement
palivizumab
Pall
P. ELD-96 Set Saver filter
P. filter PL100KL/50K
P. leukocyte removal filter
P. PL100 filter
P. RC100 filter
P. RC50 filter
P. transfusion filter
palladium-103 implantation
palliation
p. index
pure symptom p.
symptom p.
palliative
p. care
p. chemotherapy
p. esophagostomy
p. gastrojejunostomy
p. gastrostomy
p. intent
p. radiation therapy
p. radiotherapy
p. surgery
p. treatment
pallidum
direct fluorescent antibody staining for *Treponema p. (DFA-TP)*
Treponema p.
pallor
myelin p.
palm
tripe p.'s

palmar erythema
palmar-plantar erythrodysesthesia
  (PPED)
Palmaz-Schatz biliary stent
palmitate
    retinyl p.
Palmitate-A 5000
palmoplantar
    p. erythrodysesthesia syndrome
    p. keratosis
palmoplantar keratosis
palonosetron
palpable postmenopausal ovary
palpation
palpatory T-stage prostate cancer
palsy, pl. palsies
    Bell p.
    bulbar p.
    cerebral p.
    cranial nerve p.
    facial p.
    gaze p.
    hypoglossal nerve p.
    postneonatal Erb p.
    recurrent nerve p.
    vagus nerve p.
    vocal cord p.
PAM
    phenylalanine mustard
L-PAM
    L-phenylalanine mustard
    Adria + L-PAM
      Adriamycin plus L-phenylalanine
        mustard
      Adriamycin plus L-PAM
Pamelor
pamidronate disodium
p-aminobenzoic acid
pamoate
    octreotide p.
    triptorelin p.
Pamorelin
Panadol
Panafil ointment
panagglutinin
Panax ginseng
panbronchiolitis
    diffuse p.
Pancoast
    P. syndrome
    P. tumor
pancreas
    anular p.

body of p.
p. cancer
ectopic p.
intraductal papillary neoplasm of p.
  (IPNP)
pancreatic
    p. acinar cell
    p. adenocarcinoma
    p. allograft
    p. biopsy
    p. cancer
    p. cholera
    p. cyst
    p. cystic lymphangioma
    p. ductal adenocarcinoma (PDAC)
    p. ductectatic-type carcinoma
    p. endocrine tumor
    p. gland
    p. islet cell tumor
    p. oncofetal antigen
    p. polypeptide
    p. polypeptidoma (PPoma)
    p. transplant
pancreaticobiliary
    p. duct
    p. tract
pancreaticoblastoma
pancreaticoduodenectomy
pancreaticojejunostomy
    duct-to-mucosa p.
pancreatitis
    acute p.
    chronic p.
    diffuse p.
    edematous p.
    fulminant p.
    hemorrhagic p.
    hereditary p.
pancreatography
    percutaneous p.
pancreatoscopic cytology
pancreatoscopy
pancreozymin
Pancretec 2000 pump
pancuronium bromide
pancytopenia
pandemic
panel
    antibody p.
    CEA-TPA-CA15.3 tumor marker p.
    Heritage P.
    prior exposure hepatitis p.

NOTES

P

panencephalitis
  nodular p.
  subacute sclerosing p. (SSPE)
Paneth cell
Panhematin
panhematopenia
panhematopoietic cell antigen
panhypopituitarism
panimmunity
panitumumab
Panje voice button
Panmycin Oral
panmyelosis
  acute p.
panniculitis
  lymphomatoid p.
  mesenteric p. (MP)
  systemic nodular p.
panniculitis-like T-cell subcutaneous lymphoma
Panomat infusion pump
panophthalmitis
Panorex radiograph
panrenal tumor
Panretin topical gel
PANTA
  polymyxin B, amphotericin B, nalidixic acid, trimethoprim, azlocillin
Panton-Valentine leukocidin
Panvac-VF
PAP
  peroxidase-antiperoxidase
  primary atypical pneumonia
  prostatic acid phosphatase
  pulmonary alveolar proteinosis
  PAP tumor marker
Papanicolaou
  liquid-based P. (LBP)
  P. smear
  P. stain
  P. test
Papavasiliou
  P. classification
  P. classification of olecranon fractures
papaverine
paper radioimmunosorbent test (PRIST)
papilla, pl. **papillae**
  circumvallate p.
  duodenal p.
papillary
  p. adenocarcinoma
  p. blush
  p. cystadenoma lymphomatosum
  p. cystic adenoma
  p. cystic neoplasm
  p. epididymal cystadenoma
  p. hyperplasia
  p. mesothelioma

  p. microcarcinoma (PMC)
  p. serous carcinoma
  p. squamotransitional cell carcinoma
  p. syringoadenoma
  p. thyroid carcinoma (PTC)
  p. tumor
  p. urothelial neoplasm of low malignant potential (PUNLMP)
papillated
papilliferum
  hidradenoma p.
  syringocystadenoma p.
papillocarcinoma
papilloma
  basal cell p.
  choroid plexus p.
  ductal p.
  intracystic p.
  intraductal p.
  inverted p. (IP)
  inverted schneiderian p.
  penile squamous p.
  p., polyoma, vacuolating virus
  squamous cell p.
  transitional cell p.
  villous p.
  p. virus
papillomatosis
  intraductal p.
papillomavirus
  human p. (type 16, 18) (HPV)
  infectious p.
  Shope p.
papillomavirus-like particle
PAPNET system
papovavirus
  JC p.
Pappenheim
  lymphoid hemoblast of P.
Pappenheimer body
PAPS
  primary antiphospholipid antibody syndrome
PapSure cervical screening
papular
  p. eruption
  p. mucinosis
papule
  Gottron p.
papulosis
  bowenoid p.
  lymphomatoid p. (LP)
papulosquamous
  p. dermatosis
  p. disease
papulovesicular lesion
PAR
  protease-activated receptor
paraaminobenzoic acid (PABA)

paraaortic
 p. lymphadenectomy
 p. lymphadenopathy
 p. lymph node
 p. node sampling
parabiotic syndrome
paracarcinomatous myelopathy
paracardiac
 p. metastasis
 p. tumor
paracaval lymph node
paracentesis
paracervical tissue
paracetamol
parachlorophenylalanine (PCPA)
paracoccidioidal granuloma
Paracoccidioides braziliensis
paracolpos
paracrine
 p. effect
 p. loop
 p. manner
paradigm
 Halsted p.
 LENT p.
paradoxical embolus
paradoxicum
 carcinoma p.
paradoxus
 pulsus p.
paraffin
 p. block embedding
 p. cancer
 p. tissue section
 p. tumor
paraffinoma
parafollicular C cell
paraformaldehyde
paraganglioma
 intravagal p.
 jugulotympanic p.
 nonchromaffin p.
paraganglion
 aorticosympathetic p.
 branchiomeric p.
 retroperitoneal p.
 visceral p.
paraglottic space
paragon
 P. ambulatory pump
 P. immunofixation electrophoresis
 P. infuser
paragranuloma

paralaryngeal muscle
parallel
 p. arrays
 p. bones
 p. plate dialyzer
parallel-opposed
 p.-o. beams
 p.-o. fields
paralysis, pl. **paralyses**
 antigenic p.
 diaphragmatic p.
 facial nerve p.
 immunologic p.
 nerve p.
 phrenic nerve p.
 vocal cord p.
paramagnetic
 p. cation
 p. enhancement
 p. iron species
 p. microsphere
paramagnetism
 apparent p.
parameningeal rhabdomyosarcoma
parameter
 cell-cycle p.
 extrinsic cellular p.
 grading p.
 histologic p.
 pharmacokinetic p.
paramethasone acetate
parametrectomy
 radical p.
parametrium, pl. **parametria**
paranasal
 p. sinus
 p. sinus cancer
paranasopharyngeal disease
paraneoplasia
paraneoplastic
 p. acrokeratosis
 p. anemia
 p. anorexia
 p. antiphospholipid syndrome
 p. basophilia
 p. cachexia
 p. complication
 p. dermatomyositis
 p. disease
 p. ectopic ACTH production
 p. encephalomyelitis
 p. endocarditis
 p. eosinophilia

NOTES

P

paraneoplastic *(continued)*
   p. erythema
   p. erythrocytosis
   p. granulocytosis
   p. hepatopathy
   p. hypercalcemia
   p. hypercoagulability
   p. hypocalcemia
   p. malabsorption
   p. neurologic syndrome
   p. opsoclonus-myoclonus
   p. pemphigus (PNP)
   p. polymyositis
   p. retinal degeneration
   p. sensorimotor peripheral
     neuropathy
   p. sensory neuropathy
   p. thrombocytosis
paraneoplastica
   acrokeratosis p.
paranuclear body
paraparesis
   tropical spastic p. (TSP)
   X-linked spastic p.
parapharyngeal lymphatic
paraphimosis
Paraplatin
paraprotein disease
paraproteinemia
parapsilosis
     Candida p.
parapsoriasis
   large plaque p.
Paraquat poisoning
parasagittal meningioma
parasellar
   p. dermoid tumor
   p. metastasis
parasitic leiomyoma
parasympathetic ganglion
paratesticular
   p. region
   p. rhabdomyosarcoma (P-RMS)
   p. tumor
Parathar
parathormone (PTH)
parathymus gland
parathyroid
   p. adenoma
   p. biopsy
   p. carcinoma
   ectopic p.
   p. gland
   p. gland enlargement
   p. hormone (PTH)
   p. hormone-related protein (PTHrP)
   p. tumor
   p. tumor ablation
   p. vein

paratracheal
   p. adenopathy
   p. lymphadenopathy
   p. node chain
paravertebral sulcus
paregoric
parenchyma
   brain p.
   breast p.
   cerebral p.
   glandular p.
   hepatic p.
   testicular p.
   tumor p.
parenchymal
   p. blastoma
   p. brain metastasis
parent
   p. drug
   p. vector
parenteral
   p. antigen
   p. chemotherapy
   Coly-Mycin M P.
   p. nutrition
   p. phosphate therapy
   p. route
   p. site
paresthesia
   circumoral p.
   perioral p.
paricalcitol
Paris
   P. method
   P. method for radium therapy
   P. system
   P. system for brachytherapy
Parlodel
Parnate
Parodi-Irgens sarcoma virus
paromomycin
paronychial infection
parosteal
   p. osteosarcoma
   p. sarcoma
parotid
   p. cancer
   p. capsule
   p. gland
   p. gland enlargement
   p. lymph node
   p. tail
   p. tumor
parotidectomy
parotid-sparing technique
parotitis, parotiditis
   epidemic p.
parous patient

parovarian
- p. cyst
- p. cystadenocarcinoma

paroxetine

paroxysmal
- p. auricular tachycardia
- p. cold hemoglobinuria (PCH)
- p. nocturnal hemoglobinuria (PNH)
- p. nocturnal hemoglobinuria cell
- p. supraventricular tachycardia

partial
- p. duodenopancreatectomy
- p. gastrectomy
- p. hydatidiform mole (PHM)
- p. lamellar sclerouvectomy
- p. response (PR)
- p. shunt
- p. thromboplastin time (PTT)
- p. viral suppression

particle
- alpha p.
- p. beam radiation therapy
- Dane p.
- iron-dextran p.
- Ivalon p.
- neon p.
- papillomavirus-like p.
- tumor-liberated p. (TLP)
- viruslike p. (VLP)

particulate
- p. embolization
- p. radiation

Partin coefficient table

partner
- seroconcordant p.
- serodiscordant p.

parts per million (ppm)

Parvolex

parvovirus
- B19 p.
- p. B19 neutralizing antibody assay
- human p. (HPV)

parvum
- *Corynebacterium p.*

PAS
- periodic acid-Schiff
- Peripheral Access System
- physician-assisted suicide
- PAS Port Fluoro-Free catheter
- PAS stain

PASH
- pseudoangiomatous stromal hyperplasia

passage
- adiabatic fast p. (AFP)

passionflower

passive
- p. administration
- p. death wish
- p. diffusion
- p. hemagglutination
- p. humoral immunotherapy
- p. immunization
- p. shield
- p. shielding
- p. smoking

Passovoy factor

PASTA
- polarity-altered spectral selective acquisition
- PASTA imaging

Pasteurella multocida

Pasteur Institute bacillus Calmette-Guérin vaccine

past-pointing technique

patch
- ash leaf p.
- Deponit P.
- doobie derm p.
- Duragesic Transdermal p.
- Durotep p.
- marijuana p.
- Minitran P.
- mucous p.
- Nitro-Dur P.
- p. phase
- pot p.
- salmon p.
- transdermal medication p.
- Transderm-Nitro P.

PATCO
- prednisone, ara-C, 6-thioguanine, cyclophosphamide, Oncovin

patellectomy

patent blue V dye

PATEO
- periarticular thenar erythema and onycholysis

Paterson-Brown-Kelly syndrome

Paterson-Kelly syndrome

Paterson-Parker system

Paterson syndrome

Patey technique

pathlength
- effective p. (EPL)

NOTES

P

pathogen
    enteric p.
    opportunistic p.
pathogenesis
    p. dynamic
    HIV p.
    immune p.
pathognomonic sign
pathologic
    p. cell death
    p. feature
    p. fracture
    p. psychomotor slowing
pathologist
    Cancer Committee of College of
    American P.'s
pathology (PA)
    Armed Forces Institute of P.
    (AFIP)
    focal p.
    mediastinal p.
    p. specimen
    surgical p.
pathophysiology
PathVysion HER-2 DNA probe kit
pathway
    antiapoptotic signaling p.
    autonomic p.
    B7 CD28 T cell costimulatory p.
    c-fos-dependent p.
    c-fos-independent p.
    coagulation p.
    common p.
    COX p.
    cyclooxygenase p.
    Embden-Meyerhof metabolic p.
    endocytic p.
    extrinsic coagulation p.
    Fas-Fas ligand p.
    folate uptake p.
    glycolytic p.
    intrinsic coagulation p.
    ligand p.
    Luebering-Rapaport p.
    signal transduction p.
    T-cell costimulatory p.
    visual p.
patient
    adolescent nulliparous p.
    p. advocate
    cancer p.
    p. care
    chemotherapy-responsive p.
    cured p.
    p. dose monitor
    dual-diagnosis p.
    exceptional cancer p. (ECaP)
    febrile p.
    gynecologic cancer p.

    node-negative p.
    nulliparous p.
    parous p.
    postmenopausal nulliparous p.
    premenopausal p.
    receptor-negative p.
    source p.
    terminally ill p.
    tumor-free p.
patient-controlled
    p.-c. analgesia (PCA)
    p.-c. epidural analgesia (PCEA)
pattern
    airspace-filling p.
    airway p.
    alveolar p.
    antagonistic p.
    arc-beam p.
    atypical vessel colposcopic p.
    beam p.
    bony trabecular p.
    bronchovascular p.
    butterfly p.
    canalicular immunostaining p.
    cerebriform p.
    cribriform p.
    cross-resistance p.
    degenerative nuclear p.
    diffuse p.
    dissemination p.
    echolucent p.
    edema p.
    fleur-de-lis p.
    flow p.
    geographic p.
    germinal center p.
    hemangiopericytoma-like p.
    high-velocity flow p.
    insular p.
    interfollicular p.
    IRF staining p.
    leaf motion p.
    Lennert p.
    L/H nodular p.
    Likert-type response p.
    lymphatic drainage p.
    mantle zone p.
    marginal zone p.
    membranous p.
    migrant p.
    mixed p.
    morphologic p.
    mosaic p.
    mottling p.
    myxoid cell p.
    nodular p.
    onion-skinning p.
    pendulum-like swing p.
    permeative p.

pseudofollicular growth p.
ring p.
p. of spread
starry-sky p.
storiform p.
storiform-pleomorphic p.
tigroid p.
trabecular p.
tubular p.
urticaria p.
paucicellular lesion
paucimobilis
    Pseudomonas p.
paucity
pau d'arco tea
Pauli exclusion principle
paunch
    protease p.
Pautrier
    P. abscess
    P. microabscess
PAVe
    procarbazine, Alkeran, Velban
Paveral Stanley Syrup with Codeine Phosphate
PAX-5 gene
PAX-7 gene
PAXgene Blood RNA kit
paxillin protein
PB
    peripheral blood
    PB stem cell transplantation
PBD
    percutaneous biliary drainage
PBL
    peripheral blood lymphocyte
    primary brain lymphoma
    primary breast lymphoma
PBMC
    peripheral blood mononuclear cell
PBPC
    peripheral blood progenitor cell
PBPF
    primary bronchopulmonary fibrosarcoma
PBS
    phosphate-buffered saline
PBSC
    peripheral blood stem cell
PBSCR
    peripheral blood stem cell reserve
PBSCT
    peripheral blood stem cell transplant

PBTG
    Philadelphia Bone Marrow Transplant Group
PBV
    Platinol, bleomycin, vinblastine
PBX1
    PBX1 oncogene
    PBX1 protooncogene/oncogene
PC10
    monoclonal antibody PC10
PCA
    patient-controlled analgesia
P-cadherin expression
PCB
    procarbazine
PCC
    percutaneous cervical cordotomy
PCE
    Platinol, cyclophosphamide, Eldisine
    Platinol, Cytoxan, etoposide
PCEA
    patient-controlled epidural analgesia
P-cell stimulating factor
PCH
    paroxysmal cold hemoglobinuria
P-CHOP
    cisplatin, cyclophosphamide, doxorubicin, vincristine, prednisone
PCI
    prophylactic cranial irradiation
PCL
    polycation liposome
PCLI
    plasma cell labeling index
PCM
    prophylactic contralateral mastectomy
PCNA
    proliferating cell nuclear antigen
PCNHL
    primary cerebral non-Hodgkin lymphoma
PCNSL
    primary central nervous system lymphoma
        AIDS PCNSL
PCOD
    polycystic ovarian disease
PCPA
    parachlorophenylalanine
PCR
    polymerase chain reaction
        PCR detection of Hp^{del}
        RNA PCR

NOTES

P

423

PCT
  procalcitonin
PCV
  packed cell volume
  polycythemia vera
  procarbazine, CCNU, vincristine
  procarbazine, lomustine, vincristine
    PCV protocol
    PCV therapy
    PCV therapy of recurrent
      oligoastrocytoma tumor
PCZ
  procarbazine
PD-10 disposable Sephadex G-25
  column
PDAC
  pancreatic ductal adenocarcinoma
PDD
  percentage depth dose
PDE
  phosphodiesterase
PDEC
  poorly differentiated endocrine carcinoma
PD-ECGF
  platelet-derived endothelial cell growth
    factor
    PD-ECGF expression
PDET
  poorly differentiated embryonal cell
    tumor
PDGF
  platelet-derived growth factor
    PDGF-b receptor for PDGF
PDGFA
  platelet-derived growth factor A
PDGF-a receptor oncogene
PDGF-b receptor for PDGF
PdGold brachytherapy seed
PDIg
  platelet-directed immunoglobulin
PDLL
  poorly differentiated lymphocytic
    lymphoma
PDQ
  Physician Data Query
    PDQ information system
PDR
  pulsed dose rate
    PDR brachytherapy
PDT
  photodynamic therapy
    Metvix PDT
PE
  phosphatidylethanolamine
  physical examination
  pulmonary edema
  pulmonary embolism
Peacock system

peak
  Bragg p.
  photon p.
peak-dose level
peakscatter factor
peanut agglutinin
pearl
  epidermic p.
  epithelial p.
  keratin p.
  P. Omega
  p. tumor
pearly
  p. neoplasm
  p. tumor
peau d'orange
PEB
  Platinol, etoposide, bleomycin
PEC
  perivascular epithelioid cell
  Platinol, etoposide, cyclophosphamide
PECAM-1
  platelet endothelial cell adhesion
    molecule-1
pectin
  hyoscyamine, atropine, scopolamine,
    kaolin, p.
  kaolin and p.
  modified citrus p.
pectinate line
pectineus muscle
pectoral muscle
pectoris
  angina p. (AP)
Pediapred oral
pediatric
  p. brainstem glioma
  p. cancer
  p. fatty marrow
  p. fibroxanthoma
  p. hemangioma
  Lupron P.
  p. lymphoma
  p. mass
  p. multivitamin infusion
  M.V.I. P.
  P. Oncology Group (POG)
  P. RAC Registry
  p. solid tumor
Pediazole
pedicle transposition flap
pedigree
  family p.
pedis
  dorsalis p.
  tinea p.
PedTE-PAK-4
Pedtrace-4

peduncle
  cerebellar p.
  cerebral p.
pedunculated polyp
peer-to-peer discussion format
PEG
  percutaneous endoscopic gastrostomy
  polyethylene glycol
    PEG interleukin-2
    PEG r-hirudin assay
    PEG tube
peg
  p. cell
  cerebellar p.
PEG-ADA
  pegademase bovine
  polyethylene glycol-modified adenosine
    deaminase
pegademase bovine (PEG-ADA)
PEG-L-ASP
  PEG-L-asparaginase
  polyethylene glycol-conjugated L-
    asparaginase
PEG-L-asparaginase (PEG-L-ASP)
pegasparaginase
pegaspargase
PEG-camptothecin
PEG-DOXO
  pegylated liposomal doxorubicin
pegfilgrastim
  p. injection
PEG-IL-2
  polyethylene glycol-modified interleukin-
    2
PEG-Intron A
pegnology
PEG-paclitaxel
pegylated
  p. interferon
  p. liposomal doxorubicin (PEG-
    DOXO)
PEI
  percutaneous ethanol injection
PEIT
  percutaneous ethanol injection therapy
    PEIT therapy
PEJ
  percutaneous endoscopic jejunostomy
PELCA
  percutaneous excimer laser coronary
    angioplasty
Pel-Ebstein
  P.-E. disease

P.-E. fever
P.-E. pyrexia
P.-E. symptom
PELF
  cisplatin, epirubicin, folinic acid, 5-
    fluorouracil
Pelger anomaly
Pelger-Huët
  P.-H. anomaly
  P.-H. cell
  P.-H. neutrophil
pelgeroid
peliomycin
pellet
  stainless p.
  Testopel P.
pelvic
  p. ascites
  p. aspiration biopsy
  p. brim
  p. exenteration
  p. girdle
  p. irradiation
  p. lymphadenectomy
  p. lymphadenopathy
  p. lymph node
  p. lymph node dissection (PLND)
  p. malignancy
  p. malignancy in pregnancy
  p. mass
  p. and periaortic control (PPC)
  p. rest
pelvis, pl. pelves
  bifid renal p.
  bony p.
  brim of p.
  extrarenal p.
  periacetabular p.
  renal p.
  shielding of abdomen and p.
  true p.
Pembrey method
pemetrexed disodium
pemoline
pemphigoid
  bullous p.
pemphigus
  p. foliaceus
  paraneoplastic p. (PNP)
pemtumomab
pencil electron beam
penclomedine

NOTES

P

pendetide
    capromab p.
    ^{111}In-labeled capromab p.
    satumomab p.
pendulum-like swing pattern
penectomy
penetrance
penetrans
    hyperkeratosis follicularis et
      parafollicularis in cutem p.
penetration
    bowel wall p.
    transmural p.
Penetrex
penicillamine
penicillin
    p. G benzathine
    p. G benzathine and procaine
      combined
    p. G, parenteral, aqueous
    p. G procaine
    p. V potassium
Penicillium marneffei
penile
    p. bulb dosimetry
    p. bulb imaging
    p. cancer
    p. squamous papilloma
PENL
    primary extranodal lymphoma
Penrose drain
Penta/3B Plus
Pentacarinat Injection
Pentacea
pentafuside
pentagastrin-Ca stimulation test
pentagastrin stimulation test
Pentam-300 Injection
pentamethylmelamine
pentamidine
    aerosolized p.
    p. isethionate
    systemic p.
pentamustine
Pentaspan
pentastarch
Pentatrichomonas hominis
pentazocine compound
pentetreotide
pentosan
    p. polysulfate
    p. polysulfate sodium
pentostatin injection
Pentothal Sodium
pentoxifylline (PTX)
penumbra
    beam p.
    broad fuzzy p.
    sharp p.

penumbral effect
PEP
    Procytox, epipodophyllotoxin-derivative,
      prednisolone
Pepcid AC Acid Controller
peplomycin
pepper
    P. syndrome
    P. tumor
pepsinogen C
pepstatin
peptichemio
peptide
    p. activated lymphocyte
    anionic neutrophil-activating p.
      (ANAP)
    atrial natriuretic p.
    autologous T lymphocytes
      stimulated with the patient's
      tumor-specific mutated RAS p.'s
    chemotactic p.
    fusion p.
    gastrin-releasing p. (GRP)
    gp100 p.
    gp100:209-217 p.
    gp209-2M immunodominant p.
    HIV-1 gp120 C4-V-3 p.
    hybrid polyvalent synthetic p.
    immunodominant p.
    insulin-like p.
    p. major histocompatibility complex
    MART-1 p.
    neurogastrointestinal p.
    neutrophil-activating p.
    prepro-gastrin-releasing p.
      (preproGRP)
    synthetic HIV p.
    synthetic human immunodeficiency
      virus p.
    synthetic linear p.
    synthetic octameric p.
    trefoil factor p. 1 (TFF1)
    tumor antigen epitope p.
    tumor-specific mutated RAS p.
    tumor-specific mutated VHL p.
    vasoactive intestinal p. (VIP)
    vimentin p.
peptide-MHC complex
peptide-pulsed cell
peptidic MMP inhibitor
peptidomimetic inhibitor complex
Pepto-Bismol
per anum intersphincteric rectal
    dissection
percentage depth dose (PDD)
perception
    taste p.
Percocet
Percocet-Demi

Percodan
Percodan-Demi
Percogesic
Percolone
percussion and postural drainage (PPD)
percutaneous
   p. alcohol injection
   p. aspiration thromboembolectomy
   p. atherectomy
   p. biliary drainage (PBD)
   p. catheter drainage
   p. cecostomy
   p. cervical cordotomy (PCC)
   p. endoscopic gastrostomy (PEG)
   p. endoscopic gastrostomy tube
   p. endoscopic jejunostomy (PEJ)
   p. endoscopy
   p. enterostomy
   p. ethanol ablation
   p. ethanol ablation of tumor
   p. ethanol injection (PEI)
   p. ethanol injection therapy (PEIT)
   p. excimer laser coronary
      angioplasty (PELCA)
   p. excimer laser coronary
      angioplasty system
   p. exposure
   p. exposure risk
   p. fetal tissue sampling
   p. fine-needle aspiration (PFNA)
   p. fine-needle aspiration biopsy
      (PFNAB)
   p. gastroenterostomy
   p. liver biopsy
   p. localization
   p. low-stress angioplasty
   p. microwave coagulation therapy
      (PMCT)
   p. needle
   p. needle puncture
   p. nephroscope
   p. nephroscopy
   p. nephrostomy
   p. nephrostomy catheter
   p. pancreatography
   p. placement
   p. portocaval anastomosis
   p. thermal occlusion
   p. transcatheter therapy
   p. transhepatic biliary drainage
      (PTBD)
   p. transhepatic biliary procedure
   p. transhepatic catheter
   p. transhepatic cholangiography
      (PTC)
   p. transhepatic sclerosis
   p. transthoracic needle aspiration
      biopsy
   p. tumor ablation
   p. umbilical blood sampling
      (PUBS)
Perdiem Plain
per-event occupational infection
Perflex
   P. delivery system
   P. stainless steel stent
perfluorocarbon
perfluorochemical
perforating colorectal cancer
perforation
   colon p.
   colonic p.
   esophageal p.
perforator
perforin-mediated cytotoxic activity
performance status
perfosfamide
perfringens
   Clostridium p.
perfusion
   antiblastic p.
   arterial p.
   brain p.
   continuous hyperthermic
      peritoneal p. (CHPP)
   heat p.
   hepatic portal p.
   hyperthermic antiblastic p.
   hyperthermic intraperitoneal
      antiblastic p. (HIIC)
   hyperthermic limb p.
   hypothermic p.
   intraperitoneal p.
   isolated heat p.
   isolated hepatic p. (IHP)
   isolated hepatic portal and
      arterial p.
   isolated limb p. (ILP)
   limb p.
   p. study
   p. therapy
   tissue p.
Pergamid
Pergonal
periacetabular pelvis
periampullary carcinoma

NOTES

P

perianal area
periaortic
  p. lymph node
  p. mediastinal hematoma
periapical
  p. cemental dysplasia
  p. granuloma
periaquaductal stimulation
periarteriolar lymphoid sheath
periarticular
  p. fluid collection
  p. fracture
  p. margin
  p. thenar erythema and onycholysis
    (PATEO)
periauricular meningioma
pericallosal lipoma
pericardial
  p. cancer
  p. compliance
  p. drainage
  p. effusion
  p. mesothelioma
  p. rub
  p. tamponade
  p. window
pericardiectomy
  window p.
pericardiocentesis
pericardiotomy
  balloon p.
pericarditis
  chemotherapy-induced p.
  effusive p.
  radiation-induced p.
Peri-Colace
periesophageal nodal chain
perifosine
  oral p.
perihilar lymphadenectomy
perilesional white matter
perillyl alcohol
perimenopause
perinatal transmission
perineal
  p. care
  p. sphincter electromyography
  p. urethrostomy
perineoplasty
perinephric
  p. abscess drainage
  p. hematoma
  p. urinoma
perineural
  p. invasion (PNI)
  p. tumor spread
perineurioma
  intraneural p.

perinuclear
  p. CD15 antigen
  p. halo
period
  embryonic p.
  G_0 p.
  incubation p.
  postbiopsy p.
  straight-line recovery p.
  window p.
periodic
  p. acid-Schiff (PAS)
  p. acid-Schiff reaction
  p. acid-Schiff stain
  p. acid staining
periodontal
  p. bone destruction
  p. disease
periodontitis
  HIV necrotizing p.
  human immunodeficiency
    necrotizing p.
perioptic meningioma
perioral
  p. fissure
  p. paresthesia
periosteal
  p. bone
  p. fibrosarcoma
  p. osteosarcoma
  p. sarcoma
periosteum, pl. periostea
periostitis
  diaphysial p.
peripancreatic
  p. lymphadenopathy
  p. vein
peripheral
  P. Access System (PAS)
  P. Access System Port catheter
    system
  p. androgen blockade (PAB)
  p. anterior synechia
  p. blood (PB)
  p. blood lymphocyte (PBL)
  p. blood mononuclear cell (PBMC)
  p. blood mononuclear cell hepatitis
    B virus measurement
  p. blood progenitor cell (PBPC)
  p. blood progenitor cell
    mobilization regimen
  p. blood stem cell (PBSC)
  p. blood stem cell autografting
  p. blood stem cell reserve
    (PBSCR)
  p. blood stem cell support
  p. blood stem cell transplant
    (PBSCT)
  p. carcinoma

p. cholangiocarcinoma
p. chondrosarcoma
p. disciform degeneration
p. enhancement
p. injection
p. lymphoid cell
p. monocyte-derived dendritic cell immunization
p. nerve
p. nerve block
p. nerve stimulation
p. nervous system
p. neuroectodermal tumor
p. neurologic adverse effect
p. neuropathy
p. neurotoxicity
p. ossifying fibroma
p. T-cell lymphoma
p. vascular disease (PVD)
p. vein catheter
peripherally inserted central catheter (PICC)
peripherin
periprostatic fat
perirectal
p. cellulitis
p. disease
p. inflammation
perirenal lymphoma
peristalsis
esophageal p.
peritetraploid
perithelial cell
peritoneal
p. carcinomatosis
p. cytology
p. dialysis
p. dissemination
p. fluid
p. implant metastasis
p. lavage
p. lymphoma
p. macrophage
p. mesothelial cyst
p. mesothelioma
p. sampling
p. seeding
p. spill
p. washing
peritonei
carcinomatosis p.
peritoneoplasty
peritoneoscopy

peritoneoserosal
peritoneovenous
p. shunt
p. shunting
peritoneum desmoid tumor
peritonitis
sclerosing encapsulating p. (SEP)
peritrophoblastic flow
peritumoral
p. brain edema
p. tissue
periureteral disease
periurethral gland
perivascular epithelioid cell (PEC)
periventricular bright signal
periwinkle alkaloid
perlèche
permanent seed implant brachytherapy
Permapen
permeability
vascular p.
permeable collagen microcarrier
permeation
lymphatic p.
permeative
p. neuroectodermal tumor
p. pattern
permethrin
permissible exposure limit
permutation
pernicious anemia (PA)
peroral cone radiation therapy
peroxidase
horseradish p.
platelet p.
peroxidase-antiperoxidase (PAP)
peroxidation
lipid p.
peroxide
hydrogen p.
peroxisome
p. proliferator
p. proliferator activated receptor (PPAR)
perphenazine
amitriptyline and p.
Per-Q-Cath catheter
Persantine
persistence
hereditary p.
persistent
p. fetal microchimerism

NOTES

P

persistent *(continued)*
p. generalized lymphadenopathy
  (PGL)
p. hyperplastic primary vitreous
p. pulmonary hypertension
p. rhinitis
p. rhinorrhea
person with AIDS (PWA)
Perspex tube
perturbation
perturbed water motion
pertussis
  Bordetella p.
  diphtheria, tetanus, p. (DTP)
  diphtheria and tetanus toxoid with
    acellular p. (DTaP)
  Haemophilus p.
perversion
  taste p.
pes anserinus
pessary cell
PET
  positron emission tomography
    C-methionine PET
    ^{18}F-fluorodeoxyglucose PET
    MET PET
    whole body PET
petechia, pl. **petechiae**
petechial hemorrhage
Peto formula
petrosal sinus
petrositis
  apical p.
PETT
  phenethylthiazolethiourea
Peutz-Jeghers syndrome
Peyronie disease
PF4
  platelet factor 4
    Asserachrom PF4
PFA-100 testing
PFE
  Platinol, 5-fluorouracil, etoposide
Pfeiffer acrocephalosyndactyly
Pfizerpen
PFL
  Platinol, 5-fluorouracil, leucovorin
PFL-IFN
  cisplatin, 5-fluorouracil, leucovorin,
    interferon alfa-2b
PFM
  Platinol, 5-fluorouracil, methotrexate
PFNA
  percutaneous fine-needle aspiration
PFNAB
  percutaneous fine-needle aspiration
    biopsy

PFS
  progression-free survival
    Idamycin PFS
PFT
  phenylalanine, 5-fluorouracil, tamoxifen
  prednisone, 5-fluorouracil, tamoxifen
PGE
  prostaglandin E
PGF
  prostaglandin F
PGL
  persistent generalized lymphadenopathy
P-glycoprotein (P-170, P-gp)
PGM 37 antibody
P-gp
  P-glycoprotein
P-gp-negative leukemia
PgR
  progesterone receptor
  progestin receptor
PG-TXL
  polyglutamate paclitaxel
PGY1 gene
PGY3 gene
pH
  hydrogen ion concentration
    intraluminal pH
    luminal pH
phacoma, phakoma
phacomatosis, phakomatosis
phage combinatorial library
phagocyte
  p. migration
  mononuclear p.
  polymorphonuclear p.
phagocytic
  p. cell
  p. defense
  p. dysfunction disorder
    immunodeficiency
phagocytoblast
phagocytolysis
phagocytosis
  granulocyte p.
  induced p.
  spontaneous p.
phakoma *(var. of* phacoma*)*
phakomatosis *(var. of* phacomatosis*)*
phallectomy
phantom
  p. limb pain
  p. limb syndrome
  p. tumor
Pharmacal
**pharmacodynamic-pharmacokinetic
  relationship**
pharmacodynamic profile
pharmacodynamics

pharmacoendoscopy
    light-induced fluorescence endoscopy
       in combination with p.
pharmacokinetic
    Bayesian p.
    p. enhancement
    p. parameter
    p. profile
pharmacokinetic-pharmacodynamic
  relationship
pharmacologic
    p. aid
    p. maintenance erection flow
    p. method
    p. method of purging
pharmacology
pharmacotherapy
    unorthodox p.
Pharmaseal needle
PharmaSeed
    P. iodine-125 seed
    P. palladium-103 seed
Pharmorubicin RDF
pharyngeal
    p. constrictor muscle
    p. recess
    p. wall
    p. wall cancer
    p. wall carcinoma
pharynges (*pl. of* pharynx)
pharyngitis
pharyngocutaneous fistula
pharyngoepiglottic fold
pharynx, pl. **pharynges**
phase
    accelerated p.
    accumulative p.
    arterial p.
    blast p.
    blastic p.
    chronic p.
    chronic myelogenous leukemia
      blastic p. (CML-BP)
    chronic myeloid leukemia blast p.
      (CML-BP)
    convalescent p.
    dose-controlled p.
    G p.
    G_o p.
    hepatic arterial p. (HAP)
    hepatic arterial dominant p.
    p. II autologous vaccination
    p. IIb trial

    p. I–III trial
    involuting p.
    p. I protocol
    M p.
    megakaryocytic blastic p.
    patch p.
    plaque p.
    premycotic p.
    proliferative p.
    quiescent p.
    radial p.
    S p.
    slow low p.
phased-array
    p.-a. coil
    p.-a. system
phase-specific action
Ph-CML
    Philadelphia chromosome-negative
      chronic myelogenous leukemia
Phemister triad R
phenazopyridine
    sulfamethoxazole and p.
    sulfisoxazole and p.
phenelzine
Phenergan
phenethylamine
phenethylthiazolethiourea (PETT)
phenobarbital
phenol
phenomenon, pl. **phenomena**
    autoimmune p.
    dawn p.
    Denys-Leclef p.
    Dubin-Johnson p.
    embolic p.
    flare p.
    flip-flop p.
    gene-silencing p.
    Gengou p.
    Hamburger p.
    Hektoen p.
    hematocrit p.
    Herendeen p.
    iceberg p.
    Koch p.
    Leede-Rumpel p.
    Liacopoulos p.
    Lyon p.
    Matuhasi-Ogata p.
    memory p.
    Raynaud p.

NOTES

P

phenomenon *(continued)*
    Rumpel-Leede p.
    Will Rogers p.
PhenoSense GT Combination HIV Drug Resistance Assay
phenothiazine
phenotype
    Cellano p.
    lipoatrophic p.
    McLeod p.
    multidrug-resistant p.
    somatic Tax-associated mutator p.
    spindle cell p.
    syncytium-inducing p.
    T-cell p.
    viral p.
phenotypic
    p. drug resistance
    p. escape
    p. level
phenoxodiol
phenoxyacetic
    p. acid
    p. acid herbicide
phenoxybenzamine
phenpropionate
    nandrolone p.
phensuximide
phentolamine
phenylacetate
phenylalanine
    p., 5-fluorouracil, tamoxifen (PFT)
    p. mustard (PAM)
    p. mustard, methotrexate, 5-fluorouracil (PMF)
phenylbutyrate
    continuous infusion p.
phenylephrine
phenylethanolamine-N-methyltransferase
phenylhydrazine anemia
phenyloxazolone
phenylthiourea
phenyltoloxamine
    acetaminophen and p.
phenytoin-induced pseudolymphoma syndrome
pheochromocytoma
    adrenal p.
    benign p.
    extraadrenal p.
    malignant p.
pheresis
    lipid p.
Phicon
Philadelphia
    P. Bone Marrow Transplant Group (PBTG)
    P. chromosome

    P. chromosome negative (Ph-negative)
    P. chromosome-negative chronic myelogenous leukemia (Ph-CML)
    P. chromosome positive (Ph-positive)
    P. chromosome-positive chronic myelogenous leukemia
    P. translocation
Philadelphia-positive
    P.-p. acute lymphoblastic leukemia cell
    P.-p. leukemia
Philippine dengue fever
Philips Tomoscan SR 6000 CT scanner
Phillips' Milk of Magnesia
phlebitis
phlebomyomatosis
phlebotomy-related anemia
phlegmon
    mesenteric p.
PHM
    partial hydatidiform mole
    Preventive Health Model
Ph-negative
    Philadelphia chromosome negative
phobia
phonation
phorbol ester
PhosLo
phosphatase
    alkaline p. (AP)
    alkaline phosphatase-antialkaline p. (APAAP)
    heat-stable alkaline p.
    leukocyte alkaline p. (LAP)
    neutrophil alkaline p.
    phosphotyrosine p.
    placental alkaline p. (PLAP)
    prostatic acid p. (PAP)
    serine-threonine p.
    tartrate-resistant acid p. (TRAP)
    p. and tensin homologue deleted on chromosome (PTEN)
    total serum prostatic acid p. (TSPAP)
phosphatase-1
    Fas-associated p.-1 (Fap-1)
phosphate
    aluminum p.
    Aralen Phosphate With Primaquine P.
    calcium p. (CaP)
    cellulose sodium p.
    chloroquine p.
    chromic p.
    dihydroxyacetone p. (DHAP)
    estramustine p. (EMP)
    etoposide p.

fludarabine p.
Linctus With Codeine P.
nicotinamide adenine dinucleotide p.
  (NADPH, NADP)
Paveral Stanley Syrup with
  Codeine P.
potassium phosphate and sodium p.
potassium, titanyl, p. (KTP)
sodium p.
triciribine p. (TCN-P)
zidovudine p.
phosphate-buffered saline (PBS)
phosphatidylcholine
phosphatidylethanolamine (PE)
  dipalmitoyl p.
  linked to dipalmitoyl p.
  muramyl tripeptide p. (MTP-PE)
phosphatidylinositol
phosphaturic substance
Phosphocol P32
phosphodiesterase (PDE)
  p. inhibitor
phosphodiester bond
phosphoethanolamine
phosphokinase
  creatine p. (CPK)
phospholipase cyl-1 expression
phospholipid-dependent coagulation
phospholipidosis
phospholipoproteinosis
phosphomonoester (PME)
phosphonate
  acyclic nucleoside p.
  nucleoside p.
  tetraazacyclododecanetetraacetic
    tetramethylene p. (DOTP)
phosphonoformate
phosphonylmethoxyethyl
phosphonylmethoxyethyladenine (PMEA)
9-2-phosphonylmethoxyethyl adenine
  (PMEA)
phosphonylmethoxypropyl
9-R-2-phosphonylmethoxypropyl adenine
  (PMPA)
phosphoprotein
  p53 p.
phosphoramide mustard
phosphorescence
5-phosphoribosyl-1-pyrophosphate (PRPP)
phosphoribosyl transferase (PRT)
phosphorothioate
phosphorus
  colloidal chromic p.

inorganic p.
p. magnetic resonance spectroscopy
  (P-MRS)
p. trihydrazide complex
phosphorus-32 (^{32}P, P32)
phosphorylase
  polynucleotide p. (PNP, PNPase)
  thymidine p.
phosphorylation
  anabolic p.
  histone p.
  mitochondrial oxidative p.
  p. of IE
  oxidative p.
  posttranslational p.
  tyrosine p.
phosphorylcholine
phosphoserine
Phospho-Soda
  Fleet P.-S.
phosphotransferase
  nucleoside p.
phosphotriester
  thioethanol p.
phosphotyrosine phosphatase
photoactivation
photobleaching
photo cell
photochemotherapy
  extracorporeal p. (ECP)
  topical p.
photocoagulation
photodermatitis
photodynamic therapy (PDT)
photofrin
photography
  iris fluorescein p.
  Moiré p.
  monochromatic p.
photoimmunotherapy
photoirradiation
  MC-540 p.
photomicrograph
  cystic hyperplasia p.
photon
  annihilation p.
  external p.
  high-energy p.
  p. peak
  p. radiosurgery system
photon-deficient bone lesion

NOTES

P

photoneutron
2-photon excitation (TPE)
photon-radiosurgical therapy (PRS)
photopheresis
photophobia
photophoresis
    extracorporeal p.
PhotoPoint light-activated process
photoradiation
photorefractive keratectomy
photosensitivity dermatitis
photosensitization
    phthalocyanine p.
photosensitizer
photosensitizers
phototherapy
    indocyanine green-enhanced p.
phototimer
phototreatment
Ph-positive
    Philadelphia chromosome positive
phrenic
    p. nerve
    p. nerve paralysis
PHRT
    procarbazine, hydroxyurea, radiotherapy
    PHRT protocol
phrynoderma
phthalocyanine photosensitization
phthisis bulbi
phycoerythrin
phyllodes
    cystosarcoma p.
    p. tumor
phylogenetic analysis
physaliferous cell
physical
    p. examination (PE)
    p. functioning
    p. handicap
    p. restoration
physician-assisted suicide (PAS)
Physician Data Query (PDQ)
physics
    radiation p.
physiochemical effect
physiologic, physiological
    p. cell death
    p. monitoring
    p. nucleoside
    p. staging
physiotherapy
    complete decongestive p.
    complex decongestive p.
    decongestive p.
phytate colloid
phytochemical
phytoestrogen
    soy p.

phytohemagglutinin antigen
phytohemagglutinin-stimulated Jurkat T
    cell
phytonadione
PI
    protease inhibitor
pi, π
    pi meson
PIA
    Platinol, ifosfamide, Adriamycin
PIAF
    Platinol, interferon alfa, Adriamycin, 5-
    fluorouracil
PICC
    peripherally inserted central catheter
    PICC line
Picibanil
pick
    P. disease
    P. tubular adenoma
PicoGreen dsDNA Quantitation Kit
picornavirus
PICP RIA kit
PID
    primary immune deficiency
piebaldism
piecewise regression analysis
Piezo Power Microdissection
pigment
    p. change
    p. stone disease
pigmentation
    blue nail p.
    flagellate p.
    flagellation p.
pigmented
    p. dermatofibrosarcoma
    p. lesion
    p. macule
pigmenti
    incontinentia p.
pigmentosa
    urticaria p.
pigmentosum
    xeroderma p. (XP)
pigtail catheter
PIH
    pregnancy-induced hypertension
    prolactin-inhibiting hormone
pilar
    p. cyst
    p. tumor
    p. tumor of scalp
pill
    Carter's Little P.'s
pillar
    tonsillar p.
pillow
    vacuum p.

pilocarpine
　　p. chloride prognostic test
　　p. HCl
pilocytic astrocytoma
piloid astrocytoma
pilomatricoma, pilomatrixoma
pilomatrix carcinoma
pilosebaceous unit
pilot
　　Asymptomatic Cardiac Ischemia P.
　　　(ACIP)
Pima syrup
pimonidazole
pimozide
pim-1 protooncogene/oncogene
PIN
　　prostatic intraepithelial neoplasia
pin
　　Smith-Petersen p.
　　Steinmann p.
　　track of p.
pinch-off
　　p.-o. sign
　　p.-o. syndrome
PINCH protein
Pindborg tumor
pineal
　　p. cyst
　　p. dysgerminoma
　　p. germ cell tumor
　　p. germinoma
　　p. gland
　　p. gland neoplasm
　　p. gland tumor
　　p. mass
　　p. parenchymal tumor
　　p. region
　　p. region tumor
　　p. teratocarcinoma
　　p. teratoma
pinealoblastoma, pineoblastoma
pinealocytoma, pineocytoma
pinealoma
　　ectopic p.
pine cone extract
pineoblastoma (var. of pinealoblastoma)
pineocytoma (var. of pinealocytoma)
pink tetralogy
Pinkus
　　fibroepithelioma of P.
Pinocchio cell
pinocytosis
pinocytotic vacuole

PinPoint stereotactic arm
piperacillin and tazobactam sodium
piperazinedione
piperazine estrone sulfate
pipe-smokers' cancer
pipestem mandible
pipette
　　Eppendorf Repeater Pro p.
pipetting
pipobroman
piposulfan
Pipracil
pirarubicin
piriform, pyriform
　　p. sinus
　　p. sinus cancer
piriformis muscle
piritrexim isethionate
piroxantrone (PXT)
piroxicam
pitch-workers' cancer
Pitressin
pituicytoma
pituitary
　　p. adenoma (PA)
　　p. apoplexy
　　p. gland
　　p. macroadenoma
　　p. microadenoma
　　p. tumor
pivampicillin
Pivanex
pixantrone
PixCell II laser capture microdissection
　　system
Pixykine
PK110 centrifuge
PKR
　　RNA-dependent protein kinase
placebo-controlled trial
placement
　　percutaneous p.
　　transpapillary p.
placenta, pl. placentae
　　enlarged p.
　　extrachorial p.
placental
　　p. alkaline phosphatase (PLAP)
　　p. alkaline phosphatase level
　　p. metastasis
　　p. site trophoblastic tumor (PSTT)
placentitis

NOTES

P

plain
Perdiem P.
plan
comprehensive care p.
plana
vertebra p.
planar
p. gamma camera image
p. I mesh implant
plane
axial p.
calculation of p.'s
fascial p.
Frankfort horizontal p.
off-axis p.
planing
p. curve
p. curve dose
planning
3-dimensional treatment p.
discharge p.
3D radiation treatment p.
radiation treatment p. (RTP)
p. target volume (PTV)
treatment p.
plant
p. alkaloid
noni p.
p. remedy
plantain leaf
plantaris
keratosis palmaris et p.
planus
lichen p.
linear lichen p.
PLAP
placental alkaline phosphatase
plaque
atheromatous p.
atherosclerotic p.
Hollenhorst p.
infiltrative p.
Lichtheim p.
ophthalmic p.
p. phase
pleural p.
p. radiotherapy
sequential paired opposed p.
(SPOP)
plaque-forming cell
Plaquenil
Plasbumin
plasma
absorbed p.
p. antibody titer
p. AT-III level
p. cell immunocytoma
p. cell labeling index (PCLI)
p. cell leukemia

p. cell mastitis
p. cell myeloma
p. cell neoplasm
p. cell pneumonia
citrated p.
p. clot
cryopoor p.
cryoprecipitate-depleted p.
p. depletion
p. emission spectroscopy
expanded p.
p. expander
FDP p.
fresh-frozen p.
p. half-life
p. HIV RNA
p. human immunodeficiency virus
ribonucleic acid
hyperimmune p.
p. lactate
p. leptin
p. membrane
p. osteopontin
platelet-free p.
pooled p.
p. proinsulin level
p. protein C
p. protein fraction
p. protein fraction human
p. tetranectin
p. thromboplastin antecedent
p. thromboplastin component (PTC)
p. thrombospondin
p. transfusion
p. uric acid
p. uric acid level
p. viral burden
p. viral load
p. viremia
plasmablast
plasmablastic
p. differentiation
p. lymphoma
plasmacyte
plasmacytic
p. hyperplasia
p. leukemoid reaction
p. lymphadenopathy
p. polyadenopathy
p. sarcomatosis
plasmacytoid
p. differentiation
p. lymphocyte
p. lymphocytic lymphoma
p. transformation
p. variant
plasmacytoma, plasmocytoma
anaplastic p.
extramedullary p. (EMP)

extramedullary leukemic p.
p. growth factor
solitary p.
plasmacytosis
Plasmanate
plasmapheresis through a Prosorba column
plasmid construct
plasmin
plasminogen
p. activator inhibitor (PAI)
p. activator inhibitor type I
Stachrom p.
plasmocytoma (*var. of* plasmacytoma)
Plasmodium
P. falciparum
P. malariae
P. ovale
P. vivax
plasmoid reactivation assay
plastic
p. block embedding
p. lymph
p. section
p. stent
p. stent occlusion
plastica
linitis p.
plate
blood agar p.
cribriform p.
epiphysial growth p.
lawn p.
Mancini p.
Sabouraud p.
Spli-Prest p.
platelet
adhesive p.
p. agglutination
p. aggregation
p. aggregation alteration
Bizzozero p.
p. clumping
p. concentrate
p. count
p. disorder
p. distribution width
p. dysfunction
p. endothelial cell adhesion molecule-1 (PECAM-1)
p. factor 4 (PF4)
p. function analyzer testing

hemolysis, elevated liver enzymes, low p.'s (HELLP)
p. histogram
p. neutralization procedure (PNP)
p. peroxidase
p. plug
p. procoagulant activity
random donor p.'s (RDP)
random single-donor p.'s (RSDP)
p. refractoriness
single-donor apheresis p.'s (SDAP)
p. suspension immunofluorescence test (PSIFT)
thrombin-stimulated p.'s
p. transfusion
transfusion-dependent p.'s
platelet-activating factor
platelet-associated
p.-a. Ig
p.-a. immunoglobulin (PAIg)
platelet-derived
p.-d. autoantibody
p.-d. endothelial cell growth factor (PD-ECGF)
p.-d. growth factor (PDGF)
p.-d. growth factor A (PDGFA)
p.-d. growth factor B
platelet-directed
p.-d. Ig
p.-d. immunoglobulin (PDIg)
platelet-free plasma
plateletpheresis
platelet-poor blood (PPB)
platelet-rich blood
Platelia Aspergillus EIA
platinating agent
Platinol
actinomycin D, vincristine, P. (AVP)
Adriamycin and P. (AP)
P., Adriamycin, bleomycin, escalating doses of Cytoxan (PAB-Esc-C)
P., Adriamycin, cyclophosphamide (PAC, PAC-1)
P., Adriamycin, cyclophosphamide, etoposide (PACE)
Adriamycin, Solu-Medrol, ara-C, P. (ASAP)
Adriamycin, Solu-Medrol, high-dose ara-C, P. (ASHAP, A-SHAP)
ara-C and P.

NOTES

P

Platinol *(continued)*

Baker Antifol, cyclophosphamide, Adriamycin, P.

bleomycin, Eldisine, mitomycin, P. (BEMP)

bleomycin, etoposide, P. (BEP)

bleomycin, ifosfamide, P. (BIP)

bleomycin, ifosfamide with mesna rescue, P. (BIP)

bleomycin, Oncovin, P. (BOP)

bleomycin, Oncovin, mitomycin, P. (BOMP)

P., bleomycin, vinblastine (PBV)

cyclophosphamide and P. (CTX-Plat)

cyclophosphamide, Adriamycin, P. (CAP, CAP-I)

cyclophosphamide, Adriamycin, high-dose P. (CAP-II)

P., cyclophosphamide, Eldisine (PCE)

cyclophosphamide, etoposide, P. (CEP)

cyclophosphamide, Hexalen, Adriamycin, P. (CHAP)

cyclophosphamide, hexamethylmelamine, Adriamycin, P. (CHAP)

cyclophosphamide, hexamethylmelamine, 5-fluorouracil, P. (ChexUP)

Cytoxan and P. (CP)

P., Cytoxan, etoposide (PCE)

dexamethasone, high-dose ara-C, P.

dianhydrogalactitol, Adriamycin, P. (DAP)

dose-interactive cyclophosphamide, etoposide, P. (DICEP)

P. and etanidazole

etoposide and P. (EP)

etoposide, Adriamycin, P. (EAP)

P., etoposide, bleomycin (PEB)

P., etoposide, cyclophosphamide (PEC)

etoposide, dexamethasone, ara-C, P. (EDAP)

etoposide, doxorubicin, P.

etoposide, 5-fluorouracil, P. (EFP)

etoposide, Solu-Medrol, ara-C, P. (ESAP)

etoposide, Solu-Medrol, high-dose ara-C, P. (ESHAP)

5-fluorouracil, Adriamycin, P. (FAP)

5-fluorouracil, cyclophosphamide, Adriamycin, P. (FCAP)

5-fluorouracil, Cytoxan, Adriamycin, P. (FCAP)

P., 5-fluorouracil, etoposide (PFE)

P., 5-fluorouracil, leucovorin (PFL)

5-fluorouracil, leucovorin calcium, Adriamycin, P. (FLAP)

5-fluorouracil, leucovorin, etoposide, P. (FLEP)

P., 5-fluorouracil, methotrexate (PFM)

ftorafur, Adriamycin, cyclophosphamide, P. (FACP)

hexamethylenamine, Adriamycin, methotrexate, P. (HAMP)

hexamethylenamine, cyclophosphamide, Adriamycin, P. (H-CAP)

hexamethylmelamine, cyclophosphamide, Adriamycin, P. (H-CAP)

hexamethylmelamine, Cytoxan, Adriamycin, P. (H-CAP)

P., ifosfamide, Adriamycin (PIA)

P., interferon alfa, Adriamycin, 5-fluorouracil (PIAF)

mesna, ifosfamide, Novantrone, etoposide plus etoposide, Solu-Medrol, ara-C, P.

P., methotrexate, bleomycin (PMB)

P., methotrexate, vinblastine, Adriamycin, carboplatin (P-MVAC)

mitomycin, Adriamycin, P.

mitomycin C, Adriamycin, P. (MAP)

mitomycin C, etoposide, P. (MEP)

mitomycin, vinblastine, P. (MVP)

Oncovin, dianhydrogalactitol, Adriamycin, P. (O-DAP)

tamoxifen, etoposide, mitoxantrone, P. (TEMP)

triazinate, cyclophosphamide, Adriamycin, P.

Velban, ifosfamide, P. (VeIP)

VePesid and P. (VPP)

VePesid, Adriamycin, cyclophosphamide, P. (VACP)

VePesid, Adriamycin, Cytoxan, P. (VACP)

VePesid, ifosfamide, P. (VIP)

vinblastine, actinomycin D, P. (VAP, VAP-II)

P., vinblastine, bleomycin (PVB)

vinblastine, bleomycin, P. (VBP)

vinblastine, dacarbazine, P. (VDP)

vinblastine, ifosfamide, P. (VeIP, VIP)

VP-16 and P. (VPP)

P. and VP-16 (PVP)

VP-16, cyclophosphamide, P. (VCP-I)

VP-16, cyclophosphamide, Adriamycin, P. (VCAP-I)

VP-16, ifosfamide, P. (VIP)

VP-16-213, Oncovin, cyclophosphamide, Adriamycin, P. (VOCAP)

Platinol-AQ

platinum

p. analog

cis-dichlorotransdihydroxy-bis-isoprophylamine p.

cis-dichlorotransdihydroxy-bis-isoprophylamine p. IV (CHIP)

p. compound

p. diammine dichloride

p. resistant

p. sensitive

p. therapy

platinum-based

p.-b. chemotherapy

p.-b. regimen

platinum-containing

p.-c. agent

p.-c. regimen

platinum-resistant ovarian cancer

platinum-taxane chemotherapy

platybasia

Plavix

PLB

primary lymphoma of bone

PLD

potentially lethal damage

pleiotrophin

pleiotropic

p. cytokine

p. gene

Plenaxis

pleocytosis

cerebrospinal fluid p.

CSF p.

pleomorphic

p. adenoma

p. liposarcoma

p. nucleus

p. rhabdomyosarcoma

p. T-cell lymphoma

p. type

p. xanthoastrocytoma (PXA)

pleomorphism

cellular p.

cytoplasmic p.

plesiocurie therapy

plesiotherapy

plethora

conjunctival p.

pleura, pl. **pleurae**

mediastinal p.

visceral p.

pleural

p. aspergillosis

p. biopsy

p. biopsy needle

p. calcification

p. cancer

p. cytoreduction

p. effusion

p. fluid

p. fluid CEA

p. fluid hyaluronic acid

p. mesothelioma

p. plaque

p. thickening

pleurectomy

pleurisy

pleuritic pain

pleurodesis

talc p.

pleuroperitoneal shunting

pleuropneumonectomy

radical p.

pleuropneumonia-like organism

pleuropulmonary blastoma

pleuroscopy

Pleurx indwelling pleural catheter

plexiform

p. neurofibroma

p. schwannoma

plexitis

radiation p.

plexopathy

brachial p.

lower brachial p.

lumbosacral p.

radiation-induced brachial p. (RIBP)

radiation-induced lumbosacral p.

plexus, pl. **plexus, plexuses**

Auerbach p.

Batson vertebral venous p.

brachial p.

cervical p.

choroid p.

hypogastric p.

PLGA

polymorphous low-grade adenocarcinoma

plicamycin

NOTES

P

plicata
    lingua p.
PL100KL/50K
    Pall filter PL100KL/50K
PLL
    posterior longitudinal ligament
    prolymphocytic leukemia
PLND
    pelvic lymph node dissection
ploidy
    DNA p.
    flow cytometric DNA p.
    p. status
    tumor p.
plomestane
plop
    tumor p.
plot
    Weibull p.
plug
    bone p.
    dermoid p.
    echogenic p.
    platelet p.
    p. tobacco
plumbism
Plummer disease
Plummer-Vinson syndrome
plunging ranula
plurihormonal adenoma
pluripotential
    p. cell
    p. immunoproliferative syndrome
pluripotent stem cell
plus
    DHC P.
    DSMC P.
    Genasoft P.
    Lorcet P.
    Omni-Flow 4000 P.
    Penta/3B P.
    Pro-Sof P.
    Riopan P.
    Vicon P.
PM
    polymyositis
    postmortem
    prednimustine
PM-81
    PM-81 MAb
    PM-81 monoclonal antibody
PMB
    Platinol, methotrexate, bleomycin
PMC
    papillary microcarcinoma
PMCT
    percutaneous microwave coagulation
    therapy

PME
    phosphomonoester
PMEA
    phosphonylmethoxyethyladenine
    9-2-phosphonylmethoxyethyl adenine
PMF
    phenylalanine mustard, methotrexate, 5-
    fluorouracil
PMFAC
    prednisone, methotrexate, FAC
PMGCT
    primary malignant giant cell tumor
PMH
    postmenopausal hormone
PML
    promyelocytic leukemia
    HIV-associated PML
PMMA
    polymethylmethacrylate
PMN
    polymorphonuclear
PMN-elastase
PMPA
    9-R-2-phosphonylmethoxypropyl adenine
P-MRS
    phosphorus magnetic resonance
    spectroscopy
PMS-Benztropine
PMS-Bisacodyl
PMS-Carbamazepine
PMS-Cholestyramine
PMS-Clonazepam
PMS-Cyproheptadine
PMS-Desipramine
PMS-Docusate Calcium
PMS-Erythromycin
PMS-Ferrous Sulfate
PMS-Hydromorphone
PMS-Imipramine
PMS-Ketoprofen
PMS-Lactulose
PMS-Levothyroxine Sodium
PMS-Loperamide
PMS-Nystatin
PMS-Opium & belladonna
PMS-Oxazepam
PMS-Procyclidine
PMS-Progesterone
PMS-Sodium Cromoglycate
PMS-Trihexyphenidyl
PMT
    pseudosarcomatous myofibroblastic
    tumor
P-MVAC
    Platinol, methotrexate, vinblastine,
    Adriamycin, carboplatin
PNET
    primitive neuroectodermal tumor

pneumatic
  p. compression
  p. reduction
pneumatosis
  epidural p.
pneumaturia
pneumobilia
pneumococcal polysaccharide vaccine
pneumoconiosis
  barium p.
  bauxite p.
  coal workers' p.
  complicated p.
Pneumocystis
  P. carinii
  P. choroidopathy
  P. jiroveci
  P. pneumonia
Pneumocystis-**related vasculitis**
pneumocystosis
  cutaneous p.
pneumocyte hyperplasia
pneumonectomy
  p. chest
  extrapleural p.
pneumonia
  adenovirus p.
  alveolar p.
  aspiration p.
  atypical measles p.
  bacillus anthracis p.
  bacterial p.
  bilateral lower lobe p.
  caseous p.
  chronic eosinophilic p. (CEP)
  community-acquired p. (CAP)
  concomitant p.
  cytomegalovirus p.
  desquamative interstitial p.
  endogenous lipid p.
  eosinophilic p.
  extensive bilateral p.
  fungal p.
  Gram-negative p.
  Haemophilus influenzae p.
  hematogenous interstitial bacterial p.
  herpesvirus p.
  interstitial bacterial p.
  Legionella p.
  lymphocytic interstitial p.
  lymphoid interstitial p.
  Nocardia p.
  plasma cell p.

  Pneumocystis p.
  postobstructive p.
  primary atypical p. (PAP)
  staphylococcal p.
pneumoniae
  Chlamydia p.
  Diplococcus p.
  Klebsiella p.
  Mycoplasma p.
pneumonitis
  bacterial p.
  chemical p.
  cytomegalovirus interstitial p.
  desquamative interstitial p.
  infiltrating p.
  nonspecific interstitial p.
  radiation p.
  usual interstitial p.
pneumoomentum
pneumopathy
  cobalt p.
pneumophila
  Legionella p.
pneumothorax, pl. **pneumothoraces (PT)**
  tension p.
PNH
  paroxysmal nocturnal hemoglobinuria
  PNH cell
  PNH prep alloimmunization
PNI
  perineural invasion
PNP
  paraneoplastic pemphigus
  platelet neutralization procedure
  polynucleotide phosphorylase
PNPase
  polynucleotide phosphorylase
PO
  prophylactic oophorectomy
POACH
  prednisone, Oncovin, ara-C,
    cyclophosphamide, hydroxydaunomycin
POC
  procarbazine, Oncovin, CCNU
  procarbazine, Oncovin, lomustine
POCA
  prednisone, Oncovin, cytarabine,
    Adriamycin
POCC
  procarbazine, Oncovin,
    cyclophosphamide, CCNU
  procarbazine, Oncovin, Cytoxan, CCNU
pocket-sized TENS unit

NOTES

P

Pod-Ben-25
Podocon-25
Podofilm
podofilox
Podofin
podophyllin
p. and salicylic acid
topical p.
podophyllotoxin
podophyllum resin
POEMS
polyneuropathy, organomegaly, endocrine
abnormalities, M protein, skin changes
polyneuropathy, organomegaly,
endocrinopathy, monoclonal
gammopathy, skin changes
POEMS syndrome
POG
Pediatric Oncology Group
poikilocytosis
poikiloderma
point
4-p. assay
bleeding p.
choroid p.
ICRU reference p.
p. spectroscopy
point-resolved spectroscopy (PRESS)
poison
spindle p.
poisoning
arsenic p.
carbon monoxide p.
Paraquat p.
radiation p.
Poisson regression
Pokeman
POK erythroid myeloid ontogenic
POK erythroid myeloid ontogenic
(Pokeman)
pokeweed mitogen
pol
pol gene
pol protein
polar
p. anemia
p. compound
Polaris LE catheter
polarity-altered
p.-a. spectral selective acquisition
(PASTA)
p.-a. spectral selective acquisition
imaging
polarization
dynamic nuclear p.
fluorescence p.
polarographic needle electrode
policy
standardized care p.

polifeprosan
p. 20 and carmustine
p. 20 with carmustine 3.85%
implant
p. 20 with carmustine implant
wafer
polioencephalomyelopathy
poliovirus
pollicis
adductor p.
polyacrylamide
p. bead
p. gel
p. gel electrophoresis (PAGE)
polyadenopathy
angiofollicular and plasmacytic p.
plasmacytic p.
polyamine
macrocyclic p.
red blood cell p.
polyanionic sulfated compound
polyarthralgia
polyarthropathy
large-joint p.
polycarbophil
calcium p.
polycation liposome (PCL)
polychemotherapy
adjuvant p.
polychromasia
polychromatic cell
polychromatophilic
p. erythroblast
p. normoblast
polychromic erythrocyte
polychronotropism
polyclonal
p. activation
p. activator
p. CD3 antibody
p. gammopathy
p. human plasma-derived anti-HIV
immunoglobin preparation
p. population
polyclonality
Polycose
polycyclic
p. aromatic hydrocarbon (PAH)
p. compound
polycystic
p. nephroblastoma
p. ovarian disease (PCOD)
polycythemia
absolute p.
familial p.
p. hypertonica
p. rubra vera (PRV)
spurious p.
p. vera (PCV, PV)

P. Vera Study Group (PVSG)
p. vera with myeloid metaplasia
polyembryoma
polyestradiol
polyethylene
  p. balloon catheter
  p. double-pigtail stent
  p. glycol (PEG)
  p. glycol-conjugated L-asparaginase
    (PEG-L-ASP)
  p. glycol-modified adenosine
    deaminase (PEG-ADA)
  p. glycol-modified *E. coli* ASNase
  p. glycol-modified interleukin-2
    (PEG-IL-2)
  p. glycol r-hirudin mutein assay
  p. sorbitan monooleate
  p. tubing
  p. ureteral stent
Polyflux S dialyzer
Polygam S/D
polyglutamate paclitaxel (PG-TXL)
polyglutamylation
polygonal
  p. cell
  p. cell-type thymoma
polylactide copolymer
poly-*L*-lysine slide
polylobulated cell
polylysine-DOTA
polylysine-Gd-DOTA
polylysine-Gd-DTPA
polymer
  p. dosimetry
  glucose p.
  naphthalene sulfonate p.
  sulfonated p.
polymerase
  p. chain reaction (PCR)
  p. chain reaction-based method
  p. chain reaction-based method for
    acute promyelocytic leukemia
  p. chain reaction detection of
    haptoglobin gene deletion
  DNA p.
  p66/51 p.
polymeric local delivery system
polymerization of microtubule
polymerizing tissue adhesive
polymethylmethacrylate (PMMA)
polymorphic
  p. B-cell hyperplasia
  p. B-cell lymphoma

p. class I chain
p. exon
p. immunocytoma
p. midline malignant reticulosis
polymorphism
  cytokine p.
  genetic p.
  N-acetylation p.
  restriction fragment length p.
    (RFLP)
  single-strand conformation p.
    (SSCP)
  single-stranded conformational p.
    (SSCP)
polymorphocytic leukemia
polymorphonuclear (PMN)
  p. leukocyte
  p. lymphocyte
  p. neutrophil
  p. phagocyte
polymorphous
  p. low-grade adenocarcinoma
    (PLGA)
  p. low-grade carcinoma
  p. sarcoma
polymyositis (PM)
  paraneoplastic p.
polymyxin
  p. B, amphotericin B, nalidixic
    acid, trimethoprim, azlocillin
    (PANTA)
  neomycin and p. B
polyneuropathy
  chronic inflammatory
    demyelinating p.
  distal predominantly sensory p.
  distal symmetric p. (DSPN)
  distal symmetrical p.
  inflammatory demyelinating p.
  p., organomegaly, endocrine
    abnormalities, M protein, skin
    changes (POEMS)
  p., organomegaly, endocrinopathy,
    monoclonal gammopathy, skin
    changes (POEMS)
**polynuclear aromatic hydrocarbon
  (PAH)**
**polynucleotide phosphorylase (PNP,
  PNPase)**
polyostotic fibrous dysplasia
polyp
  adenomatous p. (AP)
  adenomatous colonic p.

NOTES

P

polyp *(continued)*
    antral p.
    antrochoanal p.
    choanal p.
    colonic p.
    colorectal p.
    endometrial p.
    epithelial colonic p.
    inflammatory p.
    myomatous p.
    neoplastic p.
    pedunculated p.
polypectomy
    colonoscopic p.
polypeptide
    pancreatic p.
    vasoactive p.
polypeptidoma
    pancreatic p. (PPoma)
polyphenolic compound
polyphosphate
polyploidization
polypoid
    p. adenoma
    p. fibroma
polyposis
    attenuated adenomatous p.
    attenuated familial adenomatous p. (AFAP)
    familial adenomatous p. (FAP)
    familial juvenile p.
    familial multiple p.
    juvenile p.
    lymphomatous p. (LP)
    multiple lymphomatous p.
polyprotein precursor molecule
polyradiculoneuropathy
polyradiculopathy
polyribosome
polysaccharide-iron complex
polysialic-neural cell
polysucrose
polysulfate
    pentosan p.
    sodium pentosan p.
polysulfonated naphthylurea
polytetrafluoroethylene (PTFE)
    p. graft
    p. shunt
polythiazide
polytomous logistic regression
polyuria
polyvalent melanoma cell
polyvinyl
    p. alcohol
    p. alcohol foam

    p. chloride balloon catheter
    p. sponge
polyvinyldine difluoride (PVDF)
polyvinylpyrrolidone (PVP)
    p. storage disease
pombe
    Schizosaccharomyces p.
pomegranate oil
POMP
    prednisone, Oncovin, methotrexate, 6-mercaptopurine
    prednisone, Oncovin, methotrexate, Purinethol
    POMP chemotherapy protocol
POMS
    Profile of Mood States
Pondocillin
pons, pl. **pontes**
Ponstan
Ponstel
pontes (*pl. of* pons)
ponticulus posticus
pontine, pontile
    p. angle tumor
    central p.
    p. cistern
    p. glioma
pontis
    brachium p.
Pontocaine
pool
    gene p.
    stem cell p.
pooled plasma
pooling
    neutrophil p.
poorly
    p. concentrated isotope
    p. differentiated embryonal cell tumor (PDET)
    p. differentiated endocrine carcinoma (PDEC)
    p. differentiated infiltrating duct carcinoma
    p. differentiated lymphocytic
    p. differentiated lymphocytic lymphoma (PDLL)
popcorn
    p. calcification
    p. Reed-Sternberg cell
population
    endemic p.
    high-risk p.
    occult clonal B-cell p.
    oligoclonal p.
    polyclonal p.
    predominating p.
pore
    Kohn p.

porfimer sodium
porfiromycin
porocarcinoma
porokeratosis
    linear p.
poroma
    eccrine p.
    follicular p.
porphobilinogen deaminase
porphyria
    congenital erythropoietic p. (CEP)
    p. cutanea tarda
    erythropoietic p.
    hepatoerythropoietic p.
porphyrin
    boronated p. (BOPP)
PORT
    postoperative radiation therapy
port
    Celsite implanted p.
    p. film
    implantable infusion p.
    infusion p.
    radiotherapy p.
    p. site metastasis
    totally implantable access p.
      (TIAP)
portable
    p. blood irradiator
    p. infusion pump
Port-A-Cath catheter
portacaval shunt
portal
    AP p.
    AP/PA p.
    p. of entry
    p. film
    fixed-beam p.
    p. hypertension
    p. infusion
    PA p.
    p. phase contrast-enhanced spiral
      CT
    radiation p.
    p. vein embolization (PVE)
    p. venous sampling (PVS)
    p. venous system
portion
    Fc p.
Portland
    hemoglobin P.

portography
    computed tomography during
      arterial p. (CTAP)
    CT p.
portohepatic venous shunt
porton L-asparaginase
portopulmonary venous anastomosis
portosystemic
    p. anastomosis
    p. shunt
Porvidx lung cancer screening
posaconazole
position
    catheter p.
    dwell p.
    P. Plus cushion
    prone p.
    reclining p.
    semiupright p.
    stepping-source p.
positive
    p. angiogenic molecule
    breakpoint cluster region-p. (BCR-
      positive)
    CALLA p.
    p. cerebrospinal fluid culture
    p. CSF culture
    fluorescent dye efflux p.
    IgG-ACA p.
    immunoglobulin anticardiolipin
      antibody p.
    Philadelphia chromosome p. (Ph-
      positive)
    premenopausal hormone receptor p.
      (PRP)
    replication error p. (RER+)
    Rh p.
    TRAP p.
positron
    p. emission tomography (PET)
    p. emission tomography-magnetic
      resonance imaging coregistration
postamputation neuroma
postbiopsy
    p. change
    p. period
    p. renal AV fistula
    p. skin thickening
postcricoid pharyngeal cancer
2-poster brace
posterior
    p. capsular cataract
    p. fossa boost

NOTES

P

445

posterior *(continued)*
    p. fossa tumor
    p. longitudinal ligament (PLL)
    p. mediastinal mass
    p. membranous trachea
    p. nodal chain
    p. proctotomy
    p. tibial tendon (PTT)
    p. uveal melanoma
posteroanterior (PA)
    p. projection
postexposure chemoprophylaxis
postgadolinium scan
postgastrectomy
    p. cancer recurrence
    p. carcinoma
postherpetic neuropathy
posticus
    ponticulus p.
postirradiation
    p. chondrosarcoma
    p. downstaging
    p. fracture
    p. sarcoma
    p. study
postlumpectomy skin thickening
postmastectomy lymphedema
postmenopausal
    p. adnexal cyst
    p. estrogen therapy
    p. hormone (PMH)
    p. nulliparous patient
    p. woman
postmenopause
postmortem (PM)
postnatal transmission
postneonatal Erb palsy
postobstructive pneumonia
postoperative
    p. bladder dysfunction
    p. chemotherapy
    p. complication
    p. locoregional radiotherapy
    p. pelvic radiation
    p. radiation therapy (PORT)
    p. sepsis
    p. seroma
postphlebitic syndrome
postpolycythemia
postpolycythemic myeloid metaplasia
postradiation
    p. dysplasia (PRD)
    p. therapy
postreceptor signal transduction
postrecurrence survival (PRSv)
postrenal failure
posttest counseling
posttherapy change

postthymic
    p. T-cell leukemia
    p. T-cell lymphoma
posttranscriptional step
posttransfusion purpura
posttranslation
    p. modification
    p. viral assembly
posttranslational
    p. modification
    p. phosphorylation
posttransplant
    p. IL-2
    p. lymphoproliferative disorder
      (PTLD)
posttransplantation lymphoproliferation
posttraumatic stress disorder (PTSD)
postulate
    Koch p.
postural dynamic
posture training
postvaccinial lymphadenitis
postvoiding film
postvoid residual
Potasalan
potassium (K)
    p. acetate
    p. acetate, potassium bicarbonate,
      potassium citrate
    amoxicillin and clavulanate p.
    p. bicarbonate
    p. bicarbonate and potassium
      chloride effervescent
    p. bicarbonate, potassium chloride,
      potassium citrate
    p. bicarbonate and potassium
      citrate effervescent
    p. chloride
    p. chloride and potassium
      gluconate
    p. citrate and potassium gluconate
    p. imbalance
    p. iodide
    penicillin V p.
    p. phosphate and sodium phosphate
    ticarcillin and clavulanate p.
    p., titanyl, phosphate (KTP)
potassium-39 (^{39}K)
potato tumor
potency
potent differentiating agent
potential
    leukemogenic p.
    low malignant p. (LMP)
    modulation p.
    papillary urothelial neoplasm of
      low malignant p. (PUNLMP)
    proliferating p.

prostatic stromal proliferation of uncertain malignant p. (PSPUMP)
somatosensory evoked p. (SEP)
tumoricidal p.
uncertain malignant p.
zeta p.
potentially lethal damage (PLD)
potentiator
pot patch
Pott
  P. puffy tumor
  P. shunt
pouch
  arachnoid retrocerebellar p.
  Hartmann p.
  Indiana p.
  Koch p.
  Mainz p.
  Rathke p.
  p. restorative proctocolectomy
  Studer p.
pouchogram
poudrage
povidone iodine rinse
powder
  shark p.
  zoledronic acid p.
  Zometa p.
POWER
  Preferences of Women Evaluating Risks of Tamoxifen
  POWER Study
power
  p. function
  p. law TAR method
  mass collision stopping p.
  mass radiative stopping p.
poxvirus recombinant/combination
pp65
  viral matrix protein with kinase activity pp65
PPAR
  peroxisome proliferator activated receptor
  PPAR receptor
PPB
  platelet-poor blood
p190 and p210 BCR/abl variants of Philadelphia chromosome-positive ALL
PPC
  pelvic and periaortic control
PPD
  percussion and postural drainage

purified protein derivative
  PPD test
PPED
  palmar-plantar erythrodysesthesia
Ppi
  pyrophosphate
ppm
  parts per million
PPO
  preferred provider organization
PPoma
  pancreatic polypeptidoma
p150 protein
PPTT
  prepubertal testicular tumor
PR
  partial response
  progesterone receptor
    OncoRad PR
    OncoScint PR
practice
  infection-control p.'s
PRAD-1 gene expression
praecox
  icterus p.
PrameGel
Pramosone
pramoxine and hydrocortisone
pranobex
  inosine p.
prasterone
Prax
pRB
  retinoblastoma protein
pRb
  Rb protein expression
PRD
  postradiation dysplasia
PRE
  primary resection
preadult
  p. bone marrow failure
  p. cancer
pre-B acute lymphoblastic leukemia
pre-B-cell growth factor
precancerous
  p. change
  p. condition
  p. disease
precaution
  standard p.
  universal p.
precaval lymph node

NOTES

prechiasmal optic nerve lesion
Precision 500D digital x-ray
preclinical study
precocious presentation
precursor
> abnormal localization of
>   immature p.'s (ALIP)
> p. B acute lymphoblastic leukemia
> p. B-cell lymphoma
> bone marrow myeloid p. (BMMP)
> p. B, T cell
> CD34+ derived mast cell p.
> p. cell tumor
> CTL p.
> cysteine p.
> cytotoxic T lymphocyte p. (CTLp)
> Gag-Pol p.
> granulin-epithelin p. (GEP)
> hematopoietic p.
> p. lesion
> monomeric p.
> p55 p.
> p. T acute lymphocytic leukemia

PRED
> prednisone

Predicta Human TNF-alpha ELISA kit
prediction of extracapsular prostate
cancer extension with endorectal MR
imaging
predictive
> p. assay
> p. value
> p. value of negative test
> p. value of positive test

predilection
predisposing condition
prednimustine (PM)
> CCNU, etoposide, p. (CEP)
> etoposide, mitoxantrone, p.
> VePesid, mitoxantrone, p. (VMP)

prednisolone
> Adriamycin, bleomycin,
>   cyclophosphamide, vincristine,
>   etoposide, p. I (ABCVEP-I)
> Adriamycin, bleomycin,
>   cyclophosphamide, vincristine,
>   etoposide, p. II (ABCVEP-II)
> cyclophosphamide, epirubicin,
>   vincristine, p. (CEOP)
> melphalan, p. (MP)
> Procytox, epipodophyllotoxin-
>   derivative, p. (PEP)
> systemic p.
> vincristine, epirubicin, etoposide, p.
>   (VEEP)

Prednisol TBA Injection
prednisone (PRED)
> Adriamycin, bleomycin, p. (ABP)

Adriamycin, bleomycin, dacarbazine,
  CCNU, p. (ABDIC)
Adriamycin, bleomycin, DTIC,
  CCNU, p. (ABDIC)
Adriamycin, bleomycin sulfate,
  vinblastine, p. (ABVP)
Adriamycin, bleomycin sulfate,
  vincristine, p. (ABVP)
Adriamycin, cyclophosphamide,
  Oncovin, p. (ACOP)
Adriamycin, cyclophosphamide,
  Oncovin, cytosine arabinoside, p.
  (ACOAP)
Adriamycin, cyclophosphamide,
  Oncovin, procarbazine, p.
  (ACOPP)
Adriamycin, cyclophosphamide,
  vindesine, bleomycin, p. (ACVBP)
Adriamycin, Cytoxan, Oncovin, p.
  (ACOP)
Adriamycin, Oncovin, p. (ADOP,
  AdOP)
Adriamycin, Oncovin,
  arabinosylcytosine, p. (ADOAP,
  AD-OAP, AdOAP)
AG3340 in combination with
  mitoxantrone and p.
AG3340 in combination with
  Novantrone and p.
p., ara-C, 6-thioguanine,
  cyclophosphamide, Oncovin
  (PATCO)
p., L-asparaginase, daunomycin,
  VM-26, methotrexate
BCNU, cyclophosphamide, p.
  (BCP)
BCNU, cyclophosphamide,
  Adriamycin, p. (BCAP)
BCNU, cyclophosphamide,
  Oncovin, p. (BCOP)
BCNU, cyclophosphamide,
  vinblastine, procarbazine, p.
  (BCVPP)
BCNU, cyclophosphamide,
  vincristine, p. (BCVP)
BCNU, Oncovin, p. (BOP)
BCNU, Oncovin, procarbazine, p.
  (BOPP)
BCNU, vinblastine,
  cyclophosphamide, procarbazine, p.
  (BVCPP)
BCNU, vincristine, Adriamycin, p.
  (BVAP)
BCNU, vincristine, procarbazine, p.
  (BVPP)
bleomycin, Adriamycin,
  cyclophosphamide, Oncovin, p.
  (BACOP)

bleomycin, Adriamycin, vinblastine,
imidazole carboxamide, p.
(BAVIP)
bleomycin, cyclophosphamide,
vincristine, procarbazine, p.
(BCVPP)
bleomycin, Cytoxan,
hydroxydaunomycin, Oncovin, p.
(B-CHOP)
bleomycin, etoposide, Adriamycin,
cyclophosphamide, vincristine,
procarbazine, p. (BEACOPP)
bleomycin, mechlorethamine,
Oncovin, procarbazine, p. (B-
MOPP)
bleomycin, Oncovin, Adriamycin, p.
(BOAP)
bleomycin, Oncovin, Matulane, p.
(BOMP)
CCNU, cyclophosphamide, Velban,
procarbazine, p. (CCVPP)
CCNU, Oncovin, p. (CCNU-OP)
CCNU, Oncovin, procarbazine, p.
(COPP)
chlorambucil and p. (CP)
chlorambucil, vinblastine,
procarbazine, p. (ChlVPP, CH1-
VPP)
chlorambucil, vincristine,
procarbazine, p. (LOPP)
cisplatin, cyclophosphamide,
doxorubicin, vincristine, p. (P-
CHOP)
cyclophosphamide and p. (CP)
cyclophosphamide, Adriamycin, p.
(CAP)
cyclophosphamide, Adriamycin,
bleomycin, Oncovin, p. (CABOP,
CA-BOP)
cyclophosphamide, Adriamycin, 5-
fluorouracil, p. (CAFP)
cyclophosphamide, Adriamycin, 5-
fluorouracil, vincristine, p.
(CAFVP)
cyclophosphamide, Adriamycin,
Platinol, p. (CAPPr)
cyclophosphamide, Adriamycin,
procarbazine, bleomycin,
Oncovin, p. (CAP-BOP)
cyclophosphamide, Adriamycin,
vincristine, p. (CAVP, CAVP-I)
cyclophosphamide, Adriamycin,
VM-26, p.

cyclophosphamide, doxorubicin,
vindesine, bleomycin, and p.
cyclophosphamide, epirubicin,
Oncovin, p. (CEOP)
cyclophosphamide, 5-fluorouracil, p.
(CFP)
cyclophosphamide, Halotestin,
Oncovin, p. (CHOP, CyHOP)
cyclophosphamide,
hydroxydaunomycin, Oncovin, p.
(CHOP)
cyclophosphamide,
hydroxydaunomycin, VM-26, p.
(CHVP)
cyclophosphamide,
hydroxydaunorubicin, Oncovin, p.
(CHOP)
cyclophosphamide, mechlorethamine,
Oncovin, procarbazine, p.
(CMOPP, C-MOPP)
cyclophosphamide, methotrexate, 5-
fluorouracil, p. (CMFP)
cyclophosphamide, methotrexate, 5-
fluorouracil, Adriamycin,
vincristine, p. (CMFAVP)
cyclophosphamide, methotrexate, 5-
fluorouracil, vincristine, p.
(CMFVP, CVFVP)
cyclophosphamide, Novantrone,
Oncovin, p. (CNOP, C-NOP)
cyclophosphamide, Oncovin, p.
(COP)
cyclophosphamide, Oncovin,
methotrexate, p. (COMP)
cyclophosphamide, Oncovin,
methotrexate, bleomycin,
Adriamycin, p. (COMBAP)
cyclophosphamide, Oncovin,
procarbazine, p. (COPP)
cyclophosphamide, rubidazone,
Oncovin, p. (CROP)
cyclophosphamide, Velban,
procarbazine, p. (CVPP)
cyclophosphamide, vincristine, p.
(CVP)
Cytoxan, Adriamycin, Platinol, p.
(CAPPR, CAPPr)
Cytoxan, Novantrone, Oncovin, p.
(CNOP, C-NOP)
Cytoxan, Oncovin, ara-C, p.
(COAP, mini-COAP)
daunomycin, ara-C, thioguanine,
vincristine, p.

NOTES

P

prednisone *(continued)*

daunorubicin, ara-C, 6-thioguanine, vincristine, p. (DATVP)

daunorubicin, cyclocytidine, 6-mercaptopurine, p. (DCCMP)

daunorubicin, cytarabine, 6-mercaptopurine, p. (DCMP)

daunorubicin, Oncovin, ara-C, p. (DOAP)

daunorubicin, vincristine, p. (DVP)

doxorubicin, vinblastine, mechlorethamine, vincristine, bleomycin, etoposide, p.

Eldisine, BCNU, Adriamycin, p. (EBAP)

etoposide, vinblastine, Adriamycin, p. (EVAP)

5-fluorouracil, cyclophosphamide, p. (FCP)

5-fluorouracil, methotrexate, ara-C, cyclophosphamide, Adriamycin, oncovin, p. (F-MACHOP)

p., 5-fluorouracil, tamoxifen (PFT)

leucovorin, p.

Leukeran, vinblastine, vincristine, p. (LVVP)

mechlorethamine, Oncovin, p. (MOP)

mechlorethamine, Oncovin, methotrexate, p. (MOMP)

mechlorethamine, Oncovin, procarbazine, p. (MOPP)

mechlorethamine, vinblastine, procarbazine, p. (MVPP)

mechlorethamine, vincristine, vinblastine, procarbazine, p. (MVVPP)

melphalan, Adriamycin, p. (MAP)

melphalan, cyclophosphamide, p. (MCP)

melphalan, cyclophosphamide, BCNU, p. (MCBP)

melphalan plus p. (MPL+PRED)

p., methotrexate, FAC (PMFAC)

p., methotrexate-leucovorin, Adriamycin, cyclophosphamide, etoposide (ProMACE)

p., methotrexate, leucovorin, Adriamycin, cyclophosphamide, etoposide, cytarabine

p., methotrexate-leucovorin, Adriamycin, cyclophosphamide, etoposide plus cytarabine, bleomycin, Oncovin, methotrexate (ProMACE-CytaBOM)

methotrexate, mechlorethamine, Oncovin, procarbazine, p. (MMOPP)

methotrexate, Oncovin, PEG-asparaginase, p. (MOAP)

mitoxantrone, vincristine, procarbazine, p.

Mustargen, Adriamycin, bleomycin, Oncovin, p. (MABOP)

Mustargen, Oncovin, procarbazine, p.

Novantrone, Oncovin, procarbazine, p. (NOPP)

Oncovin, ara-C, p. (OAP)

p., Oncovin, ara-C, cyclophosphamide, hydroxydaunomycin (POACH)

p., Oncovin, cytarabine, Adriamycin (POCA)

p., Oncovin, methotrexate, 6-mercaptopurine (POMP)

p., Oncovin, methotrexate, Purinethol (POMP)

Oncovin, procarbazine, p. (OPP)

Oncovin, procarbazine, prednisone, Adriamycin plus cyclophosphamide, Oncovin, procarbazine, p. (OPPA/COPP)

prednisone, methotrexate, Adriamycin, cyclophosphamide, etoposide plus mustargen, Oncovin, procarbazine, p. (ProMACE-MOPP)

procarbazine and p.

rubidazone, Oncovin, ara-C, p. (ROAP)

teniposide, procarbazine, p.

6-thioguanine, methotrexate, Oncovin, p. (T-MOP)

6-thioguanine, Oncovin, cytosine arabinoside, p. (TOAP)

6-thioguanine, rubidomycin, ara-C, p. (TRAP)

vincristine and p.

vincristine, actinomycin, methotrexate, p. (VAMP)

vincristine, Adriamycin, p. (VAP)

vincristine, Adriamycin, methotrexate, p. (VAMP)

vincristine, amethopterin, 6-mercaptopurine, p. (VAMP)

p., vincristine, L-asparaginase (PVA)

vincristine, L-asparaginase, p. (VAP)

vincristine, L-asparaginase, Adriamycin, p. (VAAP)

vincristine, BCNU, Adriamycin, p. (VBAP)

vincristine, BCNU, melphalan, cyclophosphamide, p. (VBMCP)

vincristine, carmustine, cyclophosphamide, melphalan, p. (M2) vincristine, cyclophosphamide, p. (VCP)

vincristine, cyclophosphamide, Adriamycin, p. (VCAP)

vincristine, cyclophosphamide, melphalan, p. (VCMP)

vincristine, daunorubicin, p. (VDP)

p., vincristine, daunorubicin, L-asparaginase (PVDA)

vincristine, Endoxan, 6-mercaptopurine, p. (VEMP)

vincristine, melphalan, cyclophosphamide, p. (VMCP)

predominance
monoblast p.

predominating population

preeclampsia

preepiglottic space

preference
P.'s of Women Evaluating Risks of Tamoxifen (POWER)
P.'s of Women Evaluating Risks of Tamoxifen Study

preferential
p. B-cell panhematopoietic antigen
p. T-cell panhematopoietic antigen

preferred provider organization (PPO)

PreGen-26 colorectal cancer test

pregnancy, pl. **pregnancies**
breast cancer during p.
ectopic p.
molar p.
pelvic malignancy in p.
p. test
p. tumor

pregnancy-induced hypertension (PIH)

preinvasive
p. disease
p. disease of cervix, vagina, and vulva
p. urothelial neoplasia

prekallikrein
p. deficiency
Stachrom p.

preleukemia

Prelone Oral

premalignancy
oral p.

premalignant
p. condition
p. melanosis

premature atrial contraction (PAC)

prematurity

premenopausal
p. hormone receptor positive (PRP)
p. patient

premorbid

premycotic phase

prenatal
p. testing
p. vitamin

Prenavite Forte

preneoplastic lesion

preoperative
p. chemotherapy
p. sperm banking

preovulatory proteolysis

prep
preparation
NutraPrep LoSo prep

preparation (prep)
bowel p.
buffy coat p.
immunoglobulin p.
LE p.
liposomal p.
polyclonal human plasma-derived anti-HIV immunoglobin p.
touch p.
whole virus p.

preplasma cell

preplasmacytic leukemia

prepontine white epidermoidoma

prepped and draped

prepro-gastrin-releasing peptide (preproGRP)

preproGRP
prepro-gastrin-releasing peptide

prepubertal testicular tumor (PPTT)

prerenal failure

presenilin-2

presentation
aleukemic p.
antigen p.
metachronous p.
precocious p.
synchronous p.

presenting
monocyte p.

preservation
breast p.
sphincter p.

PRESS
point-resolved spectroscopy

pressor unit

NOTES

P

451

pressure
    acoustic p.
    blood p.
    central venous p. (CVP)
    interstitial fluid p. (IFP)
    jugular venous p.
pressurized fluid jet
presurgical chemotherapy
pre-T acute lymphocytic leukemia
pretargeted antibody
pretarget lymphoma trial for non-Hodgkin lymphoma
pretherapy baseline
prethymic
pretreatment
    amifostine p.
    p. assessment
    p. evaluation
Prevacare skin care spray
Prevacid
prevalence rate
Prevalite
Prevatac
prevention
    American Stop Smoking Intervention Study for Cancer P. (ASSIST)
    hormonal p.
    nutritional p.
Preventive Health Model (PHM)
Preveon
PRH
    prolactin-releasing hormone
priapism
priliximab
Prilosec
primaquine
    chloroquine and p.
    p. phosphate antimalarial
primary
    p. amenorrhea
    p. antiphospholipid antibody syndrome (PAPS)
    p. aspergillosis
    p. atypical pneumonia (PAP)
    p. brain lymphoma (PBL)
    p. breast lymphoma (PBL)
    p. bronchopulmonary fibrosarcoma (PBPF)
    p. cancer
    carcinoma of unknown p. (CUP)
    p. cardiac lymphoma
    p. central nervous system lymphoma (PCNSL)
    p. central nervous system tumor
    p. cerebral non-Hodgkin lymphoma (PCNHL)
    p. chemotherapy (CT1)
    p. CNS lymphoma

    p. contribution
    p. effusion lymphoma
    p. extranodal lymphoma (PENL)
    p. healing
    p. healing after radiation therapy
    p. hepatocellular carcinoma
    p. herpetic stomatitis
    p. hypogammaglobulinemia
    p. immune deficiency (PID)
    p. immune response
    p. implanted tumor
    p. isolate
    p. landing zone
    p. lymphoma of bone (PLB)
    p. lymphoma of CNS
    p. lymphoma of lymphoid gland
    p. malignant giant cell tumor (PMGCT)
    p. mediastinal B-cell lymphoma
    p. melanoma
    p. myeloid metaplasia
    p. neoplasm
    p. neuroendocrine small cell carcinoma
    p. orbital lymphoma
    p. radiation
    p. refractory Burkitt lymphoma
    p. refractory Hodgkin disease
    p. resection (PRE)
    p. site
    p. surgical cytoreduction
    p. syphilis
    p. systemic amyloidosis
    p. TEP
    p. thrombocythemia
    p. thrombocytosis
    unknown p.
    p. viremia
primate model
Primaxin
PRIME
    procarbazine, ifosfamide, methotrexate
prime boost
primed lymphocyte typing
primer
    nested p.
primidone
priming
    testosterone p.
primitive
    p. neuroectoderma
    p. neuroectodermal tumor (PNET)
    p. neuroepithelial tumor
    p. neuroepithelioma
    p. stem cell
primordial
    p. cyst
    p. germ cell
Primovist

Principen
principle
    antianemia p.
    Haber toxicologic p.
    intention-to-treat p.
    isotope dilution p.
    Pauli exclusion p.
    transforming p.
principlism
prior exposure hepatitis panel
Priscoline
PRIST
    paper radioimmunosorbent test
P-RMS
    paratesticular rhabdomyosarcoma
proaccelerin
Pro-Amox
Pro-Ampi
proangiogenic molecule
proapoptotic gene
Probactrix
probe
    afterloading p.
    bcr/abl DNA p.
    blind endosonography p.
    P. brain spectroscopy
    digoxigenin-labeled
      oligonucleotide p.
    endosonography p.
    flexible endosonography p.
    gamma-detecting p.
    gamma detection p.
    genetic p.
    high-resolution p.
    HPU heat p.
    intraluminal p.
    rectal p.
    rigid endosonography p.
    sapphire-tip p.
    special p.
probenecid
    colchicine and p.
problem
    colostomy-related p.
    orgasmic p.
    sexual p.
    skin p.
procainamide
procaine
    penicillin G p.
procalcitonin (PCT)
procarbazine (PCB, PCZ)

Adriamycin, cyclophosphamide,
    Oncovin, prednisone, p. (ACOPP)
Adriamycin, vincristine, p. (AVP)
p., Alkeran, Velban (PAVe)
BCNU, methotrexate, p. (BMP)
CCNU, methotrexate, p. (CMP)
CCNU, Oncovin, methotrexate, p.
    (COMP)
CCNU, vinblastine, prednisone, p.
    (CVPP)
p., CCNU, vincristine (PCV)
cyclophosphamide, Adriamycin,
    methotrexate, p. (CAMP)
cyclophosphamide, methotrexate,
    CCNU, vincristine, Adriamycin, p.
    (CMC-VAP)
cyclophosphamide, vincristine,
    Adriamycin, BCNU,
    methotrexate, p. (CVA-BMP)
p. hydrochloride
p., hydroxyurea, radiotherapy
    (PHRT)
p., hydroxyurea, radiotherapy
    protocol
p., ifosfamide, methotrexate
    (PRIME)
p., lomustine, vincristine (PCV)
mechlorethamine, Oncovin, p.
    (MOPr)
mechlorethamine, Oncovin,
    prednisone, bleomycin,
    Adriamycin, p. (MOP-BAP)
methotrexate, doxorubicin,
    cyclophosphamide, etoposide,
    mecloretamine, vincristine, p.
p. methylhydrazine
methylprednisolone, Oncovin, p.
    (MOP)
p., Oncovin, CCNU (POC)
p., Oncovin, cyclophosphamide,
    CCNU (POCC)
p., Oncovin, Cytoxan, CCNU
    (POCC)
p., Oncovin, lomustine (POC)
p. and prednisone
vincristine, Adriamycin, p. (VAP)
vincristine, prednisone, vinblastine,
    chlorambucil, p. (VPBCPr,
    VPVCP)
procarcinogen
procedural success
procedure
    antinociceptive p.

NOTES

P

procedure *(continued)*
    Antivirogram test p.
    antral exclusion p.
    banding p.
    Bevan p.
    Bonferroni p.
    Bricker p.
    catheter-directed interventional p.
    Chamberlain p.
    Charles p.
    Devine antral exclusion p.
    DNA amplification p.
    Edman degradation p.
    endoscopic p.
    Giemsa-trypsin banding p.
    heparinization p.
    immunofluorometric p.
    implant p.
    interventional p.
    Kraske p.
    Krishan p.
    Lewis p.
    loop electrosurgical excision p.
      (LEEP)
    Meigs-Okabayashi p.
    negative selection p.
    neurostimulating p.
    Newman-Keuls p.
    nodal staging p.
    percutaneous transhepatic biliary p.
    platelet neutralization p. (PNP)
    pull-through p.
    Rashkind p.
    revascularization p.
    Roux-en-Y p.
    Sistrunk p.
    2-step p.
    Swenson pull-through p.
    test p.
    Tikhoff-Linberg p.
    transhepatic biliary p.
    transpubic p.
    transthoracic p.
    Waterhouse transpubic p.
    Whipple p.
    York-Mason p.
process
    acromion p.
    alveolar p.
    articular p.
    Cohn cold ethanol fractionation p.
    cystic p.
    ensiform p.
    freezing p.
    granulomatous p.
    infectious p.
    intracranial focal p.
    Markov p.
    neuronal apoptotic p.

    palatine p.
    PhotoPoint light-activated p.
    tumorigenic p.
processor
    COBE 2991 Cell P.
    ThinPrep 2000 p.
prochlorperazine
procoagulant
    cancer p.
procollagen
proconvertin
Procrit
proctitis
    herpetic p.
proctocolectomy
    pouch restorative p.
Proctofoam-HC
proctoperineoplasty
proctoscopic examination
proctoscopy
proctosigmoidoscopy
proctotomy
    posterior p.
Procyclid
procyclidine
Procytox, epipodophyllotoxin-derivative,
    prednisolone (PEP)
Pro-Depo
prodromal stage
prodrome
    AIDS p.
prodrug
    Combretastatin A4 P. (CA4P)
    cyclosaligenyl p.
    p. level
    lipophilic p.
    sulfonyl hydrazine p.
    tumor-activated p. (TAP)
producing
    gonadotropin p.
product
    Aloe Vesta moisturizing skin
      care p.
    BCG live p.
    bcl-2 protooncogene translocation p.
    blood p.
    cellular transfusion p.
    c-erbB2 gene p.
    cleaved polyprotein precursor
      molecule p. (p7, p9, p24)
    cytokine-mobilized blood p.
    fibrin degradation p. (FbDP, FDP)
    fibrinogen degradation p.
    fibrinogen split p.'s
    fusion p.'s
    gene p. (gp)
    gene-based p.
    hemoglobin p.
    oxygen reduction p.

recombinant subunit p.
Sensi-Care skin care p.
skeletal care p.
skin care p.
stem cell p.
tumor cell p.

production
bFGF and VEGF p.
in vitro antibody p. (IVAP)
in vitro antigen p.
lymphokine p.
paraneoplastic ectopic ACTH p.
recombinant subunit protein p.
superoxide p.
vaccine antigen p.

proerythroblast
professional antigen-presenting cell
profile
coagulation p.
fluence p.
intraluminal pressure p.
lipid p.
P. of Mood States (POMS)
neuropsychological test p.
pharmacodynamic p.
pharmacokinetic p.
urethral pressure p. (UPP)

Profilnine SD
profilometry
urethral pressure p. (UPP)

profunda
colitis cystica p.

profusion
PRO 2000 Gel
progenitalis
herpes p.

progenitor
p. cell
hematopoietic p.
human p.
leukemic blast p.
marrow p.
megakaryocyte p.
monocyte-macrophage p.
multipotent hematopoietic p.
myeloid p.

Progens
progeny
radon p.
p. virion

Progestasert
progestational agent

progesterone
p. in oil
p. receptor (PgR, PR)
p. receptor antagonist

progesterone-bound receptor
progestin receptor (PgR)
PROGINS testing
Proglycem Oral
prognosis, pl. **prognoses**
prognostic
p. factor
p. indicator
p. score (PS)
p. serum marker

prognosticator
Prograf
program
Adult Hematopoietic Stem Cell
Transplant P.
AVEU research p.
Cancer Surveillance P. (CSP)
Cancer Therapy Evaluation P.
(CTEP)
Commonweal Cancer Help P.
multimodality treatment p.
National Marrow Donor P.
(NMDP)
RISK computer p.
Society for Hematopathology p.
Solid Tumor Autologous Marrow
Transplant P. (STAMP)
stripping p.
United Nations Acquired
Immunodeficiency p. (UNAIDS)
VariSeed 7.0 software computer p.

programmable pump
programmed cell death
progranulocytic leukemia
progression
freedom from p. (FFP)
hypoxia-mediated malignant p.
hypoxia-mediated tumor p.
malignant p.
terminal p.
tumor p.

progression-free
p.-f. interval
p.-f. survival (PFS)

progressiva
encephalopathia subcorticalis p.

progressive
p. disease
p. familial cholestatic cirrhosis

NOTES

P

455

progressive *(continued)*
    p. multifocal encephalitis
    p. multifocal leukoencephalopathy
**progressively transformed germinal
  center**
Pro-Indo
proinflammatory cytokine
proinsulin
project
    Cancer Genome Anatomy P.
      (CGAP)
    Children's Art P. (CAP)
    Mayo Lung P. (MLP)
    National Collaborative
      Diethylstilbestrol Adenosis P.
      (DESAD)
    National Surgical Adjuvant
      Breast P. (NSABP)
    National Surgical Adjuvant Breast
      and Bowel P. (NSABP)
projectile vomiting
projection
    anteroposterior p.
    AP p.
    apical lordotic p.
    bony p.
    fingerlike p.
    PA p.
    posteroanterior p.
Prokine
prolactin
    p. elevation
    p. receptor
prolactin-inhibiting hormone (PIH)
prolactinoma
prolactin-producing adenoma
prolactin-releasing hormone (PRH)
prolactin-secreting
    p.-s. macroadenoma
    p.-s. microadenoma
prolapse
    mitral valve p. (MVP)
Prolastin
Prolene mesh
Proleukin
Prolieve thermodilatation system
proliferating
    p. cell nuclear antigen (PCNA)
    p. potential
    p. trichilemmal tumor
proliferation
    adnexal lymphoid p.
    angiomyoid p.
    p. area
    p. assay
    benign p.
    B-lymphocyte p.
    cell p.
    cellular p.

    endovascular p.
    extranodal p.
    fascicular p.
    histiocytic p.
    p. index
    lymphocyte p.
    lymphoid p.
    p. marker
    myofibrohistiocytic p.
    ocular adnexal lymphoid p.
    prostatic stromal p.
    p. rate
    small lymphoid cell p.
    stem cell p.
    stromal p.
    tumor p.
proliferative
    p. activity
    p. disorder
    p. phase
    p. stage
proliferator
    peroxisome p.
prolifigen TPA IRMA
Prolixin
Proloid
Proloprim
prolymphoblast
prolymphoblastic
prolymphocyte
prolymphocytic
    p. leukemia (PLL)
    p. T cell
    p. transformation
prolymphocytoid
    p. transformation
    p. variant
ProMACE
    prednisone, methotrexate-leucovorin,
    Adriamycin, cyclophosphamide,
    etoposide
ProMACE-CytaBOM
    prednisone, methotrexate-leucovorin,
    Adriamycin, cyclophosphamide,
    etoposide plus cytarabine, bleomycin,
    Oncovin, methotrexate
    ProMACE-CytaBOM regimen
ProMACE-MOPP
    prednisone, methotrexate, Adriamycin,
    cyclophosphamide, etoposide plus
    mustargen, Oncovin, procarbazine,
    prednisone
ProMaxx-100
promegakaryocyte
promethazine
    meperidine and p.
promiscuity
    lineage p.
ProMod

promonocyte
promoter
    p. element
    gene p.
    p. hypermethylation
    p. trap
ProMune
promyelocyte
promyelocytic leukemia (PML)
pronator teres (PT)
prone
    p. breast radiotherapy
    p. position
proneural gene
pronormoblast
prooxidant
Propac
Propacet
propafenone
propagation
    tumor p.
propeller technique
properitoneal fat stripe
properomine protocol
property, pl. **properties**
    antiapoptotic p.
    antiestrogenic p.
    antiproliferative p.
    estrogenic p.
    lipid-independent anti-
      atherosclerotic p.
    virulence p.
prophase
prophylactic
    p. chemotherapy
    p. contralateral mastectomy (PCM)
    p. cranial irradiation (PCI)
    p. cranial radiation
    p. oophorectomy (PO)
    p. therapy
    p. treatment
prophylaxis, pl. **prophylaxes**
    antibiotic p.
    antifungal p.
    antimycobacterial p.
    chronic antimicrobial p.
    cyclosporine p.
    G-CSF p.
    hemorrhagic cystitis p.
    immunologic p.
propionate
    dromostanolone p.
Propionibacterium

Proplex T
Propolis
proportion
    aneurysmal p.
proportional hazard model analysis
propoxyphene
    p. and acetaminophen
    p. and aspirin
propranolol
propria
    lamina p.
    muscularis p.
pro protein
propyl ketene
propylthiouracil
Propyl-Thyracil
prorubricyte
Proscar
PROSE
    prostate spectroscopy and imaging
    examination
proserum prothrombin conversion
    accelerator
prosodemic
Pro-Sof Plus
Prosorba
    P. column
    P. column platelet replenisher
prostacyclin
prostaglandin
    p. E (PGE)
    p. E_1
    p. E_2 level
    p. endoperoxide metabolism
    p. F (PGF)
    p. inhibitor
    p. synthesis
ProstaMark EPCA
prostanoic acid
ProstaScint examination
ProstaSeed I-125 seed
ProstAsure blood test
prostate
    Association for the Cure of Cancer
      of the P.
    p. brachytherapy
    p. cancer
    p. capsule
    cryosurgical ablation of p. (CSAP)
    p. gland
    p. neoplasm
    OncoRad P.
    p. seed implant

NOTES

P

457

prostate *(continued)*
    p. spectroscopy and imaging examination (PROSE)
    targeted cryoablation of p. (TCAP)
    transurethral incision of p. (TUIP)
    transurethral resection of p. (TURP)
    zonal architecture of p.
prostatectomy
    nerve-sparing radical retropubic p.
    radical p. (RP)
    radical retropubic p.
    transurethral ultrasound-guided laser-induced p. (TULIP)
prostate-specific
    p.-s. antigen (PSA)
    p.-s. antigen density (PSAD)
    p.-s. antigen doubling time (PSADT)
    p.-s. antigen velocity (PSAV)
    p.-s. membrane (PSM)
    p.-s. membrane antigen (PSMA)
    p.-s. membrane protein
prostatic
    p. acid phosphatase (PAP)
    p. adenoma
    p. bed
    p. cancer
    p. carcinoma
    p. hyperplastic nodule
    p. hyperthermia
    p. hypertrophy
    p. intraepithelial neoplasia (PIN)
    p. stent
    p. stromal proliferation
    p. stromal proliferation of uncertain malignant potential (PSPUMP)
    p. transition zone
    p. urethra
    p. urethroplasty
prostatism
prostatitis
    granulomatous p.
prostatodynia
prosthesis, pl. **prostheses**
    Ambicor inflatable p.
    aortic bifurcation p.
    ball-and-socket p.
    Becker tissue expander/breast p.
    resurgery of p.
    saddle p.
    saline-filled testicular p.
    self-expanding endovascular p.
    TEP p.
    1-way valved silicone voice p.
prosthetic
    p. buttock contour
    p. device

    p. implant
    p. replacement
Prostigmin
Prostin E2 Vaginal Suppository
ProSure nutritional therapy
protamine sulfate
protease
    CD26 p.
    p. gene
    p. inhibitor (PI)
    p. inhibitor-resistant virus
    p. paunch
    p. sequence
protease-activated receptor (PAR)
proteasome inhibitor
protection
    barrier p.
    p. factor
    radiation p.
    regions of p.
protector
    long-acting thyroid stimulator p.
Protegrin IB-367 Rinse
protein
    actin p.
    p. 1 alpha
    alpha-actinin p.
    antibodies to Epstein-Barr virus transactivator p. (ZEBRA)
    anticoagulant p.
    AP-2 gamma p.
    APL 400-047 HIV-1 core structural p.
    Bax p.
    B-cell epitope p.
    bcl-2 family p.
    Bence Jones p.
    p. 1 beta
    p. binding
    breast cancer resistance p. (BCRP)
    p. C
    p. C anticoagulant system
    p. cast precipitation syndrome
    CATA2 zinc p.
    caveolin p.
    CD4 p.
    CD5 p.
    CDK4 p.
    cell cycle-regulating p.
    cell cycle regulatory p.
    cellular retinol-binding p. (CRBP)
    c-erbB2 p.
    chemically modified p.
    chimeric p.
    clathrin p.
    c-myc p.
    core binding p.
    C-reactive p. (CRP)
    cross-reactive p. (CRP)

death-associated p. (DAP)
delta p.
desmoplakin p.
drug resistance p.
dynamin p.
dynein p.
E5 p.
E6 p.
E7 p.
ebaf p.
p. electrophoresis
endostatin p.
enhanced green fluorescent p.
  (EGFP)
env p.
envelope p.
erb A p.
exportin p.
expression of fusion p.
ezrin p.
p. factor
FHIT p.
focal adhesion kinase p.
folate-binding p.
fusion p.
G p.
Gag p.
galectin-3 p.
GATA1 zinc p.
glial fibrillary acidic p. (GFAP)
glucose transporter p. (GLUT)
glucose transporter p. 1 through
  13 (GLUT1–13)
glycosylated p.
Golgi-specific p.
green-fluorescent p. (GFP)
GTP-binding p.
guanosine triphosphatase-
  activating p.
heat shock p. 70 (hsp70)
Hektoen, Kretschmer, and
  Welker p.
HIV nucleocapsid p. (p7)
HIV-TAT p.
hRad9 p.
human endostatin p.
icosahedral coat p.
ICPO p.
IE p.
p. immunogen
immunosuppressive acidic p. (IAP)
insulin-like growth factor-binding p.
  (IGFBP)

integrase p.
128 kilodalton neuronal p.
p. kinase
p. kinase inhibitor
K1myc p.
Ku p.
laminin-5 y2 chain p.
p. level determination
lung resistance-related p. (LRP)
M p.
Mac-2 binding p. (Mac-2BP)
macrophage inflammatory p. (MIP)
macrophage inflammatory p. I
  (MIP-I)
macrophage inflammatory p. II
  (MIP-II)
mammaglobin breast cancer p.
maspin p.
p. matrix
matrix p.
Max p.
metalloproteinase-like, disintegrin-
  like, cysteine-rich p.
milk fat globule p.
monocyte chemoattractant p. 1
monocyte chemotactic p. (MCP)
monocyte inflammatory p.
morphogenetic p.
p. motif
MUC2 p.
mucin core p.
multidrug resistance p. (MRP)
murine p.
myb p.
myc p.
mycobacterial p.
myelin base p. (MBP)
myeloma p.
myoD p.
nef p.
nm23-H1 p.
novel erythropoiesis-stimulating p.
  (NESP)
nuclear matrix p. (NMP)
nucleic acid-binding p.
nucleocapsid p.
NY-ESO-1 p.
oncofetal p.
p16 p.
p24 p.
p30 p.
p53 p.
p55 p.

NOTES

P

protein *(continued)*
p150 p.
p170 p.
p185 p.
parathyroid hormone-related p.
(PTHrP)
paxillin p.
PINCH p.
plasma p. C
pol p.
pro p.
prostate-specific membrane p.
pS2 p.
purified myeloma p.
R p.
ras p.
Rb p.
recombinant fusion p.
recombinant HIV p.
recombinant human
immunodeficiency virus p.
replication p. A (RPA)
retinoblastoma p. (pRB)
Rex p.
p. S
S100-beta p.
secreted protein acidic and rich in
cysteine p.
serum-binding p.
single-chain antigen-binding p.
skeletal muscle p. (SMP)
SPARC p.
Stachrom p. C
Staclot p. (C, S)
staphylococcal p. A
synapsin Ia p.
TACI-Ig fusion p.
talin p.
Tamm-Horsfall p.
Tat p.
tax p.
T-cell receptor reactive with folate-
binding p.
telomerase-associated p. (TP1)
tensin p.
tenuin p.
TH p.
TNF receptor-associated death
domain p.
TRADD p.
transmembrane p.
trefoil factor p. (TFF)
trimeric p.
tropomyosin-binding p.
tubulin p.
p. Ty
tyrosinase p.
tyrosinase-related p.
vif p.

vinculin p.
viral envelope p.
viral matrix p.
viral p. R (vpr)
Vpu p.
whole body p. (WBP)
ZEBRA p.
protein-1
activating p.-1 (AP-1)
latent membrane p.-1 (LMP-1)
mucin core p.-1
proteinase
aspartic p.
protein-binding abnormality
ProteinChip antibody capture kit
protein-losing enteropathy
proteinosis
alveolar p.
pulmonary alveolar p. (PAP)
proteinuria
Bence Jones p.
Tamm-Horsfall p.
proteoglycan binding
proteolysis
intracellular p.
preovulatory p.
proteolytic enzyme
Prothecan
prothrombin
p. accelerator
des-carboxy p. (DCP)
des-gamma-carboxy p. (DCP)
p. time (PT)
prothrombinemia
prothrombotic disorder
prothymocyte
**ProTime microcoagulation system used
for patient self-testing**
protocol
ACE chemotherapy p.
ACIP p.
ACTG 076 p.
AIDS Clinical Treatment Group
076 p.
antineoplastic combined
chemotherapy p.
AOPE chemotherapy p.
APO chemotherapy p.
BUdR p.
CAD chemotherapy p.
CALF chemotherapy p.
Capizzi p.
CHAD p.
chemotherapy p.
Children's Hospital Medical Center
sarcoma chemotherapy p.
CoFactor trial p.
Costello p.
DECAL chemotherapy p.

DVP chemotherapy p.
FCAP chemotherapy p.
file transfer p.
freeze/thaw p.
GIMEMA p.
HDPEB p.
Intergroup Osteosarcoma p.
laboratory p.
LSA2L2 chemotherapy p.
Memorial Sloan-Kettering p.
modified Bagshawe p. (MBP)
Muenster p.
MVF chemotherapy p.
MVT chemotherapy p.
National Cancer Institute P. 89-C-41
Nigro p.
NSABP p.
NSABP p. B23
PACE chemotherapy p.
PCV p.
phase I p.
PHRT p.
POMP chemotherapy p.
procarbazine, hydroxyurea, radiotherapy p.
properomine p.
PVDA chemotherapy p.
P. 99-052 Regimen A
P. 99-052 Regimen A for nasopharyngeal carcinoma
Saltz p.
Spigos p.
Stanford V chemotherapy p.
T-2 p.
T-10 p.
Taiwan Pediatric Oncology Group acute myeloid leukemia 901 p.
telomere repeat amplification p. (TRAP)
telomeric repeat amplification p. (TRAP)
TPOG AML 901 p.
VAC chemotherapy p.
VAD chemotherapy p.
VAPE chemotherapy p.
VIC chemotherapy p.
Vokes chemotherapy p.
Wayne State p.

protocol-specified dose
proton
p. beam
p. beam radiosurgery

p. beam single-beam theory
p. beam single-dose therapy of recurrence
p. beam therapy
p. density
p. MR spectroscopy
p. pump inhibitor
proton-density axial MR scan
proton-density-weighted MRI
protooncogene
MYCN p.
protooncogene/oncogene
abl p./o.
bcl-2 p./o.
c-abl p./o.
can p./o.
c-cis p./o.
c-fms p./o.
c-myb p./o.
dek p./o.
E2A p./o.
erb A p./o.
erb B p./o.
ets-1 p./o.
ets-2 p./o.
fes p./o.
fes/fps p./o.
fgr p./o.
fms p./o.
fos p./o.
G p./o.
gip2 p./o.
gsp p./o.
hck p./o.
HER-2 p./o.
HOX11 p./o.
H-ras p./o.
hst (K-fgf) p./o.
int-2 p./o.
jun p./o.
kit p./o.
K-ras p./o.
lck p./o.
lyt-10 p./o.
lyt-10 p./o.
mas p./o.
met p./o.
mil/raf p./o.
mos p./o.
myb p./o.
myc p./o.
myl p./o.
N-ras p./o.

NOTES

P

protooncogene/oncogene *(continued)*
  PBX1 p./o.
  pim-1 p./o.
  raf-1 p./o.
  RAR-alpha p./o.
  ras p./o.
  rel p./o.
  ret p./o.
  rhombotin/Ttg-1 p./o.
  ros p./o.
  sea p./o.
  sis p./o.
  ski p./o.
  src p./o.
  tal-1 p./o.
  tan-1 p./o.
  trk p./o.
  yes p./o.
protoplasmic astrocytoma
prototype
  p. Japanese strain
  p. therapeutic
prototypic antigen-presenting cell
protracted
  p. exposure sensitization
  p. intravenous infusion therapy
protraction
protriptyline
protruding mandible
protrusio acetabuli
protrusion
  acetabular p.
  disc p.
protuberans
  dermatofibrosarcoma p. (DFSP)
prourokinase
Provenge therapeutic vaccine
Provera
  melphalan, 5-fluorouracil, P. (MFP)
provider
  conventional p.
provocation
  secretin p.
Prower factor
proximal
  p. segmental bronchus
  p. sphincter
Proxinium monotherapy
PRP
  premenopausal hormone receptor positive
PRPP
  5-phosphoribosyl-1-pyrophosphate
PRS
  photon-radiosurgical therapy
PRSv
  postrecurrence survival
PRT
  phosphoribosyl transferase

pruritus
  vulvar p.
Prussian
  P. blue
  P. blue reaction
PRV
  polycythemia rubra vera
PS
  prognostic score
pS2 protein
PSA
  prostate-specific antigen
    complex PSA
    PSA density (PSAD)
    free PSA
    free versus complexed PSA
    noncomplex PSA
    PSA prostate cancer tumor marker
    PSA slope
    PSA velocity (PSAV)
PSA4 blood test
PSAD
  prostate-specific antigen density
  PSA density
PSA-detected cancer
PSADT
  prostate-specific antigen doubling time
PSA-immunoperoxidase
psammocarcinoma
psammoma body
psammomatous
  p. calcification
  p. schwannoma
PSAV
  prostate-specific antigen velocity
  PSA velocity
PSC-833
  PSC-833 compound
  PSC-833 and vinblastine
pseudoagglutination
Pseudoallescheria boydii
pseudoanemia
pseudoaneurysm
pseudoangiomatous stromal hyperplasia (PASH)
pseudoangiosarcoma
  Masson p.
pseudoarthrosis
pseudobiopsy technique
pseudocapsule
  tumor p.
pseudocarcinoma
pseudocarcinomatous
pseudoclonality
  T-cell p.
pseudocyst
  gelatinous p.
pseudodiploidy

pseudodiverticulosis
    esophageal intramural p.
pseudoephedrine
pseudofollicle
pseudofollicular
    p. growth pattern
    p. proliferation center
pseudogene segment
pseudoglioma
pseudohermaphroditism
    male p.
pseudo-Hodgkin disease
pseudoinclusion
pseudo-Kaposi
    p.-K. sarcoma
    p.-K. syndrome
pseudoleukemia
pseudolymphoma syndrome
pseudomelanoma
pseudomembranous candidiasis
pseudomesothelioma
Pseudomonas
    P. aeruginosa
    P. paucimobilis
pseudomucinous cystadenocarcinoma
pseudoparalysis
pseudo-Pelger-Hüet change
pseudopolyposis lymphatica
pseudo-pseudohypoparathyroidism
pseudopyloric metaplasia
pseudosarcomatous
    p. fibromyxoid tumor (PSFMT)
    p. myofibroblastic tumor (PMT)
pseudostratified cell
pseudo-T-cell lymphoma
pseudotumor
    atelectatic asbestos p.
    inflammatory p.
    lymphoid inflammatory p.
    ocular adnexal inflammatory p.
pseudotype vector
pseudovirion
pseudoxanthoma
    p. cell
    p. elasticum
PSFMT
    pseudosarcomatous fibromyxoid tumor
psi
    immune cell-produced interferon p.
    p. site
PSIFT
    platelet suspension immunofluorescence test

psittaci
    Chlamydia p.
psittacosis
PSM
    prostate-specific membrane
PSMA
    prostate-specific membrane antigen
psoralen and ultraviolet A (PUVA)
psoriasiform dermatitis
psoriasis
psoriatic arthritis
^{31}**P spectroscopy**
PSPUMP
    prostatic stromal proliferation of uncertain malignant potential
PSTT
    placental site trophoblastic tumor
psychiatric comorbidity
psychoactive drug excess
psychoeducational
psychogenic water intoxication
psychological
    p. approach
    p. factor
    p. support
psychometrics
psychomimetic drug
psychomotor slowing
psychoneuroimmunology
psychooncology
psychosis, pl. psychoses
psychosocial
    p. evaluation
    p. issue
    p. oncology
psychostimulant
psychotherapist
    interpersonal p.
psychotherapy
    interpersonal p.
    supportive-expressive p.
psychotropic agent
psyllium
PT
    pneumothorax
    pronator teres
    prothrombin time
PTBD
    percutaneous transhepatic biliary drainage
PTC
    papillary thyroid carcinoma

NOTES

P

PTC *(continued)*
    percutaneous transhepatic
      cholangiography
    plasma thromboplastin component
PTCH gene
P.T.E.-4
P.T.E.-5
PTEN
    phosphatase and tensin homologue
    deleted on chromosome
      PTEN gene
pteridine chemical
pteroylglutamic acid
pterygoid
    anal p.
    p. fossa
pterygomaxillary fossa
pterygopalatine fossa
PTFE
    polytetrafluoroethylene
PTH
    parathormone
    parathyroid hormone
PTHrP
    parathyroid hormone-related protein
PTLD
    posttransplant lymphoproliferative
      disorder
ptosis
PTSD
    posttraumatic stress disorder
      chronic PTSD
PTT
    partial thromboplastin time
    posterior tibial tendon
PTV
    planning target volume
PTX
    paclitaxel
    pentoxifylline
pubertal development
PUBS
    percutaneous umbilical blood sampling
pudendi
    granuloma p.
pull-through procedure
pullup
    gastric p.
PulmoMate nebulizer
pulmonary
    p. adverse effect
    p. alveolar macrophage
    p. alveolar proteinosis (PAP)
    p. arterial hypertension
    p. artery (PA)
    p. artery hemorrhage
    p. artery intima
    p. artery sarcoma
    p. asbestosis

    p. aspergillosis
    p. blastoma
    p. cancer
    p. cavitating squamous cell
      carcinoma
    p. chondroid hamartoma
    p. complication
    p. edema (PE)
    p. embolism (PE)
    p. endocrine cell
    p. fibrosis
    p. hemosiderosis
    p. infiltration
    p. infiltration with eosinophilia
    p. lymphoid hyperplasia
    p. metastasis
    p. nocardiosis
    p. nodule
    p. reserve
    p. sequelae
    p. sling
    p. toxicity
    p. tumor
pulp
    red p.
    white p.
pulsatile
    p. mass
    p. tinnitus
pulsatility
    arterial p.
**Pulsavac Plus wound debridement
system**
pulse
    bounding peripheral p.
    p. chlorambucil
    dorsalis pedis p.
    frequency-elective p.
    jugular venous p. (JVP)
    p. labeling
    p. methotrexate
    p. oximetry
    saturation p.
    p. sequence
    p. VAC
    p. vincristine, actinomycin D,
      cyclophosphamide
pulsed
    p. brachytherapy
    p. Doppler
    p. dose rate (PDR)
    p. metal vapor laser
pulsing
    energy p.
pulsus paradoxus
pulvule
    Becotin P.'s
    Cinobac P.'s

Darvon Compound-65 P.'s
Ilosone P.'s
pump
ABCT efflux p.
ambulatory infusion p.
aortic balloon p.
balloon p.
Barron p.
Baxter p.
breast p.
CADD-PLUS external volumetric
  programmable p.
CADD-TPN p.
Deltec-Pharmacia CADD p.
drug p.
external volumetric p.
Graseby p.
Gynkotek p.
Hakim valve and p.
Imed Gemini PC-2 volumetric p.
Imed infusion p.
implantable drug p.
implantable infusion p.
implantable osmotic p.
implanted p.
Infumed p.
Infusaid p.
Infuse-A-Port infusion p.
infusion p.
Intelliject p.
IsoMed implantable drug p.
Medtronic infusion p.
Na-K exchange p.
Norport p.
osmotic p.
Pancretec 2000 p.
Panomat infusion p.
Paragon ambulatory p.
portable infusion p.
programmable p.
Sartorius breast p.
Travenol infusion p.
Travenol Infusor p.
p. twin
Verifuse ambulatory infusion p.
volumetric p.
punch
p. biopsy
Keyes dermatologic p.
punch-through
punctata
chondrodysplasia p.

punctate
p. enhancement
p. hyperintense focus
p. metastasis
puncture
antegrade p.
lumbar p. (LP)
needle p.
percutaneous needle p.
spinal p.
tracheoesophageal p. (TEP)
ultrasound-guided nephrostomy p.
PUNLMP
papillary urothelial neoplasm of low
  malignant potential
Purdue Pegboard test
pure
p. anaplastic seminoma
p. antiestrogen
p. choriocarcinoma
p. erythroid leukemia
p. red cell aplasia
p. symptom palliation
Puregene DNA Purification Kit
purged
p. marrow
p. progenitor cell
purging
bone marrow p.
immunologic method of p.
p. of marrow
pharmacologic method of p.
purified
p. human AT-III
p. myeloma protein
p. protein derivative (PPD)
p. vaccine
purine
p. analog
p. antimetabolite
p. moiety
p. nucleotide
Purinethol
prednisone, Oncovin,
  methotrexate, P. (POMP)
Purinol
Purkinje cell cytoplasm
Purlytin
purple mutation system
purpura
autoimmune thrombocytopenic p.
  (AITP)
Bateman p.

NOTES

purpura *(continued)*
    Henoch-Schönlein p.
    idiopathic thrombocytopenic p.
      (ITP)
    immune thrombocytopenic p. (ITP)
    posttransfusion p.
    thrombocytopenic p. (TP)
    thrombotic thrombocytopenic p.
      (TTP)
push-wedge method
putrescine
    methylacetylenic p.
PUVA
    psoralen and ultraviolet A
    PUVA radiation
puzzle
    substrate specificity combinatorial p.
PV
    polycythemia vera
PVA
    prednisone, vincristine, L-asparaginase
PVB
    Platinol, vinblastine, bleomycin
    PVB study
PVD
    peripheral vascular disease
PVDA
    prednisone, vincristine, daunorubicin, L-asparaginase
    PVDA chemotherapy protocol
PVDF
    polyvinyldine difluoride
PVE
    portal vein embolization
PVP
    Platinol and VP-16
    polyvinylpyrrolidone
PVS
    portal venous sampling
PVSG
    Polycythemia Vera Study Group
PWA
    person with AIDS
PXA
    pleomorphic xanthoastrocytoma
PXT
    piroxantrone
pyelogram
    antegrade p.
    intravenous p. (IVP)
pyelography
    intravenous p. (IVP)
pyelonephritis
    atrophic p.

    emphysematous p.
    xanthogranulomatous p.
pyeloureteral stent
pyemia
pyknocyte
pyknocytosis
pyknotic chromatin
pylori
    Campylobacter p.
    Helicobacter p.
pyloric gland metaplasia
pyogenic infection
pyogenicum
    granuloma p.
pyothorax-associated pleural lymphoma
pyramidine base
pyrazinamide toxicity
pyrazine diazohydroxide
pyrazofurin
pyrazoloacridine
pyretic therapy
Pyrex glass tube
pyrexia
    Pel-Ebstein p.
pyridine ring
pyridoglutethimide
pyridoxine deficiency
pyridoxine-responsive anemia
pyridoxyl-5-methyl tryptophan
pyridoxylated stroma-free hemoglobin
pyriform *(var. of* piriform*)*
pyrimethamine and sulfadiazine
pyrimidine
    p. analog
    halogenated p.
    p. metabolism
    p. nucleoside
    p. nucleoside antimetabolite
    p. nucleotide
    p. nucleotide biosynthesis
pyrogallic acid
pyronin Y
pyrophosphate (Ppi)
pyropoikilocytosis
    hereditary p. (HPP)
pyrrolizidine alkaloid
pyrrolizine
    isopropyl p. (IPP)
pyruvate
    p. kinase
    p. kinase deficiency

Q

coenzyme Q (CoQ)
compound Q
Q factor
Q fever
Formula Q

q

long arm of chromosome

5q

chromosome 5q

13q

chromosome 13q

16q

LOH at 16q

17q

chromosome 17q
isochromosome 17q

22q

chromosome 22q

QALE

quality-adjusted life expectancy

QCT

quantitative computed tomography

QIAmp tissue kit

qing dai

QLQ-C30

Quality of Life Questionnaire-C30
EORTC QLQ-C30

QOL

quality of life
QOL assessment
QOL scale

5q-syndrome

monosomy 5q-s.

QTL

quantitative trait locus

Q-TWiST

quality-adjusted time without symptoms
and toxicity

Quadramet

quadrant

quadrantectomy

quadrigeminal cistern

quadripolar 6-French diagnostic electrophysiology catheter

qualitative

q. clot retraction
q. mapping
q. platelet dysfunction

quality

q. control
q. factor
q. of life (QOL)
q. of life assessment

Q. of Life Questionnaire-C30
(QLQ-C30)

quality-adjusted

q.-a. life expectancy (QALE)
q.-a. life-year saved (QUALYS)
q.-a. time without symptoms and
toxicity (Q-TWiST)

QUALYS

quality-adjusted life-year saved

Quanta Lite ELISA autoimmune kit

quantal mitosis

Quantimet 500 analyzing system

quantitative

q. bone scan
q. cell dispersion analysis
q. computed tomography (QCT)
q. PET image
q. polymerase chain reaction assay
q. track etch autoradiography
q. trait locus (QTL)

quartet

investigational high-dose
chemotherapy q.

quasielastic laser light-scattering spectroscope

quasispecies

Quebec platelet disorder

Queckenstedt maneuver

query

Physician Data Q. (PDQ)

questionnaire

acquired immunodeficiency
syndrome health assessment q.
(AIDS-HAQ)
Cancer Needs Q. (CNQ)
McGill Pain Q. (MPQ)

questionnaire-C30

Quality of Life Q.-C30 (QLQ-C30)

Questran Light

Quetelet index

quetiapine

Queyrat

erythroplasia of Q.
Q. erythroplasia

quid

betel q.

quiescent

q. cell
q. fraction
q. phase

Quimby implant system

quinacrine

Quinamed

quinazoline

quinidine

quinine sulfate
quintana
    Bartonella q.
    Rochalimaea q.
Quinton central venous catheter

quinuclidinyl ester
quinupristin/dalfopristin
quotient
    longevity q. (LQ)
    lordosis q. (LQ)

R11 tumor suppressor gene
R5 virus
RA
  retinoic acid
²²⁶Ra
  radium-226
    ²²⁶Ra needle
Raaf catheter
RAB
  remote afterloading brachytherapy
rabbit
  r. antirat ferritin
  r. fibroma
  r. fibroma virus
rabeprazole
rabies
  r. immune globulin
  r. immune globulin human
Rabkin nitinol coil stent
racemic mixture
racemosa
  Cimicifuga r.
racemosum
  angioma venosum r.
racetrack microtron
rad
  r. fraction
  r. surface dose (RSD)
RadiaCare
  R. Cream
  R. Hydrogel Wound Dressing
  R. Klenz wound cleanser
  R. Sun Block
RadiaDres Gel Sheet
radial
  r. phase
  r. scar
radiating bone spicule
radiation
  accelerated hyperfractionated r.
  afterloading r.
  alpha r.
  r. anemia
  annihilation r.
  r. boost
  r. burden
  characteristic r.
  r. cystitis
  dactinomycin, Adriamycin,
    vincristine, cyclophosphamide, r.
  3D conformal r.
  r. dermatitis
  r. dose
  r. dosimetry
  r. duodenitis

r. effect
r. effect unit (reu)
electromagnetic r.
endocavitary r.
r. enhancement
r. enteritis
r. exposure
external beam r.
r. fibrosis
r. fractionation
fractions of r.
gamma knife r.
hemibody r.
r. hepatitis
high linear energy transfer r.
hyperfractionated r.
hypofractionated r.
r. immunity
r. injury
r. intensity
internal r.
interstitial r.
intracavitary particle r.
intraoperative r.
involved-field r.
ionizing r.
laser r.
r. liquid
local r.
low linear energy transfer r.
megavoltage r.
r. mucositis
r. myelitis
r. necrosis
r. nephritis
r. nephropathy
neuraxis r.
neutron beam r.
r. oncogenesis
r. oncologist
r. oncology
orthovoltage r.
particulate r.
r. physics
r. plexitis
r. pneumonitis
r. poisoning
r. portal
postoperative pelvic r.
primary r.
prophylactic cranial r.
r. protection
PUVA r.
radiofrequency r.
r. response

radiation *(continued)*
    r. retinopathy
    r. risk
    secondary r.
    r. seed
    r. seed treatment
    r. sensitivity testing
    r. sensitizer
    r. sickness
    r. simulator
    r. source
    superficial r.
    supervoltage r.
    r. survival curve
    r. therapy (RT)
    R. Therapy Oncology Group
      (RTOG)
    r. therapy system (RTS)
    r. therapy technique
    tissue tolerance to r.
    r. treatment planning (RTP)
    r. treatment system
    ultraviolet r.
    r. weighting factor
    whole body r. (WBR)
radiation-associated endarteritis obliterans
radiation-induced
    r.-i. brachial plexopathy (RIBP)
    r.-i. cancer
    r.-i. carcinogenesis
    r.-i. ischemia
    r.-i. leukoencephalopathy
    r.-i. lumbosacral plexopathy
    r.-i. neoplasm (RIN)
    r.-i. pericarditis
    r.-i. peripheral nerve tumor
    r.-i. pulmonary toxicity
    r.-i. sarcoma
    r.-i. transverse myelitis
    r.-i. trismus
radiation-related
    r.-r. ischemia
    r.-r. ischemic change
radiative hyperthermia device
radical
    r. abdominal hysterectomy
    r. axillary dissection
    r. cystectomy
    r. cystoprostatectomy
    r. en bloc esophagectomy
    free r.
    r. inguinal orchiectomy
    r. mastectomy
    r. neck dissection
    r. nephrectomy
    r. orchiectomy
    oxygen-reactive r.
    r. parametrectomy

    r. pleuropneumonectomy
    r. prostatectomy (RP)
    r. retropubic prostatectomy
    r. surgery
    r. vaginal hysterectomy
    r. vaginal trachelectomy
    r. vulvectomy
radicle
    biliary r.
radicular pain
radiculomyelitis
    viral r.
radiculopathy
radii (*pl. of* radius)
radioactive
    r. gold
    r. iodinated serum albumin (RISA)
    r. iodine
    r. iodine ablation
    r. iodine-125 implant
    r. iodine-125 seed
    r. isotope
    r. palladium-103 seed implant
    r. 103Pd seed implant
radiobiologic
    r. equivalent (RBE)
    r. study
radiobiology
radiocarcinogenesis
radiocephalopelvimetry
radiochemotherapy (RCT)
radiochromic film
radiocolloid
radiocurability
radiodensity
    intramedullary r.
radiofrequency
    r. ablation (RFA)
    r. coil
    r. interstitial tissue ablation (RITA)
    r. interstitial tissue ablation system
    r. radiation
Radiogardase
radiogenic breast cancer
radiograph
    axial r.
    chest r.
    digitally reconstructed r. (DRR)
    dual-energy r. (DER)
    long-bone r.
    Panorex r.
radiography
    advanced multiple-beam
     equalization r.
    air-gap r.
    bedside r.
    computed r.
    digitized chest r.
    megavoltage r.

radioimmune assay
radioimmunoassay (RIA)
    r. kit
    Nichols r.
    Truquant BR r.
radioimmunodetection (RAID)
radioimmunoelectrophoresis
radioimmunoglobulin therapy (RIT)
radioimmunoguided surgery (RIGS)
radioimmunolocalization
radioimmunoprecipitation (RIP)
    r. assay (RIPA)
radioimmunoscintigraphy
radioimmunotherapy (RAIT, RIT)
    HumaRAD compartmental r.
    IDEC-Y2B8 r.
    yttrium-90-labeled ibritumomab
    tiuxetan r.
    Zevalin r.
radioinduced sarcoma
radioiodinated metaiodobenzyl guanidine scan
radioiodine (RAI)
    r. uptake
radioisotope
    local-acting r.
radiolabeled
    r. antibody imaging
    r. antibody and VP-16 and cyclophosphamide systemic chemotherapy
    r. antibody with systemic chemotherapy using VP-16 and cyclophosphamide
    r. monoclonal antibody
    r. peptide alpha-M2
Radiological Society of North America (RSNA)
radiology
    American College of R. (ACR)
    chest r.
    r. telephone access system (RTAS)
    therapeutic r.
radiolymphoscintigraphy
radionecrosis
radionucleotide
    alpha-emitting r.
    antibody r.
radionuclide
    r. bone scan
    r. cutaneous scan
    r. imaging
    r. scanning

    r. scintigraphy
    r. study
    r. ventriculogram (RVG)
radiopaque clip
radiopharmaceutical
    r. chemistry
    r. therapy
radioprotectant
radioprotection
    Tempol-mediated r.
radioprotector
radioreceptor assay
radioresistance
radioresistant
    r. lesion
    r. tumor
radioresponsiveness
radioscintiscan
radiosensitivity
    intrinsic r.
radiosensitization
    schedule-dependent pulsed paclitaxel r.
radiosensitizer
Radiostol Forte
radiostrontium
radiosurgery (RS)
    r. and conformal radiotherapy
    dynamic stereotactic r.
    fractionated stereotactic r.
    gamma knife r.
    LINAC r.
    LINAC-based stereotactic r.
    linear accelerator r.
    linear accelerator-based r. (LINAC-RS)
    megavoltage computed tomography-assisted stereotactic r.
    megavoltage CT-assisted stereotactic r.
    proton beam r.
    STAR proton beam r.
    stereotactic r. (SRS)
radiotherapist
radiotherapy (RT, XRT)
    abdominal strip r.
    accelerated fractionated r.
    accelerated hyperfractionated r.
    accelerated hyperfractionated thoracic r. (AHFTRT)
    accelerated superfractionated r.
    altered fractionation r. (AFRT)
    combined proton-photon r.

R

NOTES

radiotherapy *(continued)*
    computer-controlled r. (CCRT, CC-RT)
    consolidative r.
    continuous-course r.
    CyberKnife SRS image-guided stereotactic radiosurgery precision r.
    cyclophosphamide, hydroxydaunomycin, Oncovin, r. (CHOR)
    3D conformal dose escalation r.
    definitive r.
    3-dimensional conformal r. (3CDRT)
    electron-arc r.
    fast-neutron r.
    fractionated extracranial stereotactic r.
    hyperfractionated r.
    hypofractionated stereotactic r.
    iceberg r.
    image-guided r. (IGRT)
    interstitial r.
    intraoperative r. (IORT)
    intraoperative electron beam r.
    intravascular r.
    large-field r.
    r. localization
    locoregional field r.
    mantle r.
    megavoltage external r.
    neuraxis r.
    orbital r.
    palliative r.
    plaque r.
    r. port
    postoperative locoregional r.
    procarbazine, hydroxyurea, r. (PHRT)
    prone breast r.
    radiosurgery and conformal r.
    ruthenium plaque r.
    salvage r.
    skeletal targeted r. (STR)
    stereotactic r.
    stereotactically guided conformal r.
    sterilizing r.
    target r.
    targeted r.
    teletherapy r.
    twice-a-day r.
    r. utilization rate
    volume-limited r.
    volume-restricted r.
    whole abdominal r.
    whole brain r. (WBRT)

radium
    intracavitary r.
    r. therapy
radium-226 (^{226}Ra)
radius, pl. **radii**
    thrombocytopenia-absent r. (TAR)
radon
    r. gas
    r. progeny
    r. seed implantation
radon-222 (^{222}Rn)
raf-1 protooncogene/oncogene
RAG-1 gene
RAG-2 gene
ragocyte
RAI
    radioiodine
Rai
    R. classification of chronic lymphocytic leukemia (stage 0–IV)
    R. classification (stage 0-IV)
    R. staging system
RAID
    radioimmunodetection
Rainier
    hemoglobin R.
RAIT
    radioimmunotherapy
Raji
    R. cell
    R. cell assay
Ralox
raloxifene
    study of tamoxifen and r. (STAR)
raltitrexed
RAMBA
    retinoic acid metabolism blocking agent
ramus, pl. **rami**
    ascending r.
    inferior pubic r.
Randall forceps
random
    r. donor platelets (RDP)
    r. high-dose chemotherapy
    r. single-donor platelets (RSDP)
randomization
randomized trial
range
    dynamic r.
    emission r.
ranimustine
ranine tumor
ranitidine hydrochloride
RANK
    receptor activator of nuclear factor kappa-beta
Ranke complex

RANKL
  receptor activator of nuclear factor
  kappa-B ligand
ranpirnase
RANTES
  regulated upon activation, normal T-cell
  expressed and secreted
  recombinant human RANTES
ranula
  plunging r.
Rapamune
rapamycin
rapeseed oil
rapid
  r. dissolution formula (RDF)
  r. high virus
  r. microbial contamination test
  r. plasma reagin (RPR)
  r. tumor lysis syndrome
rapid-fractionation irradiation
RapidScreen digital CAD
Rappaport
  R. classification
  R. classification of lymphoma
RAR
  retinoic acid receptor
RAR-alpha
  RAR-alpha oncogene
  RAR-alpha protooncogene/oncogene
rare malignant cell
ras
  ras pathway inhibitor
  Ras gene family point mutation
  ras oncogene
  ras protein
  ras protooncogene/oncogene
ras
rasburicase
rash
  butterfly r.
  drug r.
  exanthematous drug r.
  morbilliform r.
  vesiculobullous r.
Rasheed sarcoma virus
Rashkind
  R. ductus occluder device
  R. procedure
RASSF1A
  RASSF1A gene
  RASSF1A gene testing
rate
  adjusted survival r.

aldosterone secretion r. (ASR)
count r.
cure r.
dose r.
filtration r.
fixed dose r.
flow r.
glomerular filtration r. (GFR)
high dose r. (HDR)
incidence r.
low dose r. (LDR)
maximal flow r.
minimum flow r.
morbidity r.
prevalence r.
proliferation r.
pulsed dose r. (PDR)
radiotherapy utilization r.
relapse r.
Rourke-Ernstein sedimentation r.
sedimentation r.
specific absorption r. (SAR)
survival r.
ultra-low dose r. (ULDR)
utilization r.
5-year cure r.
Rathke
  R. cleft cyst
  R. pouch
  R. pouch tumor
rating
  Atkinson Life Happiness R.
ratio
  apnea/bradycardia r.
  decreased myeloid/erythroid r.
  diagnostic odd r. (DOR)
  diastolic velocity r.
  dose nonuniformity r. (DNR)
  Hybritech Tandem PSA r.
  increased M/E r.
  international normalized r. (INR)
  LQ r.
  M/E r.
  M/L r.
  monocyte/lymphocyte r.
  mortality rate r.
  myeloid/erythroid r.
  nuclear-cytoplasmic r.
  nurse-patient r.
  off-axis r. (OAR)
  off-center r. (OCR)
  oxygen enhancement r. (OER)
  risk-benefit r.

R

NOTES

ratio *(continued)*
- scatter-air r. (SAR)
- scatter-maximum r. (SMR)
- standardized incidence r. (SIR)
- target-to-nontarget r.
- thermal enhancement r. (TER)
- tissue-air r. (TAR)
- tissue-maximum r. (TMR)
- tissue-phantom r. (TPR)
- toxicity-efficacy r.
- X-axis off-axis r.

Rauscher
- R. leukemia
- R. leukemia virus

RAV
- Rous-associated virus

ravuconazole

ray
- beta r.
- grenz r.
- roentgen r.
- R. staging system of urethral cancer in males
- r. tracing approach

Raynaud phenomenon

Razi cannula introducer

razoxane

RB
- retinoblastoma

Rb
- retinoblastoma
  - Rb gene
  - Rb mutation
  - Rb protein
  - Rb protein expression (pRb)

RBE
- radiobiologic equivalent
- relative biological effectiveness

r-beta-ser interferon

Rb1 oncogene

RC
- response criteria

RCA
- red cell aplasia

RCC
- renal cell carcinoma

RCC1 gene

rCD4
- recombinant soluble human CD4

RCT
- radiochemotherapy

RCV
- red cell volume

RDF
- rapid dissolution formula
  - Adriamycin RDF
  - Pharmorubicin RDF

RDI
- relative dose intensity

rDNA
- recombinant DNA

RDP
- random donor platelets

RDW
- red cell distribution width

^{186}Re
- rhenium-186

^{188}Re
- rhenium-188

reabsorption
- bone r.

Reach to Recovery

reactant
- acute phase r.

reaction
- acute hemolytic transfusion r.
- adverse drug r. (ADR)
- allergic r.
- anaphylactic blood transfusion r.
- anaphylactoid r.
- Arthus r.
- blood transfusion r.
- citrate r.
- cytotoxic r.
- deactivating r.
- delayed hemolytic transfusion r.
- desmoplastic r.
- drug r.
- dystonic r.
- extrapyramidal r.
- fluorescent multiplexed polymerase chain r.
- galactose oxidase-Schiff r.
- giant cell r.
- GOS r.
- graft versus host r. (GVHR)
- hemolytic transfusion r.
- high-energy phosphate r.
- host r.
- human immunodeficiency virus ribonucleic acid polymerase chain r.
- hypersensitivity r.
- immune r.
- r. intramuscular myxoma
- Jarisch-Herxheimer r.
- lepra r.
- leukemoid r.
- leukoerythroblastic r.
- lichenoid r.
- long-distance polymerase chain r. (LD-PCR)
- lymphocytic leukemoid r.
- methylation-specific polymerase chain r.
- mixed lymphocyte r.
- monocytic leukemoid r.
- mucocutaneous r.

myelocytic leukemoid r.
Neufeld r.
nonspecific r.
periodic acid-Schiff r.
plasmacytic leukemoid r.
polymerase chain r. (PCR)
Prussian blue r.
reverse transcriptase-polymerase
  chain r. (RT-PCR)
ribonucleic acid polymerase
  chain r.
scirrhous r.
Shwartzman r.
spleen immune r.
r. time task
transfusion r.

reactive
r. carbonium ion
r. cyst
r. hyperemia
r. lymphoid hyperplasia
r. remodeling

reactivity
clinical cross r.
thyroglobulin r.
vimentin r.

reactor
fast-breeder r.

reagent
avidin-biotin-peroxidase r.
BN ProSpec testing r.
Coomassie protein assay r.
F r.
luciferase assay r.
reptilase r.
Schiff r.
Sickledex r.
tandem conjugate r.
TRIzol r.

reagin
rapid plasma r. (RPR)

REAL
Revised European-American Lymphoma
REAL classification

real-time
r.-t. tumor tracking radiation
  therapy (RTRT)
r.-t. ultrasonography

rearrangement
c-myc gene r.
gene r.
r. of genes

immunoglobulin gene r.
lymphocyte gene r.
Rebetron
RECAF biomarker
recanalization technique
receptive anal intercourse
receptor
r. activator of nuclear factor
  kappa-beta (RANK)
r. activator of nuclear factor
  kappa-B ligand (RANKL)
adrenergic r.
androgen r.
antiepidermal growth factor r.
antigen r.
asialoglycoprotein r.
atrial natriuretic factor r.
autocrine motility factor r.
benzodiazepine r.
beta-adrenergic r.
r. blockade
C3 r.
CCKR5 r.
CD4 cell-surface r.
chemokine r. 1-11 (CCR1–11)
chemokine r. 5 (CCR5)
chemokine-related r. (CXCR4)
CKR5 r.
complement r.
CXC chemokine r.
CX3C chemokine r.
CXCR4 r.
epidermal growth factor r. (EFGR,
  EGFR)
E rosette r.
estrogen r. (ER)
Fc r.
fibroblast growth factor r. (FGFR)
fibroblast growth factor r. 4
  (FGFR4)
FLK-1 r.
FLT1 r.
gastrin-releasing peptide r. (GRPR,
  GRP-R)
growth factor r.
histamine H1 r.
hormone r.
5-HT$_3$ r. antagonist
human androgen r.
human progesterone r. (hPR)
keratinocyte growth factor r.
  (KGFR)
laminin r.

NOTES

receptor *(continued)*
    mu r.
    neuromedin B r. (NMB-R)
    neurotensin r. type 1 (NT-R-1)
    neurotensin r. type 2 (NT-R-2)
    neurotensin r. type 3 (NT-R-3)
    NK$_1$ CNS r.
    nuclear hormone r.
    opioid r.
    overexpressed r.
    peroxisome proliferator activated r.
     (PPAR)
    PPAR r.
    progesterone r. (PgR, PR)
    progesterone-bound r.
    progestin r. (PgR)
    prolactin r.
    protease-activated r. (PAR)
    retinoic acid r. (RAR)
    retinoid X r.
    RGD recognition r.
    serotonin r.
    serum soluble r.
    soluble chemokine r.
    soluble transferrin r. (sTfR)
    r. status
    STK-1 r.
    T-cell antigen r. (TCR)
    transferrin r.
    tumor necrosis factor r. (TNFR)
    type 1 growth factor r. (T1GFR)
    r. tyrosine kinase (RTK)
    urokinase plasminogen activator r.
     (uPAR)
    urokinase-type plasminogen
     activator r. (uPAR)
receptor-negative patient
recess
    azygoesophageal r.
    cerebellopontine r.
    pharyngeal r.
recession
    gingival r.
recessive gene
recipient
    allotransplant r.
    renal allograft r.
    r. twin
reciprocal gene
recirculation
    lymphocyte r.
RECIST
    Response Evaluation Criteria in Solid
    Tumors
    RECIST criteria
Recklinghausen
    R. syndrome
    R. tumor
Recklinghausen-Appelbaum disease

reclining position
recombinant
    A/C r.
    A/C/F r.
    r. alfa-2b interferon
    r. alfa interferon
    r. anti-p185HER2 monoclonal
     antibody (rhuMAb HER-2)
    B/D r.
    B/F r.
    r. canarypox
    r. deoxyribonucleic technology
    r. disulfide stabilized immunotoxin
    r. DNA (rDNA)
    r. DNA technology
    r. engineered human anti-CD33
    factor VIIa, r.
    r. fowlpox and vaccinia viruses
     encoding the tyrosinase antigen
     immunization
    r. fowlpox virus
    r. fowlpox virus encoding the
     gp100 melanoma antigen
    r. fusion protein
    r. G-CSF
    r. glycoprotein vaccine
    r. gp160 (rgp160)
    r. hematopoietic growth factor
    r. HIV protein
    r. human erythropoietin
    r. human granulocyte colony-
     stimulating factor (rhGm-CSF,
     rHuG-CSF)
    r. human granulocyte-macrophage
     colony-stimulating factor (rGM-
     CSF)
    r. human growth factor
    r. human IL-2
    r. human IL-4
    r. human IL-10
    r. human immunodeficiency virus
     protein
    r. human interferon beta
    r. human interleukin (rhIL)
    r. human interleukin-3 (rhIL-3)
    r. human interleukin-11 (rhIL-11)
    r. human interleukin-12 (rhIL-12)
    r. humanized monoclonal antibody
     to vascular endothelial cell
     growth factor (rhuMAb-VEGF)
    r. human keratinocyte growth
     factor (rHuKGF)
    r. human macrophage colony-
     stimulating factor (rHM-CSF)
    r. human MCAF
    r. human MIP-1 alpha
    r. human RANTES
    r. interferon alfa (IFLFA, rIFN-A)
    interferon alfa-2a, r.

r. interferon-alfa-2b
interferon alfa-2b, r.
r. interferon gamma
r. interleukin-2 (rIL-2)
r. interleukin-2, dacarbazine,
  cisplatin (RIDD)
r. karyopherin
liposome-encapsulated r.
r. methionyl human granulocyte
  CSF
r. murine (rMu)
r. N-glycanase glycerol-free enzyme
NovoSeven Coagulation Factor
  VIIa r.
r. platelet factor-4 (rPF4)
r. single-chain immunotoxin
r. soluble CD4 (rsCD4)
r. soluble human CD4 (rCD4)
r. subunit product
r. subunit protein production
r. vaccine vector
r. viral vector

recombinant/combination
poxvirus r./c.

recombinase
lymphocyte r.
r. mediated cassette exchange
  (RMCE)

Recombinate

recombination
genetic r.
lox/Cre system of site-specific r.

reconstitution
hematologic r.
immune r.
immunologic r.
incomplete r.

reconstruction
analytic r.
breast r.
immediate breast r. (IBR)
mastectomy with immediate r.
  (MIR)
multiplanar r.
nipple-areolar r.
TRAM flap r.

reconstructive surgery

record
computerized patient r. (CPR)

recovery
fluid-attenuated inversion r.
  (FLAIR)
hematopoietic r.

immunologic r.
marrow r.
neutrophil r.
Reach to R.
short tau inversion r. (STIR)
stem cell r.

recruitment factor

recta (*pl. of* rectum)

rectal
r. cancer
r. carcinoma
Cortenema R.
Cortifoam R.
r. endosonography
r. fascia
Fleet Babylax R.
hydrocortisone r.
r. intussusception
r. mucosa
r. opioid
r. probe
RMS R.
r. shelf
r. stump
r. tear
r. tip

rectilinear depression

rectitis

rectocele

rectopelvic examination

rectosigmoid
r. cancer
r. irradiation tolerance
r. junction

rectum, pl. **recta, rectums**
benign lymphoma of r.
r. irradiation tolerance

rectus
r. abdominis musculocutaneous flap
r. abdominis myocutaneous flap
r. abdominis transverse flap

recurrence
contralateral breast tumor r.
  (CBTR)
free from r. (FFR)
infield r.
ipsilateral breast tumor r. (IBTR)
local r. (LR)
locoregional r.
no evidence of r. (NER)
postgastrectomy cancer r.
proton beam single-dose therapy
  of r.

NOTES

recurrence *(continued)*
  r. regimen
  stomal r.
  supraclavicular r.
  survival after r. (SAR)
  suture line r.
  Visick grading system for postgastrectomy carcinoma r.
recurrent
  r. aphthous ulcer
  r. cancer
  r. carcinoma
  r. glioblastoma
  r. glioma
  r. high-grade astrocytoma
  r. hyperparathyroidism
  r. laryngeal nerve
  r. lymphoma
  r. medulloblastoma
  r. nerve palsy
  r. oligoastrocytoma tumor
  r. relationship theme
  r. *Salmonella* septicemia
  r. sialadenitis
  r. therapy
  r. vermian oligoastrocytoma
  r. vulvovaginal candidiasis
  r. zoster
recursive partitioning analysis
red
  aniline r.
  r. blood cell
  r. blood cell antigen
  r. blood cell cast
  r. blood cell count
  r. blood cell distribution width index
  r. blood cell polyamine
  r. blood cell scintigraphy
  r. blood cell smear
  r. blood cell transfusion
  r. cell aplasia (RCA)
  r. cell distribution width (RDW)
  r. cell ghost
  r. cell volume (RCV)
  r. fluorescence
  r. marrow
  r. nucleus
  r. pulp
red-blue nodule
Redisol
redox
  r. change
  r. mediator
  r. metabolism
Redoxon
reduced
  r. folate carrier (RFC)

  r. sulfhydryl (RSH)
  r. sulfhydryl group
reductase
  dihydrofolate r. (DHFR)
  methylenetetrahydrofolate r. (MTHFR)
reduction
  hydrostatic r.
  pneumatic r.
Redutemp
Reed cell
Reed-Hodgkin disease
Reed-Sternberg (R-S)
  R.-S. cell
  Hodgkin and R.-S. (HRS)
reentrant well chamber
Reese-Ellsworth
  R.-E. classification
  R.-E. classification of retinoblastoma
ReFacto hemophilia A blood clotting factor
reference
  r. dose
  frame of r.
reflector
  diffuse r.
reflex
  Kocher-Cushing r.
reflexology
Refludan
reflux
  duodenogastroesophageal r.
  embolic r.
  esophageal r.
  gastroesophageal r.
  laryngopharyngeal r. (LPR)
refocused
  multiplanar gradient r.
refractoriness
  platelet r.
refractory
  r. anemia
  r. anemia with excess blasts
  r. anemia with excess blasts in transition
  r. anemia with ringed sideroblasts
  r. bladder cancer
  r. CD22+ B-cell lymphoma
  r. mucosal candidiasis
  r. tumor
Refsum disease
REG
  regenerating gene I
Regan isoenzyme
regenerating gene I (REG)
regenerative hyperplasia
regimen
  Atzpodien r.

BEACOPP r.
BOMP chemotherapy r.
CEVAIE r.
CEVD r.
chemotherapy r.
CIVIC chemotherapy r.
combination nucleoside analogue
 antiviral r.
Cooper r.
CY plus TBI preparative r.
cytoreductive r.
dose-intensive r.
Einhorn r.
first-generation r.
FLAG r.
FLAM r.
FOLFIRI r.
FOLFOX r.
FOLFUGEM r.
FOLFUGEM-OX r.
fractionation r.
gemcitabine plus oxaliplatin r.
GEMOX r.
Gonzalez r.
hybrid r.
hyper-CVAD r.
[131]I-labeled anti-CD45 antibody
 combined with CY and TBI r.
intensification r.
intermediate-dose salvage r.
IROX r.
Livingstone-Wheeler r.
low-intensity preparative r.
Magrath-modified r.
Melacine r.
methotrexate/arabinoside C r.
MTX/ara-C r.
multidrug r.
peripheral blood progenitor cell
 mobilization r.
platinum-based r.
platinum-containing r.
ProMACE-CytaBOM r.
Protocol 99-052 R. A
recurrence r.
Saltz r.
salvage r.
split-course r.
standard busulfan/cyclophosphamide
 preparative r.
Stanford V chemotherapy r.
taxane-based r.
transplant preparative r.

VAIA r.
VEEP r.
region
abnormally contracting r.
APOC2 r.
argyrophilic stain for nucleolar
 organizer r. (AgNOR)
axillary r.
balanopreputial r.
beta-chain variable r. (V-beta)
breakpoint cluster r. (BCR)
Broca r.
complementarity determining r.
 (CDR)
epigastric r.
Epstein-Barr early r.
Heschl r.
homogeneously staining r. (HSR)
HRC r.
hypotetraploid r.
interfollicular r.
nuclear organizing r.
nucleolar organizing r.
paratesticular r.
pineal r.
r.'s of protection
silver-stained nucleolar organizer r.
telomeric r.
regional
r. anesthesia
r. anesthetic
r. chemotherapy
r. irradiation
r. lymph nodes cannot be
 addressed (NX)
r. melanoma
r. neurolytic block
r. spread
r. tumor confinement
registrar
National Association of Tumor R.'s
 (NATR)
registry, pl. **registries**
Autologous Blood and Marrow
 Transplant R. (ABMTR)
Automated Central Tumor R.
 (ACTUR)
Bone Sarcoma R.
Breast Cancer Family R.
Breast, Ovarian and Colorectal
 Cancer Family Registries
Cancer Family R. (CFR)
Colon Cancer Family R.

NOTES

registry *(continued)*
  Eindhoven Cancer R.
  Herbst r.
  hospital-based r.
  International Bone Marrow
    Transplant R. (IBMTR)
  Kiel Pediatric Tumor R.
  Ovarian Tumor R. (OTR)
  Pediatric RAC R.
  tumor r.
Reglan
Regressin
regressing atypical histiocytosis
regression
  r. analysis
  estrogen rebound r.
  Poisson r.
  polytomous logistic r.
  tumor r.
**regulated upon activation, normal T-cell
  expressed and secreted (RANTES)**
regulation
  gene r.
  hematopoietic r.
  transcriptional r.
regulator
  cell-cycle r.
regulatory
  r. gene
  r. peptide receptor targeting
  r. T cell
Reguloid
regurgitation
  aortic r.
  mitral r.
rehabilitation
rehabilitative surgery
Reifenstein syndrome
Reiki therapy
reimbursement system
reinduction chemotherapy
reinforcement
  Wilson-Cook metal r.
reinfusion
Reinke crystal
reirradiation
Reiter syndrome
rejection
  acute cellular xenograft r.
  allograft r.
  chronic allograft r.
  graft r.
  hyperacute r.
  marrow graft r.
rel
  rel oncogene
  rel protooncogene/oncogene
Relafen

relapse
  bone marrow r.
  intraabdominal r.
  locoregional r.
  r. rate
  solitary r.
  testicular r.
relapsed chemosensitive Hodgkin disease
relapse-free survival (RFS)
related
  chemokine r.
  r. hemorrhage
relationship
  doctor-patient r.
  dose-response r.
  dose-time r.
  mutually monogamous r.
  pharmacodynamic-pharmacokinetic r.
  pharmacokinetic-pharmacodynamic r.
  structure-activity r.
  survival r.
  tumor cell-host bone r.
relative
  r. biological effectiveness (RBE)
  r. curative resection
  r. dose intensity (RDI)
  r. noncurative resection
  r. risk
relaxant
  muscle r.
relaxation
  longitudinal r.
  spin-lattice r.
  spin-spin r.
  transverse r.
release
  controlled r.
  morphine-controlled r. (MCR)
  morphine sulfate controlled r.
  slow r. (SR)
releasing
  r. factor
  hormone r.
relief
  Fleet Pain R.
ReliefBand device
relocatable stereotactic frame
remedy, pl. **remedies**
  herbal r.
  plant r.
Remeron
remifentanil
remission
  clonal r.
  complete r. (CR)
  cytogenetic r.
  r. induction
  nodular partial r. (nPR)

R

unconfirmed/uncertain complete r.
(CRu)
remission-induction chemotherapy
Remitogen
remnant
cystic duct r.
embryonal r.
thymic r.
remodeling
adaptive r.
constrictive r.
intermediate r.
reactive r.
remote afterloading brachytherapy
(RAB)
removal
endoscopic r.
surgical r.
Remune
Renagel
renal
r. abscess
r. adenocarcinoma
r. allograft
r. allograft-mediated hypertension
r. allograft recipient
r. amyloidosis
r. angiomyolipoma
r. angioplasty
r. artery embolization
r. carcinosarcoma
r. cast
r. cell cancer
r. cell carcinoma (RCC)
r. clearance
r. cortical carcinoma
r. dialysis
r. dilator
r. dysfunction
r. failure
r. function
r. function test
r. fungal infection
r. hilum
r. hypoplasia
r. impairment
r. infarction
r. infusion therapy
r. insufficiency
r. lymphoma
r. mass
r. mass cryoablation
r. medullary carcinoma

r. paraneoplastic syndrome
r. pelvis
r. pelvis carcinoma
r. replacement therapy
r. toxicity
r. transplant
r. tumor
vertebral, anal, tracheal,
esophageal, r. (VATER)
Rencarex
Rendu-Osler-Weber disease
Renese
Renova
renovascular
r. cause for hypertension
r. disease
Reolysin
ReoPro
Reosyn
reoxygenation
repair
anterior-posterior r.
AP r.
mismatch r. (MMR)
reparative giant cell granuloma
repeat
CAG trinucleotide r.
long terminal r. (LTR)
repens
erythema gyratum r.
repetition time (TR)
repifermin
replacement
fatty marrow r.
gene r.
heteroaromatic r.
prosthetic r.
replenisher
Prosorba column platelet r.
Replete
replication
DNA r.
r. error negative (RER−)
r. error positive (RER+)
gut r.
r. inhibition factor (RIF)
low-level viral r.
lytic viral r.
morphine-potentiated HIV r.
morphine-potentiated human
immunodeficiency virus r.
viral r.
replication-complete retrovirus

NOTES

replication-deficient virus
replication protein A (RPA)
replicative senescence
replicon
repolarization
reporter gene
reporting
American Joint Committee for
Cancer Staging and End
Results R.
repository
repressed gene
repressor gene
reproductive
r. function
r. toxin
r. tract embryology
reprogramming therapy
reptilase
r. reagent
r. time
repulsive force
RER–
replication error negative
RER+
replication error positive
Rescriptor
rescue
Adriamycin, 5-fluorouracil,
methotrexate with leucovorin r.
AFM with leucovorin r.
autologous bone marrow r.
(ABMR)
autologous stem cell r. (ASCR)
bone marrow r.
high-dose chemotherapy and stem
cell r. (HDC/SCR)
high-dose chemotherapy with
autologous bone marrow or stem
cell r. (HDC/ASCR)
host r.
leucovorin r.
methotrexate with r.
stem cell r.
r. technique
uridine r.
research
American Association for
Cancer R. (AACR)
American Foundation for AIDS R.
(AMFAR)
American Institute for Cancer R.
(AICR)
Institute for Cancer R. (ICR)
resectability
resectable colorectal cancer
resection
abdominoperineal r. (APR)
abdominosacral r.

absolute curative r.
absolute noncurative r.
appropriate r.
atrial septal r. (ASR)
Caldwell-Luc r.
coloanal r.
craniofacial r.
curative r.
en bloc r.
endoscopic mucosal r. (EMR)
gross total r. (GTR)
hepatic r.
International Union Against Cancer-
RO r.
limited r.
low anterior r. (LAR)
margin of r.
mucosal r.
noncurative r.
primary r. (PRE)
relative curative r.
relative noncurative r.
rim r.
subtotal r. (STR)
surgical r.
Tikhoff-Linberg r.
transurethral r. (TUR)
UICC-RO r.
wedge pulmonary r.
Whipple r.
Resectisol Irrigation Solution
resective surgery
reserve
brain perfusion r.
neutrophil r.
peripheral blood stem cell r.
(PBSCR)
pulmonary r.
reservoir
Camey r.
contiguous spinal fluid r.
ICV r.
Ommaya spinal fluid r.
Rickham r.
spinal fluid r.
viral r.
residua (*pl. of* residuum)
residual
r. disease
postvoid r.
r. tumor mass
residue
hydrophobic r.
methanol extraction r.
residuum, pl. **residua**
microscopic r.
resilience
immunoglobulin r.

R

resin
  cation exchange r.
  cholestyramine r.
  podophyllum r.
  r. sphere
resistance
  acquired drug r.
  cellular r.
  complement r.
  drug r.
  drug-induced drug r.
  end-organ r.
  extreme drug r. (EDR)
  inherent drug r.
  kinetic r.
  multidrug r. (MDR)
  multiple drug r. (MDR)
  phenotypic drug r.
  reversing drug r.
  r. wire heater
  zidovudine r.
resistance-associated mutation
resistance-conferring mutation
resistant
  isoniazid r.
  platinum r.
resistant-repellant drug
resistivity
  conductor r.
resistor
  Starling r.
resolution
  axial r.
resonance
  electron paramagnetic r. (EPR)
  electron spin r.
  magnetic r. (MR)
  nuclear magnetic r. (NMR)
  topical magnetic r. (TMR)
resorcinol spray
resorption
  bony r.
resource
  AIDS and Cancer Specimen R.
    (ACSR)
  Cooperative Breast Cancer
    Tissue R. (CBCTR)
  Cooperative Prostate Cancer
    Tissue R. (CPCTR)
respiration
  ventilator-assisted r.
respirator lung

respiratory
  r. complication
  r. enzyme complex
  r. infection
  r. status
  r. syncytial virus (RSV)
  r. and upper digestive tract
    (RUDT)
Respirgard II
response
  abrogated immune r.
  anamnestic r.
  antibody r.
  antiidiotype immune r.
  antiidiotypic immunoglobulin r.
  antitoxin r.
  apoptotic r.
  autoimmune r.
  CD4+ r.
  CD8+ r.
  clinical partial r. (CPR)
  complete r. (CR)
  complete hematologic r. (CHR)
  r. criteria (RC)
  cytotoxic T-cell lymphocyte r.
  deconditioned exercise r.
  dose r.
  elicited r.
  emetic r.
  R. Evaluation Criteria in Solid
    Tumors (RECIST)
  host r.
  human antitoxin r.
  immune r.
  inflammatory r.
  maternal humoral immune r.
  r. modifier
  mucosal immune r.
  no r. (NR)
  optimal therapeutic r.
  partial r. (PR)
  primary immune r.
  radiation r.
  secondary immune r.
  serotonergic-induced emetic r.
  systemic immune r.
  T-cell-mediated antitumor r.
  therapeutic r.
  transferred immune r.
  urokinase plasminogen activator r.
    (uPAR)
rest
  adrenal r.

NOTES

483

rest *(continued)*
    nephrogenic r.
    pelvic r.
restaging
restenosis
restitope
restoration
    physical r.
Restore hydrocolloid dressing
restriction
    antigen r.
    r. element
    r. enzyme
    r. fragment length polymorphism (RFLP)
    r. fragment length polymorphism analysis
    r. fragment length polymorphism method
    lineage r.
restructuring
result
    Surveillance Epidemiology and End R.'s (SEER)
resurgery of prosthesis
resuscitation
retardation
    mental r.
    Wilms tumor, aniridia, genitourinary abnormalities, mental r. (WAGR)
retention
    urinary r.
reticence
reticula (*pl. of* reticulum)
reticular
    r. dysgenesis
    r. type
reticulated lesion
reticulation
    coarse r.
    diffuse fine r.
reticulin
    r. deposition
    r. stain
reticulocyte count
reticulocytopenia
reticulocytosis
reticuloendothelial
    r. cell
    r. cell-origin tumor
    r. cycle
    r. system
reticuloendotheliosis
    leukemic r.
reticulohistiocytic
reticulohistiocytoma
reticulohistiocytosis
reticuloid
    actinic r.

reticulosis
    histiocytic medullary r.
    malignant r.
    midline malignant r.
    pagetoid r.
    polymorphic midline malignant r.
reticulum, pl. **reticula**
    r. cell
    r. cell sarcoma
    endoplasmic r.
Retin-A
retina
    neurosensory r.
retinaculum, gen. **retinaculi**, pl. **retinacula**
    extensor r.
retinal
    r. angiomatosis
    r. anlage tumor
    r. hamartoma
    r. hemorrhage
    r. pigmentary degeneration
    r. pigment epithelium (RPE)
    r. vasculitis
retinalis
    lipemia r.
retinamide
retinitis
    cytomegalovirus r.
    Toxoplasma r.
retinoblast
retinoblastoma (RB, Rb)
    familial r.
    r. gene
    hereditary r.
    intraocular r.
    r. protein (pRB)
    Reese-Ellsworth classification of r.
    sporadic r.
    trilateral r. (TRb)
retinoblastoma-osteosarcoma
    hereditary r.-o.
retinoic
    r. acid (RA)
    r. acid metabolism blocking agent (RAMBA)
    r. acid receptor (RAR)
    r. acid syndrome
retinoid
    synthetic r.
    r. X receptor
retinoid-related molecule
retinol
retinopathy
    radiation r.
retinyl palmitate
ret protooncogene/oncogene
retractile mesenteritis
retraction
    qualitative clot r.

R

retractor
    Rochard r.
retrievable filter
retrieval
    heat-induced epitope r. (HIER)
    heat-mediated antigen r.
retrocrural lymph node
retrogene
retrograde
    r. ejaculation
    r. transurethral prostatic
      urethroplasty
    r. urethrography (RUG)
retrolental fibroplasia
retromandibular
retromolar
    r. trigone
    r. trigone cancer
retroperitoneal
    r. leiomyosarcoma
    r. liposarcoma
    r. lymphadenectomy
    r. lymphadenopathy
    r. lymphangioma
    r. lymph node dissection (RPLND)
    r. lymphoma
    r. paraganglia
    r. residual tumor mass (RRTM)
    r. reticulum cell sarcoma
retroperitoneum
retropharyngeal lymph node
retropubic
    r. I-125 implant
    r. vesiculoprostatectomy
Retrovir
retroviral
    r. cytochrome P450
    r. replication cycle
    r. transduction
    r. transduction of *mdr-1* gene into
      peripheral blood progenitor cell
retroviremia
retrovirus
    C-type r.
    endogenous r. (ERV)
    endogenous r. 3 (ERV3)
    HTLV-I r.
    human endogenous r. (HERV)
    human endogenous r. E (HERV-E)
    human endogenous r. K (HERV-K)
    human pathogenic r.
    human T-lymphotrophic r. (HTLV)

    replication-complete r.
    r. vector
return
    anomalous pulmonary venous r.
reu
    radiation effect unit
REV
    room eye view
    REV response element (RRE)
rev
    reverse
    rev mRNA
revascularization procedure
reverse (rev)
    r. passive hemagglutination
    r. transcriptase (RT)
    r. transcriptase inhibitor (RTI)
    r. transcriptase-polymerase chain
      reaction (RT-PCR)
    r. transcriptase-polymerase chain
      reaction assay
Reversecell Ag kit
reversible polyclonal posttransplant
    lymphoproliferative disease
reversing drug resistance
revertant
    wild-type r.
Revici-guided chemotherapy
revised
    R. European-American Lymphoma
      (REAL)
    R. European-American Lymphoma
      classification
Revitalose C-1000
Revlimid immunomodulatory drug
RevM10
    gene construct RevM10
Revolution XR/d digital detector
rexinoid
Rex protein
Rex-responsive element (RXRE)
Rey Complex Figure Test
Reye syndrome
RF2000 Radiofrequency Generator
RFA
    radiofrequency ablation
RFC
    reduced folate carrier
RFLP
    restriction fragment length polymorphism
R-Frone
RFS
    relapse-free survival

NOTES

RF Vacuum Ablation System
RGD recognition receptor
R-Gel
rGM-CSF
    recombinant human granulocyte-
      macrophage colony-stimulating factor
rgp160
    recombinant gp160
RG 12915 serotonin antagonist
Rh
    Rhesus factor
      Rh agglutinin
      Rh antibody
      Rh blood group
      Rh factor
      Rh factor antigen
      Gamulin Rh
      Rh incompatibility
      Mini-Gamulin Rh
      Rh negative
      Rh positive
rhabdoid
    r. feature
    r. tumor
    r. tumor of central nervous system
    r. tumor of kidney
rhabdomyoblast
rhabdomyoma
rhabdomyosarcoma (RMS)
    alveolar r.
    botryoid embryonal r.
    embryonal r.
    extremity r.
    genitourinary r.
    ocular r.
    orbital r.
    parameningeal r.
    paratesticular r. (P-RMS)
    pleomorphic r.
    spindle cell r.
    truncal r.
    r. with rhabdoid feature
rhabdosarcoma
rhagades
rHb1.1 recombinant hemoglobin
RHD
    RHD pseudogene assay
    RHD psi test
Rh₀(D) immune globulin human
Rheaban
rhEndostatin
rhenium-186 (^{186}Re)
rhenium-186-HEDP
rhenium-188 (^{188}Re)
rheology of blood
rheolytic thrombectomy catheter
Rhesus factor (Rh)
rheumatoid arthritis
Rheumatrex

rhGm-CSF
    recombinant human granulocyte colony-
      stimulating factor
rhIL
    recombinant human interleukin
rhIL-3
    recombinant human interleukin-3
rhIL-11
    recombinant human interleukin-11
rhIL-12
    recombinant human interleukin-12
rhinitis
    persistent r.
rhinocerebral syndrome
rhinorrhea
    persistent r.
rhinotomy
    lateral r.
rhizotomy
    chemical r.
    cranial nerve r.
Rhizoxin
rHM-CSF
    recombinant human macrophage colony-
      stimulating factor
rhodesiense
    Trypanosoma r.
Rho(D) immune globulin
Rhodis
Rh(o) disease
Rhodis-EC
Rhodococcus equi
RhoGAM
rhombotin/Ttg-1
    r./Ttg-1 oncogene
    r./Ttg-1 protooncogene/oncogene
rhombotin/Ttg-2 oncogene
Rhotrimine
rhubarb
    turkey r.
rHuG-CSF
    recombinant human granulocyte colony-
      stimulating factor
rHuKGF
    recombinant human keratinocyte growth
      factor
rhuMAb HER-2
    recombinant anti-p185HER2 monoclonal
      antibody
rhuMAb-VEGF
    recombinant humanized monoclonal
      antibody to vascular endothelial cell
      growth factor
rhythm
    circadian r.
    sinus r.
RIA
    radioimmunoassay

rib
> bifid r.'s
> dense r.'s

ribavirin inhaled solution

ribbon
> hollow r.
> ^{192}Ir r.
> seed r.

riboflavin

ribonuclease (RNAse)
> r. H (RNAse H)
> oocytic r.

ribonucleic
> r. acid (RNA)
> r. acid polymerase chain reaction

riboside
> methylmercaptopurine r. (MMPR)

ribosome-lamella complex

ribozyme

RIBP
> radiation-induced brachial plexopathy

rich
> Rolaids Calcium R.
> T-cell r.

Richter
> R. syndrome
> R. syndrome-like transformation

ricin
> r. A chain
> anti-B4-blocked r.
> anti-MY9-blocked r.
> N901 blocked r.

ricin-blocked antibody

rickets
> familial hypophosphatemic r.

Rickettsia

Rickham reservoir

Rid-A-Pain

RIDD
> recombinant interleukin-2, dacarbazine, cisplatin

Ridenol

ridge
> alveolar r.
> sphenoid r.

Rieder
> R. cell
> R. cell leukemia

RIF
> replication inhibition factor

rifabutin

Rifadin
> R. Injection
> R. Oral

rifampin toxicity

rIFN-A
> recombinant interferon alfa

rIFN-gamma therapy

rigid
> r. bronchoscope
> r. endosonography probe
> r. forceps
> r. nephroscope
> r. sigmoidoscope

RigiScan

RIGS
> radioimmunoguided surgery
> RIGS system

RIGS/ACT technology

RIGScan CR49

rIL-2
> recombinant interleukin-2

Riley-Smith syndrome

rim
> dorsal r.
> r. resection
> stromal r.

Rimactane Oral

Rimadyl

rimming
> anal r.

RIN
> radiation-induced neoplasm

Rindfleisch cell

ring
> R. biliary drainage catheter
> cricoid r.
> R. drainage catheter needle
> enhancement r.
> r. of enhancement
> esophageal r.
> flocculent r.
> hemosiderin r.
> r. hydroxylation
> internal inguinal r.
> r. pattern
> pyridine r.
> r. of sideroblast
> signet r.
> stippled r.
> R. transjugular intrahepatic access set
> Waldeyer tonsillar r.

ringed sideroblast

NOTES

Ringer lactate
Ringertz-Burger grading system
Ringertz system
Ring-MacLean sump
ringworm
rinse
    Carrington oral wound r.
    glyminox oral r.
    oral wound r.
    povidone iodine r.
    Protegrin IB-367 R.
    wound r.
Riopan Plus
RIP
    radioimmunoprecipitation
RIPA
    radioimmunoprecipitation assay
RISA
    radioactive iodinated serum albumin
    RISA study
rise
    age-dependent r.
risedronate
risk
    cancer r.
    exposure r.
    r. factor
    organs at r. (OAR)
    percutaneous exposure r.
    radiation r.
    relative r.
    suicidal r.
    Weibull plot of adult T-cell
      leukemia/lymphoma r.
risk-assessment model
risk-benefit ratio
RISK computer program
risk-reduction counseling
ristocetin
    r. cofactor test
    r. von Willebrand cofactor
RIT
    radioimmunoglobulin therapy
    radioimmunotherapy
RITA
    radiofrequency interstitial tissue ablation
    RITA system
ritodrine
Rituxan and fludarabine chemotherapy
rituximab
Rivotril
RMCE
    recombinase mediated cassette exchange
RMP-7 bradykinin analog
RMS
    rhabdomyosarcoma
    RMS Rectal
rMu
    recombinant murine

rMu GM-CSF
rMu IL-6
rMu IL-7
rMu IL-1B
^{222}Rn
    radon-222
RNA
    ribonucleic acid
    Epstein-Barr early RNA (EBER)
    HIV RNA
    messenger RNA (mRNA)
    RNA PCR
    RNA PCR core kit
    plasma HIV RNA
    RNA transcription
    RNA tumor virus
RNA-dependent protein kinase (PKR)
RNA-loaded autologous dendritic cell
    vaccine
RNAse
    ribonuclease
    isoenzyme RNase
    RNAse tumor marker
RNAse H
    ribonuclease H
RNASEL gene
ROAP
    rubidazone, Oncovin, ara-C, prednisone
robertsonian translocation
robot-assisted laparoscopy
robotics
Robson
    R. classification
    R. modification of Flocks-Kadesky
      system
    R. renal cell cancer (stage I-IV)
    R. staging
Rocaltrol
Rocephin
Rochalimaea quintana
Rochard retractor
rocket
    r. immunoelectrophoresis
    r. wire
rod
    aerobic Gram-negative r.
    Auer r.'s
    r. cell
    Gram-negative r.
    Hopkins r.
rodent ulcer
RODEO
    rotating delivery of excitation off-
      resonance
    RODEO MRI
roentgenogram
roentgenography
    abdominal r.
roentgen ray

R

roentgen-ray therapy
roentgentherapy
    intraoral r.
    intravaginal r.
Rofact
rofecoxib
Roferon-A
Roferon and Accutane therapy
Rogitine
rogletimide
Rolaids Calcium Rich
role
    r. functioning
    tumorigenic r.
Rolfing structural integration
rolipram
Romanowsky stain
Römer test
roof
    acetabular r.
room eye view (REV)
root
    aortic r.
roquinimex
Rosch modification
Rosen guidewire
Rosenmüller
    fossa of R.
Rosenthal
    R. aspiration needle
    basal vein of R.
    R. fiber
    R. syndrome
rosette
    r. cell
    E r.
    Flexner-Wintersteiner r.
    Homer-Wright r.
    malarial r.
    sheep erythrocyte r.
Rose-Waaler test
rosiglitazone maleate
ros protooncogene/oncogene
rostaporfin
Rotachrom Heparin
rotamer
rotated collimators and couches
rotating delivery of excitation off-resonance (RODEO)
rotation
    r. arc
    collimator r.

    opioid r.
    r. therapy
rotational
    r. field
    r. therapy technique
rotationplasty
Rotex
    R. biopsy instrument
    R. needle
Rothmund-Thomson syndrome
Roth spot
Rotterdam
    R. Study
    R. Symptom Checklist
Rotter node
Roubac
Rouget cell
Rouleaux formation
round
    r. cell sarcoma
    r. cell tumor
roundtable
    National Colorectal Cancer R. (NCCRT)
Rourke-Ernstein sedimentation rate
Rous
    R. sarcoma
    R. sarcoma virus (RSV)
    R. tumor
Rous-associated virus (RAV)
route
    intrathecal r.
    parenteral r.
Rouviere
    nodes of R.
Roux-en-Y
    R.-e.-Y choledochojejunostomy
    R.-e.-Y procedure
Rovamycine
Rowasa enema
Roxanol SR Oral
Roxicet 5/500
Roxicodone
Roxilox
royal
    R. Jelly
    R. Marsden Hospital staging system
    R. Marsden Hospital staging system for testicular cancer
RP
    radical prostatectomy
Rp53 gene

NOTES

RPA
replication protein A
RPE
retinal pigment epithelium
rPF4
recombinant platelet factor-4
RPLND
retroperitoneal lymph node dissection
RPR
rapid plasma reagin
R protein
R-ras oncogene
RRE
REV response element
RRTM
retroperitoneal residual tumor mass
RS
radiosurgery
LINAC RS
R-S
Reed-Sternberg
rsCD4
recombinant soluble CD4
RSD
rad surface dose
RSDP
random single-donor platelets
RSH
reduced sulfhydryl
RSH group
RSNA
Radiological Society of North America
RSV
respiratory syncytial virus
Rous sarcoma virus
RSV-specific monoclonal antibody
RT
radiation therapy
radiotherapy
reverse transcriptase
RTAS
radiology telephone access system
RT-DNA-Fab complex
RTI
reverse transcriptase inhibitor
RTK
receptor tyrosine kinase
RTOG
Radiation Therapy Oncology Group
RTP
radiation treatment planning
3D RTP
RT-PCR
reverse transcriptase-polymerase chain
reaction
bcr/abl multiplex RT-PCR
RTRT
real-time tumor tracking radiation therapy

RTS
radiation therapy system
GliaSite RTS
MammoSite RTS
⁸²Ru
rubidium-82
rub
pericardial r.
Rubacell II culture
rubber
silicone r.
rubella virus
rubeosis iridis
Rubex
**rubidazone, Oncovin, ara-C, prednisone
(ROAP)**
rubidium-82 (⁸²Ru)
Rubinstein-Taybi syndrome
rubitecan
Rubramin
Rubramin-PC
rubriblast
rubricyte
rubrum
Trichophyton r.
RUDT
respiratory and upper digestive tract
ruffle
rufocromomycin
RUG
retrograde urethrography
rule
Fletcher r.
Lossen r.
modified Simpson r.
Weigert-Meyer r.
ruler
endocatheter r.
Rum-K
Rumpel-Leede
R.-L. phenomenon
R.-L. sign
R.-L. test
Rundles-Falls anemia
Runeberg anemia
runt disease
rupture
aortic r.
diaphragmatic r.
esophageal r.
intrasurgical r.
traumatic r.
ruptured capsule
Russell
R. classification
R. classification system
R. classification system for soft
tissue sarcoma

R.'s viper venom (RVV)
R.'s viper venom clotting time
Rust sign
ruthenium plaque radiotherapy
Rutledge
R. classification
R. classification of extended
hysterectomy
Rutner
R. biopsy needle
R. cannula
R. nephroscopy adapter

R-verapamil
RVG
radionuclide ventriculogram
RVV
Russell's viper venom
RXRE
Rex-responsive element
Rye classification
Rynacrom

R

NOTES

S

S phase
S subphase

S5

monoclonal antibody S5

SA

sarcoma

SAA

severe aplastic anemia

SAAND

selective apoptotic antineoplastic drug

SAB

sequential androgen blockade

Sabin vaccine
Sabouraud plate
sac

alveolar s.
endolymphatic s.
thecal s.

Saccharomyces cerevisiae
Saccomanno solution
Sacks catheter
Sacks-Malecot catheter
sacra (*pl. of* sacrum)
sacral

s. bone tumor
s. chordoma

sacrococcygeal

s. myxopapillary ependymoma
s. teratoma
s. tumor

sacrum, pl. sacra

chordoma of s.

saddle

s. block anesthesia
s. nose
s. prosthesis

S-adenosylhomocysteine (AdoHcy)

S-a. hydrolase (AdoHcyase)

S-adenosylmethionine
Saethre-Chotzen acrocephalosyndactyly
SafeCrit microhematocrit tube
safingol
sagittal thrombosis
sagrada

cascara s.

Sahli method
saimiri

Herpesvirus s.

Salagen
Salem sump tube
Salflex
salicylate

choline s.
magnesium s.

sodium s.
triethanolamine s.

salicylic acid
saline

s. cathartic
D5 half normal s.
Dulbecco phosphate-buffered s.
hypertonic s.
phosphate-buffered s. (PBS)
Tris-buffered s.

saline-enhanced radiofrequency ablation
saline-filled testicular prosthesis
Salivart
salivary

s. cotinine
s. fistula
s. gland
s. gland cancer
s. gland carcinoma
s. gland dysfunction
s. gland enlargement
s. gland infection
s. gland KS
s. gland lymphoepithelioma
s. gland pleomorphic adenoma
s. gland tumor

saliva substitute
S-allyl-L-cysteine
Salmon-Durie staging function
Salmonella

S. enteritidis
S. meningitis
S. septicemia
S. typhi
S. typhimurium

Salmonella-vectored HIV
salmonellosis
salmon patch
salpingo-oophorectomy

bilateral s.-o. (BSO)
total abdominal hysterectomy and
bilateral s.-o. (TAHBSO)

salsalate
salt

s. free (SF)
mesylate s.

Saltz

S. protocol
S. regimen

Saluron
salvage

autologous red cell s.
s. chemotherapy
limb s.
s. neck dissection

S

salvage *(continued)*
  s. radiotherapy
  s. regimen
  s. surgery
  s. therapy
  s. total laryngectomy
  s. treatment
  s. workup
salve
  cancer s.
Salzman test
SAM
  streptozocin, Adriamycin, methyl-CCNU
samarium-153 EDTMP injection
sample
  blood s.
  decalcified bone marrow s.
  fingerstick blood s.
  standard s.
sampler
  Accellon s.
  Digene Cervical S.
  Endopap endometrial s.
sampling
  asymmetric data s.
  blood s.
  chorionic villus s. (CVS)
  data s.
  fetal tissue s.
  nodal s.
  nonlinear s.
  paraaortic node s.
  percutaneous fetal tissue s.
  percutaneous umbilical blood s.
    (PUBS)
  peritoneal s.
  portal venous s. (PVS)
  tissue s.
  umbilical blood s.
Samsung
  S. Medical Center (SMC)
  S. Medical Center-type collimator
    cone
Sanctis-Cacchione syndrome
sanctuary site
sand
  hydatid s.
  s. tumor
sandbag
Sandimmune Neoral
Sandoglobulin
Sandostatin (SSTN)
  S. LAR
sandwich chemotherapy
Sanfilippo syndrome
Sanger method
sanguinaria
sanguineous
Sani-Supp Suppository

Santyl ointment
SaO$_2$
  arterial oxygen saturation
SAPK
  stress-activated protein kinase
saponin
Sappey line
sapphire-tip probe
sapremia
saquinavir
  s. hard-gel capsule
  s. mesylate
  s. soft-gel capsule
saquinavir-related toxicity
SAR
  scatter-air ratio
  specific absorption rate
  survival after recurrence
Sarasar
SarCNU
  sarcosinamide chloroethylnitrosourea
sarcocarcinoma
sarcocystosis
sarcoid
  Boeck s.
  s. granuloma
sarcoidosis
  acinar s.
  alveolar s.
  orbital s.
  Schaumann s.
sarcolectin
L-sarcolysin
sarcoma, pl. **sarcomata (SA)**
  Abernethy s.
  adipose s.
  African Kaposi s.
  AIDS-related Kaposi s. (AIDS-KS)
  alveolar soft part s. (ASPS)
  ameloblastic s.
  anaplastic s.
  angiolithic s.
  anti-Kaposi s.
  Askin s.
  bone s.
  botryoid s.
  s. botryoides
  cerebral reticulum cell s.
  cervical s.
  chloromatous s.
  chondroblastic s.
  chordoid s.
  circumscribed cerebellar
    arachnoid s.
  classical Kaposi s. (CKS)
  clear cell s. (CCS)
  deciduocellular s.
  dendritic s.
  embryonal s.

endometrial stromal s. (ESS)
epithelioid s.
Ewing s.
extraosseous Ewing s.
fascial s.
fascicular s.
fibroblastic s.
fibromyxoid s.
follicular dendritic s.
gastrointestinal s.
giant cell s.
glandular s.
granulocytic s.
hemangioendothelial s.
hepatic anaplastic s.
histiocytic s.
Hodgkin s.
idiopathic multiple pigmented
  hemorrhagic s.
immunoblastic s.
interdigitating dendritic cell s.
intracanalicular s.
irradiation-produced s.
Jensen s.
juxtacortical s.
Kaposi s. (KS)
Kupffer cell s.
leukocytic s.
low-grade fibromyxoid s.
lymphangioendothelial s.
lymphatic s.
mast cell s.
Mediterranean Kaposi s. (MEKS)
medullary s.
melanotic s.
meningeal s.
mesodermal s.
s. metastasis
mixed cell s.
mixed müllerian s.
mixed ovarian mesodermal s.
monocytic s.
müllerian s.
multiple idiopathic hemorrhagic s.
murine s.
muscle s.
myelogenic s.
myeloid s.
neurogenic s.
nonrhabdomyosarcoma soft tissue s.
osseous s.
osteoblastic s.
osteogenic s.

osteoid s.
osteolytic s.
ovarian mesodermal s.
parosteal s.
periosteal s.
s. of peripheral nerve
polymorphous s.
postirradiation s.
pseudo-Kaposi s.
pulmonary artery s.
radiation-induced s.
radioinduced s.
reticulum cell s.
retroperitoneal reticulum cell s.
round cell s.
Rous s.
Russell classification system for
  soft tissue s.
sclerotic osteogenic s.
serocystic s.
soft tissue s. (STS)
spinal synovial s.
spindle cell s.
Sternberg s.
subcutaneous murine s.
synovial s.
telangiectatic osteogenic s.
tendosynovial s.
s. of testis
T-immunoblastic s.
undifferentiated s.
uterine mixed müllerian s.
vascular s.
sarcomagenic
sarcomatoid
  s. malignant mesothelioma
  s. renal cell cancer
  s. squamous cell carcinoma
sarcomatosis
  diffuse s.
  osteogenic s.
  plasmacytic s.
  sclerosing osteogenic s.
sarcomatosum
  lipoma s.
  myxoma s.
sarcomatous degeneration
Sarcoptes scabiei
sarcosinamide chloroethylnitrosourea
  (SarCNU)
sargramostim
Sarisol invasion
Sartorius breast pump

NOTES

495

Sassone score
satellite
    s. focus
    s. focus of melanoma
    s. lesion
satiety
    early s.
satisfaction
    life s.
satraplatin
satumomab pentetide
saturated solution of potassium iodide
    (SSKI)
saturation
    arterial oxygen s. (SaO$_2$)
    s. pulse
    transferrin s.
sausage segment effect
Sauvage filamentous velour graft
Savary dilator
Savary-Gilliard dilator
saved
    quality-adjusted life-year s.
    (QUALYS)
saver
    Haemonetics Cell S.
saw
    Gigli s.
SBA
    soybean agglutinin
SBB
    Sudan Black B
    SBB stain
SBC
    skull base chordoma
SBE
    self-breast examination
S100-beta protein
SBR
    Scarf-Bloom-Richardson
SC
    sickle cell
^{47}Sc
    scandium-47
SC-68420 dual receptor agonist
SCA
    sickle cell anemia
SCAB
    streptozocin, CCNU, Adriamycin,
    bleomycin
scabicide
scabiei
    Sarcoptes s.
scabies
    Norwegian s.
scale
    Adolescent and Pediatric Pain
    Tool S.
    Affect Balance S. (ABS)

    Bauermeister s.
    Beck Hopelessness S. (BHS)
    Bethesda rating s.
    CES-D S.
    Delirium Rating S. (DRS)
    Digit Span of Wechsler Adult
    Intelligence S.
    Edmonton Symptom Assessment S.
    (ESAS)
    Flint Colon Injury S.
    gray s.
    HIV visual analog s.
    Hospital Anxiety and Depression S.
    (HADS)
    Hospital for Sick Children pain s.
    House-Brackmann grading s.
    human immunodeficiency virus
    assessment s.
    human immunodeficiency virus
    visual analog s.
    Illness Intrusiveness Rating S.
    (IIRS)
    Levi s.
    Lung Cancer Symptom S.
    Mattis Dementia Rating S.
    Memorial Delirium Assessment S.
    (MDAS)
    Memorial Symptom Assessment S.
    (MSAS)
    Memorial Symptom Assessment S.-
    Psychological (MSAS-Psych)
    Miller Behavioral Style S.
    NARS rating s.
    neuropsychiatric-acquired
    immunodeficiency syndrome
    rating s.
    Oral Mucositis Assessment S.
    QOL s.
    SOMA s.
    Total Mood Disturbance S.
    Tursky pain adjective s.
    verbal-numerical s.
    Wechsler Memory S.
    Zubrod Performance S.
    Zung Anxiety S.
scalene node biopsy
scalloped appearance
scalloping
    anterior s.
    endosteal s.
scalocephaly
    Hendel correction of s.
scalp
    pilar tumor of s.
    s. tourniquet
    s. vein needle
scan
    bone s.
    computed tomography s.

dual-phase CT s.
dynamic bone s.
^{67}Ga s.
gadolinium s.
gallium s.
head computed axial
  tomographic s.
high-resolution CT s.
HRCT s.
iodocholesterol s.
lipiodol CT s.
methydiphosphonate bone s.
MET PET s.
MIBG bone s.
MUGA s.
multiple gated acquisition s.
octreotide s.
OncoScint s.
postgadolinium s.
proton-density axial MR s.
quantitative bone s.
radioiodinated metaiodobenzyl
  guanidine s.
radionuclide bone s.
radionuclide cutaneous s.
sestamibi s.
T2-weighted s.
ZeroRad MRI s.
Scandatronix MLC system
scandium-47 (^{47}Sc)
scannable tumor
scanner
  Aloka 650 ultrasound s.
  digital slide s.
  GE Quest 300-H s.
  GF-UM3 s.
  megavoltage computed
    tomography s.
  megavoltage CT s.
  Philips Tomoscan SR 6000 CT s.
  Siemens Impact Expert MRI s.
  Siemens Impact Expert Tesla s.
  Signa superconducting magnetic
    resonance imaging s.
  Somatom Plus-S CT S.
scanning
  body s.
  Ceretec technetium-99m
    exametazime agent white blood
    cell s.
  confocal laser s.
  diffusion-weighted s.
  electrical impedance s. (EIS)

electrical impedance breast s.
external s.
laser s.
radionuclide s.
spot s.
surveillance MRI s.
scapula, pl. **scapulae**
  flaring s.
scapular
  dorsal s.
scapularis
  Ixodes s.
scar
  s. cancer
  s. carcinoma
  collagenous s.
  radial s.
  seeding of laparotomy s.
  s. tissue
Scarf-Bloom-Richardson (SBR)
  S.-B.-R. grade
  S.-B.-R. score
scarification of BCG
SCAT
  sheep cell agglutination test
  sickle cell anemia test
  SCAT test
scatter
  s. contribution
  s. dose
  s. factor
scatter-air ratio (SAR)
scattering
  coherent s.
  s. foil
  Thomson s.
scatter-maximum ratio (SMR)
scavenger cell
scavenging system
SCC
  squamous cell carcinoma
    SCC RIABEAD radioimmunoassay
      kit
    SCC tumor marker
SCC-Ag
  squamous cell carcinoma antigen
SCCHN
  squamous cell carcinoma of head and
    neck
SCCOT
  squamous cell carcinoma of oral tongue
sCD4
  soluble recombinant human CD4

NOTES

scedosporiosis
Scedosporium apiospermum
SCF
    stem cell factor
SCFA
    short-chain fatty acid
scFv
    single-chain variable fragment
SCGE
    single-cell gel electrophoresis
    SCGE assay
Schaedler blood agar
Scharff-Bloom-Richardson grading
Schaumann
    S. body
    S. disease
    S. lymphogranuloma
    S. sarcoidosis
schedule
    s. dependency
    s. dependency concept
    dose-fraction s.
    fractionation s.
schedule-dependent pulsed paclitaxel radiosensitization
Scheffe F test
Scheie syndrome
scheme
    Kauffmann-White s.
schenckii
    Sporothrix s.
Schiff
    S. base
    S. base adduct
    S. reagent
    S. stain
Schiller-Duval body
Schiller test
Schilling
    S. test
    S. type
    S. type of monocytic leukemia
Schistosoma mansoni
schistosomiasis
    hepatic s.
    urinary s.
schizocyte
schizogonic cycle
schizogony
Schizosaccharomyces pombe
schneiderian carcinoma
Schneider infusion wire
Schridde cancer hair
SC-HSV test kit
Schuco nebulizer
Schüffner dot
Schüller
    S. disease
    S. syndrome

Schüller-Christian
    S.-C. disease
    S.-C. syndrome
Schumm test
Schwann
    S. cell
    S. cell tumor
schwannian
    s. lineage
    s. spindle cell stroma
schwannoma
    acoustic s.
    bilateral vestibular s.'s
    geniculate ganglion s.
    intraaxial s.
    intracerebral s.
    malignant s.
    plexiform s.
    psammomatous s.
    vestibular s.
Schwarten Microglide LP balloon
SCID
    severe combined immunodeficiency
    severe combined immunodeficiency disease
    autosomal-recessive SCID
    Swiss-type SCID
    X-linked SCID
science
    Applied Immune S.'s (AIS)
scintigraphic evidence
scintigraphy
    adrenal s.
    bone marrow s.
    brain s.
    metaiodobenzylguanidine s.
    radionuclide s.
    red blood cell s.
    somatostatin receptor s. (SRS)
    ^{99m}Tc-DMSA s.
scintillation
scintimammography (SMM)
    ^{99m}Tc MIBI s.
    technetium-99m sestamibi s.
scirrhoid
scirrhoma
scirrhophthalmia
scirrhous
    s. adenocarcinoma
    s. carcinoma
    s. reaction
scirrhus
scission
    double-strand s.
    single-strand s.
SCLC
    small cell lung cancer
scleral ectasia

scleroderma
diffuse s.
sclerodermoid graft-versus-host disease
scleroma R
scleromyxedema R
sclerosing
s. basal cell carcinoma
s. cholangitis
s. encapsulating peritonitis (SEP)
s. osteogenic sarcomatosis
s. Sertoli cell tumor
s. stromal tumor (SST)
sclerosis
bone s.
diffuse s.
endplate s.
Mönckeberg s.
multiple s. (MS)
nodular s.
percutaneous transhepatic s.
transhepatic s.
tuberous s. (TS)
sclerostenosis R
sclerotherapy
variceal s.
sclerotic osteogenic sarcoma
sclerouvectomy
partial lamellar s.
SCLND
selective complete lymph node dissection
SCNB
stereotactically guided core needle biopsy
scopolamine
scorbutic anemia
score
Child-Pugh s.
functional independent
measurement s.
Gleason s.
International Prognostic Index s.
Johnsen s.
Lansky s.
Lung Cancer Symptom S. (LCSS)
McGill-Melzack pain s.
s. method
prognostic s. (PS)
Sassone s.
Scarf-Bloom-Richardson s.
TANIS s.
T and N integer s. (TANIS)
z s.
scoring
AMES s.

Scott syndrome
scrape cytology
screen
2-hybrid yeast s.
leukemia s.
lymphoma s.
molecular target-based s.
multicopy suppressor s.
syphilis s.
screener
AutoPap 300 QC automatic Pap s.
screening
cancer s.
cervical cancer s.
colorectal cancer s.
cytologic s.
s. flexible sigmoidoscopy
fluid s.
genetic s.
high-throughput s. (HTS)
HIV s.
lung cancer s.
s. mammography
PapSure cervical s.
single-use diagnostic system for HIV s.
s. test
urine mutagenicity s.
Scribner shunt
Scrimp technique
scrofulaceum
Mycobacterium s.
scrotal
s. abscess
s. histiocytoma
scrotum, pl. scrota, scrotums
SCT
Sertoli cell tumor
stem cell transplant
stem cell transplantation
Scully tumor
scurvy
SCWT
Stroop Color Word Test
SD
seborrheic dermatitis
single dose
AlphaNine SD
SD Plasma for elimination of risk with transfusion
Profilnine SD
S/D
solvent/detergent treated

NOTES

S/D *(continued)*
    Gammagard S/D
    Polygam S/D
SDAP
    single-donor apheresis platelets
SD-CT
    standard-dose chemotherapy
SDF
    WinRho SDF
^{75}Se
    selenium-75
sea algae extract
sea-blue
    s.-b. histiocyte
    s.-b. histiocytosis
seal
    IVA s.
sealant
    FloSeal matrix hemostatic s.
    FocalSeal-L surgical s.
sea protooncogene/oncogene
Seattle
    hemoglobin S.
sebaceous
    s. adenoma
    s. carcinoma
    s. gland
    s. gland hyperplasia
    s. lymphadenoma
    s. nevus
sebaceum
    adenoma s.
sebaceus
    nevus s.
SEBI
    stereotactic external beam irradiation
seborrhea
seborrheic dermatitis (SD)
sebum
secobarbital-hydroxyzine
second
    s. malignant neoplasm (SMN)
    s. primary cancer (SPC)
    s. primary tumor (SPT)
secondary
    s. amyloidosis
    s. axillary adenopathy
    s. axillary lymphadenopathy
    s. cancer
    s. carcinoma
    s. CD30+ anaplastic large cell lymphoma
    s. hypogammaglobulinemia
    s. immune response
    s. immunodeficiency
    s. infertility
    s. malignancy
    s. malignant giant cell tumor (SMGCT)

    s. myelodysplasia
    s. myeloid metaplasia
    s. radiation
    s. skin thickening
    s. syphilis
    s. TEP
    s. viremia
second-echelon lymph node
secondhand smoke
second-line
    s.-l. chemotherapy
    s.-l. therapy
    s.-l. treatment
second-look operation
Secran
secreted
    aminooxypentane regulated-on-activation normal T-expressed and s. (AOP-RANTES)
    s. motility-stimulating factor assay
    s. protein acidic and rich in cysteine (SPARC)
    s. protein, acidic and rich in cysteine
    s. protein acidic and rich in cysteine protein
    regulated upon activation, normal T-cell expressed and s. (RANTES)
secretin
    intraarterial s. (IAS)
    s. provocation
secretion
    adrenocortical s.
    cytokine s.
    inappropriate s.
    sinonasal s.
secretory
    s. adenocarcinoma
    s. carcinoma
    s. component
    s. diarrhea
    s. disease
    s. IgA
    s. immunoglobulin
    s. leukocyte protease inhibitor (SLPI)
    s. meningioma
section
    axial s.
    fresh-frozen tissue s.
    frozen tissue s.
    paraffin tissue s.
    plastic s.
    tissue s.
sedimentation rate
seed
    BrachySeed brachytherapy s.
    BrachySeed palladium-103 s.

EchoSeed brachytherapy s.
s. implant
s. implantation
iodine-125 brachytherapy s.
I-12t radioactive s.
PdGold brachytherapy s.
PharmaSeed iodine-125 s.
PharmaSeed palladium-103 s.
ProstaSeed I-125 s.
radiation s.
radioactive iodine-125 s.
s. ribbon
Symmetra ^{125}I brachytherapy s.
seeding
s. of biopsy tract
s. of laparotomy scar
microscopic s.
peritoneal s.
stomal s.
subarachnoid s.
subependymal s.
tumor s.
SeedNet Gold cryotherapy system
SEER
Surveillance Epidemiology and End
Results
SEGA
subependymal giant cell astrocytoma
segment
aganglionic s.
atretic s.
bronchopulmonary s.
compensator s.
hepatic s.
joining s.
pseudogene s.
s. substitution
segmental
s. hypertrophy
s. mastectomy
s. multileaf collimator
s. neurofibromatosis
segmentectomy
segmented leukocyte
Selax
SELDI
surface-enhanced laser desorption and
ionization
SELDI-MS
surface-enhanced laser desorption and
ionization mass spectrometry
Seldinger method

SELDI-TOF
surface-enhanced laser desorption and
ionization time-of-flight
SELDI-TOF analysis
SELDI-TOF-MS
surface-enhanced laser desorption and
ionization time-of-flight mass
spectrometry
SELECT
Selenium and Vitamin E Cancer
Prevention Trial
selection
clonal s.
delay time s.
site s.
selective
s. apoptotic antineoplastic drug
(SAAND)
s. complete lymph node dissection
(SCLND)
s. estrogen receptor modulator
(SERM)
s. immunoglobulin A deficiency
s. serotonin reuptake inhibitor
(SSRI)
s. serotonin reuptake inhibitor
antidepressant
Selectron system
selegiline
selenium-75 (^{75}Se)
**Selenium and Vitamin E Cancer
Prevention Trial (SELECT)**
selenomethionine
Sele-Pak
Selepen
self-assessment
linear analog s.-a. (LASA)
self-breast examination (SBE)
self-care
s.-c. concept
s.-c. deficit
self-esteem
self-examination
breast s.-e. (BSE)
genital s.-e. (GSE)
skin s.-e. (SSE)
testicular s.-e.
self-expandable
s.-e. intravascular stent
s.-e. metallic stent
self-expanding
s.-e. endovascular prosthesis

NOTES

self-expanding *(continued)*
    s.-e. metallic biliary stent
    s.-e. stainless steel stent
self-help group
self-molecule
self-renewal
self-testing
    ProTime microcoagulation system
    used for patient s.-t.
sella, pl. **sellae**
    diaphragma sellae
    s. turcica
Selrodo nebulizer
semiconductor
    complementary metal oxide s.
    (CMOS)
semiinvasive aspergillosis
seminal vesicle invasion (SVI)
seminated fungal opportunist
seminoma
    extragonadal s. (EGS)
    mediastinal s.
    pure anaplastic s.
    spermatocytic s.
    testicular s.
seminomatous tumor
semiovale
    cerebrum s.
semirigid dilator
semisynthetic
    s. anthracycline
    s. duocarmycin antibiotic
    s. taxane
semiupright position
Semliki Forest virus
semustine (MeCCNU)
senescence
    replicative s.
senile atrophic vaginitis
senna
Senna-Gen
Senographe
    S. 2000D
    S. 2000D mammography system
    S. DS mammography system
Senokot
SenoScan mammography system
SENSA
    Hemoccult II SENSA
Sensability breast self-examination aid
Sensamide
Sensi-Care
    S.-C. skin care product
    S.-C. synthetic powder-free surgical
    gloves
sensitive
    isoniazid s.
    platinum s.

sensitivity
    culture and s.
sensitization
    HLA s.
    protracted exposure s.
sensitizer
    Gd-Tex radiation s.
    hypoxic cell s.
    radiation s.
sensitometric curve
sensor
    BreastAlert differential
    temperature s.
    differential temperature s.
Sensorcaine
sensorimotor peripheral neuropathy
**SensorMedics 2200 Pulmonary Function
Test System**
sensory
    s. neuronopathy
    s. neuropathy
sentinel
    S. II
    s. clot
    s. lymphadenectomy
    s. lymph node (SLN)
    s. lymph node biopsy (SLNB)
    s. lymph node mapping and
    biopsy
    s. node biopsy
    s. node dissection
    s. node mapping
SEP
    sclerosing encapsulating peritonitis
    somatosensory evoked potential
separation
    acromioclavicular joint s.
    s. phase inhibitor
separator
    Amicus blood collection s.
Sephadex
    S. bead
    S. G-25 column
sepsis
    biliary s.
    clostridial s.
    line s.
    postoperative s.
septa (*pl. of* septum)
septal hypertrophy
Septata intestinalis
septic
    s. arthritis
    s. shock
septicemia
    bacterial s.
    recurrent *Salmonella* s.
    Salmonella s.

septicum
Clostridium *s.*
Septi-Soft skin care cleanser
septostomy
atrial s.
balloon atrial s.
Septra DS
septum, pl. **septa**
atrial s.
sequela, pl. **sequelae**
pulmonary sequelae
Sequels
Diamox S.
sequence
amino acid s.
aspargine-glycine-arginine s.
chemokine with CC s.
diffusion-sensitive s.
double inversion recovery s.
endoplasmic reticulum insertion
signal s.
fast spin-echo pulse s.
FLAIR pulse s.
gene s.
genomic s.
gradient echo s.
heptamer/nonamer s.
Japanese V3 loop s.
protease s.
pulse s.
signature s.
spatially adjacent s.
spin-echo pulse s.
trans-acting responsive s.
sequencer
automated laser-fluorescence s.
sequence-specific anti-HIV activity
sequencing
DNA s.
dye primer-based dideoxy s.
dye terminator-based dideoxy s.
full-length genome s.
gene s.
kinetic-based s.
sequential
s. androgen blockade (SAB)
s. high-dose methotrexate followed
by 5-FU in combination with
Adriamycin (FAMTX)
s. hormone therapy
s. paired opposed plaque (SPOP)
s. postremission chemotherapy

s. tomotherapy
s. transplant
sequestration
bronchopulmonary s.
disc s.
extralobar s.
extrapulmonary s.
splenic s.
sequestrum, pl. **sequestra**
button s.
SER
suppressive E-receptor
sera (*pl. of* serum)
Serax
SEREX
serological analysis of recombinant
cDNA expression
serial tomotherapy
series
small bowel s.
serine
serine-threonine
s.-t. kinase
s.-t. phosphatase
serious disease
SERM
selective estrogen receptor modulator
SERM III
seroconcordant partner
seroconversion syndrome
serocystic sarcoma
serodiagnosis
serodiscordant partner
seroincidence
higher s.
seroincident woman
serological
s. analysis of recombinant cDNA
expression (SEREX)
s. analysis of recombinant cDNA
expression library
serologic test
serology
seroma
postoperative s.
seromyectomy
duodenal s.
seronegative
HIV s.
s. individual
seropositive
HIV s.

NOTES

S

seropositivity
   HIV s.
seroprevalence
   sex-standardized s.
seroreversion (SR)
serostatus
Serostim
Sero-Strip HIV test
serotonergic blockade
serotonergic-induced emetic response
serotonin
   s. antagonist
   s. flush
   s. receptor
serotonin-producing tumor
serotype
serous
   s. adenocarcinoma
   s. borderline tumor
   s. carcinoma
   s. cystadenocarcinoma
   s. cystadenoma
   s. effusion
   s. ovarian tumor
serpiginosum
   angioma s.
serpin
Serratia marcescens **extract**
serratus anterior muscle
Sertoli
   S. cell
   S. cell-only tumor
   S. cell tumor (SCT)
   S. syncytium
Sertoli-Leydig cell tumor
Sertoli-stromal cell tumor
sertraline
serum, pl. **sera**
   aged s.
   anticrotalus s.
   antilymphocyte s. (ALS)
   s. bilirubin concentration
   s. CA125
   s. carboxyterminal telopeptide
   testing
   s. chemistry
   s. creatinine
   s. creatinine phosphokinase level
   S. CrossLaps
   s. cryoglobulin
   despeciated s.
   s. erythropoietin
   s. factor (SF)
   s. ferritin
   s. folic acid assay
   s. glutamic-oxaloacetic transaminase
   (SGOT)
   s. glutamic-pyruvate transaminase
   (SGPT)

   s. hepatitis (SH)
   s. hepatitis antigen
   immune s.
   s. immunoglobulin
   s. iron
   s. methylmalonic acid
   s. neopterin level
   s. p24 antigen concentration
   s. parathyroid hormone
   s. phenytoin level
   s. protein electrophoresis
   s. prothrombin conversion
   accelerator
   s. sickness syndrome
   s. soluble receptor
   s. syndecan-1 test
   s. Tg
   s. thymidine kinase
   s. thyroglobulin
   s. tissue polypeptide antigen (S-TPA)
   s. transferrin receptor concentration
   s. tumor marker
   Yersin s.
serumal
serum-ascites albumin gradient
serum-binding protein
serum-induced platelet procoagulant
   activity assay
service
   bereavement s.'s
   emotional support s.'s
Serzone
SES
   socioeconomic status
session
   simulation s.
sestamibi
   s. scan
   technetium-99m s. (^{99m}Tc MIBI)
set
   Amplatz dilator s.
   LifePort infusion s.
   Myelo-Nate s.
   Ring transjugular intrahepatic
   access s.
   van Sonnenberg modified coaxial
   biopsy s.
sevelamer
severe
   s. agitation
   s. aplastic anemia (SAA)
   s. combined immunodeficiency
   (SCID)
   s. combined immunodeficiency
   disease (SCID)
   s. congenital neutropenia
   s. ulcerative lesion
Sevier-Munger technique

sex
anal s.
s. cord stromal tumor
s. drive
s. hormone
s. hormone-binding globulin
(SHBG)
s. steroid
sex-linked
s.-l. gene
s.-l. hypogammaglobulinemia
s.-l. lymphoproliferative syndrome
sex-standardized seroprevalence
sextant biopsy
sexual
s. activity
s. arousal
s. dysfunction
s. function
s. problem
S. Self-Schema Scale-Male Version
(SSSS-M)
Sézary
S. lymphoma cell
S. syndrome (SS)
SF
salt free
serum factor
Kaochlor SF
SGC
sweat gland carcinoma
sGC
soluble guanylate cyclase
SGO
Society of Gynecologic Oncology
SGOT
serum glutamic-oxaloacetic transaminase
SGPT
serum glutamic-pyruvate transaminase
SH
serum hepatitis
shadow
acoustic s.
s. cell
hilar s.
shadowing
acoustical s.
s. of block
shaggy appearance
shaker
shaped mediastinal field
shaper
beam s.

shark
s. cartilage
s. powder
sharp penumbra
shave
s. biopsy
lip s.
SHBG
sex hormone-binding globulin
Shc
adopter molecule Shc
ShearBan orthotic material
sheath
arterial s.
axillary s.
bicipital tendon s.
giant cell tumor of tendon s.
intercostal nerve s.
periarteriolar lymphoid s.
Teflon s.
working s.
sheathed needle
shedding
tumor s.
sheep
s. cell agglutination test (SCAT)
s. erythrocyte rosette
s. sorrel
sheet
RadiaDres Gel S.
shelf, pl. shelves
Blumer s.
rectal s.
SHFM
split hand/split foot malformation
SHFM syndrome
shiatsu massage
shield
passive s.
shielding
s. of abdomen and pelvis
s. block
lung s.
passive s.
surface s.
shift
antigenic s.
chloride s.
colloid s.
distal s.
fluorescent s.
shigellosis

NOTES

505

Shimada
> S. system
> S. system of classification

shingles
Shirner test
shock
> fungemic s.
> septic s.

Shohl solution
Shope
> S. fibroma
> S. fibroma virus
> S. papillomavirus

short
> s. arm of chromosome (p)
> s. maxilla
> s. tau inversion recovery (STIR)

short-chain fatty acid (SCFA)
short-term nonprogressor
Sho-saiko-to
shoulder
> drooped s.
> s. girdle

shrinkage
> tumor s.

shrinking field
shrinking-field technique
shunt
> aorticopulmonary window s.
> arteriovenous s.
> Denver s.
> distal splenorenal s.
> end-to-side portacaval s.
> hexose monophosphate s.
> s. infection
> LaVeen s.
> lymphatic s.
> lymphaticovenous s.
> partial s.
> peritoneovenous s.
> polytetrafluoroethylene s.
> portacaval s.
> portohepatic venous s.
> portosystemic s.
> Pott s.
> Scribner s.
> surgical portosystemic s.
> systemic s.
> transjugular intrahepatic
>   portosystemic s. (TIPS)
> Trueta s.
> s. tubing
> s. valve
> ventriculoperitoneal s.

shunting
> arterioportal venous s.
> peritoneovenous s.
> pleuroperitoneal s.

Shwachman-Diamond syndrome

Shwartzman reaction
Shy-Drager syndrome
(S)-1-(3-hydroxy-2-
phosphonomethoxypropyl)cytosine
SI
> fusin 29
> International System of Units
> syncytium-inducing
>   Molecular Dynamics Personal
>   Densitometer SI
> SI units

SIADH
> syndrome of inappropriate secretion of
>   antidiuretic hormone

sialadenitis, sialoadenitis
> acute suppurative s.
> autoimmune s.
> myoepithelial s.
> recurrent s.

sialic
> s. acid
> s. acid tumor marker

sialoglycoprotein
sialo-type pancreatic adenocarcinoma
sialyl Lewis antigen
sialyl-Tn antigen (STn)
sialyl-Tn-KLH vaccine
SIBC
> synchronous ipsilateral breast cancer

Siberian ginseng
sibling
> s. bone marrow transplant donor
> HLA-identical s.

sibpair linkage analysis
sicca
> keratoconjunctivitis s.
> s. symptom
> s. syndrome

sick euthyroid syndrome
sickle
> s. cell (SC)
> s. cell anemia (SCA)
> s. cell anemia test (SCAT)
> s. cell crisis
> s. cell disease
> s. cell trait
> s. solubility test

Sickledex reagent
sicklemia
sicklemic
sickle-Thal disease
sickling
sickness
> decompression s.
> radiation s.

side effect
sideroblast
> refractory anemia with ringed s.'s

ring of s.
ringed s.
sideroblastic anemia
siderosis bulbi
siderotica
granulomatosis s.
siderotic nodule
sidewinder catheter
Siegel
method of Bernie S.
Siemens
S. Impact Expert MRI scanner
S. Impact Expert Tesla scanner
sievert
sigmaS tumor marker
sigmoid curve
sigmoidoscope
flexible s.
rigid s.
sigmoidoscopy
flexible s.
screening flexible s.
sign
air-crescent s.
apical cap s.
appendicular s.
Babinski s.
beak s.
bladder-within-bladder s.
bronchus s.
cervix s.
Chaussier s.
Chvostek s.
colon cutoff s.
cotton-wool s.
Courvoisier s.
crescent s.
Darier s.
differential density s.
dimple s.
drooping lily s.
flag s.
goblet s.
Grey Turner s.
Higoumenakia s.
Hoover s.
intradecidual s.
Kussmaul s.
Leser-Trélat s.
Lhermitte s.
linguine s.
localizing s.
Mercedes-Benz s.

Mexican hat s.
Mosler s.
pathognomonic s.
pinch-off s.
Rumpel-Leede s.
Rust s.
signet ring s.
Troisier s.
Trousseau s.
Signa
S. Excite 3.0T MR system
S. Excite 1.5T system
S. OpenSpeed 0.7T MR system
S. Ovation 0.35T MR system
S. superconducting magnetic
resonance imaging scanner
signal
abnormal bright s.
antimitogenic s.
bright s.
s. change
costimulatory s.'s
dark s.
hyperintense s.
increased s.
s. intensity
periventricular bright s.
s. transducing molecule STAT 5
s. transduction
s. transduction disorder
s. transduction inhibitor (STI)
s. transduction pathway
s. void
signaling
ceramide cell s.
factor-dependent mitogenic s.
s. lymphocytic activation molecule
(SLAM)
SLAM s.
suppressor of cytokine s. (SOCS)
transmembrane s.
VEGF, FGF, and PDGF
receptor s.
signature
optical s.
s. sequence
s. tumor
signet
s. ring
s. ring cell
s. ring cell carcinoma
s. ring sign

NOTES

507

significance
    atypical cell of undetermined s.
    atypical glandular cell of
        unknown s. (AGCUS, AGUS)
    atypical squamous cells of
        undetermined s. (ASCUS)
    s. level
    monoclonal gammopathy of
        undetermined s. (MGUS)
significant
    hemodynamically s.
SIL
    squamous intraepithelial lesion
Silace-C
silastic
    s. double-J stent
    s. hemodialysis catheter
    s. microsphere
    s. sphere
    s. tube
sildenafil
silencing
    transcriptional s.
silent ductus
silicone
    s. diode dosimeter
    s. rubber
silicosis
    complicated s.
silk suture
silver (Ag)
    Gomori methenamine s.
    s. stain (IFA)
silver-coated catheter
silver-stained nucleolar organizer region
simethicone
    calcium carbonate and s.
    magaldrate and s.
simian
    s. foamy virus
    s. virus 40 (SV40)
Simmond disease
Simon septic factor
Simonton method
Simplastin L
Simplate method
simple
    s. achlorhydric anemia
    s. capillary lymphangioma
simplex
    carcinoma s.
    disseminated herpes s.
    herpes s. (HS)
    hydroacanthoma s.
    toxoplasmosis, other infections,
        rubella, cytomegalovirus infection,
        herpes s. (TORCH)

Simpson
    S. classification
    S. surgical grade
Simron
simtrazene
simulated annealing
simulation
    s. film
    MCPT s.
    Monte Carlo photon transport s.
    s. session
simulator
    AcQsim CT s.
    s. film
    Nucletron s.
    radiation s.
simultaneous thermoradiotherapy (STRT)
simvastatin
Sindbis virus
Sinding-Larsen-Johansson disease
sinensis
    Clonorchiasis s.
Sinequan Oral
single
    s. balloon method
    s. dose (SD)
single-agent high-dose chemotherapy
single-cell
    s.-c. gel electrophoresis (SCGE)
    s.-c. gel electrophoresis assay
single-chain
    s.-c. antigen-binding protein
    s.-c. variable fragment (scFv)
single-day infuser
single-donor
    s.-d. apheresis
    s.-d. apheresis platelets (SDAP)
    s.-d. blood component
single-field isodose distribution
single-fraction total body irradiation
single-photon
    s.-p. emission computed
        tomography (SPECT)
    s.-p. emission tomography (SPET)
single-point acquisition
single-stick method
single-strand
    s.-s. conformation polymorphism
        (SSCP)
    s.-s. conformation polymorphism
        analysis
    s.-s. scission
single-stranded conformational
  polymorphism (SSCP)
single-tube method
single-use
    s.-u. catheter
    s.-u. diagnostic system (SUDS)

s.-u. diagnostic system for HIV screening

sinonasal
s. adenocarcinoma (SNA)
s. carcinoma
s. carcinoma with neuroendocrine differentiation (SNCD)
s. cavity
s. lesion
s. lymphoma
s. secretion
s. teratocarcinosarcoma (SNTSC)
s. tract
s. tumor
s. undifferentiated carcinoma (SNUC)

sinovaginal bulb
sinus, pl. **sinus, sinuses**
branchial s.
bronchial s.
s. cancer
cavernous s.
coronary s.
dural venous s.
endodermal s.
ethmoid s.
maxillary s.
s. occlusion
paranasal s.
petrosal s.
piriform s.
s. rhythm
s. thrombosis
venous s.

sinusitis
bacterial s.

sinusoidal large cell lymphoma
SIOP
International Society of Pediatric Oncology

Sipple syndrome
SIR
standardized incidence ratio

sirolimus
SIR-Spheres microsphere
sis protooncogene/oncogene
sister
s. chromatid exchange
S. Mary Joseph node
S. Mary Joseph nodule

Sistrunk procedure
site
antibody reaction s.

ATP binding s.
binding s.
bleeding s.
carcinoma of uncertain primary s. (CUPS)
s. of disease
donor s.
extranodal s.
fracture s.
immunologically sequestered s.
lectin-binding s.
multiple noninguinal s.'s
N-linked glycosylated s.
NNI s.
nonnucleoside reverse transcriptase inhibitor binding s.
parenteral s.
primary s.
psi s.
sanctuary s.
s. selection
tumor s.
type II estrogen-binding s.
uncertain primary s.
unknown primary s.

site-directed mutant
SiteSelect percutaneous incisional breast biopsy system
site-specific
s.-s. metastasis
s.-s. surgery
s.-s. treatment

situ
adenocarcinoma in s. (AIS)
breast carcinoma in s. (BCIS)
carcinoma in s. (CIS)
cervical carcinoma in s.
ductal carcinoma in s. (DCIS)
in s.
lobular carcinoma in s. (LCIS)
malignant melanoma in s.
nasopharyngeal carcinoma in s. (NPCIS)
transitional carcinoma in s. (TCIS)
tumor in s. (TIS)

situs, pl. **situs**
s. ambiguus
atrial s.
s. indeterminatus
s. inversus viscerum
s. solitus

sitz marker

NOTES

size
>age, distant metastases, extent, s.
>(AMES)
>fraction s.

sizofiran

SJCRH
>St. Jude Children's Research Hospital
>SJCRH staging system

Sjögren syndrome

SK
>Sloan-Kettering
>streptokinase

Skatron apparatus

skeletal
>s. biopsy
>s. care product
>s. lymphoma
>s. metastasis
>s. muscle protein (SMP)
>s. myxoid chondrosarcoma (SMC)
>s. neoplasm
>s. survey
>s. system
>s. targeted radiotherapy (STR)

skeleton
>appendicular s.
>axial s.

Skelid

skin
>s. appendage
>s. biopsy
>s. cadherin
>s. cancer
>candidiasis of glabrous s.
>s. care
>s. care product
>CD30/KI-1 positive lymphoma
>of s.
>s. depth
>s. discoloration
>s. erythema dose
>s. flap
>glabrous s.
>granulomatous slack s.
>s. hook
>s. infection
>s. lesion
>s. lesion artifact
>lymphoepithelioma-like carcinoma
>of s.
>mixed tumor of s.
>s. neurofibroma
>onion s.
>s. problem
>s. self-examination (SSE)
>s. thickening
>s. tonometry

skinning vulvectomy

skinny needle

skin-sparing
>s.-s. effect
>s.-s. mastectomy (SSM)

skip
>s. area
>s. lesion
>s. metastasis

Skipper-Schabel model

ski protooncogene/oncogene

skull
>abnormally thin s.
>s. base
>s. base chordoma (SBC)
>s. base tumor

skullcap

skyline view

SKY pain control system

slack-skin syndrome

SLAM
>signaling lymphocytic activation
>molecule
>>SLAM costimulation
>>SLAM signaling

slash defect

SLE
>systemic lupus erythematosus
>drug-induced SLE

sleep apnea

sleeve
>anterior labroligamentous
>periosteal s.
>forefoot compression s.
>s. lobectomy

slide
>Fisher-plus s.
>poly-_L_-lysine s.

slide-based test

Slidemarker/Stainer (SMS)
>Cell-Dyn S./S.

Slim-Mint

sling
>pulmonary s.

slip
>diaphragmatic s.

SLN
>sentinel lymph node

SLNB
>sentinel lymph node biopsy

Sloan-Kettering (SK)

Slo-Niacin

slope
>PSA s.

Slo-Phyllin

slough

slow
>S. Fe
>s. hemoglobin
>s. low phase
>s. release (SR)

slowing
>pathologic psychomotor s.
>psychomotor s.

Slow-K
Slow-Mag
SLPI
>secretory leukocyte protease inhibitor

sludge
>tumefactive biliary s.

slurry
>Carafate s.
>talc s.

SLX   tumor marker
Sly syndrome
SM3 antibody
SMA
>smooth muscle actin
>spinal muscular atrophy
>superior mesenteric artery

small
>s. blue cell tumor
>s. bowel
>s. bowel cancer
>s. bowel enteroscopy
>s. bowel follow-through
>   examination
>s. bowel lesion
>s. bowel series
>s. bowel tumor
>s. cell
>s. cell lung cancer (SCLC)
>s. cell neuroendocrine carcinoma
>s. cell undifferentiated carcinoma
>s. cleaved cell lymphoma
>s. intestine
>s. intestine cancer
>s. lymphocyte
>s. lymphocytic lymphoma
>s. lymphoid cell proliferation
>s. molecular weight chemical
>s. noncleaved cell lymphoma
>s. round-cell tumor (SRCT)

smart
>s. laser
>s. laser catheter tip
>s. laser system

SMART M195 antibody
SMC
>Samsung Medical Center
>skeletal myxoid chondrosarcoma

SMC-type collimator cone
smear
>Bethesda rating scale for Pap s.'s

blood s.
buffy coat s.
cytospin s.
Papanicolaou s.
red blood cell s.
Tzanck s.
vaginal cuff s. (VCS)

smegma
SMF
>streptozocin, mitomycin, 5-fluorouracil

SMGCT
>secondary malignant giant cell tumor

Smith
>S. Malecot ureteral stent
>S. Universal ureteral stent

Smith-Petersen
>S.-P. nail
>S.-P. pin

SMM
>scintimammography

SMN
>second malignant neoplasm

smoke
>environmental tobacco s. (ETS)
>secondhand s.

smokeless
>s. tobacco
>s. tobacco keratosis

smoking
>s. cessation
>cigarette s.
>passive s.

smoldering
>s. leukemia
>s. multiple myeloma

S-Monovette blood collection system
smooth
>s. muscle
>s. muscle actin (SMA)
>s. muscle cell
>s. muscle neoplasm
>s. muscle tumor

SMP
>skeletal muscle protein

SMR
>scatter-maximum ratio

SMS
>Slidemarker/Stainer
>Cell-Dyn SMS

smudge cell
SMV
>superior mesenteric vein

NOTES

SNA
sinonasal adenocarcinoma
snare
angiographic 2-wire s.
Olympus SD-9L-1 s.
s. technique
SNCB
stereotactic needle core biopsy
SNCD
sinonasal carcinoma with neuroendocrine
differentiation
sNDA
Thalomid sNDA
Snell H locus
SNM
Society of Nuclear Medicine
SNOMED
Systemized Nomenclature of Medicine
SNTSC
sinonasal teratocarcinosarcoma
SNUC
sinonasal undifferentiated carcinoma
snuff
s. dipping
moist s.
snuffbox
anatomic s.
snuff-dippers' keratosis
soak
astringent s.
soap
calcium s.
social
s. environment
s. factor
s. functioning
s. support
society
American Cancer S. (ACS)
American Musculoskeletal Tumor S.
(MSTS)
American Thoracic S. (ATS)
Canadian Cancer S.
S. of Gynecologic Oncology (SGO)
S. for Hematopathology program
Massachusetts Medical S.
S. of Nuclear Medicine (SNM)
Oncology Nursing S. (ONS)
S. of Surgical Oncology (SSO)
socioeconomic status (SES)
SOCS
suppressor of cytokine signaling
SOD2
SOD2 Val/Val gene
SOD2 Val/Val genotype
sodium (Na)
s. acetate
acyclovir s.
alendronate s.

allopurinol s.
azathioprine s.
s. bicarbonate
brequinar s.
s. chloride
cromolyn s.
s. cyanoborohydride
dalteparin s.
divalproex s.
estramustine phosphate s.
fondaparinux s.
fostriecin s.
s. heparin
ibandronate s.
s. iodide
meclofenamate s.
s. metaperiodate
methotrexate s.
Methotrexate LPF S.
oblimersen s.
pentosan polysulfate s.
s. pentosan polysulfate
Pentothal S.
s. phenylacetate and sodium
benzoate
s. phosphate
piperacillin and tazobactam s.
PMS-Levothyroxine S.
s. polystyrene sulfonate
porfimer s.
s. salicylate
suramin s.
s. tetradecyl sulfate
s. thiopental
s. thiosulfate
warfarin s.
sodium-23 (^{23}Na)
sodium-24 (^{24}Na)
sodium-hydrogen exchanger inhibitor
sodium-2-mercaptoethanesulfonate
Soflax
soft
Modane S.
s. palate cancer
s. tissue
s. tissue chondroma
s. tissue HPC
s. tissue sarcoma (STS)
s. tissue tumor
softener
D-S-S stool s.
stool s.
Softgel
DC 240 S.
DOS S.
Vita-Plus E S.
SoftScan laser mammography system
software
AdvantageSim 6.0 simulation s.

BrachyVision 6.0 s.
XKnife s.
Sokal index
solanine
solanism
Solarcaine
solar keratosis
Solcotrans drainage/reinfusion system
sole laser therapy
solid
s. cell nest
s. organ transplant
s. pilocytic astrocytoma
trabecular insular s. (TIS)
s. tumor
S. Tumor Autologous Marrow
Transplant Program (STAMP)
s. tumor malignancy
solidifier
solitary
s. bone cyst
s. fibrous tumor
s. lesion
s. lymph node
s. myeloma
s. osteochondroma
s. osteochondroma B
s. plasmacytoma
s. plasmacytoma of bone (SPB)
s. rectal ulcer syndrome (SRUS)
s. relapse
s. splenic metastasis
solitus
situs s.
Soltamox
soluble
s. antigen
s. CD4
s. chemokine receptor
s. guanylate cyclase (sGC)
s. recombinant human CD4 (sCD4)
s. transferrin receptor (sTfR)
Solu-Cortef Injection
Solu-Medrol
S.-M. injection
methotrexate, bleomycin,
Adriamycin, cyclophosphamide,
Oncovin, S.-M. (M-BACOS)
Solurex L.A.
Soluspan
Celestone S.
solution
additive s. (AS)

aqueous s.
Bretschneider HTK s.
Chloresium s.
Dakin s.
Drabkin s.
Elliott's B s.
Euro Collins s.
Fonio s.
Hanks balanced salt s.
Hayem s.
Hemopure s.
hypertonic s.
iseganan HCl oral s.
lactated Ringer s.
Lugol s.
lymph node revealing s. (LNRS)
methotrexate LFP s.
methoxsalen sterile s.
Resectisol Irrigation S.
ribavirin inhaled s.
Saccomanno s.
Shohl s.
TOBI Inhalation S.
Uvadex methoxsalen sterile s.
Xylocaine viscous s.
Zenker s.
zinc sulfate s.
solvent/detergent treated (S/D)
SOMA
subjective, objective, management,
analytic
SOMA classification
SOMA scale
somatic
s. gene therapy
s. hypermutation
s. mutation
s. mutation frequency
s. mutation theory
s. mutation theory of cancer
s. pain
s. Tax-associated mutator phenotype
SomatoKine
Somatom Plus-S CT Scanner
somatosensory evoked potential (SEP)
somatostatin
s. analog
s. receptor scintigraphy (SRS)
s. subtype testing
somatostatinoma
somatotrophic adenoma
Somatuline

NOTES

513

SOMI
  sternooccipital-mandibular
    immobilization
    SOMI brace
Somogyi unit
sonographic planning of oncology
  treatment (SPOT)
sonography
  abdominal s.
  breast s.
  color-flow Doppler s.
  Doppler s.
  endoluminal s.
  endoscopic s.
  endovaginal s.
  transcranial s.
  transrectal s.
  transvesical s.
Sopalamine/3B Plus C
Sorafenib
Sorbex hydrocolloid wound dressing
sorbitol
Sorbitrate
sorrel
  sheep s.
sorter
  FACSVantage cell s.
  fluorescence-activated cell s.
sorting
  fluorescence-activated cell s.
    (FACS)
Sorvall Discovery SE ultracentrifuge
Sotradecol
sound
  bowel s.'s
  breath s.'s
source
  AngioRad ^{192}Ir wire s.
  dummy s.
  Heyman-Simon s.
  s. patient
  radiation s.
source-film distance
source-to-skin distance (SSD)
source-tray distance (STD)
Soutar flap
southern
  S. blot
  S. blot analysis
  S. blot hybridization
  S. blot technique
Southwest Oncology Group (SWOG)
soybean agglutinin (SBA)
soy phytoestrogen
space
  abdominal s.
  acromioclavicular s.
  anterior clear s.
  arachnoid s.

buccal s.
capillary lymphatic s. (CLS)
clear s.
disc s.
epidural s.
extradural s.
leptomeningeal s.
paraglottic s.
preepiglottic s.
subarachnoid s.
subretinal s.
space-occupying lesion
spacer
  telescopic plate s. (TPS)
spacing
  interscan s.
spade field
SPARC
  secreted protein acidic and rich in
    cysteine
    SPARC glycoprotein
    SPARC protein
sparfloxacin
sparfosic acid
Sparks mandrel graft
sparsomycin
spasm
  arterial s.
spastic
  s. colitis
  s. urinary bladder
spatially adjacent sequence
SPB
  solitary plasmacytoma of bone
SPC
  second primary cancer
Spearman
  S. rank correlation method
  S. rank correlation test
special
  Lasix S.
  s. probe
specialized metaplastic epithelium
species
  electrophilic s.
  paramagnetic iron s.
  therapeutic s.
specific
  s. *abl* tyrosine kinase inhibitor
  s. absorption rate (SAR)
  s. cytoplasmic granule
  s. esterase stain
  s. factor assay
  s. granule deficiency
  s. immunotherapy
  isolate s.
  s. reverse transcriptase-polymerase
    chain reaction marker

specified
    not otherwise s. (NOS)
specimen
    catheterized barbotage s.
    gross s.
    mammary aspiration s. (MAS)
    necropsy s.
    pathology s.
SPECT
    single-photon emission computed
        tomography
        collimated SPECT
Spec-T
Spectazole
spectinomycin
spectra (*pl. of* spectrum)
spectratyping
    TCR s.
spectrin deficiency
Spectrobid Tablet
spectrometry
    imaging mass s.
    laser-desorption ionization time-of-
        flight mass s.
    matrix-assisted laser
        desorption/ionization time-of-flight
        mass s. (MALDI-TOF-MS)
    surface-enhanced laser desorption
        and ionization mass s. (SELDI-
        MS)
    surface-enhanced laser desorption
        and ionization time-of-flight
        mass s. (SELDI-TOF-MS)
spectrophotometer
    Beckman UV s.
    mass s. (MS)
spectrophotometry
    atomic absorption s.
spectroscope
    quasielastic laser light-scattering s.
spectroscopic imaging
spectroscopy
    atomic absorption s.
    diffuse reflectance s. (DRS)
    diffusion s.
    electron paramagnetic resonance s.
    electrospray ionization mass s.
    EPR s.
    fluorescence s.
    intrinsic fluorescence s. (IFS)
    laser correlational s. (LCS)
    light-scattering s. (LSS)
    magnetic resonance s. (MRS)

MR s.
multivoxel s.
NMR s.
nuclear magnetic resonance s.
^{31}P s.
phosphorus magnetic resonance s.
    (P-MRS)
plasma emission s.
point s.
point-resolved s. (PRESS)
Probe brain s.
proton MR s.
trimodal s. (TMS)
in vivo optical s. 2000 (INVOS
    2000)
spectrum, pl. **spectra, spectrums**
    electromagnetic s.
    S. Forte 29
    lissencephaly-pachygyria s.
    mutational s.
    ultraviolet s.
speech area
sperm
    s. banking
    s. count
spermatocytic seminoma
spermatogenesis
spermatogonia
spermatotoxicity
SPET
    single-photon emission tomography
SPF
    sun protection factor
S-phase
    S-p. analysis
    S-p. fraction
sphenoid
    s. ridge
    s. ridge meningioma
    s. sinus metastasis
sphere
    gelatin s.
    resin s.
    silastic s.
spherical dose distribution
sphericity
spherocytosis
    congenital s.
    hereditary s. (HS)
Spherulin
sphincter
    anal s.
    external urethral s.

S

NOTES

515

sphincter *(continued)*
    s. preservation
    proximal s.
sphincterotome
sphincterotomy
sphincter-saving surgery
sphingolipid
sphingomyelin
    lipid s.
sphingomyelinase
    activity assay s.
sphygmomanometer
    cuff s.
spiculation
    bone s.
spicule
    bone s.
    radiating bone s.
spider
    s. angioma
    s. cancer
Spigelman
    S. stage I-IV
    S. staging I-IV
Spigos protocol
spike
    monoclonal s.
spill
    peritoneal s.
spillage
    tumor s.
spin
    s. dephasing
    electron s.
spina bifida occulta
spinal
    s. accessory lymph node
    s. accessory nerve
    s. axis tumor
    s. block
    s. cord compression
    s. cord stimulation
    s. cord tumor
    s. epidural angiolipoma
    s. epidural lymphoma
    s. fluid
    s. fluid reservoir
    s. hemangioma
    s. meningioma
    s. muscular atrophy (SMA)
    s. puncture
    s. stenosis
    s. synovial sarcoma
    s. tap
spindle
    s. cell
    s. cell carcinoma
    s. cell morphology
    s. cell neoplasm

    s. cell nevus
    s. cell phenotype
    s. cell rhabdomyosarcoma
    s. cell sarcoma
    s. cell sarcoma of vagina
    s. cell stromal component
    s. cell tumor
    s. inhibitor
    s. poison
spindle-shaped tumor cell
spine
    cervical s.
    dorsal s.
spin-echo
    s.-e. pulse sequence
    turbo s.-e. (TSE)
spin-lattice relaxation
spinnbarkeit
spin-spin relaxation
spiradenocarcinoma
spiradenoma
spiral
    s. CT acquisition
    s. CT angiography
spiramycin
spiritual
    s. functioning
    s. pain
spirogermanium
spirohydantoin mustard
spiromustine
Spironazide
spironolactone
    hydrochlorothiazide and s.
spiroplatin
Spirozide
Spitzer quality of life index
Spitz-like melanoma
Spitz nevus
spitzoid malignant melanoma
splanchnicectomy
    chemical s.
splanchnic nerve block
spleen
    accessory s.
    s. colony assay
    ectopic s.
    s. immune reaction
splenectomy
splenic
    s. B-cell lymphoma
    s. bleeding
    s. flexure
    s. flexure cancer
    s. hemangioma
    s. hilus
    s. infarction
    s. leukemia

s. marginal zone lymphoma
without villous lymphocytes
s. marginal zone lymphoma with
villous lymphocytes
s. radiation therapy
s. sequestration
s. vein thrombosis

splenomegaly

splicing

gene s.

Spli-Prest

S.-P. buffer
S.-P. negative control
S.-P. plate
S.-P. positive control

split

s. beam
s. field
s. hand/split foot malformation
(SHFM)
s. hand/split foot malformation
syndrome

split-beam

s.-b. block
s.-b. technique

split-course

s.-c. irradiation
s.-c. radiation therapy
s.-c. regimen
s.-c. technique

splitter

beam s.

spoiled gradient-recalled echo MRI

spoiling

surface s.

spondylitis

ankylosing s.
cryptococcal s.

spondylosis

cervical spine s.

sponge

collagen s.
gelatin s.
polyvinyl s.

spongiform leukoencephalopathy

spongioblastoma

spontaneous

s. immortalization
s. immortalization of breast
epithelial cells
s. phagocytosis

SPOP

sequential paired opposed plaque
SPOP technique

sporadic

s. Burkitt lymphoma
s. clear cell carcinoma
s. retinoblastoma

Sporanox

sporogony

Sporothrix schenckii

sporotrichosis

sporozoite

Sportscreme

SPOT

sonographic planning of oncology
treatment
SPOT mobile 3D ultrasound
system

spot

blind s.
café au lait s.
coast of California café-au-lait s.
coast of Maine café-au-lait s.
cold s.
cotton-wool s.
Fordyce s.
Roth s.
s. scanning

spray

Miacalcin Nasal S.
Moi-Stir oral s.
nasal s.
Nitrolingual Translingual S.
Ony-Clear S.
oral s.
Prevacare skin care s.
resorcinol s.
translingual s.

spread

distant s.
extracapsular s. (ES)
halstedian concept of tumor s.
intraocular s.
locoregional s.
lymphatic s.
pattern of s.
perineural tumor s.
regional s.
subependymal s.
tumor s.

spring-tipped guidewire

NOTES

sprue
celiac s.
tropical s.
SPT
second primary tumor
superficial papillary tumor
spur
bone s.
bronchial s.
calcaneal s.
s. cell
s. cell anemia
spurious polycythemia
sputum, pl. **sputa**
s. cytology
induced s.
s. study
squalamine
squalene
squamatization
squamoid nest
squamotransitional
squamous
s. cell
s. cell carcinoma (SCC)
s. cell carcinoma antigen (SCC-Ag)
s. cell carcinoma of head and neck (SCCHN)
s. cell carcinoma of oral tongue (SCCOT)
s. cell papilloma
s. differentiation
s. epithelium
s. intraepithelial lesion (SIL)
s. metaplasia
s. odontogenic tumor
SR
seroreversion
slow release
Nitrong SR
Wellbutrin SR
src protooncogene/oncogene
SRCT
small round-cell tumor
SRS
somatostatin receptor scintigraphy
stereotactic radiosurgery
linear accelerator-based SRS
SRUS
solitary rectal ulcer syndrome
SS
Sézary syndrome
SSCP
single-strand conformation polymorphism
single-stranded conformational polymorphism
SSD
source-to-skin distance

SSE
skin self-examination
SSKI
saturated solution of potassium iodide
SSM
skin-sparing mastectomy
SSO
Society of Surgical Oncology
SSPE
subacute sclerosing panencephalitis
SSRI
selective serotonin reuptake inhibitor
SSRI antidepressant
SSSS-M
Sexual Self-Schema Scale-Male Version
SST
sclerosing stromal tumor
SSTN
Sandostatin
ST
survival time
St.
St. John's wort
St. Jude Children's Research Hospital (SJCRH)
St. Jude Children's Research Hospital staging system
St. Jude valve
St. Thomas Atherosclerosis Regression Study (STARS)
^{89}St
strontium-89
^{90}St
strontium-90
stab cell
stabilizer
Kwik Board IV and arterial line s.
stable disease
Stachrom
S. antiplasmin
S. AT-III
S. heparin
S. heparin cofactor II
S. plasminogen
S. prekallikrein
S. protein C
stack
Golgi s.
Staclot protein (C, S)
STA Compact hemostasis system
stadium, pl. **stadia**
s. caloris
s. decrementi
s. defervescentiae
s. fluorescentiae
s. frigoris
s. incrementi

s. invasionis
s. sudoris

staff cell

stage

cell cycle s.
clinical s.
Enneking s. I–III
Evans s. I–IV
incubative s.
INSS s.
s. of invasion
latent s.
Okuda s. I-III
prodromal s.
proliferative s.
Spigelman s. I-IV
tumor s.

Stagesic

staging

Ann Arbor classification of
  Hodgkin disease s.
Breslow s.
cancer s.
clinical s.
combined modality s.
disease s.
Durie s.
Durie-Salmon myeloma s.
Enneking s. I–III
Haagensen s.
Hodgkin disease s.
Jewett-Strong s.
Jewett-Strong-Marshall s.
Kadish s.
s. laparotomy
League of Nations s.
s. lymphadenectomy
lymph node s.
M.D. Anderson cancer s.
Memorial Sloan-Kettering s.
multiple myeloma s.
s. myelography
neoplasm s.
neuraxis s.
Nevin s.
Okuda s.
physiologic s.
Robson s.
Spigelman s. I-IV
surgical-pathologic s.
s. system
ultrasonographic s.

Whitmore-Jewett prostate cancer s.
wound s.

stagnant blood

stain

acid-fast s.
acid-Schiff s.
AgNOR s.
anti-Schiff s.
Bielschowsky s.
chloroacetate esterase-butyrate
  esterase s.
Cresyl violet s.
Diff-Quik s.
elastic van Gieson s.
eosin s.
fluorescent auramine-rhodamine s.
Fontana-Masson s.
Giemsa s.
Gomori trichrome s.
Gram s.
Grimelius s.
Hansel s.
Heidenhain iron hematoxylin s.
hematoxylin-eosin s.
immunocytochemical s.
immunoperoxidase s.
iron s.
Kinyoun s.
Kleihauer-Betke s.
LeDer s.
Leishman s.
leukocyte acid phosphatase s.
low-molecular keratin s.
Luxol fast blue s.
lymphocyte enzyme s.
Masson trichrome s.
May-Grunwald s.
mucicarmine s.
myeloperoxidase s.
new methylene blue N s.
nonspecific esterase s.
Papanicolaou s.
PAS s.
periodic acid-Schiff s.
reticulin s.
Romanowsky s.
SBB s.
Schiff s.
silver s. (IFA)
specific esterase s.
Sudan Black B s.
toluidine blue s.
TRAP s.

NOTES

stain *(continued)*
    trichrome s.
    Victoria blue s.
    vimentin s.
    Warthin-Starry s.
    Weigert iron hematoxylin s.
    Weigert resorcin-fuchsin s.
    Wilder reticulum s.
    Wright s.
    Wright-Giemsa s.
stainer
    Midas II automated s.
stainer/cytocentrifuge
    Aerospray hematology slide s./c.
staining
    abnormal s.
    argentaffin s.
    bone marrow s.
    CD34 s.
    chromaffin s.
    direct fluorescent antibody s.
    double-immunofluorescence s.
    ethidium bromide s.
    Feulgen s.
    HID/AB s.
    Hoechst 33342 DNA s.
    immunohistochemical s.
    immunohistologic s.
    intracellular cytokine s. (ICS)
    intravital lymphatic s.
    keratin s.
    nonspecific s.
    periodic acid s.
stainless pellet
stalk section effect
Stamey suprapubic Malecot catheter
STAMP
    Solid Tumor Autologous Marrow
      Transplant Program
    STAMP therapy
standard
    s. busulfan/cyclophosphamide
      preparative regimen
    s. FEC
    Occupational Safety and Health
      Administration bloodborne
      pathogen s.
    OSHA bloodborne pathogen s.
    s. precaution
    s. sample
    s. therapy
standard-dose chemotherapy (SD-CT)
standardized
    s. care policy
    s. CFU assay
    s. CFU-GM assay
    s. colony-forming unit assay
    s. incidence ratio (SIR)

    s. progenitor assay
    s. uptake value (SUV)
Stanford
    S. technique
    S. V chemotherapy protocol
    S. V chemotherapy regimen
staphylococcal
    s. folliculitis
    s. pneumonia
    s. protein A
Staphylococcus
    S. albus
    S. aureus
    S. epidermidis
staphyloma
stapler
    Endo-GIA s.
STAR
    study of tamoxifen and raloxifene
      STAR proton beam radiosurgery
starch
    hydroxyethyl s.
    s. microsphere
STA-R hemostasis system
Starling
    S. hypothesis
    S. resistor
Starr-Edwards valve
starry-sky pattern
STARS
    St. Thomas Atherosclerosis Regression
      Study
STart-4 clot detection system
STart-8 clot detection system
stasis
    chronic venous s.
    vascular s.
    venous s.
STAT
    signal transducing molecule STAT
      5
state
    acquired hypercoagulable s.
    acquired thrombophilic s.
    altered mental s.
    bone marrow failure s.
    congenital hypercoagulable s.
    emotional s.
    fast adiabatic trajectory in
      steady s. (FATS)
    hypercoagulable s.
    hypofibrinolytic s.
    immune s.
    neoplastic s.
    Profile of Mood S.'s (POMS)
    thrombophilic s.
State-Trait Anxiety Inventory
Statex
static image acquisition

statine
station
> lymph node s.
> mediastinal nodal s.

stationary field
statistic
> National Center for Health S.'s (NCHS)

StatSpin
> S. Express 2 centrifuge
> S. MP multipurpose centrifuge

status
> HPV DNA s.
> Karnofsky performance s. (KPS)
> nutritional s.
> performance s.
> ploidy s.
> receptor s.
> respiratory s.
> socioeconomic s. (SES)

Stauffer syndrome
staurosporine
staurosporine-induced apoptosis
stave cell
stavudine
sTCC
> superficial transitional cell carcinoma

STD
> source-tray distance

STEAM
> stimulated echo acquisition mode
> streptonigrin, 6-thioguanine, cyclophosphamide, actinomycin, mitomycin

steatorrhea
steatosis
> microvesicular hepatic s.

Steel factor
steering
> beam s.

Steinbrinck anomaly
Steinmann pin
stellate ganglion
stem
> autologous s. (AS)
> s. cell
> s. cell autograft
> s. cell concentrator
> s. cell donor antigen
> s. cell factor (SCF)
> s. cell gene therapy
> s. cell infusion
> s. cell inoculum
> s. cell leukemia
> s. cell lymphocyte
> s. cell marrow harvesting
> s. cell mobilization
> s. cell pool
> s. cell product
> s. cell proliferation
> s. cell recovery
> s. cell rescue
> s. cell support treatment
> s. cell transplant (SCT)
> s. cell transplantation (SCT)

Stemetil
Stemgen
stenosis
> acquired spinal s.
> ampullary s.
> anastomotic s.
> aortic s.
> aqueductal s.
> arterial s.
> branch pulmonary artery s.
> bronchial s.
> circumferential venous s.
> idiopathic hypertrophic subaortic s.
> membranous s.
> mitral s. (MS)
> spinal s.
> subglottic s.
> tumoral s.
> vaginal s.

Stenotrophomonas maltophilia
stent
> Amplatz double-J s.
> Amplatz tapered pyeloureteral s.
> balloon-expandable tantalum s.
> biliary s.
> Carey-Coons s.
> C-Flex double-J s.
> Cordis balloon expandable s. R
> double-J ureteral s.
> double Malecot prostatic s.
> endobiliary s.
> endobronchial s.
> EndoCoil biliary s.
> endoesophageal s.
> endoluminal s.
> Fabian prostatic s.
> intravascular s.
> luminal s.
> Palmaz-Schatz biliary s.
> Perflex stainless steel s.
> plastic s.

NOTES

S

stent *(continued)*
    polyethylene double-pigtail s.
    polyethylene ureteral s.
    prostatic s.
    pyeloureteral s.
    Rabkin nitinol coil s.
    self-expandable intravascular s.
    self-expandable metallic s.
    self-expanding metallic biliary s.
    self-expanding stainless steel s.
    silastic double-J s.
    Smith Malecot ureteral s.
    Smith Universal ureteral s.
    Strecker intravascular flexible
      tantalum s.
    Teflon s.
    tracheobronchial s.
    Ultraflex s.
    ureteral s.
    vascular s.
stenting
    airway s.
step
    posttranscriptional s.
2-step
    2-s. procedure
    2-s. technique
step-and-shoot method
stepping-source position
stercoralis
    Strongyloides s.
Sterecyt
StereoGuide
stereolithography
stereotactic
    s. biopsy
    s. boost
    s. brachytherapy
    s. core biopsy
    s. CT imaging
    s. external beam irradiation (SEBI)
    s. linear accelerator
    s. needle core biopsy (SNCB)
    s. radiation therapy
    s. radiosurgery (SRS)
    s. radiotherapy
    s. vacuum-assisted biopsy (SVAB)
    s. vacuum-assisted biopsy device
stereotactically
    s. guided conformal radiotherapy
    s. guided core needle biopsy
      (SCNB)
sterile talc insufflation
sterilizing
    s. chemotherapy
    s. immunity
    s. radiotherapy

sternal tumor
Sternberg
    S. disease
    S. sarcoma
    S. tumor
sternoclavicular thickening
sternocleidomastoid muscle
sternooccipital-mandibular
    s.-m. immobilization (SOMI)
    s.-m. immobilization brace
steroid
    anabolic s.
    s. cell tumor
    s. hormone
    s. injection
    s. myopathy
    s. refractory acute GVHD
    sex s.
    s. therapy
steroidal
    s. antiandrogen
    s. hormone
steroid-induced ulcer
steroidogenesis
steroid-refractory ITP
sterone
Stevens-Johnson syndrome
Stewart-Treves syndrome
sTfR
    soluble transferrin receptor
STI
    signal transduction inhibitor
stiffener
    wire s.
stiff-man syndrome
stiff-person syndrome
stillbirth and death model
Stilphostrol
Stimate
stimulated echo acquisition mode
   (STEAM)
stimulating
    colony s.
    s. factor granulocyte-macrophage
    granulocyte-macrophage colony s.
stimulation
    antigenic s.
    dorsal column s.
    ex vivo s.
    intracerebral s.
    mammary parenchymal s.
    periaquaductal s.
    peripheral nerve s.
    spinal cord s.
    TRH s.
stimulator
    B-lymphocyte s. (BLyS)

iodine-131-labeled B-lymphocyte s.
long-acting thyroid s. (LATS)
stimulus, pl. **stimuli**
angiogenic s.
stipple cell
stippled
s. cluster
s. ring
stippling
basophilic s.
Ziemann s.
STIR
short tau inversion recovery
STK-1 receptor
STLI
subtotal lymphoid irradiation
STn
sialyl-Tn antigen
STNI
subtotal nodal irradiation
STn-KLH
synthetic mucin vaccine STn-KLH
Stockholm
S. method
S. technique
S. technique for radium therapy
stocking
antiembolism s.'s
compression s.'s
Stokvis disease
Stokvis-Talma syndrome
stoma, pl. **stomata, stomas**
tracheal s.
Wang pleural s.
stomach
s. adenocarcinoma
body of s.
s. cancer
s. cancer metastasis
s. cell
early gastric cancer of upper s.
(EGCUS)
leather-bottle s.
stomal
s. recurrence
s. seeding
s. ulcer
s. ulceration
stomas (*pl. of* stoma)
stomata (*pl. of* stoma)
stomatitis, pl. **stomatitides**
aphthous s.
mycotic s.

necrotizing s.
nicotine s.
primary herpetic s.
Vincent s.
stomatocytosis
hereditary s.
stomatotoxicity
stone
biliary s.
cystic duct s.
extrahepatic s.
oxypurinol s.
stool
currant jelly s.
melenic s.
occult blood in s.
s. softener
storage
autologous leukapheresis,
processing, s. (ALPS)
long-term s.
s. pool disease
storiform
s. neurofibroma
s. pattern
storiform-pleomorphic pattern
S-TPA
serum tissue polypeptide antigen
STR
skeletal targeted radiotherapy
subtotal resection
strabismus
straight-line recovery period
strain
Armand-Frappier s.
macrophage-tropic HIV s.
macrophage-tropic human
immunodeficiency virus s.
monocyte-tropic s.
M-tropic s.
prototype Japanese s.
TCLA X4 HIV s.
strain-specific virus
stranding
glial s.
strandlike appearance
S-transferase
glutathione S-t.
strategy, pl. **strategies**
chemokine receptor-related s.
data evaluation s.
epidemiological surveillance s.
exposure-prevention s.

NOTES

strategy (*continued*)
    immunomodulatory s.
    mutational s.
    neurorehabilitation s.
    novel therapeutic s.
stratification
    nuclear s.
stratum corneum chymotryptic enzyme
straw-colored fluid
Strecker intravascular flexible tantalum stent
strength
    air-kerma s.
    double s. (DS)
    Excedrin, Extra S.
    extra s. (ES)
    field s.
    half s. (HS)
    Orajel Maximum S.
streptavidin-biotin amplification system
Streptococcus
    beta-hemolytic *S.*
streptococcus, pl. **streptococci**
streptokinase (SK)
    s. infusion
    s. resistance test
    s. therapy
streptolysin
Streptomyces
    S. antibioticus
    S. verticillus
streptomycin
streptonigrin, 6-thioguanine, cyclophosphamide, actinomycin, mitomycin (STEAM)
streptozocin, streptozotocin (STZ)
    Adriamycin, bleomycin sulfate, vincristine, s. (ABOS)
    s., Adriamycin, methyl-CCNU (SAM)
    bleomycin, Velban, doxorubicin, s. (BVDS)
    s., CCNU, Adriamycin, bleomycin (SCAB)
    CCNU, Adriamycin, bleomycin, s. (CABS)
    5-fluorouracil, Adriamycin, cyclophosphamide, s. (FACS)
    5-fluorouracil, Adriamycin, mitomycin C, s. (FAM-S)
    5-fluorouracil, mitomycin C, s. (FMS)
    MeCCNU, Oncovin, 5-fluorouracil plus s. (MOF-STREP)
    s., mitomycin, 5-fluorouracil (SMF)
stress
    oxidative s.
stress-activated protein kinase (SAPK)

stress-induced MHC class I-related molecule
striated muscle
striatus
    lichen s.
stricture
    anastomotic s.
    antral s.
    biliary s.
    choledochojejunostomy s.
    colonic s.
    duodenal s.
    enteric s.
    esophageal s.
    lye s.
    myopharyngeal s.
    tracheal s.
    vaginal s.
stripe
    properitoneal fat s.
stripping program
stroke
    embolic s.
    thrombotic s.
stroma
    bone marrow s.
    cervical s.
    host s.
    myxoid s.
    osteoid s.
    schwannian spindle cell s.
stromal
    s. carcinoid
    s. carcinoid of ovary
    s. cell
    s. cell tumor
    s. edema
    s. element
    s. fibroblast
    s. proliferation
    s. rim
    s. tetranectin
stromal-derived factor 1
stroma-poor tumor
stroma-rich tumor
stromelysin
stromelysin-3
stromoepithelial junction
Stronger Neo-Minophagen C
Strongyloides stercoralis
strongyloidiasis, strongyloidosis
strontium-89 (^{89}St)
strontium-90 (^{90}St)
Stroop Color Word Test (SCWT)
STRT
    simultaneous thermoradiotherapy
structure
    acidophilic s.
    basophilic s.

beta-hairpin s.
cervical s.
cystic s.
gene s.
glandular s.
helix-loop-helix s.
mosaic genome s.
müllerian s.
musculoaponeurotic s.
virion s.
Wagner-Meissnerlike s.
structure-activity relationship
structure-based
s.-b. HIV protease inhibitor
s.-b. human immunodeficiency virus
protease inhibitor
structure-directed oscillation therapy
strut
bone s.
struvite calculus
STS
soft tissue sarcoma
Stuart
S. factor
S. index
Stuart-Prower factor
stucco keratosis
Student-Newman-Keuls method
Student test
Studer pouch
studies-depression
Center for Epidemiologic S.-D.
(CES-D)
study, pl. **studies**
Alpha-Tocopherol Beta-Carotene
Cancer Prevention S.
barium s.
bone length s.
CALGB s.
cancer and leukemia group B s.
Cancer and Steroid Hormone S.
case-control s.
CASH S.
Childhood Cancer Survivor S.
(CCSS)
clinicopathologic s.
clonality s.
cohort s.
Collaborative Ocular Melanoma S.
(COMS)
Cooperative Family Registry for
Breast Cancer Studies (CFRBCS)
2-[C-11]-thymidine PET s.

DNA hybridization s.
dose-escalating s.
efficacy s.
epidemiological s.
Familial Hypercholesterolemia
Regression S. (FHRS)
gene rearrangement s.
H-NMR s.
intervention s.
Kuopio Ischemia Heart Disease
Risk Factor S.
laboratory s.
medical outcomes s. (MOS)
Mevacor Atherosclerosis
Regression S. (MARS)
Million Women S.
molecular hybridization s.
Multicenter AIDS Cohort S.
National Wilms Tumor S. (NWTS)
Optimal Atherectomy Restenosis S.
(OARS)
perfusion s.
postirradiation s.
POWER S.
preclinical s.
Preferences of Women Evaluating
Risks of Tamoxifen S.
PVB s.
radiobiologic s.
radionuclide s.
RISA s.
Rotterdam S.
sputum s.
St. Thomas Atherosclerosis
Regression S. (STARS)
s. of tamoxifen and raloxifene
(STAR)
Women's CARE s.
Women's Contraceptive and
Reproductive Experiences s.
study-2
Canadian National Breast
Screening S.-2 (CNBSS-2)
stump
s. cancer
cervical s.
gastric s.
rectal s.
Sturge-Weber
S.-W. disease
S.-W. syndrome
Sturge-Weber-Dimitri syndrome
styloglossus muscle

S

NOTES

stylomastoid foramen
Stypven time test
STZ
    streptozocin
SU101 in combination with carmustine
subacute
    s. blood
    s. encephalitis
    s. motor neuronopathy
    s. necrotizing lymphadenitis
    s. sclerosing panencephalitis (SSPE)
    s. sensory neuronopathy
subarachnoid
    s. seeding
    s. space
subareolar duct
subastrocytic tumor
subcarinal lymph node
subclavian
    s. apheresis
    s. apheresis catheter
    s. central venous catheter insertion
    s. line
    s. vein thrombosis
    s. vessel thrombosis
subclone
subcutaneous
    s. cuff
    s. emphysema
    s. fat necrosis
    s. IL-2
    s. mastectomy
    s. morphine
    s. murine sarcoma
    s. panniculitic T-cell lymphoma
    s. sacrococcygeal myxopapillary
      ependymoma
    s. tumor
subdivision
    histologic s.
subependymal
    s. giant cell
    s. giant cell astrocytoma (SEGA)
    s. oligodendroglioma
    s. seeding
    s. spread
subependymoma
subfalcine herniation
subgallate
    bismuth s.
subglottic
    s. hemangioma
    s. stenosis
subinfectious dose
subinsular mass
subjective
    s., objective, management, analytic
      (SOMA)

    s., objective, management, analytic
      classification
sublabral foramen
sublethal gene
subleukemic
    s. leukemia
    s. myelosis
Sublimaze Injection
sublingual gland
subluxation
    atlantoaxial s.
submandibular
    s. lymph node
    s. triangle
submaxillary gland
submental lymph node
submesothelial fibroma
submucosa
    vaginal s.
submucosal
    s. mass
    s. saline injection technique
    s. tumor
suboptimal
    s. examination
    s. incentive
    s. surgery
    s. virus
suboptimally debulked cancer
subpectoral implant
subphase
    G_1, G_2 s.
    S s.
subpial astrocyte
subretinal space
subsalicylate
    bismuth s.
subsegmentectomy
subset
    lymphocyte s.
    organ-restricted lymphoid s.
substance
    brain s.
    müllerian-inhibiting s. (MIS)
    s. P
    phosphaturic s.
    thyrotropic s.
substernal goiter
substitute
    blood s.
    HemAssist blood s.
    saliva s.
substituted benzamide
substitution
    segment s.
substrate-based inhibitor
substrate specificity combinatorial puzzle
subsulfate
    ferric s.

subtotal
s. lymphoid irradiation (STLI)
s. nodal irradiation (STNI)
s. resection (STR)
s. thyroidectomy
subtraction
s. cloning
s. hybridization
subtype
cytokeratin s.
E s.
genetic s.
s. heterogeneity
histologic s.
non-Burkitt s.
subungual melanoma
subunit
functional s. (FSU)
human telomerase catalytic s. (hTERT)
integrin s.
subxiphoid window
succedaneum
success
angiographic s.
device s.
lesion s.
procedural s.
succimer
succinate
hydrocortisone sodium s.
methylprednisolone sodium s.
succinic acid ester carboxorolone
sucralfate
suction
s. catheter
s. curettage
s. device
s. drainage
Sudan
S. Black B (SBB)
S. Black B stain
sudoris
stadium s.
sudotox
alvircept s.
SUDS
single-use diagnostic system
SUDS HIV-1 test
Sufenta
sufentanil
sugar
blood s.

s. permeability test
s. tumor
suicidal risk
suicide
s. gene
physician-assisted s. (PAS)
suit
hot-water circulating s.
sulbactam
ampicillin and s.
sulconazole
sulcus, pl. sulci
central s.
cerebral s.
diaphragmatic s.
gingival-buccal s.
gingival-labial s.
glossopalatine s.
paravertebral s.
sulesomab
sulfadiazine
pyrimethamine and s.
s., sulfamethazine, sulfamerazine
sulfadoxine/pyrimethamine combination
Sulfalax
sulfamerazine
sulfadiazine, sulfamethazine, s.
sulfamethoxazole and phenazopyridine
sulfanilamide
sulfate
Apo-Ferrous S.
barium s.
bleomycin s.
dehydroepiandrosterone s. (DHEAS)
dextrin s.
ferrous s.
hydrazine s.
magnesium s.
morphine s. (MS)
Mycifradin S.
piperazine estrone s.
PMS-Ferrous S.
protamine s.
quinine s.
sodium tetradecyl s.
vinblastine s.
vincristine s.
vindesine s.
zinc s.
sulfatide
Sulfatrim DS

NOTES

sulfhydryl
s. group
reduced s. (RSH)
sulfinpyrazone
sulfisoxazole
erythromycin and s.
s. and phenazopyridine
Sulfizole
sulfobromophthalein
sulfonamide hypersensitivity
sulfonate
alkane s.
methylene dimethane s. (MDMS)
sodium polystyrene s.
sulfonated polymer
sulfone
sulindac s.
sulfonyl hydrazine prodrug
sulforaphane chemical
sulfoxide
dimethyl s. (DMSO)
sulfoximine
buthionine s. (BSO)
sulfur
s. colloid
s. dioxide
s. granule
sulindac
s. sulfone
s. sulfone, FGN-1
sulofenur
sum
field-echo s.
Gleason s. 2-10
Sumacal
summation dose intensity
sump
Ring-MacLean s.
van Sonnenberg s.
Sumycin Oral
sunitinib malate
sun protection factor (SPF)
superantigen
superantigen-mediated depletion
superfamily
immunoglobulin s.
tumor necrosis factor s. (TNFSF)
superficial
s. angioma
s. bladder cancer
s. papillary tumor (SPT)
s. radiation
s. spreading carcinoma
s. spreading melanoma
s. thrombophlebitis
s. transitional cell carcinoma
(sTCC)
Superflab bolus material
superfractionated

superior
s. mesenteric artery (SMA)
s. mesenteric vein (SMV)
s. ophthalmic vein thrombosis
s. pulmonary sulcus tumor
s. sagittal sinus thrombosis
s. vena caval compression
s. vena caval obstruction (SVCO)
s. vena cava syndrome (SVCS)
Super-Leu-Dox
supernatant
supernumerary nipple
superoxide production
supervoltage radiation
supplement
Ensure nutritional s.
enteral nutritional s.
Sympt-X s.
supply
arterial s.
blood s.
tumor blood s.
support
autologous bone marrow s.
(ABMS)
autologous hematopoietic stem
cell s.
autologous peripheral hematopoietic
stem cell s. (APHSCS)
autologous stem cell s. (ASCS)
blood component s.
consolidation with peripheral blood
progenitor cell s.
s. group
hematopoietic stem cell s. (HSCS)
high-dose chemotherapy with stem
cell s.
home nutritional s.
lenograstim s.
nutritional s.
peripheral blood stem cell s.
psychological s.
social s.
supportive
s. care
S. Care Needs Survey
supportive-expressive
s.-e. psychotherapy
s.-e. theme
suppository
Anusol-HC S.
AVC s.
controlled-release morphine s.
Dilaudid S.
morphine sulfate controlled-
release s. (MS-CRS)
Prostin E2 Vaginal S.
Sani-Supp S.

suppression

androgen s.
bone marrow s.
drug-induced bone marrow s.
HPA s.
immune s.
immunologic s.
light chain isotype s.
partial viral s.
transient viral s.
viral s.

suppressive

s. E-receptor (SER)
s. thyroxine therapy

suppressor

s. of cytokine signaling (SOCS)
s. gene
immune s.
s. T cell
tumor s.

Supprettes

B&O S.

suppurative inflammation
supraclavicular

s. node involvement
s. recurrence

supraglottic

s. carcinoma
s. laryngectomy
s. larynx

supraomohyoid neck dissection
suprasellar

s. hemorrhagic germinoma
s. meningioma

supratentorial

s. extraventricular ependymal
neoplasm
s. flow compensation
s. glioblastoma multiforme
s. glioma
s. gray matter
s. pilocytic astrocytoma
s. tumor
s. white matter

supratentorium fossa
supraventricular tachycardia
Suprefact Depot
suramin

s. sodium
s. therapy
s. therapy of recurrent tumors

SureCath port access catheter
SureCell herpes test kit

Sure-Cut needle
surface

articular s.
CD20 B-lymphocyte s.
s. coil
s. epithelium vascular channel
s. irradiation
s. membrane immunoglobulin
s. osteosarcoma
s. shielding
s. spoiling

surface-dose application
surface-enhanced

s.-e. laser desorption and ionization
(SELDI)
s.-e. laser desorption and ionization
mass spectrometry (SELDI-MS)
s.-e. laser desorption and ionization
time-of-flight (SELDI-TOF)
s.-e. laser desorption and ionization
time-of-flight analysis
s.-e. laser desorption and ionization
time-of-flight mass spectrometry
(SELDI-TOF-MS)

surface-marker antigen
Surfak
surgery

abutment connection s.
breast conservation s. (BCS)
breast-conserving s. (BCS)
conservation laryngeal s.
curative s.
cytoreductive s.
debulking s.
endoscopic sinus s.
extirpative s.
gamma knife s. (GKS)
laser s.
limb-sparing s.
local s.
Mohs micrographic s.
nephron-sparing s.
palliative s.
radical s.
radioimmunoguided s. (RIGS)
reconstructive s.
rehabilitative s.
resective s.
salvage s.
site-specific s.
sphincter-saving s.
suboptimal s.
transsphincteric s.

NOTES

surgery *(continued)*
    ultraradical s.
    video-assisted thoracoscopic s.
      (VATS)
surgical
    s. debulking
    s. decompression
    s. emergency
    s. excision biopsy
    s. gloves
    s. oncologist
    s. oncology
    s. pathology
    s. portosystemic shunt
    s. removal
    s. resection
surgically created resection cavity
surgical-pathologic staging
Surgicel
surrogate marker
surveillance
    endoscopic s.
    S. Epidemiology and End Results
      (SEER)
    immune s.
    immunologic s.
    s. MRI scanning
survey
    Multicenter European
      Radiofrequency S. (MERFS)
    skeletal s.
    Supportive Care Needs S.
    Third National Cancer S.
survival
    actuarial s.
    s. after recurrence (SAR)
    biochemical recurrence-free s.
      (bRFS)
    cause-specific s. (CSS)
    cell s.
    clinical estimation of s. (CES)
    s. curve
    disease-free s. (DFS)
    disease-specific s. (DSS)
    distant disease-free s. (DDFS)
    distant metastases failure-free s.
      (DMFFS)
    event-free s. (EFS)
    failure-free s.
    s. function
    life table s.
    local recurrence-free s. (LRFS)
    locoregional failure-free s. (LRFFS)
    overall s. (OS)
    postrecurrence s. (PRSv)
    progression-free s. (PFS)
    s. rate
    relapse-free s. (RFS)
    s. relationship

    s. time (ST)
    s. trend
survivin gene
survivor
    long-term s.
survivorship
    National Coalition for Cancer S.
susceptibility
    genetic s.
suspended inspiration
suspension
    atovaquone s.
    barium s.
    Children's Advil S.
    Children's Motrin S.
    chromic phosphate ^{32}P colloidal s.
    colloidal s.
    fresh cell s.
    Fucidin Oral S.
    Megace oral s.
    monocellular s.
    Nephrox S.
    triptorelin pamoate for injectable s.
suspicion
    high index of s.
Sustacal
    S. HC
    S. Liquid
Sustiva
Sutent
suture
    s. line
    s. line cancer
    s. line recurrence
    silk s.
SUV
    standardized uptake value
SV40
    simian virus 40
    SV40 virus
SVAB
    stereotactic vacuum-assisted biopsy
    SVAB device
S-value
SVCO
    superior vena caval obstruction
SVCS
    superior vena cava syndrome
Svedberg unit
SVI
    seminal vesicle invasion
Swabsticks
    Moi-Stir S.
swallow
    barium s.
swallow-tail configuration
sweat
    s. duct adenoma
    s. gland

s. gland carcinoma (SGC)
night s.'s

sweating
gustatory s.

sweep
duodenal s.

Sweet syndrome

swelling
calf s.
leg s.

Swenson pull-through procedure
Swiss mouse leukemia virus
Swiss-type
S.-t. agammaglobulinemia
S.-t. SCID

switch
class s.
genetic s.
lineage s.

switching
gene s.

SWOG
Southwest Oncology Group

Sydenham chorea
Syed-Neblett template
Syed-Puthawala-Hedger esophageal applicator
Syed template
Syllact
Sylvius
aqueduct of S.

Symmers disease
Symmetra ^{125}**I brachytherapy seed**
symmetry-based inhibitor
sympathetic
s. dystrophy
s. ganglia tumor
s. ganglion

sympathomimetic amine
symphysectomy
symplastic leiomyoma
symptom
B s.
s. burden
extrapyramidal s.
iatropic s.
inconsequential s.
mediator-related s.
menopausal s.
mononucleosis-like s.
s. palliation
Pel-Ebstein s.
sicca s.

symptomatic
s. myeloid metaplasia
s. neurosyphilis

Sympt-X supplement
Synagis
Synalgos-DC
synapsin Ia protein
synaptophysin
Synchron LX20 pro chemical analyzer
synchronous
s. adenoma
s. bilateral Wilms tumors
s. carcinoma
s. colonic adenocarcinoma
s. colorectal cancer
s. disease
s. ipsilateral breast cancer (SIBC)
s. malignancy
s. presentation
s. primary bilateral breast lymphoma

synchrotron
syncytia (*pl. of* syncytium)
syncytial
s. meningioma
s. variant

syncytiotrophoblast cell
syncytiotrophoblastic giant cell
syncytium, pl. **syncytia**
Sertoli s.

syncytium-inducing (SI)
s.-i. ability
s.-i. phenotype
s.-i. virus

syndecan-1 test
syndrome
acquired cellular immune deficiency s. (ACIDS)
acquired immunodeficiency s. (AIDS)
acute chest s.
acute radiation bone marrow s.
acute respiratory distress s. (ARDS)
acute retroviral s.
acute seroconversion s.
acute tumor lysis s.
Addison s.
adenomatous polyposis s.
adrenal feminizing s.
adrenal virilizing s.
adrenogenital s.
adult respiratory distress s. (ARDS)

NOTES

531

syndrome *(continued)*
afferent loop s.
Aicardi s.
Aldrich s.
aminopterin s.
analgesic s.
androgen insensitivity s.
angioosteohypertrophy s.
anomalous innominate artery
  compression s.
anterior spinal artery s.
antibody deficiency s.
anti-Ri s.
apallic s.
Apert s.
asplenia s. R
ataxia-hemiparesis s.
ATL s.
autoerythrocyte sensitization s.
autoimmune polyendocrine-
  candidiasis s.
Bard s.
bare lymphocyte s.
basal cell nevus s.
Bassen-Kornzweig s.
Bateman s.
Bazex s.
Beckwith-Wiedemann s. (BWS)
Bernard-Soulier s.
biliary obstruction s.
Birt-Hogg-Dubé s.
Bloch-Sulzberger s.
Bloom s.
blueberry muffin s.
bone marrow failure s.
breast-ovarian cancer s.
Brown-Sequard s.
cancer, anorexia, cachexia s.
  (CACS)
cancer-hemolytic uremic s. (C-HUS)
capillary leak s.
carcinoid s.
carcinoma s.
Carney s.
Carpenter s.
Cassidy-Scholte s.
cellular immunity deficiency s.
  (CIDS)
central cord s.
cerebrohepatorenal s.
cervical disc s.
cervical pain s.
Chédiak-Higashi s.
chemotherapy-hemolytic uremic s.
  (C-HUS)
chronic fatigue s. (CFS)
chronic fatigue and immune
  dysfunction s. (CFIDS)
chronic pain s.

chronic pluripotential
  immunoproliferative s.
chronic venous statis s.
Churg-Strauss s.
cleft face s.
Cockayne s.
community-acquired
  immunodeficiency s. (CAIDS)
Conn s.
constitutional bone marrow s.
Cowden s.
Cronkhite-Canada s.
Cushing s.
Cushing virilizing s. (CVS)
De Toni-Debré-Fanconi s.
Debré-De Toni-Fanconi s.
defibrination s.
Denny-Brown s.
Denys-Drash s. (DDS)
Diamond-Blackfan s.
diarrheogenic s.
diencephalic s.
DiGeorge s.
Di Guglielmo s.
disuse s.
Drash s.
Dresbach s.
Dressler s.
dumping s.
Duncan s.
Dyke-Young s.
dysarthria s.
dysmyelopoietic s.
dysplastic nevus s. (DNS)
Eaton-Lambert myasthenic s.
ectopic ACTH s.
ectopic Cushing s.
empty sella s.
encephalotrigeminal s.
Epstein-Barr virus-associated
  lymphoproliferative s.
euthyroid-sick s.
Evans s.
extrapyramidal s. (EPS)
Faber s.
failing ovary s.
Fallot s.
familial adenomatous polyposis s.
familial atypical multiple mole
  melanoma s.
familial dysplastic nevus s. (FDNS)
familial-type dysplastic nevus s.
FAMMM s.
Fanconi s.
Felty s.
feminization s. (FS)
Fetty s.
Frey s.
Froin s.

Gardner s.
Gasser s.
Gianotti-Crosti s.
Glanzmann s.
glucagonoma s.
Goltz s.
Good s.
Goodpasture s.
Gorlin s.
Gorlin-Pindborg s.
Gradenigo s.
granulomatous slack skin s.
gray platelet s.
Greig s.
Hakim s.
Hedinger s.
Heerfordt s.
HELLP s.
hemichorea-hemiballismus s.
hemolytic transfusion s.
hemolytic uremic s. (HUS)
hemophagocytic s.
hereditary familial cancer s.
hereditary papillary renal
  carcinoma s.
Hermansky-Pudlak s.
Horner s.
HPRC s.
Hunter s.
Hurler s. (HS)
Hutchinson-Boeck s.
Hutchison-Gilford s.
hypereosinophilic s.
hyperviscosity s.
hypoperistalsis s.
Imerslünd s.
Imerslünd-Graesbeck s.
immotile cilia s.
s. of inappropriate secretion of
  antidiuretic hormone (SIADH)
infantile choriocarcinoma s.
infantile monosomy 7 s.
infusion-related cytokine release s.
  (IRCRS)
inherited class II HLA
  deficiency s.
Ivemark s.
Job s.
juvenile polyposis s.
Kallmann s.
Karroo s.
Kasabach-Merritt s.
Kast s.

Kaznelson s.
Ketron-Goodman s.
Klinefelter s. (KS)
Klippel-Trenaunay-Weber s.
Knobloch s.
Kostmann s.
Kozlowski-Tsuruta s.
Lambert-Eaton myasthenic s.
Langer-Giedion s. (LGS)
Launois-Cléret s.
lazy leukocyte s. (LLS)
Lemierre s.
Lesch-Nyhan s.
Lhermitte s.
Li-Fraumeni s. (LFS)
Li-Fraumeni familial cancer s.
lipodystrophy s.
Lloyd s.
Lucey-Driscoll s.
lymphadenopathy s. (LAS)
lymphoproliferative s.
Lynch cancer family s. (I, II)
macrocephaly-cutis marmorata
  telangiectatica congenita s.
Maffucci s.
malignant carcinoid s.
Malin s.
Marfan s.
Maroteaux-Lamy s.
marrow failure s.
May-Hegglin s.
McLeod s.
M-CMTC s.
Meigs s.
melanoma/astrocytoma s.
metastatic carcinoid s.
Mikulicz s.
Mikulicz-Radecki s.
Mikulicz-Sjögren s.
misery perfusion s.
monosomy 7 s.
Morquio s.
Mosse s.
mucocutaneous lymph node s.
  (MLNS)
Muir-Torre s. (MTS)
multiple basal cell neuroma s.
multiple hamartoma s.
murine-acquired
  immunodeficiency s. (MAIDS)
myasthenic s. (MS)
mycosis fungoides/Sézary s.
myelodysplastic s. (MDS)

NOTES

S

syndrome *(continued)*

Nelson s.
nephrotic s.
neurocutaneous s.
neuroleptic malignant s.
neurologic paraneoplastic s.
neuropsychiatric-acquired
  immunodeficiency s. (NARS)
nevoid basal cell cancer s.
nevoid basal cell carcinoma s.
  (NBCCS)
Nezelof s.
Nijmegen breakage s. (NBS)
Noonan s.
numb chin s.
oculoectodermal s.
Omenn s.
opsomyoclonus s.
palmoplantar erythrodysesthesia s.
Pancoast s.
parabiotic s.
paraneoplastic antiphospholipid s.
paraneoplastic neurologic s.
Paterson s.
Paterson-Brown-Kelly s.
Paterson-Kelly s.
Pepper s.
Peutz-Jeghers s.
phantom limb s.
phenytoin-induced
  pseudolymphoma s.
pinch-off s.
Plummer-Vinson s.
pluripotential immunoproliferative s.
POEMS s.
postphlebitic s.
primary antiphospholipid antibody s.
  (PAPS)
protein cast precipitation s.
pseudo-Kaposi s.
pseudolymphoma s.
rapid tumor lysis s.
Recklinghausen s.
Reifenstein s.
Reiter s.
renal paraneoplastic s.
retinoic acid s.
Reye s.
rhinocerebral s.
Richter s.
Riley-Smith s.
Rosenthal s.
Rothmund-Thomson s.
Rubinstein-Taybi s.
Sanctis-Cacchione s.
Sanfilippo s.
Scheie s.
Schüller s.
Schüller-Christian s.

Scott s.
seroconversion s.
serum sickness s.
sex-linked lymphoproliferative s.
Sézary s. (SS)
SHFM s.
Shwachman-Diamond s.
Shy-Drager s.
sicca s.
sick euthyroid s.
Sipple s.
Sjögren s.
slack-skin s.
Sly s.
solitary rectal ulcer s. (SRUS)
split hand/split foot malformation s.
Stauffer s.
Stevens-Johnson s.
Stewart-Treves s.
stiff-man s.
stiff-person s.
Stokvis-Talma s.
Sturge-Weber s.
Sturge-Weber-Dimitri s.
superior vena cava s. (SVCS)
Sweet s.
TAR s.
therapy-related myelodysplastic s.
  (T-MDS)
Thorson-Bioerck s.
thrombocytopenia-absent radius s.
TORCH s.
toxic oil s.
transfusion s.
transient myelopathic s.
Troisier s.
Trousseau s.
tumor lysis s.
Turcot s.
twin-twin transfusion s.
vascular leak s.
vena cava s.
Verner-Morrison s.
VIPoma s.
virilization s. (VS)
von Hippel-Lindau s.
von Mikulicz s.
Waardenburg s.
WAGR s.
wasting s.
Waterhouse-Friderichsen s.
WDHA s.
Weismann-Netter s.
Well s.
Wermer s.
Werner s.
white clot s.
Wiskott-Aldrich s.
Woringer-Kolopp s.

X-linked hyperimmunoglobulin M s.
X-linked IgM s.
X-linked lymphoproliferative s.
XLP s.
yellow nail s.
Zieve s.
Zollinger-Ellison s. (ZES)
synechia, pl. **synechiae**
peripheral anterior s.
Synercid
synergism
therapeutic s.
synergistic cytotoxicity
synergy
s. peptide synthesizer
therapeutic s.
Synflex
syngeneic
s. bone marrow transplant
s. tissue
s. transplantation
syngraft
Syn-Minocycline
synovial
s. cartilaginous focus
s. sarcoma
synovioma
synovitis
s. tumor
villonodular s.
synthase
(2′-deoxy)thymidylate s. (TS)
deoxythymidylic acid s.
fatty acid s.
nitric oxide s.
thymidylate s. (TS)
synthesis
ceramide s.
collagen s.
dihydropteroate s.
heme s.
IgA s.
inhibitor s.
prostaglandin s.
synthesizer
synergy peptide s.
synthetase
argininosuccinate s. (ASS)
fatty acyl-Co-A s.
folylpolyglutamate s.
glutamylcysteine s.
oligoadenylate s.

synthetase/lyase
adenylosuccinate s./l.
synthetic
s. analog
s. analogue of fumagillin
s. bisphosphonate
s. HIV peptide
s. HIV peptide complex
s. human immunodeficiency virus peptide
s. human immunodeficiency virus peptide complex
s. inhibitor
s. linear peptide
s. mucin vaccine STn-KLH
s. octameric peptide
s. retinoid
Synthroid
syphilis
cardiovascular s.
congenital s.
gummatous s.
latent s.
primary s.
s. screen
secondary s.
tertiary s.
syphilitic
s. aortitis
s. gumma
syringe
syringoadenoma
papillary s.
syringocarcinoma
syringocystadenoma papilliferum
syringoid eccrine carcinoma
syringoma
chondroid s.
syrup
Pima s.
system
ABS2000 blood typing s.
AccuProbe s.
ACIT s.
Advanced Interventional S.'s (AIS)
Advantx LC/LP cardiac biplane s.
air filtration s.
Alexa 1000 breast diagnostic s.
AlloMune s.
Androderm Transdermal S.
Anger gamma camera s.
Ann Arbor staging s. I-IV
anterolateral s.

NOTES

S

system *(continued)*

antibody-based detection s.
aortoiliac inflow s.
Apogee 800 ultrasound s.
Architect ci8200 immunoassay s.
Architect i2000 immunoassay s.
Arizona Cancer Center multiple myeloma staging s.
Aspen ultrasound s.
Astler-Coller staging s.
Atec TriMark marker s.
Atrigel drug delivery s.
Aurora MR breast imaging s.
AutoCyte PREP S.
automated cellular imaging s. (ACIS)
AutoPap 300 QC S.
Aviva mammography s.
Baculovirus Expression Vector S. (BEVS)
BAT s.
Behavioral Risk Factor Surveillance S. (BRFSS)
Bethesda s.
Bevalac s.
BIAcore s.
bifid collecting s.
biliary s.
Binet staging s.
BioLogic-HT s.
Bio-Rad Model 5000 Titanium s.
Black nuclear grading s.
blood group s. (A, AB, B, O)
blood typing s.
Bodin-Gibb staging s.
Borrmann gastric cancer typing s.
Bosniak classification s.
Breast Imaging Reporting and Data S. (BI-RADS)
BreastScan IR s.
Breslow microstaging s.
Broders s.
CADD-TPN ambulatory infusion s.
Cancer Rehabilitation Evaluation S. (CARES)
CellFIT acquisition s.
CellQuest acquisition s.
central nervous s. (CNS)
Centrica rotational core biopsy s.
cervical cap delivery s.
Chachoua staging s.
Chang staging s.
ChemoBloc vial venting s.
Clark classification s.
Clark staging s.
CMSI warming s.
coagulation s.
COBE Spectra apheresis s.

Composite Laryngeal Recurrence Staging S. (CLRSS)
comprehensive health enhancement support s. (CHESS)
Conforma 3000 Proton Beam Treatment S.
Cotrel-Dubousset s.
CryoGuide ultrasound guidance s.
cryotherapy s.
CS-5 cryosurgical s.
CyberKnife SRS image-guided stereotactic radiosurgery precision radiotherapy s.
CYP3A4 enzyme s.
cytochrome enzyme s.
cytochrome P450 s.
DebioClip single-dose delivery s.
Denver chromosome identification s.
diagnostic s.
diffuse neuroendocrine s. (DNES)
digestive s.
Discovery LS imaging s.
DOBI s.
drug delivery s.
Durie-Salmon staging s.
dye laser s.
Dynal CELLection s.
Dynamic Optical Breast Imaging S.
Edmondson-Steiner grading s.
Edmonton Staging S.
electrostatic imaging s.
endocrine s.
Enzinger and Weiss s.
epicardial s.
Evans-D'Angio staging s.
ExAblate 2000 ultrasound s.
extrapyramidal s.
FastPack s.
fibrinolytic s.
fiducial alignment s.
FIGO staging s.
First Warning s.
Fletcher-Suit s.
Fletcher-Suit-Delclos s.
Flocks-Kadesky s.
folate polyglutamylation s.
free radical scavenging s.
Fuhrman grading s.
fully automated blood typing s.
gated irradiation s.
GenESA s.
Gleason tumor grading s.
GliaSite radiation therapy s.
GliaSite RTS s.
Gunderson-Sosin staging s.
Hardy-Vezine classification s.
Hemasure r/LS red blood cell filtration s.

hematopoietic s.
hepatic P450 cytochrome s.
Hewlett-Packard SONOS 1500 s.
HIMAC s.
host vector s.
human immunodeficiency virus
  overview of problems
  evaluation s. (HOPES)
Hyams grading s.
2-hybrid s.
immune s.
immunoregulatory effector s.
implantable drug delivery s.
Infinia Hawkeye nuclear
  medicine s.
Innova 4100 flat-panel x-ray s.
Intensified Radiographic Imaging S.
  (IRIS)
International Neuroblastoma
  Staging S. (INSS)
International Staging S.
IS1000 gel documentation
  imaging s.
Isolex 300i magnetic stem cell
  selection s.
IsoMed Constant-Flow Infusion S.
Jackson staging s.
Jass grading s.
Jewett-Marshall staging s.
Kadesky staging s.
Kadish staging s.
Kagan staging s.
Kernohan grading s. I-IV
Kernohan histologic grading s.
Krigel staging s.
Leksell stereotactic s.
Leukotrap RC s.
Leukotrap red cell storage s.
light collection s.
lymphatic s.
lymphatic and hematopoietic s.
  (LHS)
Mammex TR computer-aided
  mammography diagnosis s.
MammoReader computer-aided
  detection s.
MammoSite Radiation Therapy S.
Mammotest Plus breast biopsy s.
Manchester LDR implant s.
Masaoka staging s.
M.D. Anderson grading s.
M.D. Anderson tumor score s.
MDS s.

medication event monitoring s.
  (MEMS)
MIBB breast biopsy s.
micromultileaf collimator s.
microscopic angiogenesis grading s.
  (MAGS)
microtiter blood typing s.
Mini Quant D-dimer test s.
MIR s.
Mirels scoring s.
Mitsuyasu staging s.
Mobetron intraoperative radiation
  therapy treatment s.
model s.
Murphy staging s.
musculoskeletal s.
NEAD s.
near-UV excited autofluorescence
  diagnosis s.
nervous s.
Neurostat Mark II cryoanalgesia s.
New International Staging S.
Node Seeker surgical radiation
  detection s.
Novoste Beta-Cath delivery s.
ON-Q pain management infusion s.
OPAL knowledge-entry s.
Optical Biopsy S.
OutBound disposable syringe
  infusion s.
oxygen-based therapeutic s.
PadKit sample collection s.
PAPNET s.
Paris s.
Paterson-Parker s.
PDQ information s.
Peacock s.
percutaneous excimer laser coronary
  angioplasty s.
Perflex delivery s.
Peripheral Access S. (PAS)
Peripheral Access System Port
  catheter s.
peripheral nervous s.
phased-array s.
photon radiosurgery s.
PixCell II laser capture
  microdissection s.
polymeric local delivery s.
portal venous s.
Prolieve thermodilatation s.
protein C anticoagulant s.

S

NOTES

system *(continued)*
    Pulsavac Plus wound debridement s.
    purple mutation s.
    Quantimet 500 analyzing s.
    Quimby implant s.
    radiation therapy s. (RTS)
    radiation treatment s.
    radiofrequency interstitial tissue ablation s.
    radiology telephone access s. (RTAS)
    Rai staging s.
    reimbursement s.
    reticuloendothelial s.
    RF Vacuum Ablation S.
    rhabdoid tumor of central nervous s.
    RIGS s.
    Ringertz s.
    Ringertz-Burger grading s.
    RITA s.
    Robson modification of Flocks-Kadesky s.
    Royal Marsden Hospital staging s.
    Russell classification s.
    Scandatronix MLC s.
    scavenging s.
    SeedNet Gold cryotherapy s.
    Selectron s.
    Senographe 2000D mammography s.
    Senographe DS mammography s.
    SenoScan mammography s.
    SensorMedics 2200 Pulmonary Function Test S.
    Shimada s.
    Signa Excite 1.5T s.
    Signa Excite 3.0T MR s.
    Signa OpenSpeed 0.7T MR s.
    Signa Ovation 0.35T MR s.
    single-use diagnostic s. (SUDS)
    SiteSelect percutaneous incisional breast biopsy s.
    SJCRH staging s.
    skeletal s.
    SKY pain control s.
    smart laser s.
    S-Monovette blood collection s.
    SoftScan laser mammography s.
    Solcotrans drainage/reinfusion s.
    SPOT mobile 3D ultrasound s.
    STA Compact hemostasis s.
    staging s.
    STA-R hemostasis s.
    STart-4 clot detection s.
    STart-8 clot detection s.
    St. Jude Children's Research Hospital staging s.
    streptavidin-biotin amplification s.
    television s.
    ThermoChem s.
    ThermoChem-HT s.
    TIS staging s.
    1.5-T MR imaging s.
    TNM staging s.
    Tod and Meredith s.
    transposon insertion s.
    TransScan TS2000 electrical impedance scanning s.
    Trilogy image-guided radiosurgery s.
    tumor, immune, systemic staging s.
    Uni-frame patient immobilization s.
    University of Florida staging s.
    Unopette s.
    Varian MLC s.
    Visica Treatment S.
    Visick grading s.
    Warm-Up wound care s.
    Xillix LIFE-GI fluorescence endoscopy s.
    Xillix LIFE-Lung s.
    Zolla-Pazner immunological staging s.

systematic desensitization
systematized epidermal nevus
systemic
    s. amyloidosis
    s. antibiotic therapy
    s. chemotherapy
    s. immune response
    s. infusion
    s. Langerhans cell histiocytosis
    s. LCH
    s. lupus erythematosus (SLE)
    s. lymphoma
    s. lymphoproliferative disorder
    s. mastocytosis
    s. micrometastasis
    s. model
    s. nodular panniculitis
    s. pentamidine
    s. prednisolone
    s. radioimmunoglobulin therapy
    s. shunt
    tumor, immune, s. (TIS)
Systemized Nomenclature of Medicine (SNOMED)
Sytobex
SYT-SSX fusion gene detection

τ (*var. of* tau)

T
    temperature
    tocopherol
    torque
        Autoplex T
        T helper cell (Th)
        T helper cell 1 (Th1)
        T helper cell 2 (Th2)
        T helper suppressor cell (Ts)
        T lymphocyte
        T and N integer score (TANIS)
        T suppressor cell
        thioflavin T

T-2 protocol

T$_3$
    triiodothyronine
        T$_3$ uptake

T4
    T4 cell
    T4 enolase V, liposome
        encapsulated
    T4 helper cell
    WHO classification for transitional
        cell carcinoma of the urinary
        bladder (stages Ta through T4)

T-10 protocol
T-101 therapy
t(14,18) chromosomal translocation
t(15;17) cytogenic subtypes of acute
    myeloid leukemia
^{178}Ta
    tantalum-178
^{182}Ta
    tantalum-182
TAA
    tumor-associated antigen
tab
    Apo-Doxy T.'s
table
    Partin coefficient t.
tablet
    BD glucose t.
    Dialose T.
    Diatx t.
    DiatxFe t.
    Equalactin Chewable T.
    Fucidin T.
    Kytril t.
    Methitest t.
    Mitrolan Chewable T.
    Mylocel t.
    Nitrong Oral T.
    Nolvadex t.
    orally disintegrating t. (ODT)
    Spectrobid T.
    tamoxifen citrate t.
    Tums E-X Extra Strength T.

TAC
    transient aplastic crisis
Tac-3 Injection
Tac-40 Injection
Tac-expressing malignancy
tachycardia
    auricular t.
    paroxysmal auricular t.
    paroxysmal supraventricular t.
    supraventricular t.
tachykinin
tachyphylaxis
tachypnea
TACI-Ig fusion protein
tacrolimus
TAD
    6-thioguanine, ara-C, daunomycin
    6-thioguanine, ara-C, daunorubicin
TADG-15
    tumor-associated differentially expressed
        gene 15
TAE
    transcatheter arterial embolization
TAG
    tumor-associated glycoprotein
TAG-72
    tumor-associated glycoprotein-72
Tagamet
Tagamet-HB
tagging
    bolus t.
TAH
    total abdominal hysterectomy
TAHBSO
    total abdominal hysterectomy and
        bilateral salpingo-oophorectomy
taheebo tea
TA-HPV vaccine
Taifun
    Fentanyl T.
tail
    axillary t.
    t. of breast
    cytoplasmic t.
    dural t.
    lipid t.
    parotid t.
    1-t. test
    2-t. test
tailgut cyst
tailored FEC

tailoring
custom t.

Taiwan
T. Pediatric Oncology Group (TPOG)
T. Pediatric Oncology Group acute myeloid leukemia 901
T. Pediatric Oncology Group acute myeloid leukemia 901 protocol

TAL
tumor-associated lymphocyte

tal-1
tal-1 oncogene
tal-1 protooncogene/oncogene

talabostat

Talacen

talc
baked t.
intrapleural t.
t. pleurodesis
t. slurry

talin protein

talipes equinovarus (TEV)

talisomycin

tall cell variant

tallimustine

tal oncogene

talotrexin

tal-1/SIL fusion gene

Talwin
T. Compound
T. NX

TAM
tamoxifen
tumor-associated macrophage

Tamm-Horsfall (TH)
T.-H. mucoprotein
T.-H. protein
T.-H. proteinuria

Tamofen

tamoxifen (TAM, TMX)
cisplatin, BCNU, dacarbazine, t. (CBDT)
t. citrate
t. citrate tablet
cyclophosphamide, methotrexate, 5-fluorouracil, t. (CMFT, CMF-TAM)
cyclophosphamide, methotrexate, 5-fluorouracil, prednisone, t. (CMFPT)
Cytoxan, methotrexate, 5-fluorouracil, prednisone, t. (CMFPT)
dimethyltriazenoimidazole carboxamide, bischloroethylnitrosourea, Platinol, t. (DBPT)

t., etoposide, mitoxantrone, Platinol (TEMP)
phenylalanine, 5-fluorouracil, t. (PFT)
prednisone, 5-fluorouracil, t. (PFT)
Preferences of Women Evaluating Risks of T. (POWER)

tamp
inflatable bone t. (IBT)

tampon

tamponade
balloon t.
cardiac t.
t. needle tract
pericardial t.

tan-1
tan-1 oncogene
tan-1 protooncogene/oncogene

tandem
t. applicator
t. conjugate reagent
t. double dose
Fletcher-Suit-Delclos t.
t. high-dose chemotherapy
MIR intrauterine t.
t. and ovoid
t. stem cell transplant
t. technique
t. transplant (TAT)

tangent
t. fields
t. screen testing

TANIS
T and N integer score
TANIS score

tank volumetry

tanned red cell

tannic acid fixative

tantalum-178 (^{178}Ta)

tantalum-182 (^{182}Ta)

Tantaphen

T-antigen

tanycyte

TAP
tumor-activated prodrug

tap
spinal t.

Tapanol

Tapazole

tape
Bioflex 647 t.
Bioflex 648 t.
Bioflex Rx222P t.
Bioflex Rx216V t.
Bioflex Rx232V t.
clonidine transdermal t.
genetic masking t.
Johnson & Johnson waterproof t.
Megazinc Pink adhesive t.

Micropore t.
Omnifix t.
tapered-tip dilator
TAPET
tumor-amplified protein expression therapy
tapioca melanoma
TaqMan analysis
TAR
thrombocytopenia-absent radius
tissue-air ratio
transactivator
TAR inhibitor
TAR syndrome
Tarceva
tarda
porphyria cutanea t.
target
antigenic t.
aspartate t.
assay t.
t. cell
t. depth
t. dose
t. erythrocyte
intracellular t.
t. lesion
t. organ
t. radiotherapy
t. volume
targeted
t. alpha-particle therapy
t. cryoablation
t. cryoablation device
t. cryoablation of prostate (TCAP)
t. cryosurgery
t. radiotherapy
t. radiotherapy using ¹³¹I anti-CD20 antibody
targeting
t. agent
B-mode acquisition and t. (BAT)
magnetite in tumor t.
regulatory peptide receptor t.
tumor t.
target-to-nontarget ratio
Targretin
T. capsule
T. gel
tariquidar
Taro-Ampicillin
Taro-Cloxacillin
tart cell

tartrate
butorphanol t.
vinorelbine t.
tartrate-resistant
t.-r. acid phosphatase (TRAP)
t.-r. acid phosphatase assay
task
t. activation
fingertapping t.
reaction time t.
Tasmar
taste
t. abnormality
foul t.
t. perception
t. perversion
TAT
tandem transplant
TAT III complex
tat
human immunodeficiency virus tat
Tat protein
TATA
tumor-associated transplantation antigen
TATA box
TATE
tumor-associated tissue eosinophilia
tattoo
tau, τ
t. interferon
Taub test
tauromustine (TCNU)
tautomer
Tavocept
tax
t. gene
t. protein
taxane
t.'s class of anticancer drugs
t. refractory non-small-cell lung carcinoma
t. resistant non-small-cell lung carcinoma
semisynthetic t.
taxane-based regimen
taxane-resistant breast cancer
Taxol
T., cisplatin, gemcitabine (TCG)
mesna, ifosfamide, Novantrone, T. (MINT)
Taxol-resistant tumor
Taxoprexin DHA-paclitaxel

NOTES

Taxotere
  Doxil and T.
  T. and doxorubicin neoadjuvant
    therapy
  T., Platinol, 5-fluorouracil (TPF)
tax-responsive element
Taxus brevifolia
Tazicef
Tazidime
tazobactam
Tazocin
Tazorac
TB
  tuberculosis
    TB antigen
T-bar immobilization device
TBBMC
  total body bone mineral content
TBC-CEA vaccine
TBI
  total body irradiation
  tracheobronchial injury
    ^{131}I-labeled anti-CD45 antibody
      combined with CY and TBI
TBSA
  total body surface area
TC
  6-thioguanine and cytarabine
  typical carcinoid
3TC
  2′,3′-dideoxy-3′thiacytidine
TC62
  oligonucleotide probe TC62
^{99m}Tc
  technetium-99m
    ^{99m}Tc anti-CEA
    ^{99m}Tc Tetrofosmin
TCA
  thymic carcinoma
  tricyclic antidepressant
TCAP
  targeted cryoablation of prostate
3TC/AZT
  lamivudine triphosphate and
    azidothymidine
TCC
  transitional cell carcinoma
Tc-diethylenetriamine pentaacetic acid
^{99m}Tc-DMSA scintigraphy
^{99m}Tc-DTPA
  technetium-99m diethylenetriamine
    pentaacetic acid
T-cell
  T-c. acute lymphoblastic leukemia
  T-c. anergy
  T-c. antigen receptor (TCR)
  T-c. antigen receptor Vb
  T-c. costimulatory pathway
  T-c. deletion

T-c. differentiation
T-c. line
T-c. line-adapted isolate
T-c. lymphoblastic lymphoma
T-c. lymphoma variant
T-c. malignancy
T-c. marker
T-c. neoplasm
T-c. phenotype
T-c. prolymphocytic leukemia
T-c. pseudoclonality
T-c. receptor reactive with folate-
  binding protein
T-c. receptor V-alpha
T-c. receptor V-beta
T-c. rich
T-c. stimulating factor
T-cell-mediated antitumor response
T-cell-rich
  T-c.-r. B cell
  T-c.-r. B-cell lymphoma
T-cell-tropic
  T-c.-t. HIV-1
  T-c.-t. human immunodeficiency
    virus 1
TCG
  Taxol, cisplatin, gemcitabine
^{99m}Tc-HMPAO
  technetium-99m
    hexamethylpropyleneamine oxime
    ^{99m}Tc-HMPAO cerebral perfusion
      SPECT imaging
    ^{99m}Tc-HMPAO SPECT imaging
TCIS
  transitional carcinoma in situ
TCLA
  TCLA X4
  TCLA X4 HIV strain
tcl-1 oncogene
tcl-2 oncogene
tcl-3 oncogene
tcl-4 oncogene
^{99m}Tc-MAA
  technetium-99m macroaggregated
    albumin
^{99m}Tc macroaggregated albumin
^{99m}Tc MIBI
  technetium-99m
    methoxyisobutylisonitrile
  technetium-99m sestamibi
    ^{99m}Tc MIBI scintimammography
TCN-P
  triciribine phosphate
TCNU
  tauromustine
TCR
  T-cell antigen receptor
    TCR spectratyping
    TCR Vb

TCRT
thoracic conformal radiation therapy
T-cytotoxic cell
T_d
diffusion time
TDLN
tumor-draining lymph node
TDM
therapeutic drug monitoring
TDR
thymidine deoxyriboside
TdT
terminal deoxynucleotidyl transferase
TE
echo-time
tracheoesophageal
tea
chaparral t.
Essiac t.
herbal t.
Kombucha t.
pau d'arco t.
taheebo t.
valerian t.
white t.
team
interdisciplinary t.
nutrition support t. (NST)
transplant t.
tear
anulus fibrosus t.
esophageal t.
rectal t.
TEC
thiotepa, etoposide, carboplatin
teceleukin
technetium H2 autoanalyzer
technetium-labeled nanocolloid
technetium-99m (^{99m}Tc)
t.-99m diethylenetriamine pentaacetic acid (^{99m}Tc-DTPA)
t.-99m hexamethylpropyleneamine oxime (^{99m}Tc-HMPAO)
t.-99m macroaggregated albumin (^{99m}Tc-MAA)
t.-99m methoxyisobutylisonitrile (^{99m}Tc MIBI)
t.-99m sestamibi (^{99m}Tc MIBI)
t.-99m sestamibi scintimammography
technique
afterloading t.
air-gap t.
Alexander t.

arc therapy t.
assay t.
balloon catheter t.
BAT radiation therapy t.
bilateral t.
Bolton-Hunter t.
boost t.
bougienage t.
catheter-securing t.
chemical shift imaging t.
cognitive t.
Cox proportional hazard modeling t.
cytopreparatory t.
Dixon t.
DNA microinjection t.
dose-delayed t.
double dose-delayed t.
dynamic bolus tracking t.
electron arc t.
endofluoroscopic t.
endovascular t.
enzyme-multiplied immunoassay t. (EMIT)
external looping t.
3-field arc t.
3-field isocentric t.
4-field t.
fluorescent antibody t.
flushing t.
Hahnemann University Hospital t.
hairpin t.
hanging-block t.
hybridoma t.
immersion t.
immune monitoring t.
immunoadsorption t.
immunodetection t.
immunofluorescence t.
immunohistochemical t.
inside-out t.
intraoral swage t.
ISH EBER t.
Laurell t.
low-dose helical scanning t.
marking t.
Martinez t.
matchline t.
mathematical modeling t.
McWhirter t.
microwave epitope retrieval t.
mixed photon-electron t.
molecular genetic t.

NOTES

543

technique *(continued)*
- monitoring t.
- monoisocentric t.
- moving-strip t.
- multicoil array t.
- 2-needle t.
- neuroablative t.
- neutron t.
- nonaxial beam t.
- noncoplanar beam t.
- no-touch t.
- Oakley-Fulthorpe t.
- parotid-sparing t.
- past-pointing t.
- Patey t.
- propeller t.
- pseudobiopsy t.
- radiation therapy t.
- recanalization t.
- rescue t.
- rotational therapy t.
- Scrimp t.
- Sevier-Munger t.
- shrinking-field t.
- snare t.
- Southern blot t.
- split-beam t.
- split-course t.
- SPOP t.
- Stanford t.
- 2-step t.
- Stockholm t.
- submucosal saline injection t.
- tandem t.
- thermal debulking t.
- tissue-sparing t.
- tourniquet t.
- T-Pouch t.
- trocar t.
- trocar-cannula t.
- wedged-pair t.
- whole blood lysis t.

technology, pl. **technologies**
- acoustic response t.
- Arrhythmia Research T. (ART)
- cell imaging t.
- column or bead t.
- combinatorial Array T.
- focused heat t.
- lymphochip t.
- National Institute of Standards and T. (NIST)
- recombinant deoxyribonucleic t.
- recombinant DNA t.
- RIGS/ACT t.
- XenoMouse t.

tectal glioma

teeth (*pl. of* tooth)

TEF
- tracheoesophageal fistula

Teflon
- T. catheter
- T. dilator
- T. sheath
- T. stent

Teflon-coated needle

Tegaderm
- T. dressing
- T. TFD

tegafur
- uracil, 5-fluorouracil, t. (UFT)

Tegretol

Tegretol-XR

Teichmann crystal

telangiectasia
- ataxia t.
- hemorrhagic t.
- hereditary hemorrhagic t.

telangiectasis

telangiectatic
- t. angioma
- t. cancer
- t. fibroma
- t. osteogenic
- t. osteogenic sarcoma
- t. osteosarcoma

telangiectaticum
- granuloma t.

Telcyta

telecobalt therapy

telescopic plate spacer (TPS)

teletherapy radiotherapy

television system

telogen effluvium

telolysosome

telomerase
- t. activity
- t. activity assay
- enzyme t.
- human t. (hTR)
- t. reverse transcriptase (TERT)

telomerase-active stem cell

telomerase-associated protein (TP1)

telomerase-expressing cancer cell

telomere repeat amplification protocol (TRAP)

telomeric
- t. association
- t. DNA
- t. region
- t. repeat amplification protocol (TRAP)

telophase

telosome

teloxantrone hydrochloride

TEM
> Temodal
> transmission electron microscopy

temazepam
Temno biopsy needle
Temodal (TEM)
> Gliadel plus CPT-11 or T.

Temodar capsule
temoporfin
temozolomide (TMZ)
> t. plus thalidomide

TEMP
> tamoxifen, etoposide, mitoxantrone,
> Platinol

temperature (T)
> mean perfusate t.

template
> amplicon t.
> homopolymeric t.
> Kuske breast t.
> Martinez Universal Perineal
>   Interstitial T. (MUPIT)
> Syed t.
> Syed-Neblett t.

Tempol-mediated radioprotection
temporal
> t. bone tumor
> t. meningioma

temporary diverting colostomy
temporoinsular astrocytoma
temporooccipital glioma
Tenckhoff catheter
tendon
> Achilles t.
> anterior tibial t.
> biceps brachii t.
> brachioradialis t.
> central t.
> extensor t.
> posterior tibial t. (PTT)

tendosynovial sarcoma
tenecteplase
tenesmus
teniposide, procarbazine, prednisone
Tenju-gann
Ten-K
tenofovir
tenosynovial giant cell tumor
tenosynovitis
> de Quervain t.

Tensilon
tensin protein
tension pneumothorax

tensor veli palatini muscle
tentorial meningioma
tentorium cerebelli
tenuin protein
TEP
> tracheoesophageal puncture
> primary TEP
> TEP prosthesis
> secondary TEP

TER
> thermal enhancement ratio

teratoblastoma of ovary
teratocarcinoma
> t. of ovary
> pineal t.

teratocarcinosarcoma
> sinonasal t. (SNTSC)

teratogen
teratogenic effect
teratogenicity
teratoid
> t. carcinosarcoma
> t. tumor

teratologic
teratological
teratologist
teratoma, pl. **teratomata**
> cystic t.
> embryonal t.
> immature mediastinal t.
> malignant t. (MT)
> malignant ovarian t.
> mature cystic t.
> mature mediastinal t.
> mature ovarian t.
> mediastinal t.
> ovarian cystic t.
> ovarian embryonal t.
> pineal t.
> sacrococcygeal t.

terazosin
terbinafine
> topical t.

terbutaline
terephthalamide
terephthalamidine
teres
> pronator t. (PT)

terfenadine
teriparatide
terlipressin
terminal
> t. care

NOTES

T

terminal *(continued)*
- t. deoxynucleotide transferase UTP nick-end labeling
- t. deoxynucleotidyl transferase (TdT)
- t. deoxynucleotidyl transferase-mediated digoxigenin-dUTP nick-end labeling (TUNEL)
- t. differentiation
- t. duct lobular unit
- t. leukocytosis
- t. progression
- t. transferase-mediated dUTP-biotin nick-end labeling
- t. ureterectasis

terminally ill patient
terminator
- DNA chain t.
- obligate chain t.

terminus
- amino t.
- cytoplasmic carboxy t.

teroxirone
terpene
Terra-Cortril ointment
Terramycin
- T. I.M. Injection
- T. Oral

terreus
- *Aspergillus* t.

Terry-Mayo needle
TERT
- telomerase reverse transcriptase

tertiary syphilis
Terumo guidewire
Tesamone Injection
TESE
- testicular sperm extraction

Teslac
1.5 tesla MRI
Teslascan contrast
tesmilifene
TESPA
- triethylenethiophosphoramide

test
- acid t.
- acidified serum lysis t.
- ACPA blood t.
- ACS:180 BR breast cancer screening t.
- Actalyke activated clotting time t.
- activated clotting time t.
- Alexagram breast lesion diagnostic t.
- Ames t.
- ANA t.
- anergy t.
- anthropometric t.
- anti-B19 antibody t.

- anticytoplasmic antibody t.
- antigliadin IgA ELISA autoimmune t.
- antigliadin IgG ELISA autoimmune t.
- APC stool t.
- aspirin tolerance t.
- AuraTek rapid cancer t.
- automated complete blood t.
- automated factor V Leiden mutation t.
- Aware AccuMeter rapid HIV t.
- Bayer HER-2/neu serum t.
- *bcr/abl* protein t.
- beta-hCG t.
- biceps brachii tendon reflex t.
- bilirubin t.
- BladderScan t.
- bleeding time t.
- blood urea nitrogen t.
- Bonferroni t.
- brachioradialis tendon reflex t.
- BreastAlert t.
- BTA stat t.
- B/T Blue Gene Rearrangement t.
- California Verbal Learning T. (CVLT)
- *Campylobacter* 16S-23S rRNA ISR t.
- CA15-2 RIA t.
- Casoni skin t.
- c-erbB2 p185 t.
- cerebrospinal fluid Venereal Disease Research Laboratory t.
- clearance t.
- Coat-A-Count PSA IRMA t.
- coccidioidin skin t.
- Cochran-Mantel-Haenszel t.
- Colaris genetic susceptibility t.
- complement fixation t.
- Complex Figure T. (CFT)
- conglutinating complement absorption t.
- Coombs t.
- Cortrosyn-stimulating t.
- CSF VDRL t.
- Dako HercepTest immunohistochemical t.
- D-Di t.
- delayed-type hypersensitivity t.
- demethylation t.
- dexamethasone suppression t.
- Dick t.
- DR-70 tumor marker t.
- dye reduction spot t.
- EBNA t.
- ethanol gelation t.
- factor V Leiden mutation t.
- Farr t.

fecal occult blood t. (FOBT)
FlexSure OBT t.
Fouchet t.
FS unit t.
GeneAmp PCR t.
genetic t.
germ tube t.
HA-HAase urine t.
Hammarsten t.
HC2 t.
Heartscan heart attack prediction t.
Hema-Strip HIV t.
HemeSelect t.
Hemoccult t.
hepaplastin t.
HercepTest immunohistochemical t.
Herp-Check antibody t.
Hicks-Pitney thromboplastin
  generation t.
Hinton t.
Hoppe-Seyler t.
Hybrid Capture 2 t.
Hybrid Capture 2 HPV DNA t.
Hybritech Free PSA t.
immunobead-binding assay t.
immunoblot t.
Immuno1 Complexed PSA t.
ImmunoCyt urine t.
immunohistochemical diagnostic t.
indirect fluorescent antibody t.
indocyanine green retention t.
induced sputum t.
Inform HER-2/neu breast cancer t.
INNO-LIA syphilis t.
Integra PBS Pageblot t.
iron-binding capacity t.
Kaiser ninhydrin t.
Kitzmiller t.
Kleihauer t.
Kobert t.
Kolmer t.
Kowarsky t.
Kveim t.
La Bross spot t.
Ladendorff t.
LAP t.
liver function t. (LFT)
log-rank t.
low-range heparin management t.
  (LHMT)
Luria-Delbruck fluctuation t.
Machado t.
Machado-Guerreiro t.

mammary aspiration specimen
  cytology t. (MASCT)
MAS cytology t.
McNemar t.
Middlebrook-Dubos
  hemagglutination t.
Moloney t.
Molulsky dye reduction t.
Monospot t.
multipuncture t.
National Adult Reading T. (NART)
Nippe t.
Noguchi t.
Northern blot t.
omeprazole stimulation t.
OraQuick t.
OraSure t.
osmotic fragility t.
Papanicolaou t.
paper radioimmunosorbent t.
  (PRIST)
pentagastrin-Ca stimulation t.
pentagastrin stimulation t.
pilocarpine chloride prognostic t.
platelet suspension
  immunofluorescence t. (PSIFT)
PPD t.
predictive value of negative t.
predictive value of positive t.
PreGen-26 colorectal cancer t.
pregnancy t.
t. procedure
ProstAsure blood t.
PSA4 blood t.
Purdue Pegboard t.
rapid microbial contamination t.
renal function t.
Rey Complex Figure T.
RHD psi t.
ristocetin cofactor t.
Römer t.
Rose-Waaler t.
Rumpel-Leede t.
Salzman t.
SCAT t.
Scheffe F t.
Schiller t.
Schilling t.
Schumm t.
screening t.
serologic t.
Sero-Strip HIV t.
serum syndecan-1 t.

T

NOTES

test *(continued)*
  sheep cell agglutination t. (SCAT)
  Shirner t.
  sickle cell anemia t. (SCAT)
  sickle solubility t.
  slide-based t.
  Spearman rank correlation t.
  streptokinase resistance t.
  Stroop Color Word T. (SCWT)
  Student t.
  Stypven time t.
  SUDS HIV-1 t.
  sugar permeability t.
  syndecan-1 t.
  1-tail t.
  2-tail t.
  Taub t.
  ThinPrep Pap T.
  Thrombo-Wellco t.
  thyroperoxidase antibody t.
  Trail Making T. (TMT)
  Triboulet t.
  Trichophyton skin t.
  tuberculin skin t. (TST)
  Tukey t.
  Tuttle t.
  ultrastructural platelet peroxidase t.
  uPM3 urine t.
  urine t.
  Urovision urine t.
  van den Bergh t.
  Voges-Proskauer t.
  Vysis PathVysion genomic disease management t.
  Waaler-Rose t.
  water-loading t.
  water-siphon t.
  Welch *t* t.
  Widmark t.
  Williamson blood t.
  Winn t.
  Word Fluency T.
  Zaleski t.
  Zelen exact t.
  zinc turbidity t. (ZTT)
Testamone
Testandro
Testaqua
testes (*pl. of* testis)
Testex
testicle
testicular
  t. biopsy
  t. cancer
  t. cyst
  t. germ cell carcinoma (TGCC)
  t. germ cell tumor (TGCT)
  t. leukemia
  t. metastasis

  t. non-Hodgkin lymphoma
  t. parenchyma
  t. relapse
  t. self-examination
  t. seminoma
  t. sperm extraction (TESE)
  t. thymoma
  t. torsion
  t. tubular adenoma
  t. tumor
testiculoepididymal groove
testing
  antiphosphatidylserine-prothrombin complex antibody t.
  aPS antibody t.
  bcl-10 gene t.
  BRCA1 genetic t.
  BRCA genetic t.
  CD44H t.
  CD95 breast cancer t.
  CD137 t.
  cyclooxygenase-1 t.
  cyclooxygenase-2 t.
  D-dimer t.
  delta-aminolevulinate dehydratase t.
  fecal occult blood t.
  genetic t.
  guaiac t.
  HEK293-p53-EGFP cellular t.
  histocompatibility t.
  HPV DNA t.
  human papillomavirus DNA t.
  human progesterone receptor gene polymorphism t.
  hyal-1 t.
  hyal-2 t.
  hyaluronic acid t.
  hyaluronidase t.
  hypothesis t.
  lung function t.
  manometric t.
  microsatellite instability t.
  MSI t.
  neurodevelopment t.
  nucleic acid t. (NAT)
  occult blood t.
  PFA-100 t.
  platelet function analyzer t.
  prenatal t.
  PROGINS t.
  radiation sensitivity t.
  RASSF1A gene t.
  serum carboxyterminal telopeptide t.
  somatostatin subtype t.
  tangent screen t.
  visual acuity t.
testis, pl. **testes**
  t. cancer
  cryptorchid t.

ectopia t.
interstitial cell tumor of t.
maldescended t.
mediastinum t.
sarcoma of t.
tunica vaginalis t.
testolactone
Testopel Pellet
testosterone
T. Aqueous
cyclophosphamide, methotrexate, 5-
fluorouracil, vincristine,
Adriamycin, t. (CMFVAT)
t. cypionate
t. enanthate
free t.
t. priming
Testred
Testrin
TET
thymic epithelial tumor
tetanus
t. antigen
t. immune globulin
t. immune globulin human
tetanus-pertussis
tetany
tetraacetate
ethylene diamine t.
tripotassium ethylene diamine t.
tetraazacyclododecanetetraacetic
t. acid (DOTA)
t. tetramethylene phosphonate
(DOTP)
tetracaine
tetracycline
intrapleural t.
Tetracyn
tetradecanoyl phorbol acetate
tetradiploid tumor
tetrahydrate
disodium clodronate t.
tetrahydrofolate
tetrahydrouridine (THU)
tetralogy
pink t.
tetramer
tetranectin
plasma t.
stromal t.
tetraphenylborate
tetraplatin
tetraploid tumor

tetrazolium
t. bromide
nitroblue t.
tetrofosmin
^{99m}Tc t.
TEV
talipes equinovarus
texaphyrin
gadolinium t. (Gd-Tex)
lutetium t.
Texas
T. Cancer Genetics Consortium
T. cocktail
tezacitabine
Tf
transferrin
TFD
thin film dressing
Bioclusive TFD
OpSite TFD
Tegaderm TFD
Uniflex TFD
TFF
trefoil factor protein
TFF1
trefoil factor peptide 1
TfR concentration
6-TG
6-thioguanine
Tg
thyroglobulin
serum Tg
T-gamma
T-g. lymphoma
T-g. lymphoproliferative disorder
T-g. proliferative disease
TGCC
testicular germ cell carcinoma
TGCT
testicular germ cell tumor
T-Gesic
TGF
therapeutic gain factor
TGFa
transforming growth factor a
TGF-alpha
transforming growth factor alpha
TGF-beta
transforming growth factor beta
T1GFR
type 1 growth factor receptor
TGI
tumor gene index

NOTES

549

TH
  Tamm-Horsfall
  tyrosine hydroxylase
    TH mucoprotein
    TH protein
Th
  T helper cell
Th1
  T helper cell 1
Th2
  T helper cell 2
Th1-associated cytokine
Th1-type T cell
Th2-type T cell
thalamic-hypothalamic mass
thalamic infiltrating glioma
thalassemia
  t. intermedia
  t. major
thalidomide
  t. analog
  BCNU and t.
  carboplatin and t.
  temozolomide plus t.
Thalitone
thallium-201 (^{201}Tl)
Thalomid sNDA
THE
  transhiatal esophagectomy
theca, pl. thecae
  t. cell tumor
thecal sac
thecoma
  luteinized t.
  t. of ovary
Theelin Aqueous
Theiler
  T. murine encephalomyelitis virus
  T. virus infection
theme
  recurrent relationship t.
  supportive-expressive t.
thenylidene
theophylline
theorem
theory, pl. theories
  cellular immunity t.
  clonal deletion t.
  clonal selection t.
  darwinian t.
  decision t.
  Ehrlich t.
  Fisher-Race t.
  Frerich t.
  Jerne t.
  lattice t.
  Metchnikoff cellular immunity t.
  natural selection t.
  network t.

  proton beam single-beam t.
  somatic mutation t.
  unitarian t.
Therabid
theraccine
  melanoma t.
TheraCys
Theradex
Theradigm-HBV
Theragran
  T. Hematinic
  T. Liquid
Theragran-M
Theragyn
therapeutic
  t. approach
  t. bronchoscopy
  t. colonoscopy
  t. drug monitoring (TDM)
  t. gain factor (TGF)
  hemoglobin glutamer-250 oxygen-
    based t.
  t. lymph node dissection (TLND)
  t. microsphere
  oxygen t.
  prototype t.
  t. radiology
  t. response
  t. species
  t. synergism
  t. synergy
therapy, pl. therapies
  ablation t.
  ablative t.
  accelerated fractionated radiation t.
  accelerated hyperfractionated
    radiation t.
  accelerated radiation t.
  adeno p53 t.
  adjuvant postradiation t.
  adoptive cell transfer t.
  adoptive cellular t. (ACT)
  alkylator t.
  allogeneic cellular immune t.
    (ACIT)
  all-*trans*-retinoic acid, daunomycin,
    arsenic trioxide sequential t.
  alternating triple T. (ATT)
  amino acid t.
  5-aminolevulinic acid
    photodynamic t. (ALA-PDT)
  androgen ablation t.
  androgen deprivation t. (ADT)
  androgen suppression t. (AST)
  angiostatin with radiation t.
  anthracycline-based t.
  antiangiogenesis gene t.
  antiangiogenic t.
  antibiotic t.

antibody-directed enzyme prodrug t. (ADEPT)
antiestrogen t.
antifungal t.
antineoplastic t.
antineoplaston A10 and As2-1 t.
antiplatelet t.
antipleiotrophin t.
antiretroviral t. (ART)
anti-T-cell t.
anti-toxo t.
antitoxoplasma t.
antiviral t.
arc t.
autologous cellular t.
autolymphocyte t.
B1 t.
Berlin-Frankfurt-Munster t.
beta-ray ophthalmic plaque t.
Bexxar t.
biochemopreventive t.
biologic t.
blood component t.
bone-targeted t.
boost t.
boron neutron capture t. (BNCT)
brain tumor t.
breast-conserving t. (BCT)
calcium antagonist t.
Cancell t.
cellular immune t.
cesium t.
chelation t.
chemoendocrine t.
chemohormonal t.
chemoradiation t.
cognitive t.
cognitive-behavioral t.
combination antiretroviral t.
combination hormone t.
combined antiretroviral t. (CART)
combined modality t. (CMT)
compartmental radioimmunoglobulin t.
complex decongestive t.
complex lymphedema t.
composite cyclic t. (CCT)
computer-controlled conformal radiation t. (CCRT, CC-RT)
concomitant antiviral t.
concomitant triple antiretroviral t.
conformal proton t.
conformal radiation t. (CRT)

consolidation t.
continuous hyperfractionated accelerated radiation t. (CHART)
continuous renal replacement t.
craniosacral t.
crossfire radiation t.
cyclosporine t.
cytokine t.
decongestive lymphatic t. (DLT)
definitive radiation t.
dendritic cell t.
diet t.
dietary t.
differentiation-inducing t.
3-dimensional conformal t.
directly observed t. (DOT)
dose escalated and tailored FEC t.
dose-escalation BCNU t.
3-drug antiviral t.
electroconvulsive t. (ECT)
electron beam intraoperative radiation t. (EB-IORT)
electron beam radiation t.
empiric t.
endocrine t.
endourological t.
estrogen replacement t. (ERT)
experimental t.
extended-field irradiation t.
external beam radiation t. (EBRT, ERT)
external x-ray t.
ex vivo gene t.
fast neutron radiation t.
fibrinolytic t.
first-line salvage t.
Fletcher-Suit system for radium t.
focal cranial radiation t. (FCRT)
Foscan mediated photodynamic t.
fractionated radiation t.
Functional Assessment of Cancer T. (FACT)
ganciclovir t.
gene replacement t.
gene transfer t.
Gerson t.
Gliadel wafer t.
hadron t.
half-body radiation t.
HBO t.
HDR intracavitary radiation t.
helium ion t.
hematoporphyrin t.

NOTES

therapy *(continued)*

- heparin-fragment t.
- Herceptin antineoplasm t.
- herpes viral t.
- high-dose t. (HDT)
- high dose rate intracavitary t.
- highly active antiretroviral t. (HAART)
- hormonal ablative t.
- hormone replacement t. (HRT)
- HS-tk gene t.
- HSV-tk with ganciclovir t.
- hyperbaric oxygen t.
- hyperthermia t.
- hypofractionated radiation t.
- IFNa and CRA t.
- ImmTher t.
- immune-mediated t.
- immunoaugmentative t.
- immunomodulatory t.
- immunosuppressive t.
- individualized mutant p53 peptide-pulsed cultured autologous dendritic cell t.
- induction t.
- innovative t.
- instillational t.
- intensity-modulated arc t.
- intensity-modulated radiation t. (IMRT)
- interferon alpha t.
- interlesional t.
- internal radiation t.
- interstitial photon-radiosurgical t.
- interstitial radiation t.
- intraarterial t.
- intracavernous injection t.
- intracavitary t.
- intralesional t.
- intraoperative radiation t. (IORT)
- intrathecal t.
- intravascular radiation t.
- intravenous ozone t.
- intraventricular t.
- intravesical t. (IVT)
- invasive t.
- isolation perfusion t.
- laser t.
- late intensive t.
- LDR intracavitary radiation t.
- lens-sparing external beam radiation t. (LSRT)
- liver-directed t.
- local radiation t.
- low dose rate intracavity t.
- low-level laser t. (LLLT)
- magnetic t.
- Manchester system for radium t.
- medical t.
- megavitamin t.
- methylprednisolone pulse t. (MPPT)
- microwave coagulation t.
- modified systemic Berlin-Frankfurt-Munster t.
- mold t.
- monoclonal antibody t.
- movement t.
- multimodality t.
- multimodal physical t.
- multiple agent t. (MAT)
- music t.
- mutant Ras peptide-pulsed dendritic cell t.
- myoablative t.
- NanoInvasive t.
- NDV t.
- neoadjuvant t.
- neutron capture t.
- new approaches to brain tumor t. (NABTT)
- Newcastle disease virus t.
- nonpharmacologic t.
- nonsealed radionuclide t.
- nutritional t.
- ocular radiation t. (ORT)
- oral rehydration t.
- oscillation t.
- oxygen t.
- palliative radiation t.
- parenteral phosphate t.
- Paris method for radium t.
- particle beam radiation t.
- PCV t.
- PEIT t.
- percutaneous ethanol injection t. (PEIT)
- percutaneous microwave coagulation t. (PMCT)
- percutaneous transcatheter t.
- perfusion t.
- peroral cone radiation t.
- photodynamic t. (PDT)
- photon-radiosurgical t. (PRS)
- platinum t.
- plesiocurie t.
- postmenopausal estrogen t.
- postoperative radiation t. (PORT)
- postradiation t.
- primary healing after radiation t.
- prophylactic t.
- ProSure nutritional t.
- proton beam t.
- protracted intravenous infusion t.
- pyretic t.
- radiation t., radiotherapy (RT)
- radioimmunoglobulin t. (RIT)
- radiopharmaceutical t.
- radium t.

real-time tumor tracking radiation t. (RTRT)
recurrent t.
Reiki t.
renal infusion t.
renal replacement t.
reprogramming t.
rIFN-gamma t.
roentgen-ray t.
Roferon and Accutane t.
rotation t.
salvage t.
second-line t.
sequential hormone t.
sole laser t.
somatic gene t.
splenic radiation t.
split-course radiation t.
STAMP t.
standard t.
stem cell gene t.
stereotactic radiation t.
steroid t.
Stockholm technique for radium t.
streptokinase t.
structure-directed oscillation t.
suppressive thyroxine t.
suramin t.
systemic antibiotic t.
systemic radioimmunoglobulin t.
T-101 t.
targeted alpha-particle t.
Taxotere and doxorubicin neoadjuvant t.
telecobalt t.
thoracic conformal radiation t. (TCRT)
TNP-470 and BCNU t.
total B t.
total skin electron beam t. (TSEBT)
transplantation t.
transpupillary thermal t. (TTT)
trimodal t.
trimodality t.
Trinam gene t.
triple intrathecal t. (TIT)
tumor t.
tumor-amplified protein expression t. (TAPET)
ultraviolet irradiation t.
unconventional t.
unorthodox t.
unproven t.
unsealed internal radiation t.
vaccine t.
ventilator t.
warfarin t.
whole body radiation t.
whole brain radiation t. (WBRT)
wide-field radiation t. (WFRT)
wide-range radiation t.
XKnife software for stereotatic radiation t.
x-ray t. (XRT)

therapy-bladder
    Functional Assessment of Cancer T.-B. (FACT-BL)
therapy-fatigue
    Functional Assessment of Cancer T.-F. (FACT-F)
therapy-related myelodysplastic syndrome (T-MDS)
TheraSeed
Theratope-STn
Theratope vaccine
thermal
    t. ablation
    t. debulking technique
    t. enhancement ratio (TER)
    t. modeling
Thermistor catheter
ThermoChem-HT system
thermochemotherapy
    intraperitoneal t.
ThermoChem system
thermocouple
thermography
    liquid crystal t.
thermoluminescence dosimeter
thermoluminescent dosimeter (TLD)
thermometer
    Distress t.
    First Temp Genius tympanic t.
    Thermoscan Pro-1 instant t.
thermometry
    invasive t.
    magnetic resonance imaging t.
    MRI t.
    noninvasive t.
thermoradiosensitization
thermoradiotherapy (TRT)
    simultaneous t. (STRT)
thermorhizotomy
    gasserian t.
Thermoscan Pro-1 instant thermometer

NOTES

thermotherapy
 transurethral microwave t. (TUMT)
thermotolerance
theta herpesvirus
thiacytidine
thiamine
thiamiprine
thickening
 antral mucosal t.
 apical pleural t.
 bladder wall t.
 diffuse t.
 mucosal t.
 nasal t.
 nodular t.
 pleural t.
 postbiopsy skin t.
 postlumpectomy skin t.
 secondary skin t.
 skin t.
 sternoclavicular t.
thickness
 bladder wall t.
 Breslow t.
 endometrial t.
thiethylperazine maleate
thin
 t. film dressing (TFD)
 t. melanoma
thinning
 white matter t.
ThinPrep
 T. Pap Test
 T. 2000 processor
thioethanol phosphotriester
thioflavin T
6-thioguanine (6-TG)
 6-t., ara-C, daunomycin (TAD)
 6-t., ara-C, daunorubicin (TAD)
 ara-C plus 6-t.
 6-t., asparaginase, BCNU,
  hydroxyurea
 BCNU, ara-C,
  cyclophosphamide, 6-t. (BACT)
 cyclophosphamide, vincristine,
  prednisone, daunomycin,
  methotrexate, cytarabine, 6-t.
 6-t. and cytarabine (TC)
 cytarabine and 6-t. (CT)
 cytarabine, Adriamycin, 6-t. (CAT)
 cytarabine plus 6-t.
 cytosine arabinoside and 6-t.
  (CAT)
 cytosine arabinoside,
  Adriamycin, 6-t. (CAT)
 daunomycin, cytarabine, 6-t.
 daunorubicin, ara-C, 6-t. (DAT)
 daunorubicin, cytarabine, 6-t. (DCT)

 6-t., methotrexate, Oncovin,
  prednisone (T-MOP)
 6-t., Oncovin, cytosine arabinoside,
  prednisone (TOAP)
 6-t., procarbazine, CCNU,
  hydroxyurea (TPCH)
 6-t., procarbazine, DBC, CCNU,
  vincristine (TPDCV)
 6-t., procarbazine, dibromodulcitol,
  CCNU, 5-fluorouracil, hydroxyurea
 6-t., procarbazine, dibromodulcitol,
  CCNU, vincristine (TPDCV)
 6-t., rubidomycin, ara-C,
  methotrexate, prednisolone,
  cyclophosphamide, Oncovin
 6-t., rubidomycin, ara-C, prednisone
  (TRAP)
 vincristine, ara-C, 6-t. (VAT)
thiol compound
thionamide
thiopental
 sodium t.
Thioplex
thioridazine
thiosemicarbazone
thiosulfate
 sodium t.
thiotepa (TSPA)
 busulfan, melphalan, t.
 t. and carboplatin
 t., etoposide, carboplatin (TEC)
 melphalan and t.
 mitoxantrone, VePesid, t. (MVT)
 mitoxantrone, VP-16, t. (MVT)
 vinblastine, Adriamycin, t. (VAT)
Third National Cancer Survey
thistle
 milk t.
Thoma-Zeiss counting cell
Thomsen-Friedenreich T antigen
Thomson scattering
ThoraCath catheter
thoracentesis
thoraces (*pl. of* thorax)
thoracic
 t. cancer
 t. conformal radiation therapy
  (TCRT)
 t. esophagectomy
 t. gibbus
 t. inlet
 t. spinal neoplasm
thoracoscope
thoracoscopic lobectomy
thoracoscopy
 video-assisted t.
thoracostomy
 tube t.
 t. tube

thoracotomy
thorax, pl. **thoraces**
    bony t.
Thorazine
Thoreus #3 filter
Thorotrast
    T. contrast agent
    T. contrast medium
Thorson-Bioerck syndrome
threat
    home, education, abuse, drugs,
      safety, friends, image, recreation,
      sexuality, t.'s (HEADS FIRST)
threatened pathologic fracture
threonine 215 tyrosine mutation
threshold dose
thrive
    failure to t.
throat
    Vicks Chloraseptic Sore T.
thrombasthenia
    Glanzmann t.
Thrombate III
thrombi (*pl. of* thrombus)
thrombin-antithrombin III complex
thrombin-stimulated platelets
thromboanoic acid
thrombocyte
thrombocythemia
    essential t.
    hemorrhagic t.
    idiopathic t.
    primary t.
thrombocytic leukemia
thrombocytopathic
thrombocytopathy
thrombocytopenia
    amegakaryocytic t.
    autoimmune neonatal t.
    heparin-induced t. (HIT)
    HIV-associated t.
    hypoproliferative t.
    idiopathic t.
    immune t.
    immune-mediated t.
    isoimmune neonatal t.
    malignant t.
    thrombotic t.
thrombocytopenia-absent
    t.-a. radius (TAR)
    t.-a. radius syndrome
thrombocytopenic purpura (TP)

thrombocytosis
    paraneoplastic t.
    primary t.
thromboembolectomy
    percutaneous aspiration t.
thromboembolic
    t. disease
    t. pulmonary arterial hypertension
thromboembolism
    venous t.
Thrombogen
thrombogenic coil
thrombolytic time
thrombomodulin antibody
thrombopenia
thrombopenic anemia
thrombophilia
    genetic t.
thrombophilic state
thrombophlebitis
    deep vein t.
    superficial t.
thromboplastin
thrombopoiesis
thrombopoietin (TPO)
    t. growth factor
thrombosis, pl. **thromboses**
    aortic t.
    ascending medullary vein t.
    atrial t.
    axillosubclavian vein t.
    calf vein t.
    catheter-induced subclavian vein t.
    catheter-related t.
    coronary t.
    deep venous t. (DVT)
    dural sinus t.
    European Concerted Action on T.
     (ECAT)
    idiopathic venous t.
    intervillous t.
    sagittal t.
    sinus t.
    splenic vein t.
    subclavian vein t.
    subclavian vessel t.
    superior ophthalmic vein t.
    superior sagittal sinus t.
    venous t.
thrombospondin
    Asserachrom t.
    plasma t.
thrombotherapy

NOTES

thrombotic
    t. microangiopathy (TMA)
    t. occlusion
    t. stroke
    t. thrombocytopenia
    t. thrombocytopenic purpura (TTP)
Thrombo-Wellco test
thromboxane
thrombus, pl. thrombi
    anechoic t.
    ball t.
    mural t.
    tumor t.
thrush
    oral t.
THU
    tetrahydrouridine
thymalfasin
thymectomy
thymic
    t. alymphoplasia
    t. carcinoid
    t. carcinoma (TCA)
    t. cortex
    t. enlargement
    t. epithelial neoplasm
    t. epithelial tumor (TET)
    t. humoral factor
    t. interdigitating dendritic cell
    t. involution
    t. leukemia
    t. lymphocyte
    t. lymphocyte antigen
    t. lymphoma
    t. remnant
thymic-dependent deficiency
thymidine
    t. analog
    2-[C-11]-t. PET study
    t. deoxyriboside (TDR)
    hypoxanthine aminopterin t. (HAT)
    t. kinase (TK)
    t. labeling index (TLI)
    t. phosphorylase
    t. triphosphate
thymidylate
    t. complex
    t. kinase
    t. synthase (TS)
    t. synthase expression
thymine dimer
Thymitaq
thymocyte
Thymoglobulin
thymolipoma
thymolipomatous hamartoma
thymoma
    atypical t.
    t. cancer

cortical t.
epithelial-rich t.
invasive t.
Masaoka staging system for t.
medullary t.
mixed t.
polygonal cell-type t.
testicular t.
thymopentin
thymosin
thymostimulin (TP-1)
thymus-dependent lymphopoiesis
Thyro-Block
thyrocalcitonin hormone
Thyrogen
thyroglobulin (Tg)
    athyreotic t.
    t. reactivity
    serum t.
thyrohyoid membrane
thyroid
    t. adenoma
    t. cancer
    t. carcinoma
    t. cartilage
    t. cystadenoma
    follicular adenocarcinoma of t.
    t. function
    t. gland
    t. hormone
    insular carcinoma of t.
    t. lymphoma
    medullary carcinoma of t. (MCT)
    t. needle biopsy
    t. nodule ablation
    t. notch
    t. tracheal tumor
thyroidectomy
    near-total t.
    subtotal t.
    total t. (TT)
thyroiditis
    acute suppurative t.
    de Quervain t.
    Hashimoto t.
    lymphocytic t.
**thyroid-peroxidase autoantibody
  (TPO.Ab)**
thyroid-stimulating hormone (TSH)
Thyrolar
thyroperoxidase (TPO)
    t. antibody test
thyrotoxicosis
thyrotropic substance
thyrotropin alfa
thyrotropin-producing adenoma
thyrotropin-releasing
    t.-r. factor
    t.-r. hormone (TRH)

thyroxin-binding globulin
thyroxine
tiagabine
TIAP
  totally implantable access port
tiazofurin
Tiazole
TIBC
  total iron-binding capacity
tibia
  t. aplasia
  t. aplasia association
tibial agenesis
Ticar
ticarcillin and clavulanate potassium
TICE BCG
tidal volume
tie-on needle
tigroid pattern
Tikhoff-Linberg
  T.-L. procedure
  T.-L. resection
TIL
  tumor-infiltrating lymphocyte
  TIL cell
tilorone
tiludronate
time
  acquisition t.
  activated clotting t. (ACT)
  activated coagulation t. (ACT)
  activated partial thromboplastin t.
    (APTT)
  background equivalent radiation t.
  bleeding t.
  carcinoembryonic antigen
    doubling t. (CEA-DT)
  cerebral circulation t.
  circulation t.
  closure t.
  clot retraction t.
  clotting t.
  cycle t.
  Dale-Laidlaw clotting t.
  delay t.
  diffusion t. (T_d)
  Duke bleeding t.
  ecarin clotting t. (ECT)
  effective transverse relation t.
  efficient relaxation t.
  euglobulin lysis t.
  hematologic recovery t.
  Ivy bleeding t.

  Lee-White clotting t.
  median survival t. (MST)
  partial thromboplastin t. (PTT)
  prostate-specific antigen doubling t.
    (PSADT)
  prothrombin t. (PT)
  repetition t. (TR)
  reptilase t.
  Russell's viper venom clotting t.
  survival t. (ST)
  thrombolytic t.
  tumor doubling t.
  t. without symptoms and toxicity
    (TwiST)
Timecelles
  Cebid T.
Timentin
time-of-flight
  surface-enhanced laser desorption
    and ionization t.-o.-f. (SELDI-
    TOF)
time-release
  t.-r. ara-C
  t.-r. form
time-resolved imaging
time-to-treatment failure (TTF)
T-immunoblastic sarcoma
TIMP
  tissue inhibitor of metalloproteinase
TIMP-1
  tissue inhibitor of matrix
    metalloproteinase-1
Timunox
Tinactin
tincture
  Fungoid T.
  opium t.
tinea
  t. capitis
  t. corporis
  t. cruris
  t. pedis
tin ethyl etiopurpurin
tinnitus
  pulsatile t.
tinzaparin
  t. sodium injectable
  t. sodium injection
tioconazole
tip
  catheter t.
  Combitip Plus pipette t.

NOTES

557

tip *(continued)*
    rectal t.
    smart laser catheter t.
tipifarnib
TIPS
    transjugular intrahepatic portosystemic
    shunt
tirapazamine
tiratricol
Tirazone
TIS
    trabecular insular solid
    tumor, immune, systemic
    tumor in situ
        TIS carcinoma
        TIS staging system
tissue
    t. adhesive
    adipose t.
    anisotropic t.
    t. autotransplantation
    t. bank
    t. block
    t. blocking
    bronchial-associated lymphoid t.
      (BALT)
    bronchus-associated lymphoid t.
      (BALT)
    central lymphoid t.
    connective t.
    core of t.
    ectopic t.
    engrafted allogenic t.
    t. factor
    formalin-fixed t.
    freeze-dried paraffin-embedded t.
    glandular t.
    gut-associated lymphoid t. (GALT)
    t. heterogeneity
    histiocytic t.
    human hemopoietic t.
    t. hyperplasia
    t. inhibitor
    t. inhibitor of matrix
      metalloproteinase-1 (TIMP-1)
    t. inhibitor of metalloproteinase
      (TIMP)
    t. inhibitor of metalloproteinase-2
      assay
    t. iron
    Late Effects of Normal T. (LENT)
    t. lymph
    lymphoid t.
    malignant fibrous histiocytoma of
      soft t.
    mesothelial t.
    microscopically normal t.
    mucosa-associated lymphoid t.
      (MALT)

    mutation in hematopoietic t.
    neural t.
    normal t.
    paracervical t.
    t. perfusion
    peritumoral t.
    t. plasminogen activator (TPA)
    t. polypeptide antigen (TPA)
    t. sampling
    scar t.
    t. section
    soft t.
    syngeneic t.
    t. tolerance
    t. tolerance to radiation
    t. trauma
    tumoral t.
    vasculoconnective t.
    visceral adipose t. (VAT)
tissue-air ratio (TAR)
tissue-equivalent bolus
tissue-maximum ratio (TMR)
tissue-phantom ratio (TPR)
tissue-sparing technique
TIT
    triple intrathecal therapy
titer
    antibody t.
    antigen t.
    anti-HHV8 antibody t.
    anti-human herpesvirus 8
      antibody t.
    antistreptolysin O titer
    ASO t.
    CEA t.
    cerebrospinal fluid cryptococcal
      antigen t.
    CSF cryptococcal antigen t.
    fungal immunodiffusion t.
    hemagglutination t.
    log infectious virus t.
    nontreponemal antibody t.
    plasma antibody t.
    vaccine antigen-specific antibody t.
Titralac Plus Liquid
tiuxetan
    ibritumomab t.
    Y ibritumomab t.
TK
    thymidine kinase
^{201}Tl
    thallium-201
TLD
    thermoluminescent dosimeter
    tumor lethal dose
TLI
    thymidine labeling index
    total lymphoid irradiation
    tritiated thymidine labeling index

TLND
therapeutic lymph node dissection
TLP
tumor-liberated particle
TM
transmembrane
TM gp41
TMA
thrombotic microangiopathy
T-MDS
therapy-related myelodysplastic
syndrome
TME
total mesorectal excision
TMIF
tumor cell migration-inhibition factor
T-MOP
6-thioguanine, methotrexate, Oncovin,
prednisone
TMP
trimethoprim
TMP-SMX
trimethoprim-sulfamethoxazole
TMP-SMX-intolerant individual
TMQ
trimetrexate
TMR
tissue-maximum ratio
topical magnetic resonance
TMS
trimodal spectroscopy
TMT
Trail Making Test
TMTX
trimetrexate
TMX
tamoxifen
TMZ
temozolomide
TND
twenty-nail dystrophy
TNF
tumor necrosis factor
TNF receptor-associated death
domain
TNF receptor-associated death
domain protein
TNFa
tumor necrosis factor a
TNF-alpha
tumor necrosis factor-alpha
TNF-alpha kinoid
TNF-alpha mRNA

TNF-beta
tumor necrosis factor-beta
TNFerade
TNFR
tumor necrosis factor receptor
TNF-related apoptosis-inducing ligand
TNFSF
tumor necrosis factor superfamily
TNKase
TNM
tumor, node, metastasis
TNM classification
TNM staging system
TNP-470 and BCNU therapy
TOAP
6-thioguanine, Oncovin, cytosine
arabinoside, prednisone
tobacco
black t.
blond t.
loose-leaf t.
plug t.
t. pouch keratosis
smokeless t.
twist t.
tobacco-specific nitrosamine (TSNA)
TOBI Inhalation Solution
tobramycin
Tobrex Ophthalmic
Tocantins bone marrow biopsy needle
tocopherol (T)
alpha t.
Tocosol Paclitaxel
Tod and Meredith system
Tofranil
Tofranil-PM
toilet
bronchopulmonary t.
Tolectin DS
tolerance
antigen t.
drug t.
Fletcher rule of irradiation t.
immune t.
immunologic t.
rectosigmoid irradiation t.
rectum irradiation t.
tissue t.
tolerogen
tolmetin
tolnaftate
toluene

NOTES

toluidine
    t. blue
    t. blue stain
tomato tumor
tomodensitometric examination
tomography
    automated computerized axial t. (ACAT)
    t. cine CT
    computed t. (CT)
    computed tomography-single photon emission computed t. (CT/SPECT)
    computerized axial t.
    cone-beam computed t.
    contrast-enhanced computed t. (CECT)
    3-dimensional computed t.
    dynamic computed t. (DCT)
    electrical impedance t. (EIT)
    emission computed t. (ECT)
    expiratory computed t.
    F-fluorodeoxyglucose dual-head positron emission t. (FDG-PET)
    fluorodeoxyglucose positron emission t. (FDG-PET)
    high-resolution computed t. (HRCT)
    megavoltage computed t.
    optical coherence t. (OCT)
    positron emission t. (PET)
    quantitative computed t. (QCT)
    single-photon emission t. (SPET)
    single-photon emission computed t. (SPECT)
tomosynthesis
tomotherapy
    helical t.
    sequential t.
    serial t.
Tomudex
tongue
    t. base
    squamous cell carcinoma of oral t. (SCCOT)
    t. of tumor
Tonnesen catheter
tonometry
    skin t.
tonsil
    t. cancer
    cerebellar t.
tonsillar
    t. area cancer
    t. pillar
tonsurans
    Trichophyton t.
tooth, pl. **teeth**
    t. abrasion
    carious teeth

    high-arched teeth
    Hutchinson teeth
Topamax
topical
    t. anesthetic
    Canesten T.
    t. chemotherapy
    Cleocin T T.
    Clinda-Derm T.
    Corticaine T.
    Dalacin C T.
    t. 4,4′-dihydroxybenzophenone-2,4-dinitrophenylhydrazone (A-007) 0.25% gel
    t. effect
    Efudex T.
    Exelderm T.
    Fluoroplex T.
    t. 5-FU
    Gelfoam T.
    t. magnetic resonance (TMR)
    Micatin T.
    t. microbicide
    Monistat-Derm T.
    Mycelex-G T.
    Mycogen II T.
    Mycolog-II T.
    Myconel T.
    Mytrex F T.
    Oxistat T.
    t. photochemotherapy
    t. podophyllin
    t. terbinafine
topiramate
topoisomerase (I-II) inhibitor
Toposar Injection
topotecan (TPT)
    cyclophosphamide, cytosine arabinoside, t. (CAT)
    t. HCl
    t. hydrochloride
    t. plus BCNU
    t., vincristine, doxorubicin (TVD)
Toradol
TORCH
    toxoplasmosis, other infections, rubella, cytomegalovirus infection, herpes simplex
    TORCH syndrome
Torecan
toremifene citrate
torpedo
    Gelfoam t.
torque (T)
torsemide
torsion
    acute testicular t.
    extravaginal testicular t.
    testicular t.

Toshiba SSA-380A ultrasound
tositumomab
^{131}I t.
total
  t. abdominal hysterectomy (TAH)
  t. abdominal hysterectomy and
   bilateral salpingo-oophorectomy
   (TAHBSO)
  t. adenine deoxyribonucleotide
   (dAXP)
  t. androgen ablation
  t. androgen blockade
  t. bilirubin
  t. body aromatization
  t. body bone mineral content
   (TBBMC)
  t. body irradiation (TBI)
  t. body surface area (TBSA)
  t. B therapy
  t. dose over time concept
  t. enteral nutrition
  t. gastrectomy
  t. glossectomy
  t. hormonal ablation
  t. iron-binding capacity (TIBC)
  t. lymphoid irradiation (TLI)
  t. mesorectal excision (TME)
  T. Mood Disturbance Scale
  t. nodal irradiation
  t. parenteral nutrition (TPN)
  t. pelvic exenteration (TPE)
  t. reference air-kerma (TRAK)
  t. serum prostatic acid phosphatase
   (TSPAP)
  t. simple prophylactic mastectomy
  t. skin electron beam therapy
   (TSEBT)
  t. thoracic esophagectomy (TTE)
  t. thyroidectomy (TT)
  t. vaginal hysterectomy
  t. white cell count
totally
  t. implantable access port (TIAP)
  t. implantable catheter
toto
  in t.
touch preparation
tourniquet
  scalp t.
  t. technique
Touton giant cell
toxic
  t. agranulocytosis

  t. granulation
  t. methemoglobinemia
  t. oil syndrome
toxicity
  amphotericin B t.
  bone marrow t.
  chemotherapy-induced pulmonary t.
  cyclosporine t.
  delayed acute radiation t.
  digitalis t.
  dose-limiting t. (DLT)
  drug t.
  endocrine t.
  epithelial t.
  ethambutol t.
  extramedullary t.
  hematologic t.
  isoniazid t.
  itraconazole t.
  late central nervous system t.
   (LCNST)
  mucosal t.
  myocardial t.
  neuromuscular t.
  nonhematologic t.
  nonmyelosuppressive t.
  ocular t.
  organ t.
  pulmonary t.
  pyrazinamide t.
  quality-adjusted time without
   symptoms and t. (Q-TWiST)
  radiation-induced pulmonary t.
  renal t.
  rifampin t.
  saquinavir-related t.
  time without symptoms and t.
   (TwiST)
toxicity-efficacy ratio
toxin
  bacterial t.
  Coley t.
  DABIL-2 t.
  interleukin-4 fusion t.
  reproductive t.
toxinic
Toxoplasma
  T. encephalitis
  T. *gondii*
  T. IgG antibody
  T. retinitis
toxoplasmosis
  cerebral t.

NOTES

toxoplasmosis *(continued)*
  t. lymphadenopathy
  ocular t.
  t., other infections, rubella,
    cytomegalovirus infection, herpes
    simplex (TORCH)
TP
  thrombocytopenic purpura
TP1
  telomerase-associated protein
TP-1
  thymostimulin
TPA
  tissue plasminogen activator
  tissue polypeptide antigen
    TPA tumor marker
TPCH
  6-thioguanine, procarbazine, CCNU,
    hydroxyurea
TPDCV
  6-thioguanine, procarbazine, DBC,
    CCNU, vincristine
  6-thioguanine, procarbazine,
    dibromodulcitol, CCNU, vincristine
TPE
  2-photon excitation
  total pelvic exenteration
TPF
  Taxotere, Platinol, 5-fluorouracil
TPI
  trigger point injection
TPN
  total parenteral nutrition
TPO
  thrombopoietin
  thyroperoxidase
TPO.Ab
  thyroid-peroxidase autoantibody
TPOG
  Taiwan Pediatric Oncology Group
    TPOG AML 901 protocol
T-Pouch technique
TPR
  tissue-phantom ratio
TPS
  telescopic plate spacer
TPT
  topotecan
TR
  repetition time
TRA
  trans-retinoic acid
trabecular
  t. carcinoma
  t. insular solid (TIS)
  t. insular solid carcinoma
  t. meshwork
  t. pattern
trabeculated bone lesion

trace metals
tracer
  t. accumulation
  carbon dioxide t.
  deposition of t.
trachea
  posterior membranous t.
tracheal
  t. deviation
  t. stoma
  t. stricture
  t. tumor
tracheitis
trachelectomy
  radical vaginal t.
tracheobronchial
  t. injury (TBI)
  t. stent
  t. tree
tracheobronchitis
  necrotizing superficial t.
tracheoesophageal (TE)
  t. fistula (TEF)
  t. puncture (TEP)
tracheostomy tube
Trach-Eze closed suction catheter
trachomatis
  Chlamydia t.
tracing
  direct ray t.
  M-mode t.
track
  needle t.
  t. of pin
Tracker-18 Unibody catheter
Tracker coaxial infusion catheter
tracking
  anterior t.
  bolus t.
  lymphatic t.
  tumor t.
tract
  abnormal fetal urogenital t.
  aerodigestive t.
  alimentary t.
  association t.
  biliary t.
  biopsy t.
  bronchial t.
  dermal sinus t.
  t. dilatation
  internodal t.
  pancreaticobiliary t.
  respiratory and upper digestive t.
    (RUDT)
  seeding of biopsy t.
  sinonasal t.
  tamponade needle t.

upper aerodigestive t. (UADT)
uveal t.
traction
breast t.
t. fracture
t. retinal t. (TRD)
TRADD
tumor necrosis factor receptor-associated
death domain
TRADD protein
TRAF
tumor necrosis factor receptor-associated
factor
Trager approach
tragus, pl. tragi
TRAIDS
transfusion-related AIDS
TRAIL
tumor necrosis factor-related apoptosis-
inducing ligand
Trail Making Test (TMT)
training
posture t.
trait
Lepore t.
sickle cell t.
trajectory
dying t.
TRAK
total reference air-kerma
TRAM
transverse rectus abdominis muscle
transverse rectus abdominis
myocutaneous
TRAM flap
TRAM flap reconstruction
tramadol
tranexamic acid
trans-acting responsive sequence
transactivator (TAR)
transaminase
aspartate t.
elevated t.
hepatic t.
liver t.
serum glutamic-oxaloacetic t.
(SGOT)
serum glutamic-pyruvate t. (SGPT)
transaminitis
transarticular skip metastasis
transaxillary needle

transbronchial
t. biopsy
t. needle aspiration
transbronchoscopic biopsy
transcarbamylase
ornithine t. (OTC)
transcatheter
t. arterial chemoembolization
t. arterial embolization (TAE)
t. brachytherapy
t. closure
t. occlusion
t. splenic embolization
t. therapeutic infarction
transcobalamin II
transcranial sonography
transcript
bcr/abl t.
genomic viral messenger ribonucleic
acid t.
genomic viral mRNA t.
leukemia t.
multigene t.
transcriptase
HIV reverse t.
human immunodeficiency virus
reverse t.
human telomerase reverse t.
(hTERT)
reverse t. (RT)
telomerase reverse t. (TERT)
transcription
t. factor
gene t.
RNA t.
transcriptional
t. activation
t. activator
t. mutation
t. regulation
t. silencing
transcubital approach
transcutaneous embolization
transcytosis
epithelial t.
transdermal
Alora T.
Climara T.
Duragesic T.
Esclim T.
Estraderm T.
t. estradiol

NOTES

transdermal *(continued)*
    t. medication patch
    Vivelle T.
Transderm-Nitro Patch
transduced cell
transducer
    Acuson linear array t.
    biopsy t.
    ultrasound t.
transduction
    p53-dependent signal t.
    postreceptor signal t.
    retroviral t.
    signal t.
transdural herniation
transection
    aortic t.
transfectant
    K1myc t.
transfected cell
transfection
    DNA t.
    gene t.
    locoregional t.
transfemoral venous catheterization
transfer
    activated T-cell t.
    adoptive cell t.
    cell t.
    t. characteristic
    embryo t. (ET)
    t. factor
    gene t.
    immunity t.
    linear energy t. (LET)
    magnetization t. (MT)
    osteomyocutaneous free-tissue t.
    transplacental t.
    in vivo gene t.
transferase
    adenine phosphoribosyl t.
    adenosine diphosphoribosyl t.
      (ADPRT)
    t. enterocyte
    farnesyl t. (FT)
    glutathione t.
    hypoxanthine-guanine
      phosphoribosyl t. (HxGPRT)
    N-myristoyl t.
    phosphoribosyl t. (PRT)
    terminal deoxynucleotidyl t. (TdT)
transferred immune response
transferrin (Tf)
    t. receptor
    t. saturation
transformation
    blastic t.
    lymphoblastic t.

    lymphocyte t.
    murine fibroblast t.
    plasmacytoid t.
    prolymphocytic t.
    prolymphocytoid t.
    Richter syndrome-like t.
    t. zone
transforming
    t. gene
    t. growth factor a (TGFa)
    t. growth factor alpha (TGF-alpha)
    t. growth factor beta (TGF-beta)
    t. growth factor beta4
    t. principle
transfused blood
transfusion
    allogeneic blood t.
    blood t.
    erythrocyte t.
    fetomaternal t.
    granulocyte t.
    t. hemosiderosis
    leukocyte t.
    matched lymphocyte t.
    plasma t.
    platelet t.
    t. reaction
    red blood cell t.
    SD Plasma for elimination of risk
      with t.
    t. syndrome
    white blood cell t.
transfusion-dependent
    t.-d. packed red blood cells
    t.-d. platelets
transfusion-related
    t.-r. AIDS (TRAIDS)
    t.-r. hemosiderosis
transgene
transgluteal approach
transhepatic
    t. biliary procedure
    t. sclerosis
transhiatal esophagectomy (THE)
transient
    t. angiolymphoid hyperplasia
    t. aplastic crisis (TAC)
    t. equilibrium
    t. erythroblastopenia
    t. hypogammaglobulinemia of
      infancy
    t. infection
    t. myelopathic syndrome
    t. myeloproliferative disease
    t. viral suppression
transit
    delayed small bowel t.
    t. volume

transition
  refractory anemia with excess blasts in t.
  t. zone
transitional
  t. carcinoma in situ (TCIS)
  t. cell cancer
  t. cell carcinoma (TCC)
  t. cell neoplasm
  t. cell papilloma
  t. leukocyte
  t. meningioma
transjugular intrahepatic portosystemic shunt (TIPS)
translation
  nick t.
translingual spray
translocation
  bacterial t.
  chromosomal t.
  nonreciprocal t.
  Philadelphia t.
  robertsonian t.
  t(14,18) chromosomal t.
translucency
translumbar access
transluminal brachytherapy
transmembrane (TM)
  t. domain
  t. glucoprotein
  gp41 t.
  t. protein
  t. receptor tyrosine kinase
  t. signaling
TransMID
transmissibility
transmissible venereal tumor
transmission
  airborne t.
  t. electron microscopy (TEM)
  enzootic t.
  horizontal t.
  intrafamilial t.
  male-to-female t.
  maternal-fetal t.
  mother-to-child t. (MTCT)
  occupational t.
  perinatal t.
  postnatal t.
  vertical t.
transmucosal
  Actiq Oral T.

transmural
  t. invasion
  t. penetration
transnasal intraduodenal feeding catheter
transpapillary placement
transparent film dressing
transpeptidase
  gamma-glutamyl t.
transperineal
  t. implant
  t. prostate brachytherapy
transplacental
  t. carcinogenicity
  t. transfer
transplant
  allogeneic bone marrow t. (ABMT)
  allogeneic peripheral cell t.
  autologous t. (AT)
  autologous bone marrow t. (ABMT)
  bone marrow t. (BMT)
  double t.
  high-dose chemotherapy and autologous stem cell t.
  HLA-identical sibling t.
  human-leukocyte-antigen-identical t.
  kidney t.
  marrow t.
  MUD t.
  nonmyeloablative allogeneic stem cell t.
  organ t.
  pancreatic t.
  peripheral blood stem cell t. (PBSCT)
  t. preparative regimen
  renal t.
  sequential t.
  solid organ t.
  stem cell t. (SCT)
  syngeneic bone marrow t.
  tandem t. (TAT)
  tandem stem cell t.
  t. team
  twin donor t.
transplantation
  allogeneic bone marrow t. (ABMT)
  allogeneic stem cell t.
  t. antigen
  autologous and allogeneic marrow t.
  autologous blood stem cell t.

NOTES

transplantation *(continued)*
    autologous bone marrow t.
        (ABMT, AuBMT)
    autologous hematopoietic progenitor
        cell t. (AHPCT)
    autologous hematopoietic stem
        cell t. (AHSCT)
    autologous ovarian t.
    autologous peripheral blood stem
        cell t. (APBSCT)
    blood cell allogeneic t.
    bone marrow t. (BMT)
    growth factor mobilized autologous
        peripheral blood stem cell t.
    hematopoietic stem cell t. (HSCT)
    HLA-matched peripheral blood
        mobilized hematopoietic progenitor
        cell t.
    IL-2 after allogeneic t.
    t. immunity
    t. immunology
    PB stem cell t.
    stem cell t. (SCT)
    syngeneic t.
    t. therapy
    tumor-associated t.
    tumor-specific t.
    unrelated donor bone marrow t.
        (UD-BMT)
transplatin
transport
    iron t.
    Monte Carlo photon t. (MCPT)
transporter
    ABC t.
    ATP-binding cassette t. (ABCT)
transposition
    t. flap
    laparoscopic ovarian t.
transposon insertion system
transpubic procedure
transpupillary thermal therapy (TTT)
transrectal
    t. sonography
    t. ultrasonography (TRUS)
    t. ultrasound (TRUS)
    t. ultrasound biopsy
trans-**retinoic acid (TRA)**
**TransScan TS2000 electrical impedance
    scanning system**
transscrotal orchiectomy
transseptal catheterization
transsphincteric surgery
transtentorial herniation
transthoracic
    t. esophagectomy
    t. needle aspiration (TTNA)
    t. needle biopsy

    t. percutaneous fine-needle
        aspiration biopsy
    t. procedure
transurethral
    t. balloon dilatation
    t. incision
    t. incision of prostate (TUIP)
    t. microwave (TURM)
    t. microwave thermotherapy
        (TUMT)
    t. needle ablation (TUNA)
    t. resection (TUR)
    t. resection of bladder (TURB)
    t. resection of bladder tumor
        (TUR-Bt)
    t. resection of prostate (TURP)
    t. resection of prostate ulceration
    t. ultrasound-guided laser-induced
        prostatectomy (TULIP)
transvaginal
    t. approach
    t. implant
    t. ultrasonography (TVS)
transverse
    t. colon carcinoma
    t. flap
    t. myelitis
    t. rectus abdominis muscle
        (TRAM)
    t. rectus abdominis myocutaneous
        (TRAM)
    t. relaxation
transversus
transvesical sonography
tranverse flap
TRAP
    tartrate-resistant acid phosphatase
    telomere repeat amplification protocol
    telomeric repeat amplification protocol
    6-thioguanine, rubidomycin, ara-C,
        prednisone
    TRAP assay
    TRAP positive
    TRAP stain
trap
    promoter t.
    VEGF t.
trapped lung
trapping
    air t.
trastuzumab
    Evacet and t.
Trasylol
trauma, pl. **traumata, traumas**
    abdominal t.
    tissue t.
traumatic
    t. bone cyst
    t. injury

t. lipid cyst
t. lung cyst
t. rupture
t. rupture of diaphragm (TRD)
traveler's diarrhea
Travenol
T. biopsy needle
T. Infusor pump
TRb
trilateral retinoblastoma
TRD
traction retinal detachment
traumatic rupture of diaphragm
iatrogenic TRD
treated
solvent/detergent t. (S/D)
treatment
add-on t.
adjuvant t.
allocation of t.
autolymphocyte-based t.
cancer t.
conservative t.
coumarin t.
crossfire t.
curative t.
3-dimensional-assisted conformal t.
etoposide chemotherapy t.
experimental t.
ex vivo marrow t.
first-line t.
fixed-schedule t.
hematopoietic stem cell t.
Hoxsey t.
hyperthermia t.
hypothermia t.
indomethacin t.
manual lymphedema t.
multimodal t.
oncology t.
t. option
ozone t.
palliative t.
^{32}P intraperitoneal t.
t. planning
prophylactic t.
radiation seed t.
salvage t.
second-line t.
site-specific t.
sonographic planning of
oncology t. (SPOT)
stem cell support t.

treatment-related
t.-r. mortality (TRM)
t.-r. secondary cancer
treatment-resistant mycosis fungoides
tree
biliary t.
bronchial t.
Classification and Regression T.
(CART)
decision t.
tracheobronchial t.
trefoil
t. factor peptide 1 (TFF1)
t. factor protein (TFF)
Treitz
ligament of T.
Trelstar
T. Depot
T. LA
Tremytoine
TREND
Trial on Reversing Endothelial
Dysfunction
trend
t. line analysis
survival t.
Trental
Trentin hematopoietic-inductive
microenvironment model
treosulfan
trephine biopsy
Treponema pallidum
trestolone
tretinoin
t. emollient cream
liposomal t.
Trexall
TRG
tumor regression grade
TRH
thyrotropin-releasing hormone
TRH stimulation
Triacana
triad
Carney t.
Cushing t.
fragile histidine t. (FHIT)
Hutchinson t.
Osler t.
Phemister t. R
Triadapin
trial
t. accrual

NOTES

trial *(continued)*
    Arimidex, Tamoxifen, Alone or in
      Combination t.
    ATAC t.
    Breast Cancer Prevention T.
      (BCPT)
    Cetus t.
    clinical t.
    Cooperative Colorectal Cancer
      Combination Chemotherapy
      Clinical T.
    crossover t.
    Gothenburg Breast Screening T.
    IDEC-Y2B8 radioimmunotherapy t.
    intermediate-sized t.
    Ludwig T.
    MORE t.
    multicenter t.
    Multiple Outcomes of Raloxifene
      Evaluation t.
    T. on Reversing Endothelial
      Dysfunction (TREND)
    phase IIb t.
    phase I–III t.
    placebo-controlled t.
    randomized t.
    Selenium and Vitamin E Cancer
      Prevention T. (SELECT)
Triam-A Injection
triamcinolone
    intralesional t.
    nystatin and t.
Triam Forte Injection
Triamonide Injection
triamterene
    hydrochlorothiazide and t.
triangle
    anal t.
    cervical t.
    Codman t.
    submandibular t.
triangulation
    daily t.
Triapine
triazinate, cyclophosphamide,
  Adriamycin, Platinol
triazolam
triazole
Triboulet test
trichilemmal
    t. cyst
    t. tumor
trichilemmoma
    t. carcinoma
    facial t.
trichlormethiazide
trichloroacetic acid
trichodiscoma

trichoepithelioma
    dermoplastic t.
trichofolliculoma
Trichomonas vaginalis
Trichophyton
    T. rubrum
    T. skin test
    T. tonsurans
Trichosanthes kirilowii
trichosanthin
Trichosporon
    T. beigelii
    T. cutaneum
trichosporonosis
trichothiodystrophy
trichrome stain
triciribine phosphate (TCN-P)
TriCor
tricyclic antidepressant (TCA)
tridentata
    Larrea t.
Tridil Injection
triethanolamine salicylate
triethylenemelamine
triethylenethiophosphoramide (TESPA)
trifluoperazine
trifluridine
trigeminal
    t. nerve
    t. neuroma
    t. neuropathy
TriGem vaccine
trigger
    t. point injection (TPI)
    t. zone
triggering
triglyceride
    medium chain t.'s
trigone
    retromolar t.
trigonum, pl. trigona
Trihexy
trihexyphenidyl
triiodothyronine (T_3)
Tri-K
Tri-Kort Injection
trilateral retinoblastoma (TRb)
trilineage
    t. engraftment
    t. hematopoiesis
Trilisate
Trilog Injection
Trilogy image-guided radiosurgery
  system
Trilone Injection
trilostane
trimer
trimeric protein

trimethadione
trimethoprim (TMP)
    dapsone and t. (DAP/TMP)
trimethoprim-sulfamethoxazole (TMP-SMX)
    t.-s. intolerant individual
trimetrexate (TMQ, TMTX)
    t. gluconate
    t. glucuronate
trimipramine
trimodal
    t. spectroscopy (TMS)
    t. therapy
trimodality therapy
Trimox
Trimpex
Trinam gene therapy
trinitrate
    glyceryl t. (GTN)
trinucleotide
Triosil
Triostat Injection
trioxide
    arsenic t. (AsO₃, ATO)
tripartite duodenal carcinoma
tripelennamine hydrochloride
tripe palms
tripeptide
    intracellular t.
    muramyl t. (MTP)
triphosphate
    t. analog
    deoxyadenosine t. (dATP)
    deoxycytidine t. (dCTP)
    deoxyguanosine t. (dGTP, GTP)
    2′-deoxythymidine 5′-t. (dTTP)
    thymidine t.
    uradine t. (UTP)
    zidovudine t.
5′-triphosphate
    adenosine 5′-t. (ATP)
    ara-C 5′-t.
    2-deoxycytidine 5′-t.
triple-color
    t.-c. flow cytometric assay
    t.-c. flow cytometry
    t.-c. fluorochrome labeling
triple intrathecal therapy (TIT)
triple-lumen catheter
triple-peak-angle camera visualization
triplet
    amino acid t.
triploidy

tripotassium ethylene diamine
    tetraacetate
Triptil
triptorelin
    t. pamoate
    t. pamoate for injectable suspension
trisalicylate
    choline magnesium t.
Tris-buffered saline
trisegmentectomy
Trisenox
trismus
    radiation-induced t.
trisomy 12
tritiated thymidine labeling index (TLI)
triton tumor
Trizivir
TRIzol reagent
trkA expression
trkC expression
trk protooncogene/oncogene
TRM
    treatment-related mortality
Trobicin
Trocaine
trocar
    t. catheter
    t. drainage method
    t. needle
    t. technique
trocar-cannula technique
troche
    Mycelex T.
trochlear
    t. nerve
    t. nerve neoplasm
troglitazone
Troisier
    T. ganglion
    T. node
    T. sign
    T. syndrome
troleandomycin
Trombovar
tromethamine
    carboprost t.
    ketorolac t.
    lodoxamide t.
Tronolane
tropane
trophoblast
trophoblastic
    t. disease

NOTES

T

trophoblastic *(continued)*
    malignant teratoma, t. (MTT)
    t. neoplasm
    t. tumor
trophozoite
tropica
    Leishmania t.
tropical
    t. eosinophilia
    t. hemobilia
    t. macrocytic anemia
    t. spastic paraparesis (TSP)
    t. sprue
tropicalis
    Candida t.
tropicum
    granuloma t.
tropisetron
tropism
    infection t.
tropomyosin-binding protein
Trousseau
    T. sign
    T. syndrome
TroVax
troxacitabine
Troxatyl
TRT
    thermoradiotherapy
Tru-Cut
    T.-C. liver biopsy needle
    T.-C. needle biopsy
true
    t. desmosome
    t. histiocytic lymphoma
    t. pelvis
    t. vocal cord
Trueta shunt
truncal rhabdomyosarcoma
trunk
    brachiocephalic t.
    celiac t.
    lymphatic t.
Truquant BR radioimmunoassay
TRUS
    transrectal ultrasonography
    transrectal ultrasound
    TRUS biopsy
Tru-Scint AD imaging agent
Trypanosoma
    T. gambiense
    T. rhodesiense
trypanosomiasis
    African t.
trypsinization
tryptophan
    pyridoxyl-5-methyl t.
TS
    (2′-deoxy)thymidylate synthase

    thymidylate synthase
    tuberous sclerosis
        TS gene
Ts
    T helper suppressor cell
TSA
    tumor-specific antigen
    tyramide signal amplification
TSC
    tuberous sclerosis complex
TSC2 gene
T-Scan 2000 breast imaging device
TSE
    turbo spin-echo
TSEBT
    total skin electron beam therapy
TSG
    tumor suppressor gene
TSH
    thyroid-stimulating hormone
TSH-displacing antibody
TSNA
    tobacco-specific nitrosamine
TSP
    tropical spastic paraparesis
TSPA
    thiotepa
TSPAP
    total serum prostatic acid phosphatase
TST
    tuberculin skin test
TSTA
    tumor-specific transplantation antigen
TT
    total thyroidectomy
TTE
    total thoracic esophagectomy
TTF
    time-to-treatment failure
TTNA
    transthoracic needle aspiration
TTP
    thrombotic thrombocytopenic purpura
TTT
    transpupillary thermal therapy
tube
    Amersham J t.
    Argyle feeding t.
    Atkinson t.
    auditory t.
    Celestin t.
    chest t.
    collection t.
    Dobbhoff feeding t.
    double-lumen endotracheal t.
    endotracheal t.
    enteral feeding t.
    Eppendorf t.
    ET t.

eustachian t.
fallopian t.
feeding t.
field emission t.
t. formation assay
gastrostomy t.
Hemagard collection t.
Hemochron P214 glass-activated
  ACT t.
jejunostomy t.
MIC t.
nasobiliary t. (NBT)
Newvicon camera t.
PEG t.
percutaneous endoscopic
  gastrostomy t.
Perspex t.
Pyrex glass t.
SafeCrit microhematocrit t.
Salem sump t.
silastic t.
thoracostomy t.
t. thoracostomy
tracheostomy t.
Vacutainer collection t.
Wintrobe t.
Xomed endotracheal t.
tubercidin
tubercle
adductor t.
dorsal t.
tuberculin
new t.
t. skin test (TST)
tuberculoma
tuberculosis (TB)
anorectal t.
t. antigen
atypical t.
disseminated t.
endobronchial t.
exudative t.
multidrug-resistant t. (MDR-TB)
Mycobacterium t.
typical t.
tuberculous meningitis
tuberculum sellae meningioma
tuberosity
ischial t.
tuberous
t. sclerosis (TS)
t. sclerosis complex (TSC)

tubing
polyethylene t.
shunt t.
tubular
t. adenocarcinoma
t. adenoma
t. carcinoma
t. pattern
tubulin
depolymerization of t.
t. protein
tubulointerstitial nephritis
tubulopapillary
t. adenoma
t. tumor
tubulovillous adenoma
Tucks Wipes
TUIP
transurethral incision of prostate
Tukey test
TULIP
transurethral ultrasound-guided laser-
  induced prostatectomy
tumefactive
t. amyloid deposit
t. biliary sludge
tumor
abdominal wall desmoid t.
t. ablation
Abrikosov t.
acinar cell t.
acoustic nerve sheath t.
t. activity marker
acute splenic t.
adenoid t.
adenomatoid odontogenic t.
adipose t.
adnexal t.
adrenal t.
adrenocortical rest cell t.
t. allograft
amelanotic t.
ameloblastic adenomatoid t.
amyloid t.
aneuploid NBX t.
t. aneuploidy
t. angiogenesis
t. angiogenesis factor
t. angiogenic factor
angiomatoid t.
angiosarcoma bone t.
t. antigen
t. antigen epitope peptide

NOTES

tumor *(continued)*

t. antigenicity
aortic body t.
argentaffin carcinoid t.
Armed Forces Institute of Pathology classification of testicular t.'s
Askin t.
atypical teratoid rhabdoid t. (ATRT)
autochthonous t.
t. autocrine mobility factor
autologous t.
Azzopardi t.
B-cell lymphoplasmacytic t.
t. bed
Bednar t.
benign lymphoepithelial parotid t.
benign ovarian t.
benign pulmonary and esophageal t.'s
benign salivary gland t.
t. biology
bipotential precursor cell t.
bladder t. (BT)
blood t.
t. blood supply
blue cell t.
t. blush
bone t.
bone-forming t.
borderline ovarian t.
brain t. (BT)
Brenner t.
bronchial carcinoid t.
Brooke t.
t. bulb
bulky mediastinal t.
t. burden
Burkitt t.
burned-out t.
Buschke-Löwenstein t.
cake of t.
carcinoid t.
cardiac t.
carotid body t.
cartilage t.
cartilage-containing giant cell t.
cartilage-forming t.
cartilaginous t.
Castleman t.
t. cavity
cell t.
t. cell
t. cell aggressiveness
t. cell-host bone relationship
t. cell line
t. cell migration-inhibition factor (TMIF)

t. cell necrosis
t. cell product
cellular t.
central nervous system t.
central neuroepithelial cell-origin t.
cerebellopontine angle t.
cervical t.
chemoreceptor t.
chemoresistant t.
chemosensitive brain t.
chest wall and sternal t.
childhood brain t. (CBT)
chromaffin t.
clear cell t.
Codman t.
collision t.
combined germ cell t. (CGCT)
confluent t.
congenital cardiac t.
connective tissue t.
cutaneous Merkel cell t.
cystic t.
t. cytoreduction
debulking of t.
dedifferentiated t.
deep t.
t. defect
dermal duct t.
dermoid t.
desmoid t.
desmoplastic small cell t.
desmoplastic small round-cell t. (DSRCT)
diploid t.
t. doubling time
drug-resistant t.
ductectatic mucinous t.
dumbbell t.
dumbbell-shaped t.
dysembryoplastic neuroepithelial t. (DNET, DNT)
dysgerminoma germ cell t.
ear t.
eighth cranial nerve t.
t. embolism
embryonal t.
embryonic t.
endocrine pancreatic t. (EPT)
endodermal sinus t.
endolymphatic sac t.
endometrioid t.
endophytum-type t.
Enneking stage of bone t.'s (I–III)
t. enucleation
epidermoid t.
epithelial t.
Erdheim t.
t. erosion
esophageal t.

estrogen-receptor positive t.
Ewing family of t.'s (EFT)
Ewing sarcoma family of t.'s (ESFT)
exophytum-type t.
extraaxial t.
extracranial nontesticular germ cell t.
extragonadal germ cell t. (EGCT)
extrahepatic primary malignant t.
extratesticular t.
extrinsic t.
familial Wilms t.
fatty t.
fecal t.
fibrous t.
t. fixation
t. flare
follicular dendritic cell t.
fungating t.
gastrointestinal stromal t. (GIST)
t. gene index (TGI)
germ cell t. (GCT)
germ cell testicular t.
gestational trophoblastic t.
giant cell t.
Glazunov t.
glial brain t.
glomus caroticum t.
glomus jugulare t. (GJT)
glomus malignant t.
t. grade
granular cell t.
granulosa-stromal cell t.
Grawitz t.
t. growth
growth hormone-releasing factor neuroendocrine t. (GRFoma)
gynecologic t.
haarscheibe t.
hepatic t.
HER-2 overexpressing breast t.
HER-2 overexpressing ovarian t.
heterologous t.
high-grade cartilaginous t.
hilar cell t.
histoid t.
homologous t.
hourglass-shaped t.
human t.
Hürthle cell t.
hyaline cartilage matrix t.
hylic t.

hyperdiploid t.
hypervascularized t.
hypopharyngeal t.
hypothalamic t.
t. hypoxia
t., immune, systemic (TIS)
t., immune, systemic staging system
immunogenic t.
t. immunology
immunoperoxidase t.
t. immunotherapy
t. implant
t. imprint cytology
infiltrating t.
t. infiltration
inflammatory myofibroblastic t.
infratentorial t.
innocent t.
INSS stage 1 t.
interstitial cell t.
intestinal carcinoid t.
intraaabdominal desmoplastic small round cell t.
intraaxial t.
intracapsular t.
intracerebral nerve sheath t.
intracranial t.
intraductal papillary mucinous t. (IPMT)
intralesional curettage of t.
intramural t.
intranodal hemorrhagic spindle cell t.
intraorbital granular cell t.
intraparenchymal nerve sheath t.
intravascular t.
intraventricular t.
ipsilateral t.
iris melanocytic t.
islet cell t.
juxtaglomerular t.
Keasby t.
Klatskin t.
Koenen t.
Krukenberg t.
Landschutz t.
large cell calcifying Sertoli cell t. (LCCSCT)
leiomyomatous t.
leptomeningeal t.
t. lethal dose (TLD)
Leydig cell t. (LCT)

NOTES

tumor *(continued)*
    Lindau t.
    liver t.
    localized t.
    low malignant potential epithelial
      ovarian t.
    Lugano classification for
      testicular t.
    lymphoepithelial t.
    lymphoid t.
    lymphoreticular t.
    t. lysis
    t. lysis syndrome
    male germ line t.
    t. malignancy
    malignant giant cell t. (MGCT)
    malignant mixed mesodermal t.
      (MMMT)
    malignant mixed müllerian t.
    malignant ovarian t.
    malignant peripheral nerve sheath t.
      (MPNST)
    malignant salivary gland t. (MST)
    malignant small round cell t.
    malignant trichilemma t.
    t. margin
    t. mass
    mediastinal germ cell t.
    mediastinal mesenchymal t.
    mediorenal t.
    melanotic neuroectodermal t.
    Merkel cell t.
    mesenchymal bone t.
    mesenchymal sex cord stromal t.
    mesonephroid t.
    metachronous testicular germ cell t.
    metastatic lymph node t.
    Middeldorpf t.
    migrated t.
    migratory t.
    mixed germ cell t.
    mixed histology t.
    mixed mesodermal t.
    mixed müllerian t. (MMT)
    mixed sex cord-stromal t.
    t. M2-pyruvate kinase
    t. M2-pyruvate kinase assay
    mucinous t.
    mucin-producing t.
    mucoepidermoid t.
    müllerian t.
    müllerian peritoneal t.
    t. multifocality
    multiploid t.
    t. mycosis fungoides d'emblée
    myofibroblastic t.
    nasal fossa t.
    t. necrosis factor (TNF)
    t. necrosis factor a (TNFa)

    t. necrosis factor-alpha (TNF-alpha)
    t. necrosis factor-alpha messenger
      ribonucleic acid
    t. necrosis factor-beta (TNF-beta)
    t. necrosis factor-beta-lymphotoxin
    t. necrosis factor receptor (TNFR)
    t. necrosis factor receptor-associated
      death domain (TRADD)
    t. necrosis factor receptor-associated
      factor (TRAF)
    t. necrosis factor receptor family
    t. necrosis factor-related apoptosis-
      inducing ligand (TRAIL)
    t. necrosis factor superfamily
      (TNFSF)
    Nelson t.
    t. neovasculature
    nerve cell t.
    nerve sheath malignant t.
    neuraxial desmoplastic
      neuroepithelial t.
    neuraxis t.
    neuroectodermal t.
    neuroendocrine t. (NET)
    neuroepithelial t.
    neurogenic t.
    neuronal t.
    neuronal-glial t.
    t. neurooncology
    t., node, metastasis (TNM)
    t., node, metastasis classification
    node-negative primary t.
    nonencapsulated sclerosing t.
    nonepithelial t.
    nongerminoma germ cell t.
    nonimmunogenic t.
    nonsclerosing t.
    nonseminomatous germ cell t.
      (NSGCT)
    nonseminomatous testicular germ
      cell t. (NSTGCT)
    oat cell t.
    odontogenic t.
    oil t.
    oligoastrocytoma t.
    oligodendroglial t.
    oncocytic hepatocellular t.
    organoid t.
    osteoclastoma giant cell t.
    t. osteoid
    ovarian carcinoid t.
    ovarian epithelial t. (OVET)
    ovarian granulosa-stromal cell t.
    ovarian granulosa-theca cell t.
    ovarian hilar cell t.
    t. oxygenation
    paclitaxel-resistant t.
    Pancoast t.
    pancreatic endocrine t.

pancreatic islet cell t.
panrenal t.
papillary t.
paracardiac t.
paraffin t.
parasellar dermoid t.
paratesticular t.
parathyroid t.
t. parenchyma
parotid t.
PCV therapy of recurrent
  oligoastrocytoma t.
pearl t.
pearly t.
pediatric solid t.
Pepper t.
percutaneous ethanol ablation of t.
peripheral neuroectodermal t.
peritoneum desmoid t.
permeative neuroectodermal t.
phantom t.
phyllodes t.
pilar t.
Pindborg t.
pineal germ cell t.
pineal gland t.
pineal parenchymal t.
pineal region t.
pituitary t.
placental site trophoblastic t.
  (PSTT)
t. ploidy
t. plop
pontine angle t.
poorly differentiated embryonal
  cell t. (PDET)
posterior fossa t.
potato t.
Pott puffy t.
precursor cell t.
pregnancy t.
prepubertal testicular t. (PPTT)
primary central nervous system t.
primary implanted t.
primary malignant giant cell t.
  (PMGCT)
primitive neuroectodermal t.
  (PNET)
primitive neuroepithelial t.
t. progression
proliferating trichilemmal t.
t. proliferation
t. propagation

t. pseudocapsule
pseudosarcomatous fibromyxoid t.
  (PSFMT)
pseudosarcomatous
  myofibroblastic t. (PMT)
pulmonary t.
radiation-induced peripheral nerve t.
radioresistant t.
ranine t.
Rathke pouch t.
t. receptor protein negative
Recklinghausen t.
recurrent oligoastrocytoma t.
refractory t.
t. registry
t. regression
t. regression grade (TRG)
renal t.
Response Evaluation Criteria in
  Solid T.'s (RECIST)
reticuloendothelial cell-origin t.
retinal anlage t.
rhabdoid t.
round cell t.
Rous t.
sacral bone t.
sacrococcygeal t.
salivary gland t.
sand t.
scannable t.
Schwann cell t.
sclerosing Sertoli cell t.
sclerosing stromal t. (SST)
Scully t.
secondary malignant giant cell t.
  (SMGCT)
second primary t. (SPT)
t. seeding
seminomatous t.
serotonin-producing t.
serous borderline t.
serous ovarian t.
Sertoli cell t. (SCT)
Sertoli cell-only t.
Sertoli-Leydig cell t.
Sertoli-stromal cell t.
sex cord stromal t.
t. shedding
t. shrinkage
signature t.
sinonasal t.
t. site
t. in situ (TIS)

NOTES

tumor *(continued)*
  skull base t.
  small blue cell t.
  small bowel t.
  small round-cell t. (SRCT)
  smooth muscle t.
  soft tissue t.
  solid t.
  solitary fibrous t.
  t. spillage
  spinal axis t.
  spinal cord t.
  spindle cell t.
  t. spread
  squamous odontogenic t.
  t. stage
  sternal t.
  Sternberg t.
  steroid cell t.
  stromal cell t.
  stroma-poor t.
  stroma-rich t.
  subastrocytic t.
  subcutaneous t.
  submucosal t.
  sugar t.
  superficial papillary t. (SPT)
  superior pulmonary sulcus t.
  t. suppressor
  t. suppressor gene (TSG)
  t. suppressor gene inactivation
  supratentorial t.
  suramin therapy of recurrent t.'s
  sympathetic ganglia t.
  synchronous bilateral Wilms t.'s
  synovitis t.
  t. targeting
  Taxol-resistant t.
  temporal bone t.
  tenosynovial giant cell t.
  teratoid t.
  testicular t.
  testicular germ cell t. (TGCT)
  tetradiploid t.
  tetraploid t.
  theca cell t.
  t. therapy
  t. thrombus
  thymic epithelial t. (TET)
  thyroid tracheal t.
  tomato t.
  tongue of t.
  tracheal t.
  t. tracking
  transmissible venereal t.
  transurethral resection of bladder t.
    (TUR-Bt)
  trichilemmal t.
  triton t.

  trophoblastic t.
  tubulopapillary t.
  turban t.
  tympanic body t.
  t. type
  ulcerative t.
  urethral t.
  uroepithelial t.
  t. vaccine
  vagal body t.
  vaginal t.
  vanishing t.
  vascular t.
  t. vascularity
  vasoactive intestinal peptide-
    secreting t. (VIPoma)
  vasoactive intestinal polypeptide t.
    (VIPoma)
  t. viability imaging
  villous t.
  t. virus
  t. volume
  t. volumetrics
  von Hippel t.
  Warthin t.
  t. water diffusion
  well-differentiated polycystic
    Wilms t.
  Wilms t.
  Yaba t.
  yolk sac t.
  Zollinger-Ellison t.
tumor-activated prodrug (TAP)
tumoral
  t. calcinosis
  t. fat
  t. melanin
  t. microcalcification
  t. stenosis
  t. tissue
tumor-amplified protein expression
  therapy (TAPET)
tumor-associated
  t.-a. antigen (TAA)
  t.-a. differentially expressed gene
    15 (TADG-15)
  t.-a. glycoprotein (TAG)
  t.-a. glycoprotein-72 (TAG-72)
  t.-a. glycoprotein-72 antigen
  t.-a. lymphocyte (TAL)
  t.-a. macrophage (TAM)
  t.-a. tissue eosinophilia (TATE)
  t.-a. transplantation
  t.-a. transplantation antigen (TATA)
tumor-bearing host
tumor-derived
  t.-d. activated cell
  t.-d. antigen

t.-d. immunoglobulin idiotype/QS-21
adjuvant combination vaccination
tumor-dose weighting
tumor-draining lymph node (TDLN)
tumorectomy
tumor-free patient
tumoricidal
    t. activity
    t. effect
    t. potential
tumorigenesis
    mammary t.
tumorigenic
    t. cell
    t. mechanism
    t. process
    t. role
tumorigenicity
tumor-induced hypercalcemia
tumor-infiltrating lymphocyte (TIL)
tumor-liberated
    t.-l. particle (TLP)
    t.-l. particle antigen expression
tumorlike
    t. amyloid deposit
    t. bone condition
tumor-limiting factor
tumor-matrix degradation
tumor-specific
    t.-s. antigen (TSA)
    t.-s. mutated RAS peptide
    t.-s. mutated VHL peptide
    t.-s. peptide vaccination
    t.-s. transplantation
    t.-s. transplantation antigen (TSTA)
tumor-suppressor gene expression
tumor-targeting ability
Tums
    T. E-X Extra Strength Tablet
    T. Extra Strength Liquid
tumstatin
TUMT
    transurethral microwave thermotherapy
TUNA
    transurethral needle ablation
TUNEL
    terminal deoxynucleotidyl transferase-
mediated digoxigenin-dUTP nick-end
labeling
        TUNEL method
tungstate
tungsten-188 (^{188}W)

tunica
    t. adventitia
    t. albuginea
    t. intima
    t. vaginalis
    t. vaginalis testis
tunnel
    carpal t.
tunneled catheter
TUR
    transurethral resection
TURB
    transurethral resection of bladder
turban tumor
turbo
    t. spin-echo (TSE)
TUR-Bt
    transurethral resection of bladder tumor
turcica
    sella t.
Turcot
    T. gene
    T. syndrome
Türk
    T. cell
    T. leukocyte
Turkel needle
turkey rhubarb
TURM
    transurethral microwave
turnover
    collagen t.
    viral t.
TURP
    transurethral resection of prostate
Tursky pain adjective scale
Tuttle test
TVCa
    high-dose etoposide, thiotepa, dose-
adjusted carboplatin
TVD
    topotecan, vincristine, doxorubicin
TVS
    transvaginal ultrasonography
T2-weighted
    T2-w. image
    T2-w. scan
twenty-nail dystrophy (TND)
twice-a-day radiotherapy
twin
    donor t.
    t. donor
    t. donor transplant

NOTES

twin *(continued)*
    pump t.
    recipient t.
Twin-K
twin-twin transfusion syndrome
TwiST
    time without symptoms and toxicity
twist tobacco
Tworek bone marrow-aspirating needle
Ty
    protein Ty
tylectomy
Tylenol with Codeine
tylosis, pl. **tyloses**
Tylox
tympanic
    t. body
    t. body tumor
tympanicum jugulare
type
    blood t.
    centrocyte-like t.
    columnar cell t.
    diffuse fibrosis t.
    dysplastic nevus syndrome,
     familial t.
    giant pore t.
    t. 1 growth factor receptor
     (T1GFR)
    hand-mirror cell t.
    human T-cell leukemia virus t. I
     (HTLV-I)
    human T-cell leukemia virus t. II
     (HTLV-II)
    human T-cell leukemia virus t. III
     (HTLV-III)
    5-hydroxytryptamine t. 3 (5-HT$_3$)
    t. I glycogen storage disease
    t. II estrogen-binding site
    L/H t.

    lymphomatous t.
    major histocompatibility t.
    mixed-cellularity t.
    Naegeli t.
    nonconvoluted t.
    pleomorphic t.
    reticular t.
    Schilling t.
    tumor t.
typhi
    live-attenuated recombinant
     Salmonella t.
    Salmonella t.
typhimurium
    Salmonella t.
typhlitis
typical
    t. carcinoid (TC)
    t. nephropathy
    t. tuberculosis
typing
    blood t.
    HLA t.
    Mostofi histologic t.
    primed lymphocyte t.
tyramide signal amplification (TSA)
Tyr^5,1^2,Lys^7-polyphemusin II
tyrosinase
    t. melanoma antigen
    t. protein
tyrosinase-related protein
tyrosine (Y)
    t. hydroxylase (TH)
    t. kinase
    t. kinase inhibitor
    t. phosphorylation
tyrosinemia
Tzanck smear
T-zone lymphoma

U

 U fiber
 U fiber damage

UA

 urinalysis

UAD

 upper aerodigestive

UADT

 upper aerodigestive tract

ubenimex

U-BFP

 urinary basic fetoprotein

ubiquitin

UC

 ulcerative colitis
 undifferentiated carcinoma

U-cell lymphoma

Ucephan

UCN-01 and fludarabine

UD-BMT

 unrelated donor bone marrow
 transplantation

UDCA

 ursodeoxycholic acid

UDP

 uridine 5'-diphosphate

UESL

 undifferentiated embryonal sarcoma of
 liver

UFT

 uracil, 5-fluorouracil, tegafur
 uracil plus Ftorafur
 uracil-tegafur

UFT/leucovorin calcium

UICC

 International Union Against Cancer
 Union Internationale Contre le Cancer
 UICC classification

UICC-RO resection

UK

 urokinase

ulcer

 antral u.
 aphthous u.
 atherosclerotic u.
 benign gastric u.
 Buruli u.
 colonic u.
 u. dressing
 duodenal u.
 esophageal u.
 gastric u.
 herpetic u.
 leg u.
 oral u.

recurrent aphthous u.
rodent u.
steroid-induced u.
stomal u.

ulcerans

 Mycobacterium u.

ulcerated melanoma

ulcerating lesion

ulceration

 aphthous u.
 esophageal u.
 necrotic u.
 stomal u.
 transurethral resection of
 prostate u.

ulcerative

 u. colitis (UC)
 u. lesion
 u. tumor

Ulcerease

ulceroglandular

ULDR

 ultra-low dose rate
 ULDR brachytherapy

Ulex europaeus I lectin

ulnaris

 extensor carpi u.

U-loop nephrostomy catheter

Ultiva

ultracentrifuge

 Sorvall Discovery SE u.

ultrafast MRI

Ultraflex stent

ultra-low

 u.-l. dose IL-2
 u.-l. dose rate (ULDR)
 u.-l. dose rate brachytherapy

Ultram

Ultramop

ultraradical surgery

ultrasmall superparamagnetic iron oxide

ultrasonic hyperthermia

ultrasonographic

 u. modeling
 u. staging

**ultrasonographically guided core needle
 biopsy (USCNB)**

ultrasonography

 axillary u.
 B-mode u.
 continuous-wave Doppler u.
 endorectal u. (EUS)
 endoscopic u. (EUS)
 endovaginal u.
 intraductal u.

ultrasonography *(continued)*
 intraoperative u. (IOUS)
 laparoscopic u. (LUS)
 real-time u.
 transrectal u. (TRUS)
 transvaginal u. (TVS)
ultrasound
 color Doppler u.
 compression u.
 Doppler u.
 endoluminal u.
 endorectal u.
 endoscopic u. (EUS)
 u. hyperthermia
 intravascular u.
 MR-guided focused u.
 Toshiba SSA-380A u.
 u. transducer
 transrectal u. (TRUS)
ultrasound-guided
 u.-g. needle aspiration
 u.-g. needle core biopsy (UNCB)
 u.-g. nephrostomy puncture
ultrastructural platelet peroxidase test
ultrastructure
ultraviolet
 u. detector
 u. irradiation therapy
 psoralen and u. A (PUVA)
 u. radiation
 u. spectrum
UM
 uracil mustard
umbilical
 u. blood sampling
 u. cord blood
 u. cord cyst
 u. cord hematoma
 u. human cord blood
UMP
 uradine monophosphate
UNAIDS
 Joint United Nations Programme on
 HIV/AIDS
 United Nations Acquired
 Immunodeficiency program
Unasyn
UNCB
 ultrasound-guided needle core biopsy
uncertain
 u. malignant potential
 u. primary site
unconfirmed/uncertain complete
 remission (CRu)
unconventional therapy
uncoordinated cell growth
undersampling
undertreatment

undifferentiated
 u. carcinoma (UC)
 u. carcinoma of ovary
 u. cell adenoma
 u. embryonal sarcoma of liver
 (UESL)
 u. nasopharyngeal carcinoma
 (UNPC)
 u. sarcoma
 u. sarcomatous component
undiversion
 urinary u.
unexplained fever
unfavorable histology
unfractionated lymphocyte
ungual fibroma
Unguentine
unicameral bone cyst
Unicap
unicentricity
unicryptal adenoma
unidermatomal zoster
Uniflex
 U. dressing
 U. TFD
uniformity
 differential u.
 extrinsic field u.
 field u.
 integral u.
Uni-frame patient immobilization system
unilobar disease
unilocular lesion
unintegrated
 u. HIV
 u. human immunodeficiency virus
unintentional injury
Union Internationale Contre le Cancer
 (UICC)
Uni-Pro
Uniserts
 Bisacodyl U.
unit
 adapted standard mammography u.
 AIDS Vaccine Evaluation U.
 (AVEU)
 Bethesda u.
 blast colony-forming u.
 burst-forming u.
 colony-forming u. (CFU)
 fibrinogen equivalent u. (FEU)
 granulocyte colony-forming u. (G-
 CFU)
 granulocyte-macrophage colony-
 forming u. (GM-CFU)
 heater probe u. (HPU)
 Hounsfield u. (H)
 International System of U.'s (SI)
 kallikrein-inhibiting u.

King-Armstrong u.
Lf u.
megakaryocyte colony-forming u.
monitor u. (MU)
murine colony-forming u.
pilosebaceous u.
pocket-sized TENS u.
pressor u.
radiation effect u. (reu)
SI u.'s
Somogyi u.
Svedberg u.
terminal duct lobular u.

unitarian theory
unit-culture
colony-forming u.-c. (CFU-C)
United Nations Acquired
Immunodeficiency program (UNAIDS)
unit-eosinophil
colony-forming u.-e. (CFU$_{EOS}$)
unit-erythrocyte
colony-forming u.-e. (CFU-E)
unit-fibroblast
colony-forming u.-f. (CFU-F)
unit-granulocyte-macrophage
colony-forming u.-g.-m. (CFU-GM)
universal
u. donor
u. life energy
u. precaution
University of Florida staging system
unknown
u. origin
u. primary
u. primary site
unmasking
antigen u.
unmodified
u. G-CSF mobilized peripheral
blood stem cell
u. marrow
Unopette system
unorthodox
u. pharmacotherapy
u. therapy
UNPC
undifferentiated nasopharyngeal
carcinoma
unproven therapy
unrelated
u. bone marrow donor
u. donor (URD)

u. donor bone marrow
transplantation (UD-BMT)
unresectable colorectal cancer
unresponsiveness
immunologic u.
unrest
nuclear u.
unsaturated fat
unsealed internal radiation therapy
unstable electrophile
uPA
urokinase-type plasminogen activator
uPAR
urokinase plasminogen activator receptor
urokinase plasminogen activator response
urokinase-type plasminogen activator
receptor
uPM3 urine test
UPP
urethral pressure profile
urethral pressure profilometry
upper
u. aerodigestive (UAD)
u. aerodigestive tract (UADT)
u. clivus
u. respiratory infection
upregulate
upregulated
upregulation
COX-2 u.
UPSC
uterine papillary serous carcinoma
uptake
amine precursor u.
radioiodine u.
T$_3$ u.
UR-2 sarcoma virus
urachal carcinoma
urachus
embryonal remnant of u.
uracil
u., 5-fluorouracil, tegafur (UFT)
u. mustard (UM)
u. plus Ftorafur (UFT)
uracil-tegafur (UFT)
uradine
u. monophosphate (UMP)
u. triphosphate (UTP)
uramustine
uranium mining
URD
unrelated donor
uredepa

NOTES

U

ureidopenicillin
uremia
uremic
   u. follicular hyperkeratosis
   u. medullary cystic disease
ureter
   beaded u.
   bifid u.
   extravesical infrasphincteric
     ectopic u.
ureteral
   u. carcinoma
   u. obstruction
   u. stent
ureterectasis
   terminal u.
ureterocele
   ectopic u.
ureterolysis
ureteroneocystostomy
ureteropyelostomy
ureterorenoscopy
ureterostomy
ureteroureteral anastomosis
ureteroureterostomy
urethra
   prostatic u.
urethral
   u. pressure profile (UPP)
   u. pressure profilometry (UPP)
   u. tumor
   u. warming
urethritis
urethrography
   retrograde u. (RUG)
urethroplasty
   prostatic u.
   retrograde transurethral prostatic u.
urethroscopy
urethrostomy
   perineal u.
urethrotomy
uric
   u. acid
   u. acid nephropathy
uridine
   u. 5'-diphosphate (UDP)
   u. 5'-diphosphate
     glucuronosyltransferase
   u. 5'-diphosphate
     glucuronosyltransferase deficiency
   u. rescue
Uridon
urinalysis (UA)
urinary
   u. basic fetoprotein (U-BFP)
   u. bladder
   u. cast
   u. catecholamine assay

   u. catheterization
   u. diversion
   u. dysfunction
   u. retention
   u. schistosomiasis
   u. tract infection (UTI)
   u. undiversion
urine
   u. hemosiderin
   u. leak
   u. mutagenicity screening
   u. test
urinoma
   perinephric u.
Uritol
urodynamics
   eyeball u.
   video u. (VUDS)
uroepithelial
   u. malignancy
   u. tumor
uroflow
urogenital
   u. diaphragm
   u. embryology
   u. malignancy
urography
   excretory u. (EU)
urokinase (UK)
   u. plasminogen activator receptor
     (uPAR)
   u. plasminogen activator response
     (uPAR)
urokinase-type
   u.-t. plasminogen activator (uPA)
   u.-t. plasminogen activator receptor
     (uPAR)
Uro-KP-Neutral
urolagnia
Urolene Blue
urologic emergency
uropathy
   chronic obstructive u.
   obstructive u.
uroporphyrinogen
uroprotection
   u. and etoposide
   mesna u.
UroScore staging algorithm
urosepsis
urothelial
   u. cancer
   u. transitional cell
urothelium
   neoplastic u.
Urovision urine test
UroVysion
   U. bladder cancer kit
   U. test kit

Urozide
ursodeoxycholic acid (UDCA)
ursodiol
urticaria
    u. pattern
    u. pigmentosa
usage
    ethanol u.
USCNB
    ultrasonographically guided core needle
    biopsy
user
    injection drug u. (IDU)
    intravenous drug u. (IVDU)
Ussing equation
usual interstitial pneumonitis
uterine
    u. angiosarcoma
    u. aplasia
    u. bleeding
    u. carcinosarcoma
    u. cervical cancer
    u. cervix
    u. chondrosarcoma
    u. corpus
    u. corpus lymphoma
    u. enlargement
    u. leiomyosarcoma

    u. mixed müllerian sarcoma
    u. papillary serous carcinoma
    (UPSC)
    u. sarcoma metastasis
uterus, pl. **uteri**
    adenocarcinoma of u.
    anteflexed u.
    anteverted u.
    u. arcuatus
    body of u.
    liposarcoma of u.
    müllerian sarcoma of u.
UTI
    urinary tract infection
utilization rate
UTP
    uradine triphosphate
utricle cyst
Uvadex methoxsalen sterile solution
uveal
    u. melanocyte
    u. melanoma
    u. tract
uveitis
UV irradiation
uvulae
    musculus u.

NOTES

U

V

V bypass
V factor
V gene

V-2 carcinoma

V3

V3 domain
V3 loop of gp120

VA

vincristine and actinomycin D

VAAP

vincristine, L-asparaginase, Adriamycin,
prednisone

VAB

vacuum-assisted breast biopsy
vinblastine, actinomycin D, bleomycin

VAB 2, VAB-II

vinblastine, actinomycin D, bleomycin,
cisplatin

VAB 3, VAB-III

vinblastine, actinomycin D, bleomycin,
cisplatin, cyclophosphamide,
chlorambucil

VAB 4, VAB-IV

vinblastine, actinomycin D, bleomycin,
cisplatin, cyclophosphamide

VAB 5, VAB-V

vinblastine, actinomycin D, bleomycin,
cyclophosphamide, cisplatin

VAB 6, VAB-VI

vinblastine, actinomycin D, bleomycin,
cyclophosphamide, cisplatin

VABCD

vinblastine, Adriamycin, bleomycin,
CCNU, DTIC

VAB-II (*var. of* VAB 2)
VAB-III (*var. of* VAB 3)
VAB-IV (*var. of* VAB 4)
Vabra aspirator
VAB-V (*var. of* VAB 5)
VAB-VI (*var. of* VAB 6)

VAC

vincristine, actinomycin D,
cyclophosphamide
vincristine, Adriamycin,
cyclophosphamide
VAC chemotherapy protocol
pulse VAC

VACA

vincristine, actinomycin A,
cyclophosphamide, Adriamycin
vincristine, actinomycin D,
cyclophosphamide, Adriamycin

VACAD

vinblastine, Adriamycin, Cytoxan,
actinomycin D, dacarbazine
vincristine, actinomycin D,
cyclophosphamide, Adriamycin,
dacarbazine

vaccination

dendritic cell v.
Detox adjuvant v.
GD2-KLH v.
idiotype v.
nucleic acid v.
phase II autologous v.
tumor-derived immunoglobulin
idiotype/QS-21 adjuvant
combination v.
tumor-specific peptide v.

vaccine

AC v.
AIDSVAX B/B v.
allogeneic tumor cell v.
anticancer v.
v. antigen production
v. antigen-specific antibody titer
antitumor v.
autologous cell v.
bacille Calmette-Guérin v.
BCG v.
BioHepB recombinant hepatitis
B v.
breast cancer v.
Canvaxin cancer v.
DC anti-tumor v.
dendritic tumor cell v.
diphtheria, tetanus, pertussis,
Haemophilus influenzae type b v.
DTP-Hib v.
enhanced inactivated polio v.
(EIPV)
GMK v.
gonadotropin-releasing hormone v.
GVAX pancreatic cancer v.
human diploid cell strain rabies v.
(HDRV)
killed virus v.
live-attenuated lentiviral v.
live vector v.
L-Vax v.
Lyme disease v.
measles v.
melanoma cell lysate v.
melanoma whole cell v.
methanol extraction residue of
bacillus Calmette-Guérin v.
monoclonal antibody anticancer v.

V

vaccine *(continued)*
>murine monoclonal anticancer v.
>M-Vax v.
>Mylovenge therapeutic v.
>naked DNA vector v.
>Oncophage cancer v.
>O-Vax v.
>Pasteur Institute bacillus Calmette-Guérin v.
>pneumococcal polysaccharide v.
>Provenge therapeutic v.
>purified v.
>recombinant glycoprotein v.
>RNA-loaded autologous dendritic cell v.
>Sabin v.
>sialyl-Tn-KLH v.
>TA-HPV v.
>TBC-CEA v.
>v. therapy
>Theratope v.
>TriGem v.
>tumor v.
>varicella virus v.
>Vaxid v.
>VaxSyn HIV-1 v.
>whole cell v.

vaccine-induced
>v.-i. noncytolic CD8
>v.-i. noncytolic cytarabine daunorubicin

vaccinia
>v. melanoma oncolysate (VMO)
>v. vaccine vector
>v. virus

vaccinia/BHK-21 cell
vaccinia-gp160
vaccinia-HIV env/gag/pol
vaccinia/vero cell
VACP
>VePesid, Adriamycin, cyclophosphamide, Platinol
>VePesid, Adriamycin, Cytoxan, Platinol

vacuolar myelopathy
vacuolated-appearing cell
vacuolated megakaryocyte
vacuole
>pinocytotic v.

vacuolization
>basal cytoplasmic v.

VACURG
>Veterans Administration Cooperative Urological Research Group

Vacutainer
>V. collection tube
>V. needle

vacuum
>v. constriction device (VCD)
>v. drain

>v. erection device
>v. pillow

vacuum-assisted breast biopsy (VAB)
VAD
>vincristine, Adriamycin, dexamethasone
>vincristine, doxorubicin, Decadron
>VAD chemotherapy protocol

VAdCA + I/E
>vincristine, doxorubicin, cyclophosphamide, dactinomycin plus ifosfamide with mesna

VAD/V
>vinblastine, Adriamycin, dexamethasone, verapamil
>vincristine, Adriamycin, dexamethasone plus verapamil

VAFAC
>vincristine, amethopterin, 5-fluorouracil, Adriamycin, cyclophosphamide

vagal body tumor
vagina
>apical v.
>intraepithelial neoplasia of v.
>in situ carcinoma of v.
>spindle cell sarcoma of v.

vaginal
>v. atrophy
>v. bleeding
>v. cancer
>Canesten V.
>v. carcinoma
>v. cuff
>v. cuff smear (VCS)
>v. cylinder
>v. discharge
>v. epithelium
>v. hysterectomy
>v. intraepithelial neoplasm (VAIN)
>v. microbicide
>v. stenosis
>v. stricture
>v. submucosa
>v. tumor
>v. webbing

vaginalis
>*Gardnerella* v.
>*Trichomonas* v.
>tunica v.

vaginectomy
vaginitis
>senile atrophic v.

vaginoperineoplasty
vaginosis
>bacterial v.

vagotomy
vagus
>v. nerve
>v. nerve palsy

VAI
  vincristine, actinomycin D, ifosfamide
VAIA
  vincristine, actinomycin D, ifosfamide,
    Adriamycin
      VAIA regimen
VAIN
  vaginal intraepithelial neoplasm
valacyclovir, valaciclovir
valerate
      estradiol v.
valerian tea
valganciclovir
validation
      histopathologic v.
VALOP-B
  etoposide, doxorubicin,
    cyclophosphamide, vincristine,
    prednisone, bleomycin
V-alpha
      T-cell receptor V-a.
valproate
valproic
      v. acid
      v. acid and derivatives
valrubicin
valspodar
Valstar
Valsuani disease
Valtrex
value
      absolute lymphocyte v.
      CADD v.
      central axis v.
      dose v.
      OAR v.
      predictive v.
      standardized uptake v. (SUV)
      Z v.
valve
      aortic v.
      atrioventricular v.
      attenuation v.
      esophageal Z-stent with dual anti-
        reflux v.
      homograft v.
      shunt v.
      Starr-Edwards v.
      St. Jude v.
valvuloplasty
      balloon dilation v.

VAM
  vinblastine, Adriamycin, mitomycin C
  VP-16-213, Adriamycin, methotrexate
VAMP
  vincristine, actinomycin, methotrexate,
    prednisone
  vincristine, Adriamycin, methotrexate,
    prednisone
  vincristine, Adriamycin,
    methylprednisolone
  vincristine, amethopterin, 6-
    mercaptopurine, prednisone
van
      v. den Bergh test
      v. der Waal interaction
      V. Nuys classification
      V. Nuys Prognostic Index in
        breast cancer
      v. Sonnenberg modified coaxial
        biopsy set
      v. Sonnenberg sump
Vancocin
      V. CP
      V. Injection
      V. Oral
Vancoled Injection
vancomycin
vanillylmandelic
      v. acid (VMA)
      v. acid level
vanishing tumor
Vantin
VAP
  vinblastine, actinomycin D, Platinol
  vincristine, Adriamycin, prednisone
  vincristine, Adriamycin, procarbazine
  vincristine, L-asparaginase, prednisone
VAPA
  vincristine, Adriamycin, prednisone, ara-
    C
VAPE
  vincristine, Adriamycin, procarbazine,
    etoposide
      VAPE chemotherapy protocol
VAP-II
  vinblastine, actinomycin D, Platinol
Vapocet
vaporization
      laser v.
vapreotide
Vaquez-Osler disease
variability
      genetic v.

NOTES

variability *(continued)*
    interindividual v.
    ventricular rate v. (VRV)
variable region of Ig
Varian
    V. accelerator
    V. MLC system
variance
variant
    anatomical v.
    blastic v.
    fibroblastic v.
    fibrolamellar v.
    fibrosarcoma v.
    hyaline-vascular v.
    Japanese v.
    Ketron-Goodman v.
    L-phase v.
    lymphohistiocytic v.
    macrophage v.
    MAT-LyLu v.
    normal v.
    NSI v.
    plasmacytoid v.
    prolymphocytoid v.
    syncytial v.
    tall cell v.
    T-cell lymphoma v.
variation
    coefficient of v.
    ethnic v.
    natural v.
variceal
    v. bleeding
    v. sclerotherapy
varicella virus vaccine
varicella-zoster virus (VZV)
varices (*pl. of* varix)
varicoid
    v. carcinoma
    v. esophageal cancer
VariSeed 7.0 software computer program
Varivax
varix, pl. **varices**
    colonic v.
    duodenal v.
    esophageal v.
vascular
    v. brachytherapy
    v. cell adhesion molecule-1 (VCAM-1)
    v. elastosis
    v. endothelial cell
    v. endothelial factor
    v. endothelial growth factor (VEFG, VEGF)
    v. endothelial growth factor-C (VEGF-C)

    v. leak syndrome
    v. lesion
    v. obstruction
    v. permeability
    v. permeability factor (VPF)
    v. sarcoma
    v. stasis
    v. stent
    v. tumor
vascular-disrupting agent (VDA)
vascularity
    tumor v.
vasculature
    cerebral v.
    extracranial cerebral v.
vasculitis
    bacterial v.
    leukocytoclastic v.
    Pneumocystis-related v.
    retinal v.
vasculoconnective tissue
vasculopathy
    lupus v.
vasoactive
    v. intestinal peptide (VIP)
    v. intestinal peptide-secreting tumor (VIPoma)
    v. intestinal polypeptide tumor (VIPoma)
    v. polypeptide
vasomotor instability
vasoocclusive crisis
vasopermeation enhancement agent (VEA)
vasopressin (VP)
    v. infusion
vasoreactivity
    cerebral v.
vasorum
VAT
    vinblastine, Adriamycin, thiotepa
    vincristine, ara-C, 6-thioguanine
    visceral adipose tissue
VATD
    vincristine, ara-C, 6-thioguanine, daunorubicin
VATER
    vertebral, anal, tracheal, esophageal, renal
    VATER association
    VATER complex
Vater
    ampulla of V.
VATH
    vinblastine, Adriamycin, thiotepa, Halotestin
VATS
    video-assisted thoracoscopic surgery
VAV
    VP-16-213, Adriamycin, vincristine

Vaxid vaccine
VaxSyn HIV-1 vaccine
VB
>vinblastine
>vinblastine and bleomycin

Vb
>>T-cell antigen receptor Vb
>>TCR Vb

VBA
>vincristine, BCNU, Adriamycin

VBAP
>vincristine, BCNU, Adriamycin, prednisone

VBC
>VePesid, BCNU, cyclophosphamide
>vinblastine, bleomycin, cisplatin

VBD
>vinblastine, bleomycin, DDP

V-beta
>beta-chain variable region
>T-cell receptor V-beta

VBH
>Vogele-Bale-Hohner
>VBH head holder

VBL
>vinblastine

VBM
>vincristine, bleomycin, methotrexate

VBMCP
>vincristine, BCNU, melphalan, cyclophosphamide, prednisone

VBMF
>vinblastine, bleomycin, methotrexate, 5-fluorouracil
>vincristine, bleomycin, methotrexate, 5-fluorouracil

VBMPC
>vinblastine, BCNU, melphalan, prednisone, Cytoxan

VBP
>vinblastine, bleomycin, Platinol

VC
>VePesid and carboplatin
>vincristine
>vinorelbine and cisplatin
>vital capacity

VCAM-1
>vascular cell adhesion molecule-1

VCAP
>vincristine, cyclophosphamide, Adriamycin, prednisone

VCAP-I
>VP-16, cyclophosphamide, Adriamycin, Platinol

VCD
>vacuum constriction device

VCF
>vincristine, cyclophosphamide, 5-fluorouracil

VCMP
>vincristine, cyclophosphamide, melphalan, prednisone

VCP
>vincristine, cyclophosphamide, prednisone

VCP-I
>VP-16, cyclophosphamide, Platinol

VCR
>vincristine

VCS
>vaginal cuff smear

VDA
>vascular-disrupting agent
>vincristine, daunorubicin, ʟ-asparaginase

VDBCC
>vincristine, dactinomycin, bleomycin, cisplatin, cyclophosphamide

VDD
>vincristine, doxorubicin, dexamethasone

VDP
>vinblastine, dacarbazine, Platinol
>vincristine, daunorubicin, prednisone

VDRL
>Venereal Disease Research Laboratory
>CSF VDRL

VDS
>vindesine

VEA
>vasopermeation enhancement agent

Vectastain Elite ABC kit
vector
>>adenoassociated virus v.
>>adenovirus v.
>>attenuated bacterial v.
>>bacterial v.
>>canarypox v.
>>cosmid cloning v.
>>gene delivery v.
>>lentiviral v.
>>live viral v.
>>v. magnitude (VM)
>>nucleic acid v.
>>parent v.
>>pseudotype v.

NOTES

V

vector *(continued)*
    recombinant vaccine v.
    recombinant viral v.
    retrovirus v.
    v. transfectant control
    vaccinia vaccine v.
VEE
    Venezuelan equine encephalitis
Veenema-Gusberg prostatic biopsy needle
VEEP
    vincristine, epirubicin, etoposide, prednisolone
    VEEP regimen
Veetids
VEFG
    vascular endothelial growth factor
vegetable
    cruciferous v.
vegetarianism
VEGF
    vascular endothelial growth factor
    VEGF, FGF, and PDGF receptor signaling
    FLKk-1 receptor for VEGF
    FLT1 receptor for VEGF
    VEGF receptor signal blocker
    VEGF trap
VEGF-C
    vascular endothelial growth factor-C
vehicle
    citrate-phosphate v.
veiled cell
vein
    accessory hepatic v.
    adrenal v.
    antecubital v.
    axillary v.
    azygos v.
    basilic v.
    basivertebral v.
    brachial v.
    cephalic v.
    cerebral v.
    dorsal penile v.
    epigastric v.
    esophageal v.
    Labbé v.
    parathyroid v.
    peripancreatic v.
    superior mesenteric v. (SMV)
VeIP
    Velban, ifosfamide, Platinol
    vinblastine, ifosfamide, Platinol
Velban
    bleomycin, CCNU, Adriamycin, V. (BCAVe, B-CAVe)
    CCNU, Adriamycin, V. (CAVe, CA-Ve)

cyclophosphamide, Adriamycin, V. (CAV)
    V., ifosfamide, Platinol (VeIP)
    procarbazine, Alkeran, V. (PAVe)
Velbe
Velcade
velocity
    acoustic v.
    average peak v. (APV)
    blood v.
    prostate-specific antigen v. (PSAV)
    PSA v. (PSAV)
Velosef
VEMP
    vincristine, Endoxan, 6-mercaptopurine, prednisone
vena cava syndrome
Vena-Tech filter
venereal
    V. Disease Research Laboratory (VDRL)
    v. lymphogranuloma
venereum
    granuloma v.
    lymphogranuloma v.
Venezuelan
    V. equine encephalitis (VEE)
    V. equine encephalitis virus
venipuncture
venlafaxine
Venofer
Venoglobulin-S
venography
    antegrade v.
    contrast v.
venom
    Russell's viper v. (RVV)
venoocclusive
    v. disease (VOD)
    v. disease of liver
venosus
    ductus v.
venous
    v. access device
    v. angioma
    v. blood
    v. cutdown
    v. hum
    v. hypertension
    v. NIVA
    v. obstruction
    v. oozing
    v. sinus
    v. stasis
    v. thromboembolism
    v. thrombosis
Ventana
    V. 320 automated immunostainer
    V. Immuno-automated machine

ventilation
    controlled mechanical v. (CMV)
ventilator-assisted respiration
ventilator therapy
ventricle
    cerebral v.
    colloid cyst of third v.
    laryngeal v.
    left v. (LV)
ventricular
    v. encasement
    v. hemangioblastoma
    v. rate variability (VRV)
ventriculitis
    cytomegalovirus v.
ventriculogram
    radionuclide v. (RVG)
ventriculography
    cerebral v.
ventriculoperitoneal shunt
Venturi effect
VEPA
    vinblastine, etoposide, prednisone,
      Adriamycin
VEPA-M
    vincristine, etoposide, prednisone,
      Adriamycin, methotrexate
VePesid
    etoposide
    VP-16
    VP-16-213
    VePesid, Adriamycin,
      cyclophosphamide, Platinol
      (VACP)
    VePesid, Adriamycin, Cytoxan,
      Platinol (VACP)
    VePesid, BCNU, cyclophosphamide
      (VBC)
    VePesid and carboplatin (VC)
    cisplatin and VePesid (CV)
    cyclophosphamide, BCNU, VePesid
      (CBV)
    DDP, 5-fluorouracil, VePesid
      (DFV)
    VePesid, ifosfamide, Platinol (VIP)
    mitoxantrone, ifosfamide, VePesid
      (MIV)
    VePesid, mitoxantrone,
      prednimustine (VMP)
    VePesid and Platinol (VPP)
    VePesid, 6-thioguanine, ara-C,
      daunorubicin (V-TAD)

vera
    polycythemia v. (PCV, PV)
    polycythemia rubra v. (PRV)
verapamil (VPAM)
    vinblastine, Adriamycin,
      dexamethasone, v. (VAD/V)
    vincristine, Adriamycin,
      dexamethasone plus v. (VAD/V)
verbal-numerical scale
Veress needle
verge
    anal v.
Verifuse ambulatory infusion pump
Verluma diagnostic imaging agent
vermian oligoastrocytoma
vermicularis
    Enterobacter v.
vermilionectomy
Verner-Morrison syndrome
vernier
    couch v.
vero vector with IL2 gene
verruca
    filiform v.
    v. vulgaris
verruciformis
    epidermodysplasia v.
verrucosis
    nevus v.
verrucous squamous cell carcinoma
Versed
Versenate
    Calcium Disodium V.
version
    Sexual Self-Schema Scale-Male V.
      (SSSS-M)
    Ways of Coping, Cancer V.
      (WOC-CA)
vertebra, pl. **vertebrae**
    anterior scalloping of vertebrae
    bone-within-bone v.
    cervical v.
    v. plana
vertebral
    v., anal, tracheal, esophageal, renal
      (VATER)
    v. hemangioma
vertebroplasty
verteporfin
vertical
    v. partial laryngectomy
    v. transmission

V

NOTES

verticillus
  Streptomyces v.
vertigo
Vesanoid
vesicle
  brain region v.
  lipid-containing v.
vesicular nucleus
vesiculobullous rash
vesiculoprostatectomy
  retropubic v.
vessel
  abdominal great v.
  axillary v.
  blood v.
  brachiocephalic v.
  capsular v.
  cerebral blood v.
  v. encasement
  feeding v.
  great v.
vestibular schwannoma
vestibule
  esophageal v.
  nasal v.
Veterans Administration Cooperative Urological Research Group (VACURG)
veto
  v. activity
  v. cell
Vfend
VH
  viral hepatitis
  VH gene
VHL
  von Hippel-Lindau
  VHL disease
  VHL tumor suppressor gene
viable donor lymphocyte infusion
Viadur implant
Viagra
Vibramycin
VIBRANT
  volume imaging for breast assessment
  VIBRANT breast imaging
Vibra-Tabs
vibrio
  V. cholerae
  El Tor v.
VIC
  vinblastine, ifosfamide, CCNU
  VP-16, ifosfamide, carboplatin
  VIC chemotherapy protocol
VICE
  vincristine, ifosfamide, carboplatin, etoposide

Vicks
  V. Children's Chloraseptic
  V. Chloraseptic Sore Throat
Vicodin ES
Vicon
  V. Forte
  V. Plus
Vicoprofen
Victoria blue stain
vidarabine
Vi-Daylin
Vi-Daylin/F
Vidaza
video
  v. endoscopy
  v. urodynamics (VUDS)
video-assisted
  v.-a. thoracoscopic surgery (VATS)
  v.-a. thoracoscopy
videolaparoscopy
videostroboscopy
video urodynamics (VUDS)
Videx EC
VIE
  vinblastine, ifosfamide, etoposide
  vincristine, ifosfamide, etoposide
view
  air contrast v.
  apical lordotic v.
  axial v.
  axillary v.
  beam's eye v. (BEV)
  circular field of v. (CFOV)
  expiratory v.
  extended field of v.
  extension v.
  external rotation v.
  field of v.
  1-v. mammography
  2-v. mammography
  orthogonal v.
  room eye v. (REV)
  skyline v.
vif protein
VIG
  vinblastine, ifosfamide, gallium nitrate
VigiFOAM dressing
Vigilon gel dressing
VII:Ag
  factor VII antigen
  Asserachrom VII:Ag10000
villi (*pl. of* villus)
villoglandular adenocarcinoma
villonodular synovitis
villotubular adenoma
villous, villose
  v. adenoma
  v. carcinoma
  v. lymphocyte

v. papilloma
v. tumor
villus, pl. **villi**
arachnoid villi
Vilona
VIMB
VP-16, ifosfamide, mitoxantrone,
bleomycin
vimentin
v. immunostaining
v. peptide
v. reactivity
v. stain
VIMRxyn
Vim-Silverman needle
VIN
vulvar intraepithelial neoplasia
vulvar intraepithelial neoplasm
vinblastine (VB, VBL)
v., actinomycin D, bleomycin
(VAB)
v., actinomycin D, bleomycin,
cisplatin (VAB 2, VAB-II)
v., actinomycin D, bleomycin,
cisplatin, chlorambucil,
cyclophosphamide
v., actinomycin D, bleomycin,
cisplatin, cyclophosphamide (VAB
4, VAB-IV)
v., actinomycin D, bleomycin,
cisplatin, cyclophosphamide,
chlorambucil (VAB 3, VAB-III)
v., actinomycin D, bleomycin,
cyclophosphamide, cisplatin (VAB
5, VAB-V, VAB 6, VAB-VI)
v., actinomycin D,
cyclophosphamide
v., actinomycin D, Platinol (VAP,
VAP-II)
Adriamycin, bleomycin, v. (ABV)
v., Adriamycin, bleomycin, CCNU,
DTIC (VABCD)
Adriamycin, bleomycin, DTIC, v.
(ABDV)
v., Adriamycin, Cytoxan,
actinomycin D, dacarbazine
(VACAD)
v., Adriamycin, dexamethasone,
verapamil (VAD/V)
v., Adriamycin, mitomycin C
(VAM)
v., Adriamycin, procarbazine,
etoposide

v., Adriamycin, thiotepa (VAT)
v., Adriamycin, thiotepa, Halotestin
(VATH)
amifostine, cisplatin, v. (ACV)
v., BCNU, melphalan, prednisone,
Cytoxan (VBMPC)
v. and bleomycin (VB)
v., bleomycin, cisplatin (VBC)
v., bleomycin, DDP (VBD)
v., bleomycin, methotrexate, 5-
fluorouracil (VBMF)
v., bleomycin, Platinol (VBP)
CCNU, Adriamycin, v. (CAVe,
CA-Ve)
cisplatin, methotrexate, v. (CMV)
cyclophosphamide, Adriamycin, v.
(CAV)
cyclophosphamide, Oncovin,
procarbazine,
prednisone/Adriamycin,
bleomycin, v.
v. and dacarbazine
v., dacarbazine, Platinol (VDP)
epirubicin, bleomycin, v. (EBV)
v., etoposide, prednisone,
Adriamycin (VEPA)
v., ifosfamide, CCNU (VIC)
v., ifosfamide, cisplatin
v., ifosfamide, etoposide (VIE)
v., ifosfamide, gallium nitrate
(VIG)
v., ifosfamide, Platinol (VeIP, VIP)
mechlorethamine, Oncovin,
procarbazine, prednisone plus
Adriamycin, bleomycin, v.
(MOPP/ABV)
methotrexate, cisplatin, v. (MCV)
mitomycin and v. (MV)
v. and mitomycin (VM)
nitrogen mustard, vincristine,
procarbazine,
prednisone/doxorubicin,
bleomycin, v.
v., Platinol, bleomycin (VPB)
Platinol, bleomycin, v. (PBV)
PSC-833 and v.
v. sulfate
Vinca alkaloid
vincaleucoblastine
Vinca-related neuropathy
Vincent stomatitis
vincristine (VC, VCR)

NOTES

V

vincristine *(continued)*
v., actinomycin A, cyclophosphamide, Adriamycin (VACA)
v. and actinomycin D (VA)
actinomycin D, bleomycin, v. (ABV)
v., actinomycin D, cyclophosphamide (VAC)
v., actinomycin D, cyclophosphamide, Adriamycin (VACA)
v., actinomycin D, cyclophosphamide, Adriamycin, dacarbazine (VACAD)
v., actinomycin D, ifosfamide (VAI)
v., actinomycin D, ifosfamide, Adriamycin (VAIA)
v., actinomycin, methotrexate, prednisone (VAMP)
Adriamycin and v. (AV)
v., Adriamycin, cisplatin
v., Adriamycin, cyclophosphamide (VAC)
v., Adriamycin, dexamethasone (VAD)
v., Adriamycin, dexamethasone plus verapamil (VAD/V)
v., Adriamycin, methotrexate, prednisone (VAMP)
v., Adriamycin, methylprednisolone (VAMP)
v., Adriamycin, prednisone (VAP)
v., Adriamycin, prednisone, ara-C (VAPA)
v., Adriamycin, procarbazine (VAP)
v., Adriamycin, procarbazine, etoposide (VAPE)
v., amethopterin, 5-fluorouracil, Adriamycin, cyclophosphamide (VAFAC)
v., amethopterin, 6-mercaptopurine, prednisone (VAMP)
v., ara-C, 6-thioguanine (VAT)
v., ara-C, 6-thioguanine, daunorubicin (VATD)
v., L-asparaginase, Adriamycin, prednisone (VAAP)
v., L-asparaginase, prednisone (VAP)
v., BCNU, Adriamycin (VBA)
v., BCNU, Adriamycin, prednisone (VBAP)
BCNU, hydroxyurea, dacarbazine, v. (BHD-V)
v., BCNU, melphalan, cyclophosphamide, prednisone (VBMCP)

bleomycin, etoposide, prednimustine, procarbazine, cyclophosphamide, doxorubicin, v.
v., bleomycin, methotrexate (VBM)
v., bleomycin, methotrexate, 5-fluorouracil (VBMF)
v., carmustine, cyclophosphamide, melphalan, prednisone (M2)
CCNU, cyclophosphamide, v. (CCV)
cyclophosphamide, Adriamycin, v. (CAV)
v., cyclophosphamide, Adriamycin, prednisone (VCAP)
cyclophosphamide, etoposide, v. (CEV)
v., cyclophosphamide, 5-fluorouracil (VCF)
cyclophosphamide, 5-fluorouracil, epirubicin, v. (CFEV)
v., cyclophosphamide, melphalan, prednisone (VCMP)
cyclophosphamide, methotrexate, epirubicin, v. (CMEV)
cyclophosphamide, methotrexate, 5-fluorouracil, v. (CMFV)
cyclophosphamide, methotrexate, 5-fluorouracil, Adriamycin, v. (CMF-AV)
v., cyclophosphamide, prednisone (VCP)
dacarbazine, BCNU, v. (DBV)
dacarbazine, CCNU, v. (DCV)
v., dactinomycin, bleomycin, cisplatin, cyclophosphamide (VDBCC)
v., daunorubicin, L-asparaginase (VDA)
v., daunorubicin, prednisone (VDP)
dibromodulcitol, Adriamycin, v. (DAV)
dibromodulcitol, doxorubicin, v.
v., doxorubicin, cyclophosphamide, dactinomycin plus ifosfamide with mesna (VAdCA + I/E)
doxorubicin, cyclophosphamide, 5-fluorouracil, methotrexate, v.
v., doxorubicin, Decadron (VAD)
v., doxorubicin, dexamethasone (VDD)
v., doxorubicin, prednisone, asparaginase, 6-mercaptopurine, methotrexate
DTIC, CCNU, v. (DCV)
v., Endoxan, 6-mercaptopurine, prednisone (VEMP)
v., epirubicin, etoposide, prednisolone (VEEP)

etoposide, Cytoxan, methotrexate, v. (ECMV)
v., etoposide, prednisone, Adriamycin, methotrexate (VEPA-M)
v., ifosfamide, carboplatin, etoposide (VICE)
v., ifosfamide, etoposide (VIE)
liposomal v.
v., melphalan, cyclophosphamide, prednisone (VMCP)
v., methotrexate, Adriamycin, actinomycin D (VMAD)
methotrexate, 5-fluorouracil, epirubicin, v. (MFEV)
v. and prednisone
v., prednisone, L-asparaginase (VP+A)
v., prednisone, cyclophosphamide, ara-C (VPCA)
v., prednisone, cyclophosphamide, methotrexate, 5-fluorouracil (VPCMF)
v., prednisone, vinblastine, chlorambucil, procarbazine (VPBCPr, VPVCP)
procarbazine, CCNU, v. (PCV)
procarbazine, lomustine, v. (PCV)
v. sulfate
v. sulfate liposome
6-thioguanine, procarbazine, DBC, CCNU, v. (TPDCV)
6-thioguanine, procarbazine, dibromodulcitol, CCNU, v. (TPDCV)
VP-16-213, Adriamycin, v. (VAV)
vinculin protein
vindesine (VDS)
v. sulfate
vindoline
vinepidine
vinglycinate
vinleurosine
vinorelbine (VNR, VRL)
vinorelbine and cisplatin (VC)
vinorelbine tartrate
vinrosidine
vinzolidine
violaceous nodule
violet
aniline gentian v.
gentian v.
Vioxx

VIP
vasoactive intestinal peptide
VePesid, ifosfamide, Platinol
vinblastine, ifosfamide, Platinol
VP-16, ifosfamide, Platinol
VIP-B
VP-16, ifosfamide, Platinol, bleomycin
VIPoma
vasoactive intestinal peptide-secreting tumor
vasoactive intestinal polypeptide tumor
VIPoma syndrome
Viprinex
Vira-A Ophthalmic
Viracept
viral
v. envelope protein
v. expression
v. gene ICP47
genomic v.
v. hemagglutination
v. hepatitis (VH)
v. hepatitis coinfection
v. host cell interaction
v. load
v. matrix protein
v. matrix protein with kinase activity pp65
v. oncogenesis
v. phenotype
v. protease inhibitor
v. protein R (vpr)
v. radiculomyelitis
v. replication
v. reservoir
v. suppression
v. turnover
viral-induced atypical squamous metaplasia
viral-mediated cellular activation
Viramune
Virazole Aerosol
Virchow
V. cell
V. metastasis
V. node
Virchow-Hassall body
Virchow-Trosier node
VircoGEN genotyping
Viread
viremia
high-titer v.
plasma v.

NOTES

viremia (*continued*)
    primary v.
    secondary v.
viricidal (*var. of* virucidal)
viricide (*var. of* virucide)
virilism
virilization syndrome (VS)
Virilon
virion
    filamentous v.
    infectious v.
    progeny v.
    v. structure
Viroptic Ophthalmic
virtual
    v. bronchoscopy
    v. colonoscopy
virucidal, viricidal
virucide, viricide
virulence property
viruliferous
Virulizin
virus
    Abelson murine leukemia v.
    adenoassociated v. (AAV)
    AIDS-related v. (ARV)
    A-P-C v.
    avian E26 v.
    avian leukosis-sarcoma v.
    avian sarcoma v.
    B v.
    Balb/C sarcoma v.
    BK v.
    v. blockade
    Brunhilde v.
    Bwamba v.
    CA v.
    Cache Valley v.
    California v.
    Catu v.
    chimeric v.
    circulating free v.
    Coe v.
    Colorado tick fever v.
    community-acquired respirator v.
      (CRV)
    croup-associated v.
    dengue v.
    Ebola v.
    Ebola-Marburg v.
    ECHO v., echovirus
    ECMO v.
    Epstein-Barr v. (EBV)
    feline ataxia v.
    feline immunodeficiency v. (FIV)
    feline leukemia v.
    feline leukemia-sarcoma v.
    fluorescent treponemal antibody v.
    Friend leukemia v.

    Gardner-Rasheed sarcoma v.
    Germiston v.
    gibbon ape leukemia v. (GALV)
    gibbon ape lymphosarcoma v.
    gp160 recombinant vaccinia v.
    Graffi v.
    Gross leukemia v.
    Guama v.
    Guaroa v.
    Hardy-Zuckerman 2 feline
      sarcoma v.
    Harvey sarcoma v.
    hepatitis A v. (HAV)
    hepatitis B v. (HBV)
    hepatitis C v. (HCV)
    hepatitis D v. (HDV)
    hepatitis delta v. (HDV)
    hepatitis E v. (HEV)
    hepatitis G v. (HGV)
    hepatotropic v.
    herpes simplex v. (HSV)
    herpes simplex v. type 1 (HSV-1)
    herpes simplex v. type 2 (HSV-2)
    herpes simplex v. type 6 (HSV-6)
    herpes simplex v. type 7 (HSV-7)
    herpes zoster v.
    horizontal transmission of v.
    v. HTLV-III
    human breast carcinoma v.
    human immunodeficiency v. (HIV)
    human immunodeficiency v. type 1
      (HIV-1)
    human immunodeficiency v. type
      1E (HIV-1E)
    human immunodeficiency v. type 2
      (HIV-2)
    human mammary tumor v.
      (HMTV)
    human T-cell leukemia v. (HTLV)
    human T-cell
      leukemia/lymphoma v.
    human T-cell leukemia v. (type 1-
      5)
    human T-cell lymphotropic v.
    human T-lymphotrophic v. type I
      (HTLV-I)
    human T-lymphotrophic v. type II
      (HTLV-II)
    human T-lymphotrophic v. type III
      (HTLV-III)
    Ilhéus v.
    immunodeficiency v.
    influenza v.
    Itaqui v.
    Japanese B encephalitis v.
    JC v.
    Jeryl Lynn mumps v.
    Junin v.
    Kaposi sarcoma-associated v.

Kemerovo v.
killed v.
Kirsten sarcoma v.
KS-associated v.
Langat v.
Lassa fever v.
Latino v.
LCM v.
Lepore v.
lipid-coated v.
live-attenuated human
   immunodeficiency v.
Lucké v.
Lunyo v.
lymphadenopathy-associated v.
   (LAV)
lymphogranuloma venereum v.
Machupo v.
Makonde v.
Marburg v.
Marituba v.
masked v.
Mason-Pfizer monkey v.
Mayaro v.
McDonough sarcoma v.
McKrae herpes simplex v.
medical outcomes study-human
   immunodeficiency v. (MOS-HIV)
Mengo v.
Molony murine leukemia v.
Mossuril v.
Multidimensional Quality of Life
   Questionnaire for Persons with
   Human Immunodeficiency V.
   (MQOL-HIV)
mumps v.
murine lymphocytic
   choriomeningitis v.
murine sarcoma v.
Murray Valley encephalitis v.
myeloproliferative leukemia v.
   (MPLV)
nef-deleted v.
nef gene-deleted v.
Newcastle disease v. (NDV)
nonsyncytia-forming human
   immunodeficiency v.
Ntaya v.
oncogenic v.
papilloma v.
papilloma, polyoma, vacuolating v.
Parodi-Irgens sarcoma v.
protease inhibitor-resistant v.

R5 v.
rabbit fibroma v.
rapid high v.
Rasheed sarcoma v.
Rauscher leukemia v.
recombinant fowlpox v.
replication-deficient v.
respiratory syncytial v. (RSV)
RNA tumor v.
Rous-associated v. (RAV)
Rous sarcoma v. (RSV)
rubella v.
Semliki Forest v.
Shope fibroma v.
simian v. 40 (SV40)
simian foamy v.
Sindbis v.
strain-specific v.
suboptimal v.
SV40 v.
Swiss mouse leukemia v.
syncytium-inducing v.
T-cell-tropic human
   immunodeficiency v. 1
Theiler murine encephalomyelitis v.
tumor v.
unintegrated human
   immunodeficiency v.
UR-2 sarcoma v.
vaccinia v.
varicella-zoster v. (VZV)
Venezuelan equine encephalitis v.
woodchuck hepatitis v.
Yamaguchi sarcoma v.

viruslike particle (VLP)
virus-neutralization laboratory assay
virus-neutralizing antibody
virus-positive antibody-negative
   individual
viscera (*pl. of* viscus)
visceral
   v. adipose tissue (VAT)
   v. larva migrans
   v. pain
   v. paraganglia
   v. pleura
viscerum
   situs inversus v.
viscosimeter
   capillary tube plasma v.
viscus, pl. **viscera**
   abdominal v.
Visica Treatment System

NOTES

Visick
> V. gastric cancer grading
> V. grading system
> V. grading system for postgastrectomy carcinoma recurrence

Visipaque
Vistaril
Vistide
visual
> v. acuity testing
> v. imagery
> v. pathway
> v. pathway glioma

visualization
> double-peak-angle camera v.
> triple-peak-angle camera v.

Vita-C
Vita cuff
vital
> v. blue dye
> v. capacity (VC)

vitamin
> v. A
> v. B complex
> v. B_{12} deficiency
> v. C
> v. C drops
> v. D analog
> v. E
> intermittent high-dose v. C
> prenatal v.

Vita-Plus E Softgel
Vitaxin
Vitec lotion
Vitrasert implant
Vitravene
vitreous
> v. hemorrhage
> v. opacity
> persistent hyperplastic primary v.

vitro
> in v.

vitronectin
vivax
> *Plasmodium v.*

Vivelle Transdermal
vivo
> in v.

VLP
> viruslike particle

VM
> vector magnitude
> vinblastine and mitomycin

VMA
> vanillylmandelic acid

VMAD
> vincristine, methotrexate, Adriamycin, actinomycin D

VMC
> VP-16, methotrexate, citrovorum factor

VMCP
> vincristine, melphalan, cyclophosphamide, prednisone

VMO
> vaccinia melanoma oncolysate

VMP
> VePesid, mitoxantrone, prednimustine

VNR
> vinorelbine

VOCA
> VP-16, Oncovin, cyclophosphamide, Adriamycin

vocal
> v. cord
> v. cord cancer
> v. cord keratosis
> v. cord palsy
> v. cord paralysis

vocalis muscle
VOCAP
> VP-16-213, Oncovin, cyclophosphamide, Adriamycin, Platinol

VOD
> venoocclusive disease
> VOD of liver

Vogele-Bale-Hohner (VBH)
> V.-B.-H. head holder

Voges-Proskauer test
void
> flow v.
> signal v.

Vokes chemotherapy protocol
volemic hyponatremia
volt
> electron v. (eV)
> kiloelectron v. (keV, kev)
> megaelectron v. (MeV)

Voltaren Ophthalmic
Voltaren-XR Oral
volume
> aortic flow v.
> cerebral blood v.
> cerebrospinal fluid v.
> clinical target v. (CTV)
> clinical tumor v. (CTV)
> cytosolic v.
> electron boost v. (EBV)
> v. element
> erythrocyte v.
> gross tumor v. (GTV)
> v. imaging for breast assessment (VIBRANT)
> mean corpuscular v. (MCV)
> mean plasma v. (MPV)
> mean platelet v. (MPV)
> organ v.
> v. overload

packed cell v. (PCV)
v. of packed cells (VPC)
planning target v. (PTV)
red cell v. (RCV)
target v.
tidal v.
transit v.
tumor v.
volume-limited radiotherapy
volume-restricted radiotherapy
volumetric pump
volumetrics
tumor v.
volumetry
tank v.
water-displacement v.
volvulus
cecal v.
colonic v.
vomiting
anticipatory v.
chemotherapy-induced nausea
and v. (CINV)
delayed v.
projectile v.
von
v. Hippel-Lindau (VHL)
v. Hippel-Lindau complex
v. Hippel-Lindau disease
v. Hippel-Lindau gene
v. Hippel-Lindau syndrome
v. Hippel tumor
v. Jaksch anemia
v. Mikulicz syndrome
v. Recklinghausen disease
v. Recklinghausen neurofibromatosis
v. Willebrand disease
v. Willebrand factor (vWF)
voriconazole
vorozole
vortex keratopathy
votumumab
voxel element
VP
vasopressin
VP-16 (VePesid)
CCNU, cyclophosphamide, Adriamycin,
vincristine, VP-16
CCNU, cyclophosphamide,
Adriamycin, vincristine, VP-16
(CCAVV, VP-16)
cisplatin and VP-16 (CV)

cyclophosphamide, Adriamycin, VP-
16 (CAVP16)
VP-16, cyclophosphamide,
Adriamycin, Platinol (VCAP-I)
cyclophosphamide, Adriamycin,
vincristine, VP-16
VP-16, cyclophosphamide, Platinol
(VCP-I)
cyclophosphamide, Platinol, VP-16
(CPV)
Cytoxan, Adriamycin, VP-16
(CAVP16)
Cytoxan, BCNU, VP-16 (CBV)
daunomycin, cytosine, arabinoside,
VP-16
daunorubicin, ara-C, VP-16 (DAV)
5-fluorouracil, Adriamycin,
cyclophosphamide, VP-16
(FACVP)
high-dose cyclophosphamide,
mitoxantrone, VP-16 (HD-CNVp)
VP-16, ifosfamide, carboplatin
(VIC)
VP-16, ifosfamide, mitoxantrone,
bleomycin (VIMB)
VP-16, ifosfamide, Platinol (VIP)
VP-16, ifosfamide, Platinol,
bleomycin (VIP-B)
VP-16, methotrexate, citrovorum
factor (VMC)
mitoxantrone and VP-16 (MV)
VP-16, Oncovin, cyclophosphamide,
Adriamycin (VOCA)
oral VP-16
VP-16 and Platinol (VPP)
Platinol and VP-16 (PVP)
VP-16-213 (VePesid)
VP-16-213, Adriamycin,
methotrexate (VAM)
VP-16-213, Adriamycin, vincristine
(VAV)
cyclophosphamide, BCNU, VP-16-
213 (CBV)
VP-16-213, Oncovin,
cyclophosphamide, Adriamycin,
Platinol (VOCAP)
VP+A
vincristine, prednisone, L-asparaginase
VPAM
verapamil
VPB
vinblastine, Platinol, bleomycin

NOTES

V

VPBCPr
  vincristine, prednisone, vinblastine, chlorambucil, procarbazine
VPC
  volume of packed cells
VPCA
  vincristine, prednisone, cyclophosphamide, ara-C
VPCMF
  vincristine, prednisone, cyclophosphamide, methotrexate, 5-fluorouracil
VPF
  vascular permeability factor
VPP
  VePesid and Platinol
  VP-16 and Platinol
vpr
  viral protein R
    vpr gene
Vpu protein
VPVCP
  vincristine, prednisone, vinblastine, chlorambucil, procarbazine
VRL
  vinorelbine
VRV
  ventricular rate variability
VS
  virilization syndrome
V-TAD
  VePesid, 6-thioguanine, ara-C, daunorubicin
VUDS
  video urodynamics
vulgaris
    verruca v.
vulva, pl. **vulvae**

bowenoid papulosis of v.
epidermoid carcinoma of v.
intraepithelial neoplasia of v.
nevus of v.
preinvasive disease of cervix, vagina, and v.
vulvar
  v. adenocystic adenocarinoma
  v. atrophy
  v. biopsy
  v. cancer
  v. carcinoma
  v. intraepithelial neoplasia (VIN)
  v. intraepithelial neoplasm (VIN)
  v. malignancy
  v. melanoma
  v. pruritus
vulvectomy
  radical v.
  skinning v.
vulvovaginal
  v. carcinoma
  v. lesion
Vumon
vWF
  von Willebrand factor
  Assera vWF
  Asserachrom vWF
Vysis
  V. PathVysion genomic disease management test
  V. PathVysion HER-2 DNA Probe Kit
  V. UroVysion DNA probe assay
VZV
  varicella-zoster virus

tungsten-188
Waaler-Rose test
Waardenburg syndrome
wafer
    BCNU-impregnated w.
    carmustine w.
    chemotherapy w.
    Gliadel w.
    interstitial BCNU administered
        via w.
    polifeprosan 20 with carmustine
        implant w.
Wagner-Meissnerlike structure
WAGR
    Wilms tumor, aniridia, genitourinary
        abnormalities, mental retardation
    WAGR syndrome
waiting
    watchful w.
Waldenström
    W. macrogammaglobulinemia
    W. macroglobulinemia
Waldeyer
    W. ring lesion
    W. ring lymphoma
    W. tonsillar ring
Waldmar link
Walker
    W. carcinoma
    W. carcinosarcoma
walking
    labyrinth w.
wall
    abdominal w.
    anterolateral abdominal w.
    arterial w.
    bladder w.
    bowel w.
    chest w.
    hypopharyngeal w.
    lateral pharyngeal w.
    pharyngeal w.
wallerian degeneration
Wallner interstitial prostate implanter
Wallstent biliary endoprosthesis
Walthard nest
Wan
    Danggui Longhui W.
wandering cell
Wang
    W. applicator
    W. needle biopsy
    W. pleural stoma

WAP
    whole abdominopelvic irradiation
Warburg apparatus
warfarin
    w. sodium
    w. therapy
**warm-and-cold-type autoimmune
    hemolytic anemia**
**warm-antibody acquired autoimmune
    hemolytic anemia**
warmer
    blood w.
warming
    urethral w.
warm-reactive antibody
**warm-type autoimmune hemolytic
    anemia**
Warm-Up wound care system
wart
    anal w.
    anogenital w.
Warthin
    W. cell
    W. tumor
Warthin-Finkeldey giant cell
Warthin-Starry stain
warty dyskeratoma
washed red cell
washing
    bronchial w.
    endometrial jet w.
    peritoneal w.
wasting syndrome
watchful waiting
water
    w. cancer
    free w.
    hydration layer w.
water-bottle heart
water-displacement volumetry
Waterfield needle
Waterhouse-Friderichsen syndrome
Waterhouse transpubic procedure
water-in-oil-in-water (W/O/W)
water-loading test
water-siphon test
**Waters M-440 fixed wavelength
    detector**
watery
    w. diarrhea, hypokalemia,
        achlorhydria (WDHA)
    w. diarrhea with hypokalemic
        alkalosis (WDHA)
wave
    acoustic w.

W

wave *(continued)*
    electromagnetic w.
    extracorporeal shock w.
    mucosal w.
waveform
    arterial w.
way
    W.'s of Coping (WOC)
    W.'s of Coping, Cancer Version
      (WOC-CA)
    1-w. valved silicone voice
      prosthesis
Wayne State protocol
WBC
    white blood cell
      WBC count
WBP
    whole body protein
WBR
    whole body radiation
WBRT
    whole brain radiation therapy
    whole brain radiotherapy
WDHA
    watery diarrhea, hypokalemia,
      achlorhydria
    watery diarrhea with hypokalemic
      alkalosis
      WDHA syndrome
WDLL
    well-differentiated lymphocytic
      lymphoma
weakness
    Eaton-Lambert muscular w.
    muscle w.
web
    antral w.
    esophageal w.
webbing
    vaginal w.
Weber-Fergusson incision
Webster cheek advancement flap
Wechsler Memory Scale
wedge
    dynamic w.
    w. factor
    w. filter
    w. pulmonary resection
wedged field
wedged-pair technique
Wegener granulomatosis
Weibull
    W. plot
    W. plot of adult T-cell
      leukemia/lymphoma risk
Weigert
    W. iron hematoxylin stain
    W. resorcin-fuchsin stain
Weigert-Meyer rule

weight
    w. estimation and assessment
    w. loss
    molecular w.
weighting
    beam w.
    tumor-dose w.
Weismann-Netter syndrome
Welch *t* test
Wellbutrin SR
well-circumscribed
    w.-c. carcinoma
    w.-c. lesion
Wellcovorin
well-demarcated lesion
well-differentiated
    w.-d. lymphocytic
    w.-d. lymphocytic lymphoma
      (WDLL)
    w.-d. polycystic Wilms tumor
Wellferon lymphoblastoid interferon IFN alfa-n
Well syndrome
Werlhof disease
Wermer syndrome
Werner syndrome
Wernicke
    W. aphasia
    W. area
    W. encephalopathy
Wertheim hysterectomy
Wertheim-Okabayashi radical hysterectomy
Westcott needle
Westergren method
western
    W. ligand blot (WLB)
    W. yew
WFRT
    wide-field radiation therapy
Wharton duct
Whatmann filter
wheat
    w. bran
    w. germ agglutinin
Wheaton tissue homogenizer
Whipple
    W. disease
    W. operation
    W. procedure
    W. resection
white
    w. blood cell (WBC)
    w. blood cell contamination
    w. blood cell count
    w. blood cell depletion
    w. blood cell engraftment
    w. blood cell function
    w. blood cell transfusion

w. clot syndrome
w. matter demyelination
w. matter edema
w. matter hyperintensity
w. matter hypodensity
w. matter thinning
w. pulp
w. sponge nevus
w. tea

whitlow

herpes w.
herpetic w.

Whitmore-Jewett prostate cancer staging
WHO

World Health Organization
WHO classification for transitional
cell carcinoma of the urinary
bladder (stages Ta through T4)
WHO grade I-IV

whole

w. abdominal irradiation
w. abdominal radiotherapy
w. abdominopelvic irradiation
(WAP)
w. blood
w. blood lysis technique
w. body hyperthermia
w. body PET
w. body protein (WBP)
w. body radiation (WBR)
w. body radiation therapy
w. brain
w. brain radiation therapy (WBRT)
w. brain radiation therapy without
stereotactic boost
w. brain radiation therapy with
stereotactic boost
w. brain radiotherapy (WBRT)
w. cell vaccine
w. lung irradiation
w. pelvic irradiation
w. pelvis irradiation
w. virus preparation

whorling

cellular w.

wide-field radiation therapy (WFRT)
wide local excision (WLE)
widely invasive follicular carcinoma
(WIFC)
wide-range radiation therapy
Widmark test

width

platelet distribution w.
red cell distribution w. (RDW)

Wiener filter
WIFC

widely invasive follicular carcinoma

Wilder reticulum stain
wild-type

w.-t. allele
w.-t. cell
w.-t. gene
w.-t. p53
w.-t. revertant

Williamson blood test
Will Rogers phenomenon
Wills factor
Wilms

W. tumor
W. tumor, aniridia, genitourinary
abnormalities, mental retardation
(WAGR)

Wilson-Cook metal reinforcement
wimp mutation
Winckel disease
window

acquisition w.
aortic w.
aorticopulmonary w.
aortic-pulmonary w.
biologic w.
cortical w.
w. of opportunity
pericardial w.
w. pericardiectomy
w. period
subxiphoid w.

wing

ambient w.
iliac w.

Winn test
Winpred
WinRho

W. SDF
W. SDF immune globulin

Wintrobe

W. index
W. and Landsberg method
W. tube

wipe

Tucks W.'s

wire

Amplatz stiffening w.
atherolytic reperfusion w.

NOTES

W

wire *(continued)*
- guide w.
- infusion w.
- ^{192}Ir w.
- rocket w.
- Schneider infusion w.
- w. stiffener

Wisconsin Brief Pain Inventory

wish
- death w.
- passive death w.

Wiskott-Aldrich syndrome

witch hazel

withdrawal
- antiandrogen w.
- opiate w.

withdrawn alive

Witts anemia

Witzel jejunostomy

WLB
- Western ligand blot

WLE
- wide local excision

Wnt-1 expression

Wobe-Mugos

WOC
- Ways of Coping

WOC-CA
- Ways of Coping, Cancer Version

Wolfe
- W. breast carcinoma classification
- W. classification of breast carcinoma
- W. grade

wolffian
- w. duct
- w. duct carcinoma

Wolman disease

woman, pl. **women**
- antibody-positive w.
- Women's CARE Study
- Women's Contraceptive and Reproductive Experiences Study
- postmenopausal w.
- seroincident w.

woman's

woodchuck hepatitis virus

Wood light

Word Fluency Test

Woringer-Kolopp
- W.-K. disease
- W.-K. syndrome

working
- W. Formula classification
- W. Formulation of non-Hodgkin lymphoma
- w. sheath

workstation
- GENS-S Cell hematology w.
- Mayfield/ACCISS stereotactic w.

workup
- salvage w.

world
- W. Health Organization (WHO)
- W. Health Organization classification

wort
- St. John's w.

wound
- w. breakdown
- w. healing
- w. infection
- oral w.
- w. rinse
- w. staging

W/O/W
- water-in-oil-in-water
- W/O/W emulsion

Wright-Giemsa
- W.-G. evaluation
- W.-G. stain

Wright stain

W-shaped ileoneobladder

WT1
- WT1 gene
- WT1 transcription factor

wtp53 cell

Wuchereria bancrofti

Wycillin

Wymox

X
magnification
X factor
X gradient
X4
TCLA X4
Xact positioning cushion
X:Ag
factor X antigen
Asserachrom X:Ag
xanthemia
xanthine
xanthinuria
xanthoastrocytoma
pleomorphic x. (PXA)
xanthochromia
xanthochromic cerebrospinal fluid
xanthogranuloma
intramuscular juvenile x.
juvenile x.
necrobiotic x.
xanthogranulomatous pyelonephritis
xanthoma, pl. xanthomata, xanthomas
neutrophilic x.
xanthomatosis
familial x.
Xanthomonas maltophilia
xanthosarcoma
X-axis off-axis ratio
Xcytrin
^{127}Xe
xenon-127
^{133}Xe
xenon-133
Xeloda
xemilofiban
xenograft
human-murine x.
orthotopic x.
XenoMouse technology
xenon
x. arc
x. flash lamp
xenon-127 (^{127}Xe)
xenon-133 (^{133}Xe)
xenopi
Mycobacterium x.
xenotransplantation
cellular x.
Xerecept
xerocytosis
hereditary x.
xeroderma pigmentosum (XP)

xerophthalmia
xeroradiography
xerorhinia
xerosis
xerostomia
Xillix
X. LIFE-GI fluorescence endoscopy
system
X. LIFE-Lung system
ximelagatran
Xinlay
XKnife
X. software
X. software for stereotatic radiation
therapy
X-linked
X-l. agammaglobulinemia
X-l. gene
X-l. hyperimmunoglobulin M
syndrome
X-l. hypogammaglobulinemia
X-l. IgM syndrome
X-l. lymphoproliferative (XLP)
X-l. lymphoproliferative syndrome
X-l. SCID
X-l. spastic paraparesis
XLP
X-linked lymphoproliferative
XLP syndrome
XMG
x-ray mammogram
Xomed endotracheal tube
XP
xeroderma pigmentosum
X-Prep Liquid
x-ray
chest x-r.
x-r. mammogram (XMG)
x-r. mammography
Precision 500D digital x-r.
x-r. therapy (XRT)
XRCC1 gene
XRT
radiotherapy
x-ray therapy
Xyctrin
xylazine
Xylocaine viscous solution
xylol, xylene
Xyotax

X

Y
tyrosine
yttrium
   Y adapter
   Y gradient
   Y ibritumomab tiuxetan
^{50}Y
yttrium-50
^{90}Y
yttrium-90
Yaba tumor
YAC
yeast artificial chromosome
Yakima
hemoglobin Y.
Yale brace
Yamaguchi sarcoma virus
$[^{90}$Y]-DOTA-D-Ph^{1}1-Tyr^3 octreotide
ye
da qing y.
year
5-y. cure rate
yeast
y. artificial chromosome (YAC)
budding y.
yellow
y. dock
y. fever
y. nail syndrome
Yersin serum

yes protooncogene/oncogene
yew
Himalayan y.
Pacific y.
Western y.
yield
fluorescence y.
Y-jaws
YLF
yttrium lithium fluoride
Yocon
Yodoxin
yoga
yohimbine
yolk sac tumor
Yondelis
York-Mason procedure
You-Bend hemodialysis catheterization kit
yttrium (Y)
y. lithium fluoride (YLF)
yttrium-50 (^{50}Y)
yttrium-90 (^{90}Y)
y.-90 radiolabeled humanized anti-Tac and calcium-DTPA
yttrium-90-labeled
y.-90-l. anti-B2 immunoconjugate
y.-90-l. antiferritin
y.-90-l. ibritumomab tiuxetan radioimmunotherapy

Y

ζ (*var. of* zeta)
Zadaxin
Zagam
Zahn infarct
zalcitabine (ddC)
Zaleski test
Zamyl
Zanosar
zanoterone
Zantac
ZAP-70
    zeta-associated protein 70
Zarnestra
Zarontin
Zaroxolyn
Zavala lung biopsy needle
z-dependent dose-volume histogram (zDVH)
ZDV
    zidovudine
zDVH
    z-dependent dose-volume histogram
zearalenone
ZEBRA
    antibodies to Epstein-Barr virus
    transactivator protein
        ZEBRA artifact
        ZEBRA protein
Zeis
    glands of Z.
Zeiss Axioskop microscope
Zelen exact test
zellballen cell
Zemplar
Zenapax
Zenker solution
Zen macrobiotic diet
Zerit
    didehydrodideoxythymidine,
    stavudine, Z. (d4T)
ZeroRad MRI scan
ZES
    Zollinger-Ellison syndrome
zeta, ζ
    zeta potential
zeta-associated protein 70 (ZAP-70)
zetacrit
Zevalin radioimmunotherapy
zhi
    ling z.
Ziagen
ziconotide
zidovudine (ZDV)
    z. and lamivudine
    z. phosphate

z. phosphate secondary to negative
    feedback
z. resistance
z. triphosphate
Ziemann stippling
Zieve syndrome
Zilactin-B Medicated
Zinacef Injection
zinc
    z. chelation
    z. chelation complex
    z. chloride
    z. finger motif
    z. sulfate
    z. sulfate solution
    z. turbidity test (ZTT)
Zinca-Pak
zindoxifene
Zinecard
zinostatin
zipper
    leucine z.
ziprasidone
Zithromax Z-Pak
Zocor
Zofran ODT
Zoladex
    flutamide and Z. (FZ)
    Z. implant
zoledronate
zoledronic
    z. acid
    z. acid for injection
    z. acid powder
zolimomab aritox
Zolla-Pazner immunological staging system
Zollinger-Ellison
    Z.-E. syndrome (ZES)
    Z.-E. tumor
zolpidem
Zometa powder
zonal
    z. anatomy
    z. architecture
    z. architecture of prostate
zone
    chemoreceptor trigger z. (CTZ)
    follicular mantle z.
    high-intensity z. (HIZ)
    hypointense z.
    junctional z.
    landing z.
    large loop excision of
        transformation z. (LLETZ)

Z

zone *(continued)*
    mantle z.
    marginal z.
    noninfarct z. (NIZ)
    primary landing z.
    prostatic transition z.
    transformation z.
    transition z.
    trigger z.
Zone-A Forte
zooagglutinin
ZORprin
zorubicin hydrochloride
zoster
    dermatomal z.
    herpes z.
    multidermatomal herpes z.
    z. ophthalmicus
    recurrent z.
    unidermatomal z.
Zostrix
Zostrix-HP
zosuquidar
Zosyn

Zovirax
Z-Pak
    Zithromax Z-P.
Z-plasty
z score
ZTT
    zinc turbidity test
Zubrod Performance Scale
Zuckerkandl
    organ of Z.
Zung
    Z. Anxiety Scale
    Z. Depression Inventory
Z value
Zyban
Zydone
Zyflamend
zygomycosis
zygosity
Zyloprim
Zymogen
zymography
    gelatin z.

Contents: The Appendices

Contents: The Appendices

Appendix 1
Anatomical Illustrations

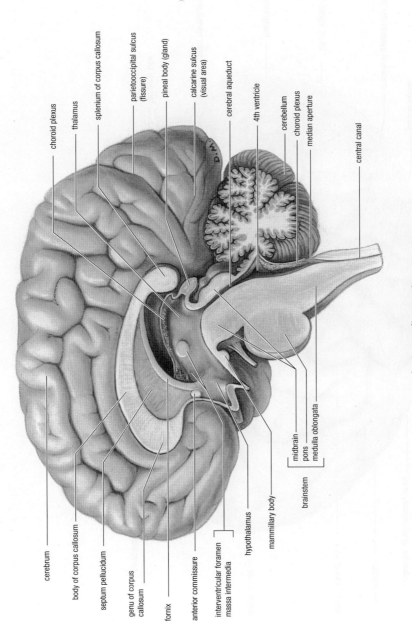

brain, median section

choroid plexus

thalamus

splenium of corpus callosum

parietooccipital sulcus (fissure)

pineal body (gland)

calcarine sulcus (visual area)

cerebral aqueduct

4th ventricle

cerebellum

choroid plexus

median aperture

central canal

cerebrum

body of corpus callosum

septum pellucidum

genu of corpus callosum

fornix

anterior commissure

interventricular foramen

massa intermedia

hypothalamus

mammillary body

brainstem

midbrain

pons

medulla oblongata

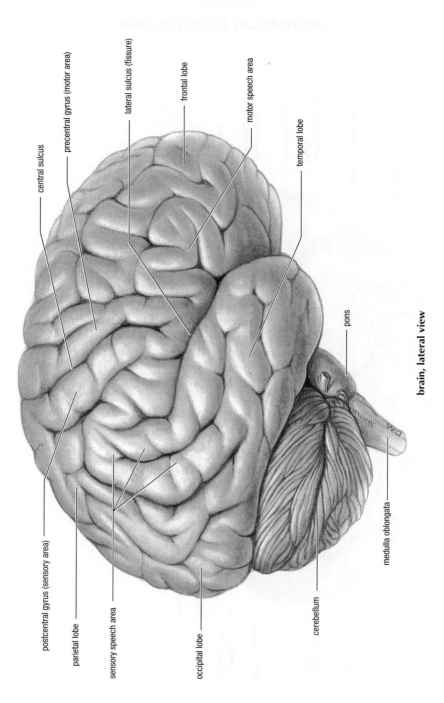

central sulcus

precentral gyrus (motor area)

lateral sulcus (fissure)

frontal lobe

motor speech area

temporal lobe

pons

medulla oblongata

cerebellum

occipital lobe

sensory speech area

parietal lobe

postcentral gyrus (sensory area)

brain, lateral view

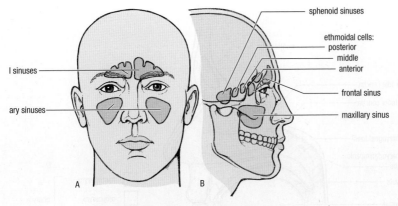

sphenoid sinuses

ethmoidal cells:
posterior
middle
anterior

frontal sinus

maxillary sinus

l sinuses

ary sinuses

A

B

paranasal sinuses: anterior (A) and lateral (B) views of the head

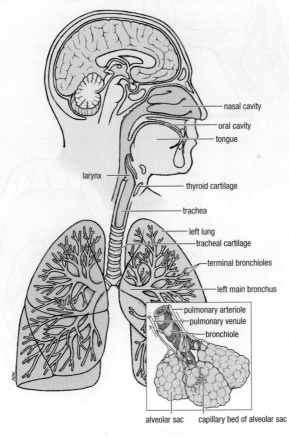

nasal cavity

oral cavity

tongue

larynx

thyroid cartilage

trachea

left lung

tracheal cartilage

terminal bronchioles

left main bronchus

pulmonary arteriole
pulmonary venule
bronchiole

alveolar sac   capillary bed of alveolar sac

lungs and respiratory anatomy

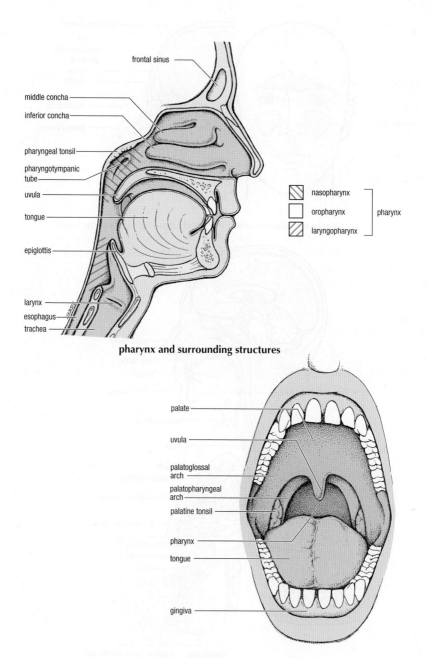

pharynx and surrounding structures

oral cavity

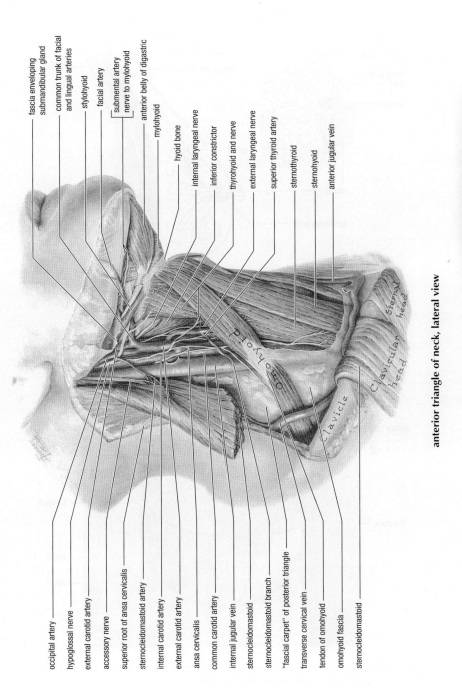

fascia enveloping submandibular gland

common trunk of facial and lingual arteries

stylohyoid

facial artery

submental artery
nerve to mylohyoid

anterior belly of digastric

mylohyoid

hyoid bone

internal laryngeal nerve

inferior constrictor

thyrohyoid and nerve

external laryngeal nerve

superior thyroid artery

sternothyroid

sternohyoid

anterior jugular vein

occipital artery

hypoglossal nerve

external carotid artery

accessory nerve

superior root of ansa cervicalis

sternocleidomastoid artery

internal carotid artery

external carotid artery

ansa cervicalis

common carotid artery

internal jugular vein

sternocleidomastoid

sternocleidomastoid branch

"fascial carpet" of posterior triangle

transverse cervical vein

tendon of omohyoid

omohyoid fascia

sternocleidomastoid

Omohyoid

Sternal head

Clavicular head

Clavicle

anterior triangle of neck, lateral view

A5

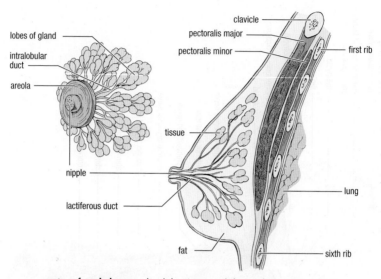

mature female breast: glandular tissue and ducts of mammary gland

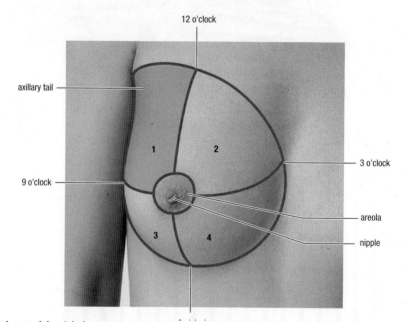

quadrants of the right breast: (1) upper outer (50% of cancerous breast tumors are found in this quadrant), (2) upper inner, (3) lower outer, (4) lower inner

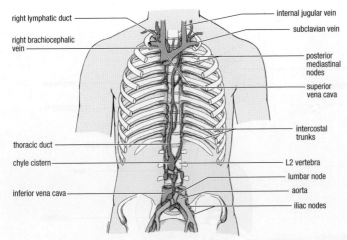

right lymphatic duct

right brachiocephalic
vein

thoracic duct

chyle cistern

inferior vena cava

internal jugular vein

subclavian vein

posterior
mediastinal
nodes

superior
vena cava

intercostal
trunks

L2 vertebra

lumbar node

aorta

iliac nodes

thoracic and right lymphatic ducts: deep lymphatic vessels and nodes are also shown

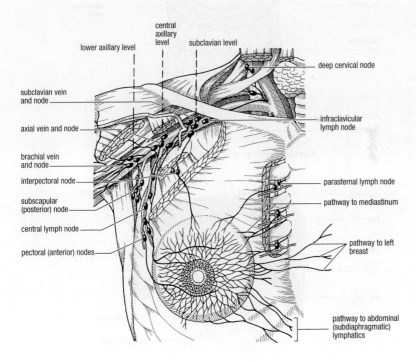

central
axillary
level

lower axillary level

subclavian level

deep cervical node

subclavian vein
and node

axial vein and node

brachial vein
and node

interpectoral node

subscapular
(posterior) node

central lymph node

pectoral (anterior) nodes

infraclavicular
lymph node

parasternal lymph node

pathway to mediastinum

pathway to left
breast

pathway to abdominal
(subdiaphragmatic)
lymphatics

lymphatic drainage of breast

A7

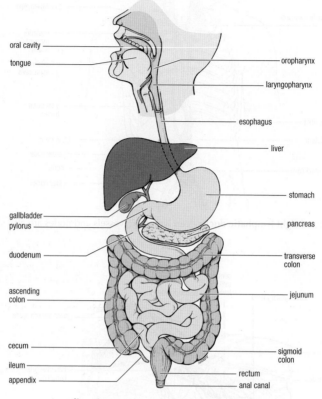

oral cavity

tongue

oropharynx

laryngopharynx

esophagus

liver

stomach

gallbladder

pylorus

pancreas

duodenum

transverse colon

ascending colon

jejunum

cecum

sigmoid colon

ileum

rectum

appendix

anal canal

digestive system and associated structures

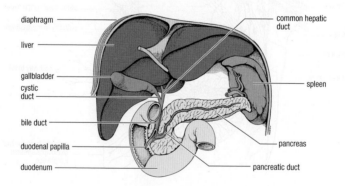

diaphragm

common hepatic duct

liver

gallbladder

cystic duct

spleen

bile duct

duodenal papilla

pancreas

duodenum

pancreatic duct

gallbladder, liver, and biliary system

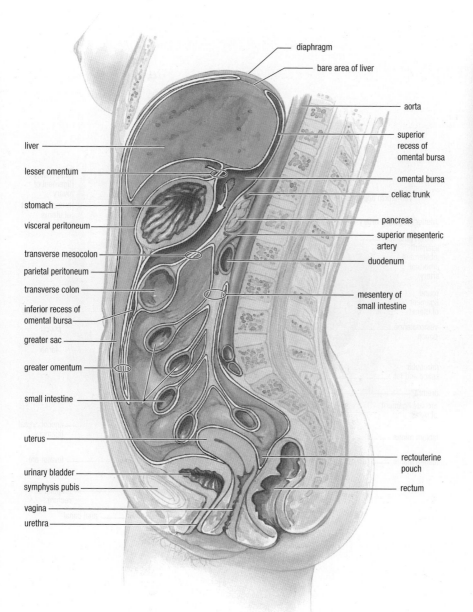

diaphragm

bare area of liver

aorta

superior
recess of
omental bursa

omental bursa

celiac trunk

liver

lesser omentum

pancreas

superior mesenteric
artery

stomach

visceral peritoneum

duodenum

transverse mesocolon

parietal peritoneum

mesentery of
small intestine

transverse colon

inferior recess of
omental bursa

greater sac

greater omentum

small intestine

uterus

rectouterine
pouch

urinary bladder

rectum

symphysis pubis

vagina

urethra

peritoneal cavity of the female: greater sac and omental bursa (lesser sac), median section

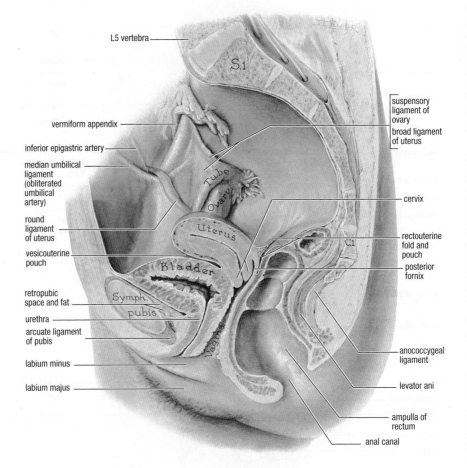

L5 vertebra

S.1

suspensory ligament of ovary

broad ligament of uterus

vermiform appendix

inferior epigastric artery

median umbilical ligament (obliterated umbilical artery)

Tube

Ovary

cervix

round ligament of uterus

Uterus

vesicouterine pouch

Bladder

C.1

rectouterine fold and pouch

posterior fornix

retropubic space and fat

Symph. pubis

urethra

arcuate ligament of pubis

Vagina

anococcygeal ligament

labium minus

levator ani

labium majus

ampulla of rectum

anal canal

female pelvis, median section

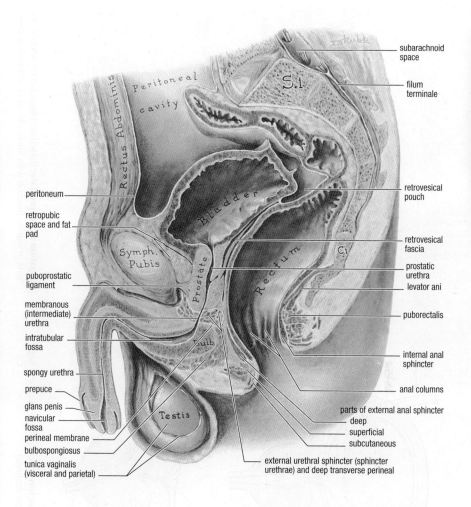

peritoneum

retropubic space and fat pad

puboprostatic ligament

membranous (intermediate) urethra

intratubular fossa

spongy urethra

prepuce

glans penis

navicular fossa

perineal membrane

bulbospongiosus

tunica vaginalis (visceral and parietal)

subarachnoid space

filum terminale

retrovesical pouch

retrovesical fascia

prostatic urethra

levator ani

puborectalis

internal anal sphincter

anal columns

parts of external anal sphincter

deep

superficial

subcutaneous

external urethral sphincter (sphincter urethrae) and deep transverse perineal

male pelvis, median section

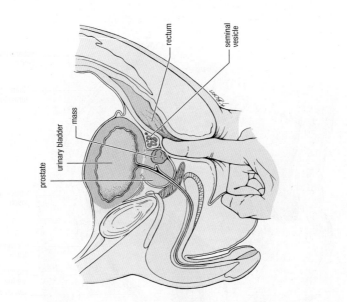

palpation of the prostate: (based on physician preference, patient is either lying in supine position with knees elevated, or bending over at the waist)

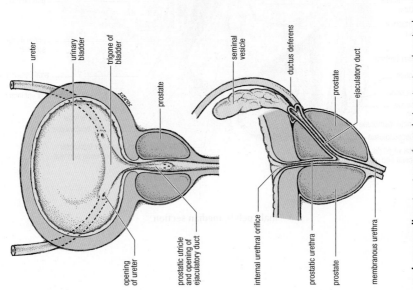

prostate and surrounding structures: frontal view (top) and sagittal view (bottom)

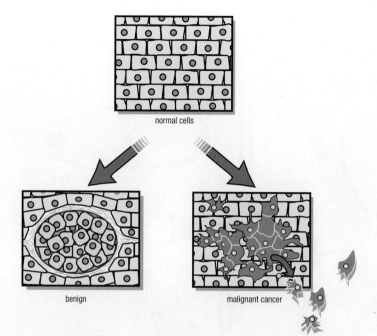

normal cells

benign

malignant cancer

tissues at the histological level to show normal (top), benign (lower left), and cancerous (lower right) growth

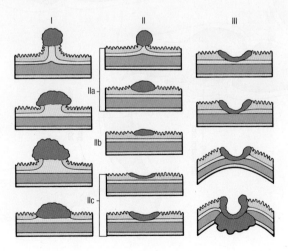

I

II

III

IIa

IIb

IIc

carcinoma: patterns of development in carcinomas of the stomach; (I) polypoid or fungating; (II) superficial extension (a) elevated, (b) plaquelike, (c) depressed; (III) ulcerating

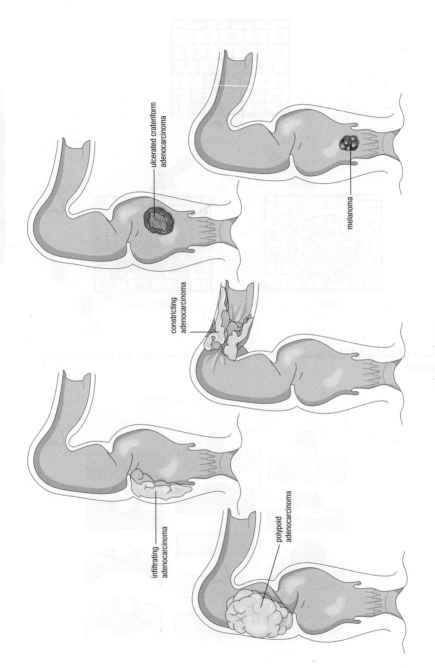

ulcerated crateriform
adenocarcinoma

melanoma

constricting
adenocarcinoma

infiltrating
adenocarcinoma

polypoid
adenocarcinoma

colorectal cancers

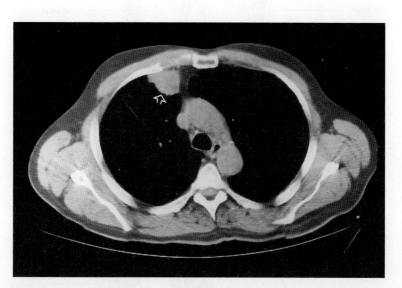

lung carcinoma: CT section shows mass to be located in anterior segment of right upper lobe (arrow) adjacent to pleura

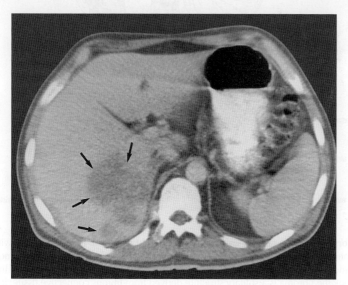

liver metastases: CT image of patient with renal carcinoma showing lucent areas within the liver (arrows)

A15

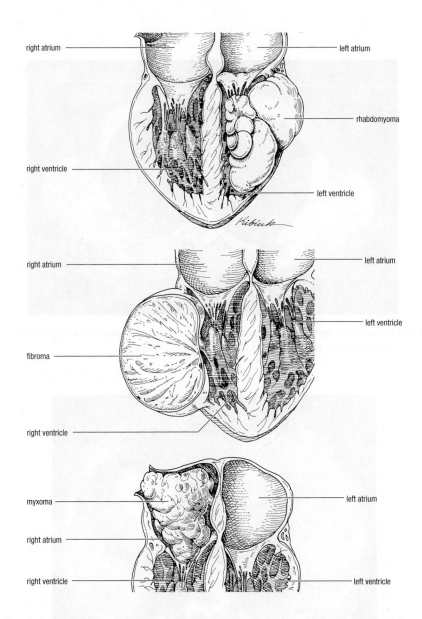

right atrium — — left atrium

— rhabdomyoma

right ventricle — — left ventricle

right atrium — — left atrium

— left ventricle

fibroma —

right ventricle —

myxoma — — left atrium

right atrium —

right ventricle — — left ventricle

cardiac tumors in children: primary cardiac tumors in children appear to be associated with familial syndromes with autosomal dominant inheritance; rhabdomyoma is the most common benign tumor and is derived from striated muscle elements; it is located within the walls of the myocardium (top); the fibroma is a solitary structure derived from fibrous connective tissue; it occurs in children under 10 years of age (middle); the myxoma arises from the lining of the atrium and resembles a polyp; it is a benign tumor (bottom)

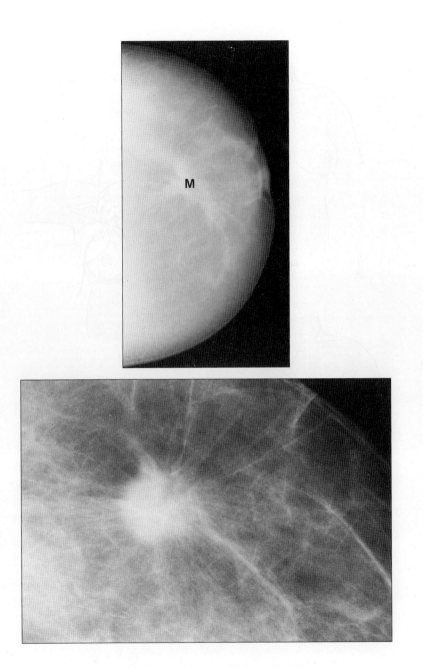

breast carcinomas: top, mammogram revealing deep-seated carcinoma (M), bottom, mammogram shows infiltrating duct carcinoma as a spiculated breast mass

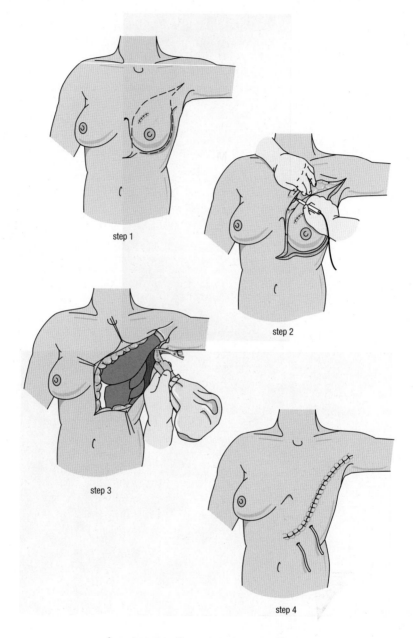

step 1

step 2

step 3

step 4

four-step operative mastectomy procedure

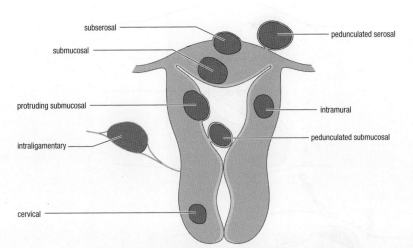

subserosal
submucosal
protruding submucosal
intraligamentary
cervical

pedunculated serosal
intramural
pedunculated submucosal

common types of uterine myomas

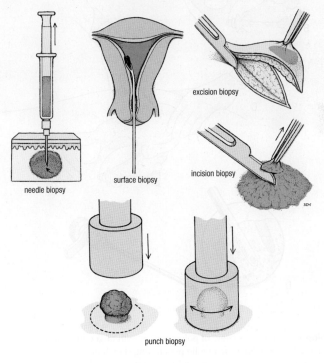

excision biopsy

surface biopsy

incision biopsy

needle biopsy

punch biopsy

biopsy methods

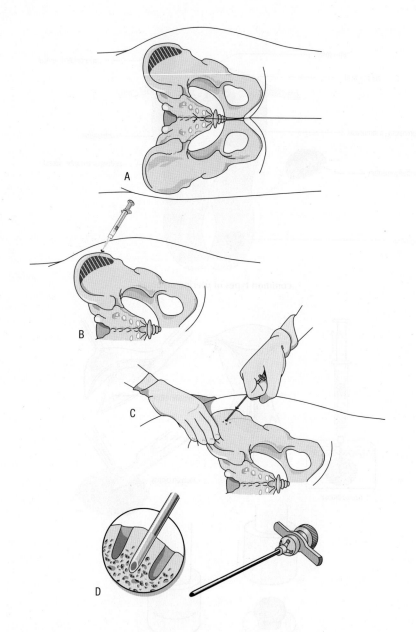

bone marrow biopsy: (A) posterior view of pelvic region with target area for bone marrow transplant highlighted; (B) hypodermic needle penetrating skin at an angle to reach ilium and just below the iliac crest; (C) bone marrow sample aspirated through a needle; (D) close-up of technique used to aspirate bone marrow sample

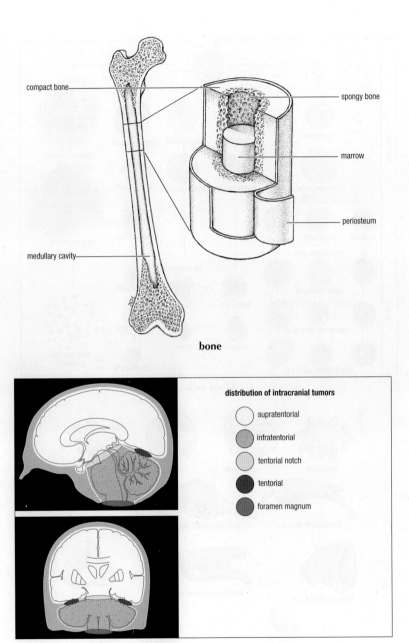

compact bone

spongy bone

marrow

periosteum

medullary cavity

bone

distribution of intracranial tumors

supratentorial

infratentorial

tentorial notch

tentorial

foramen magnum

distribution of intracranial tumors

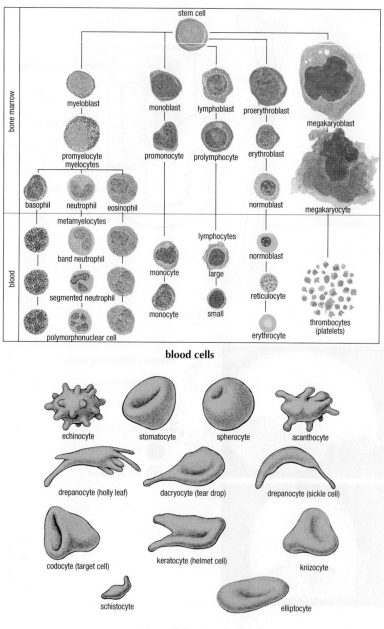

blood cells

poikilocytes

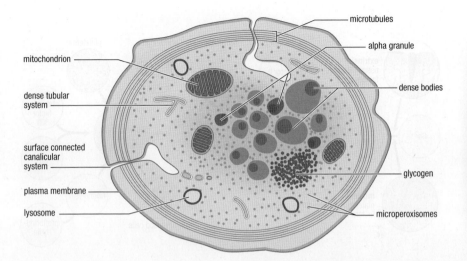

microtubules

alpha granule

mitochondrion

dense bodies

dense tubular
system

surface connected
canalicular
system

plasma membrane

glycogen

lysosome

microperoxisomes

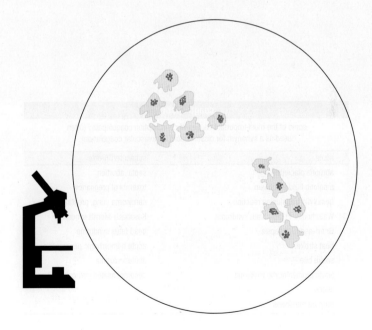

platelet: top, cellular structure; bottom, microscopic view

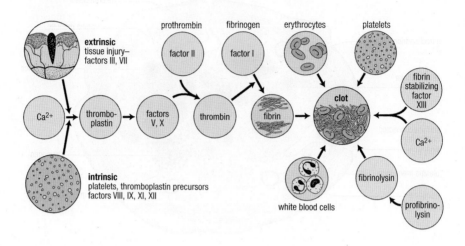

blood clotting

coagulopathy	
some of the most important causes of consumption coagulopathy (often used as a synonym for disseminated intravascular coagulation)	
acute	subacute/Chronic
abruptio placentae	septic abortion
amniotic fluid embolism	toxemia of pregnancy
hemolytic transfusion reaction	carcinoma (lung, prostate)
Waterhouse-Friderichsen syndrome	Kasabach-Merritt syndrome
Gram-negative sepsis	dead fetus syndrome
heat stroke	acute hemorrhagic pancreatitis
snake bite	acute leukemia
acute promyelocytic leukemia	decompensated cirrhosis of liver
shock	
purpura fulminans	

coagulopathy

some common lasers used in medicine		
continuous wave lasers	wavelength (nm)	some common uses
argon	488/514	trabeculoplasty; dental surface preparation
CO_2	10,600	dermatology; otologic surgery; laryngeal surgery
He-Ne *	632.8	nephelometry; guide for invisible lasers
krypton	647	ophthalmic photocoagulation
quasicontinuous wave lasers		
copper vapor/bromide	510/578	pigmented or vascular skin lesions
dye argon	577/585	vascular skin lesions
KTP †	532	vascular skin lesions; otologic surgery
XeCl °	308	phacoablation
pulsed lasers		
erbium: YAG ‡	2940	skin resurfacing; ophthalmic procedures
flashlamp-pumped pulsed dye	585	vascular skin lesions
holmium: YAG	2100	urologic surgery
HF •	2900	dental surface preparation
Q-switched lasers		
alexandrite	755	pigmented skin lesions
Nd: YAG	1064	dermatology; endotracheal surgery; aerodigestive tumors
ruby	694	pigmented skin lesions; button removal

* helium, neon
† potassium, titanyl, phosphate
° xenon, chlorine

‡ yttrium, aluminum, garnet
• hydrogen fluoride

some common lasers used in medicine

oncogenic viruses			
virus family	**virus**	**host of origin**	**associated tumors**
Herpesviridae	frog, herpesvirus	leopard frog	adenocarcinomas
	Marek disease virus	fowl	neurolymphomatosis (T-cell)
	herpesvirus	monkey	lymphoma, leukemia
	Epstein-Barr virus (EBV)	human	Burkitt lymphoma, nasopharyngeal carcinoma
	herpes simplex type 2	human	cervical neoplasia
	herpes simplex type 8 (HHV8)	human	kaposi sarcoma
Poxviridae	shope fibroma	rabbit	fibroma
	yaba virus	monkey	nodular fibromatous hyperplasia
	molluscum contagiosum	human	nodular epidermal hyperplasia
Hepadnaviridae	hepatitis B group	human, ape, rodent, duck	primary hepatocellular carcinoma
Papovaviridae	polyoma	mouse	various carcinomas and sarcomas
	SV40	monkey	sarcoma (in rodents)
	BK and JC	human	none in humans; neural tumors in rodents and monkeys
	papilloma	human	genital, laryngeal, and skin warts; may progress to cervical carcinoma, laryngeal carcinoma, and skin carcinoma
		cattle	genital, alimentary, and skin warts; may progress to alimentary carcinoma and skin carcinoma
		other mammals	papillomas; may progress to carcinomas

oncogenic viruses

Appendix 2
Normal Lab Values

Tests	Conventional Units	SI Units
Acetone		
Serum		
Qualitative	Negative	Negative
Quantitative	0.3–2.0 mg/dL	0.05–0.34 mmol/L
Urine		
Qualitative	Negative	Negative
*Alanine aminotransferase (ALT, SGPT), serum		
Male	13–40 U/L (37°C)	0.22–0.68 µkat/L (37°C)
Female	10–28 U/L (37°C)	0.17–0.48 µkat/L (37°C)
Albumin		
Serum		
Adult	3.5–5.2 g/dL	35–52 g/L
>60 y	3.2–4.6 g/dL	32–46 g/L
	Avg. of 0.3 g/dL higher in upright individuals	Avg. of 3 g/dL higher in upright individuals
Urine		
Qualitative	Negative	Negative
Quantitative	50–80 mg/24 h	50–80 mg/24 h
CSF	10–30 mg/dL	100–300 mg/dL
*Aldolase, serum (30°C)	1.0–7.5 U/L (30°C)	0.02–0.13 µkat/L
Aldosterone		
Serum		
Supine	3–16 ng/dL	0.08–0.44 nmol/L
Standing	7–30 ng/dL	0.19–0.83 nmol/L
Urine	3–19 µg/24 h	8–51 nmol/24 h
Ammonia		
Plasma (Hep)	9–33 µmol/L	9–33 µmol/L
*Amylase		
Serum	27–131 U/L	0.46–2.23 µkat/L
Urine	1–17 U/h	0.017–0.29 µkat/h
Amylase/creatine clearance ratio	1–4%	0.01–0.04
*Aspartate aminotransferase (AST, SGOT), serum	10–59 U/L (37°C)	0.17–1.00 –2 to +3 kat/L (37°C)

Appendix 2

Tests	Conventional Units	SI Units
Base excess, blood (Hep)	−2 to +3 mmol/L	−2 to +3 mmol/L
Bicarbonate, serum (venous)	22–29 mmol/L	22–29 mmol/L
*Bilirubin		
Serum		
Adult		
Conjugated	0.0–0.3 mg/dL	0–5 µmol/L
Unconjugated	0.1–1.1 mg/dL	1.7–19 µmol/L
Delta	0–0.2 mg/dL	0–3 µmol/L
Total	0.2–1.3 mg/L	3–22 µmol/L
Neonates		
Conjugated	0–0.6 mg/dL	0–10 µmol/L
Unconjugated	0.6–10.5 mg/dL	10–180 µmol/L
Total	1.5–12 mg/dL	1.7–180 µmol/L
Urine, qualitative	Negative	Negative
Bone marrow, differential cell count		
Adult		
Undifferentiated cells	0–1%	0–0.01
Myeloblast	0–2%	0–0.02
Promyelocyte	0–4%	0–0.04
Myelocytes		
Neutrophilic	5–20%	0.05–0.20
Eosinophilic	0–3%	0–0.03
Basophilic	0–1%	0–0.01
Metamyelocytes and bands		
Neutrophilic	5–35%	0.05–0.35
Eosinophilic	0–5%	0–0.05
Basophilic	0–1%	0–0.01
Segmented neutrophils	5–15%	0.05–0.15
Pronormoblast	0–1.5%	0–0.015
Basophilic normoblast	0–5%	0–0.05
Polychromatophilic normoblast	5–30%	0.05–0.30
Orthochromatic normoblast	5–10%	0.05–0.10
Lymphocytes	10–20%	0.10–0.20
Plasma cells	0–2%	0–0.02
Monocytes	0–5%	0–0.05
CA 125, serum	<35 U/mL	<35 kU/L
CA 15–3, serum	<30 U/mL	<30 kU/L
CA 19–9, serum	<37 U/mL	<37 kU/L
Calcium, serum	8.6–10.0 mg/dL (Slightly higher in children)	2.15–2.50 mmol/L (Slightly higher in children)

Tests	Conventional Units		SI Units
Calcium, ionized, serum	4.64–5.28 mg/dl		1.16–1.32 mmol/L
Calcium, urine			
Low calcium diet	50–150 mg/24 h		1.25–3.75 mmol/24 h
Usual diet; trough	100–300 mg/24 h		2.50–7.50 mmol/24 h
Carbon dioxide, total			
serum/plasma (Hep)	22–28 mmol/L		22–28 mmol/L
Carbon dioxide (PCO_2), Male	35–48 mmHg		4.66–6.38 kPa
blood arterial Female	32–45 mmHg		4.26–5.99 kPa
Carbon monoxide as carboxy-Hemoglobin (HbCO), whole blood (EDTA)			
Nonsmokers	0.5–1.5% total Hb		0.005–0.015 HbCO fraction
Smokers			
1–2 packs/d	4–5% total Hb		0.04–0.05 HbCO fraction
>2 packs/d	8–9% total Hb		0.08–0.09 HbCO fraction
Toxic	>20% total Hb		>0.20 HbCO fraction
Lethal	>50% total Hb		>0.50 HbCO fraction
*Cell counts, adult			
RBC			
Male	4.7–6.1 x 10⁶/4L		4.7–6.1 x 10¹²/L
Female	4.2–5.4 x 10⁶/4L		4.2–5.4 x 10¹²/L
Leukocytes			
Total	4.8–10.8 x 10³/4L		4.8–10.8 x 10⁶/L
Differential	Percentage	Absolute	Absolute (SI)
Myelocytes	0	0/μL	0/L
Neutrophils			
bands	3–5	150–400/μL	150–400 * 10⁶/L
Segmented	54–62	3000–5800/μL	3000–5800 * 10⁶/L
Lymphocytes	20.5–51.1	1.2–3.4 * 10³/μL	1.2–3.4 * 10⁹/L
Monocytes	1.7–9.3	0.11–0.59 * 10³/μL	0.11–0.59 x 10⁹/L
Granulocytes	42.2–75.2	1.4–6.5 * 10³/μL	1.4–6.5 x 10⁹/L
Eosinophils		0.07 x 10³/μL	0.07 x 10⁹/L
Basophils		0.02 x 10³/μL	0.11–0.59 x 10⁹/L
			0.02 x 10⁹/L
Platelets	130–400 x 10³/μL		1340–400 x 10⁹/L
Reticulocytes	0.5–1.5% red cells		0.005–0.015 of RBC
	24,000–84,000/μL		24–84 x 10⁹/L
Cells, CSF	0–10 lymphocytes/mm³		0–10 lymphocytes/ mm³
	0 RBC/ mm³		0 RBC/ mm³

Tests	Conventional Units	SI Units
Ceruloplasmin, serum	20–60 mg/dL	0.2–6.0 g/L
Chloride		
Serum or plasma	98–107 mmol/L	98–107 mmol/L
Sweat		
Normal	5–35 mmol/L	5–35 mmol/L
Cystic fibrosis	60–200 mmol/L	60–200 mmol/L
Urine, 24 h (varies greatly with Cl intake)		
Infant	2–10 mmol/24 h	2–10 mmol/24 h
Child	15–40 mmol/24 h	15–40 mmol/24 h
Adult	110–250 mmol/24 h	110–250 mmol/24 h
CSF	118–332 mmol/L	118–332 mmol/L
	(20 mmol/L higher than serum)	(20 mmol/L higher than serum)
Cholesterol, serum		
Adult		
desirable	<200 mg/dL	<5.2 mmol/L
borderline	200–239 mg/dL	5.2–6.2 mmol/L
high risk	≥240 mg/dL	≥6.2 mmol/L
Coagulation tests		
Antithrombin III (synthetic substrate)	80–120% of normal	0.8–1.2 of normal
Bleeding time (Duke)	0–6 min	0–6 min
Bleeding time (Ivy)	1–6 min	1–6 min
Bleeding time (template)	2.3–9.5 min	2.3–9.5 min
Clot retraction, qualitative	50–100% in 2 h	0.5–1.0/2 h
Coagulation time (Lee-White)	5–15 min (glass tubes)	5–15 min (glass tubes)
	19–60 min (siliconized tubes)	19–60 min (siliconized tubes)
Corpuscular values of erythrocytes (values are for adults; in children values vary with age)		
Mean corpuscular hemoglobin (MCH)	27–31 pg	0.42–0.48 fmol
Mean corpuscular hemoglobin concentration (MCHC)	33–37 g/dL	330–370 g/L
Mean corpuscular volume (MCV)	Male 80–94 µ3	80–94 fL
	Female 81–99 µ3	81–99 fL
Cortisol, serum		
Plasma (Hep, EDTA, Ox)		
8 a.m.	5–23 µg/dL	138–635 nmol/L
4 p.m.	3–16 µg/dL	83–441 nmol/L
10 p.m.	<50% of 8 a.m. value	<0.5 of 8 a.m. value
Free, urine	<50 µg/24 h	<138 mmol/24 h

Tests	Conventional Units	SI Units
*1Creatine kinase (CK), serum		
Male	15–105 U/L (30°C)	0.26–1.79 µkat/L (30°C)
Female	10–80 U/L (30°C)	0.17–1.36 µkat/L (30°C)

Note: Strenuous exercise or intramuscular injections may cause transient elevation of CK.

*Creatine kinase MB		
isoenzyme, serum	0–7 ng/mL	0–7 µg/L
*Creatinine		
Serum or plasma, adult		
Male	0.7–1.3 mg/dL	62–115 4mol/L
Female	0.6–1.1 mg/dL	53–97 4mol/L
Urine		
Male	14–26 mg/kg body weight/24 h	124–230 4mol/kg body weight/24 h
Female	11–20 mg/kg body weight/24 h	97–177 4mol/kg body weight/24 h
Ferritin, serum		
Male	20–150 ng/mL	20–250 µg/L
Female	10–120 ng/mL	10–120 µg/L

Ferritin values of <20 ng/mL (20 4g/L) have been reported to be generally associated with depleted iron stores.

*Fibrinogen, plasma (NaCit)	200–400 mg/dL	2–4 g/L
*Folate,		
Serum	3–20 ng/mL	7–45 nmol/L
Erythrocytes	140–628 ng/mL RBC	317–1422 nmol/L RBC
Glucose (fasting)		
Blood	65–95 mg/dL	3.5–5.3 mmol/L
Plasma or serum	74–106 mg/dL	4.1–5.9 mmol/L
Glucose, 2 h postprandial, serum	<120 mg/dL	<6.7 mmol/L
Glucose, urine		
Quantitative	<500 mg/24 h	<2.8 mmol/24 h
Qualitative	Negative	Negative
Glucose, CSF	40–70 mg/dL	2.2–3.9 mmol/L
*Glucose-6–phosphate dehydrogenase (G-6–PD) in erythrocytes, whole blood	12.1 ± 2.1 U/g Hb (SD) 351 ± 60.6 U/10^{12} RBC	0.78 ± 0.13 mU/mol Hb 0.35 ± 0.06 nU/RBC
(ACD, EDTA, or Hep)	4.11 ± 0.71 U/mL RBC	4.11 ± 0.71 kU/L RBC

Tests	Conventional Units	SI Units
Glycosylated hemoglobin (Hemoglobin A1c), whole blood (EDTA)	4.2–5.9%	0.042–0.059
HDL-cholesterol (HDL-C), serum or plasma (EDTA)		
Adult		
desirable	>40 mg/dL	>1.04 mmol/L
borderline	35–40 mg/dL	0.78–1.04 mmol/L
high risk	<35 mg/dL	<0.78 mmol/L
Hematocrit		
Male	42–52%	0.42–0.52
Female	37–47%	0.37–0.47
Newborn	53–65%	0.53–0.65
Child (varies with age)	30–43%	0.30–0.43
Hemoglobin (Hb)		
Male	14.0–18.0 g/dL	2.17–2.79 mmol/L
Female	12.0–16.0 g/dL	1.86–2.48 mmol/L
Newborn	17.0–23.0 g/dL	2.64–3.57 mmol/L
Child (varies with age)	11.2–16.5 g/dL	1.74–2.56 mmol/L
Hemoglobin, fetal	≥1 y old: <2% of total Hb	≥1 y old: <0.02% of total Hb
Hemoglobin, plasma	<3 mg/dL	<0.47 µmol/L
*Iron, serum		
Males	65–175 µg/dL	11.6–31.3 µmol/L
Females	50–170 µg/dL	9.0–30.4 µol/L
Iron binding capacity, serum total (TIBC)	250–425 µg/dL	44.8–71.6 µmol/L
Iron saturation, serum		
Male	20–50%	0.2–0.5
Female	15–50%	0.15–0.5
*Isoenzymes, serum by agarose gel electrophoresis		
Fraction 1	14–26% of total	0.14–0.26 fraction of total
Fraction 2	29–39% of total	0.29–0.39 fraction of total
Fraction 3	20–26% of total	0.20–0.26 fraction of total
Fraction 4	8–16% of total	0.08–0.16 fraction of total
Fraction 5	6–16% of total	0.06–0.16 fraction of total

Tests	Conventional Units	SI Units
*Lactate dehydrogenase, CSF	10% of serum value	0.10 fraction of serum value
*Lactate dehydrogenase (LDH) Total (LBP), 37°C, serum		
Newborn	290–775 U/L	4.9–13.2 μkat/L
Neonate	545–2000 U/L	9.3–34 μkat/L
Infant	180–430 U/L	3.1–7.3 μkat/L
Child	110–295 U/L	1.9–5 μkat/L
Adult	100–190 U/L	1.7–3.2 μkat/L
>60 y	110–210 U/L	1.9–3.6 μkat/L
*Lipase, serum	23–300 U/L (37°C)	0.39–5.1 μkat/L (37°C)
Magnesium		
Serum	1.3–2.1 mEq/L 1.6–2.6 mg/dL	0.65–1.07 mmol/L 16–26 mg/L
Urine	6.0–10.0 mEq/24 h	3.0–5.0 mmol/24 h
Methemoglobin, (metHb, hemoglobin), whole blood [EDTA], Hep or ACD)	0.06–0.24 g/dL or 0.78 ± 0.37% of total Hb (SD)	9.3–37.2 μmol/L or mass fraction of total Hb:0.008 ± 0.0037 (SD)
Occult blood, feces, random	Negative (<2 mL blood/ 150 g stool/d)	Negative (<13.3 mL stool/d)
Osmolality		
Serum	275–295 mOsm/kg serum water	275–295 mmol/kg serum water
Urine	50–1200 mOsm/kg water	50–1200 mmol/kg water
Ratio, urine/serum	1.0–3.0, 3.0–4.7 after 12 h fluid restriction	1.0–3.0, 3.0–4.7 after 12 h fluid restriction
Oxygen, blood		
Capacity	16–24 vol% (varies with hemoglobin)	7.14–10.7 mmol/L (varies with hemoglobin)
Content		
Arterial	15–23 vol%	6.69–10.3 mmol/L
Venous	10–16 vol%	4.46–7.14 mmol/L
Saturation		
Arterial and capillary	95–98% of capacity	0.95–0.98 of capacity
Venous	60–85% of capacity	0.60–0.85 of capacity
Tension		
PO2 arterial and capillary	83–108 mmHg	11.1–14.4 kPa
Venous	35–45 mmHg	4.6–6.0 kPa

Tests	Conventional Units	SI Units
Partial thromboplastin time activated (APTT)	<35 sec	<35 sec
pH		
Blood, arterial	7.35–7.45	7.35–7.45
Urine	4.6–8.0 (depends on diet)	Same
*Phosphatase, alkaline, total, serum	38–126 U/L (37°C)	0.65–2.14 µkat/L
Phosphate, inorganic, serum		
Adult	2.7–4.5 mg/dL	0.87–1.45 mmol/L
Child	4.5–5.5 mg/dL	1.45–1.78 mmol/L
Potassium		
Serum		
Premature		
Cord	5.0–10.2 mmol/L	5.0–10.2 mmol/L
48 h	3.0–6.0 mmol/L	3.0–6.0 mmol/L
Newborn cord	5.6–12.0 mmol/L	5.6–12.0 mmol/L
Newborn	3.7–5.9 mmol/L	3.7–5.9 mmol/L
Infant	4.1–5.3 mmol/L	4.1–5.3 mmol/L
Child	3.4–4.7 mmol/L	3.4–4.7 mmol/L
Adult	3.5–5.1 mmol/L	3.5–5.1 mmol/L
Urine, 24 h	25–125 mmol/d; varies with diet	25–125 mmol/d; varies with diet
CSF	70% of plasma level or 2.5–3.2 mmol/L; rises with plasma hyperosmolality	0.70 of plasma level; rises with plasma hyperosmolality
Prealbumin (transthyretin), serum	10–40 mg/dL	100–400 mg/L
Progesterone receptor		
*Prostate-specific antigen (PSA), serum		
Male	<4.0 ng/mL	<4.0 µg/L
*Protein, serum		
Total	6.4–8.3 g/dL	64–83 g/L
Albumin	3.9–5.1 g/dL	39–51 g/L
Globulin		
α_1	0.2–0.4 g/dL	2–4 g/L
α_2	0.4–0.8 g/dL	4–8 g/L
β	0.5–1.0 g/dL	5–10 g/L
γ	0.6–1.3 g/dL	6–13 g/L
Urine		
Qualitative	Negative	Negative
Quantitative	50–80 mg/24 h (at rest)	50–80 mg/24 h (at rest)
CSF, total	8–32 mg/dL	80–320 mg/dL

Tests	Conventional Units	SI Units
*Prothrombin time (PT)	12–14 sec	12–14 sec
Sodium		
Serum or plasma (Hep)		
Premature		
Cord	116–140 mmol/L	116–140 mmol/L
48 h	128–148 mmol/L	128–148 mmol/L
Newborn, cord	126–166 mmol/L	126–166 mmol/L
Newborn	133–146 mmol/L	133–146 mmol/L
Infant	139–146 mmol/L	139–146 mmol/L
Child	138–145 mmol/L	138–145 mmol/L
Adult	136–145 mmol/L	136–145 mmol/L
Urine, 24 h	40–220 mEq/d (diet dependent)	40–220 mmol/d (diet dependent)
Sweat		
Normal	10–40 mmol/L	10–40 mmol/L
Cystic fibrosis	70–190 mmol/L	70–190 mmol/L
Specific gravity, urine	1.002–1.030	1.002–1.030
*Thyroid-stimulating hormone (TSH), serum	0.4–4.2 µU/mL	0.4–4.2 mU/L
Thyroxine (T4) serum	5–12 µg/dL (varies with age, higher in children and pregnant women)	65–155 nmol/L (varies with age, higher in children and pregnant women)
*Thyroxine, free, serum	0.8–2.7 ng/dL	10.3–35 pmol/L
Thyroxine binding globulin (TBG), serum	1.2–3.0 mg/dL	12–30 mg/L
Triglycerides, serum, fasting		
Desirable	<250 mg/dL	<2.83 mmol/L
Borderline high	250–500 mg/dL	2.83–5.67 mmol/L
Hypertriglyceridemic	>500 mg/dL	>5.65 mmol/L
*Triiodothyronine, total (T3) serum	100–200 ng/dL	1.54–3.8 nmol/L
*Troponin-I, cardiac, serum	undetectable	undetectable
Urobilinogen, urine	0.1–0.8 EU/2 h\n0.5–4.0 EU/d	0.1–0.8 EU/2 h\n0.5–4.0 EU/d
Valproic acid, serum or plasma (Hep or EDTA); trough		
Therapeutic	50–100 µg/mL	347–693 µmol/L
Toxic	>100 µg/mL	>693 µmol/L

Normal Lab Values

A35

Tests	Conventional Units	SI Units
Vancomycin, serum or plasma (Hep or EDTA)		
Therapeutic		
Peak	20–40 µg/mL	14–28 µmol/L
Trough	5–10 µg/mL	3–7 µmol/L
Toxic	>80–100 µg/mL	>55–69 µmol/L
Urea nitrogen, serum	6–20 mg/dL	2.1–7.1 mmol urea/L
*Uric acid		
Serum, enzymatic		
Male	4.5–8.0 mg/dL	0.27–0.47 mmol/L
Female	2.5–6.2 mg/dL	0.15–0.37 mmol/L
Child	2.0–5.5 mg/dL	0.12–0.32 mmol/L
Urine	250–750 mg/24h (with normal diet)	1.48–4.43 mmol/24h (with normal diet)
Vitamin B12, serum	110–800 pg/mL	81–590 pmol/L

* Test values are method dependent.
†Test values are race dependent.
‡Actual therapeutic range should be adjusted for individual patient.
§ "Fatty acids" include a mixture of different aliphatic acids of varying molecular weight; a mean molecular weight of 284 daltons has been assumed.

Chemotherapy Treatments

Regimen Name	Drug Content of Regimen	Cancer Treated
ABV	doxorubicin, bleomycin, vinblastine	Kaposi sarcoma
ABV	doxorubicin, bleomycin, vincristine	Kaposi sarcoma
ABVD	doxorubicin, bleomycin, vinblastine, dacarbazine	Hodgkin lymphoma
AC	doxorubicin, cisplatin	Sarcoma (bony)
AC	doxorubicin, cyclophosphamide	Breast
AC	doxorubicin, cyclophosphamide	Neuroblastoma
ACE	doxorubicin, cyclophosphamide, etoposide	Small cell lung
AC(e)	doxorubicin, cyclophosphamide	Breast
AD	doxorubicin, dacarbazine	Sarcoma
AP	doxorubicin, cisplatin	Endometrial Ovarian
ARAC-DNR	cytarabine, daunorubicin	Acute myelocytic leukemia (AML)
B-CAVe	bleomycin, lomustine, doxorubicin, vinblastine	Hodgkin lymphoma
BCVPP	carmustine, cyclophosphamide, vinblastine, procarbazine, prednisone	Hodgkin lymphoma
BEACOPP	bleomycin, etoposide, doxorubicin, cyclophosphamide, vincristine, procarbazine, prednisone, filgrastim	Hodgkin lymphoma
BEP	bleomycin, etoposide, cisplatin	Testicular
BIP	bleomycin, cisplatin, ifosfamide, mesna	Cervical
BOMP	bleomycin, vincristine, cisplatin, mitomycin	Cervical
CA	cytarabine, asparaginase	Acute myelocytic leukemia (AML)
CABO	cisplatin, methotrexate, bleomycin, vincristine	Head and neck
CAF	cyclophosphamide, doxorubicin, fluorouracil	Breast
CAL-G	cyclophosphamide, daunorubicin, vincristine, prednisone, asparaginase	Acute lymphocytic leukemia (ALL)
CAMP	cyclophosphamide, doxorubicin, methotrexate, procarbazine	Non-small-cell lung
CAP	cyclophosphamide, doxorubicin, cisplatin	Non-small-cell lung
Carbo-Tax (CaT)	carboplatin, paclitaxel	Adenocarcinoma Endometrial Ovarian
CAV	cyclophosphamide, doxorubicin, vincristine	Small cell lung

Regimen Name	Drug Content of Regimen	Cancer Treated
CAVE	cyclophosphamide, doxorubicin, vincristine, etoposide	Small cell lung
CA-VP16	cyclophosphamide, doxorubicin, etoposide	Small cell lung
CC	carboplatin, cyclophosphamide	Endometrial Ovarian
CDDP/VP-16	cisplatin, etoposide	Brain
CEF	cyclophosphamide, epirubicin, fluorouracil	Breast
CEPP	cyclophosphamide, etoposide, prednisone	Non-Hodgkin lymphoma
CEPP(B)	cyclophosphamide, etoposide, prednisone, bleomycin	Non-Hodgkin lymphoma
CEV	cyclophosphamide, etoposide, vincristine	Small cell lung
CF	carboplatin, fluorouracil	Head/neck
CF	cisplatin, fluorouracil	Adenocarcinoma Head/neck
CFM	cyclophosphamide, fluorouracil, mitoxantrone	Breast
CEP	lomustine, etoposide, prednimustine	Hodgkin lymphoma
CFPT	cyclophosphamide, fluorouracil, prednisone, tamoxifen	Breast
CHAP	cyclophosphamide, altretamine, doxorubicin, cisplatin	Endometrial Ovarian
ChlVPP	chlorambucil, vinblastine, procarbazine, prednisone	Hodgkin lymphoma
CHlVPP/EVA	chlorambucil, vinblastine, procarbazine, prednisone, etoposide, vincristine, doxorubicin	Hodgkin lymphoma
CHOP	cyclophosphamide, doxorubicin, vincristine, prednisone	Non-Hodgkin lymphoma
CHOP-BLEO	cyclophosphamide, doxorubicin, vincristine, prednisone, bleomycin	Non-Hodgkin lymphoma
CISCA	cisplatin, cyclophosphamide, doxorubicin	Bladder
CLD-BOMP	bleomycin, vincristine, mitomycin, cisplatin	Cervical
CMF	cyclophosphamide, methotrexate, fluorouracil	Breast
CMFP	cyclophosphamide, methotrexate, fluorouracil, prednisone	Breast
C-MOPP	cyclophosphamide, vincristine, procarbazine, prednisone	Hodgkin lymphoma Non-Hodgkin lymphoma
CMV	cisplatin, methotrexate, vinblastine	Bladder
CNF	cyclophosphamide mitoxantrone, fluorouracil	Breast

Regimen Name	Drug Content of Regimen	Cancer Treated
CNOP	cyclophosphamide, mitoxantrone vincristine, prednisone	Non-Hodgkin lymphoma
COB	cisplatin, vincristine, bleomycin	Head/neck
CODE	cisplatin, vincristine, doxorubicin, etoposide	Small cell lung
CODOX-M/IVAC	cyclophosphamide, vincristine, doxorubicin, methotrexate, ifosfamide, mesna, etoposide, cytarabine	Non-Hodgkin lymphoma
COMLA	cyclophosphamide, vincristine, methotrexate, leucovorin, cytarabine	Non-Hodgkin lymphoma
COMP	cyclophosphamide, vincristine, methotrexate, prednisone	Hodgkin lymphoma
COP	cyclophosphamide, vincristine, prednisone	Non-Hodgkin lymphoma
COP-BLAM	cyclophosphamide, vincristine, prednisone, bleomycin, doxorubicin, procarbazine	Large cell lymphoma
COPP	cyclophosphamide, vincristine, procarbazine, prednisone	Hodgkin lymphoma Non-Hodgkin lymphoma
CP	cyclophosphamide, cisplatin	Endometrial Ovarian
CP	chlorambucil, prednisone	Chronic lymphocytic leukemia (CLL)
CT	cisplatin, paclitaxel	Endometrial Non-small-cell lung Ovarian
CVD	cisplatin, vinblastine, dacarbazine	Melanoma
CVD+IL-21	cisplatin, vinblastine, dacarbazine, aldesleukin, interferon alfa	Malignant melanoma
CVI	carboplatin, etoposide, ifosfamide, mesna	Non-small-cell lung
CVP	cyclophosphamide, vincristine, prednisone	Chronic lymphocytic leukemia (CLL) Non-Hodgkin lymphoma
CVPP	lomustine, vinblastine, procarbazine, prednisone	Hodgkin lymphoma
CYVADIC	cyclophosphamide, vincristine, doxorubicin, dacarbazine	Sarcoma
DA	daunorubicin, cytarabine	Acute myelocytic leukemia (AML)
DA+ATRA	daunorubicin, cytarabine, tretinoin	Acute promyelocytic leukemia (APL)
DAT	daunorubicin, cytarabine, thioguanine	Acute myelocytic leukemia (AML)

Regimen Name	Drug Content of Regimen	Cancer Treated
DAV	daunorubicin, cytarabine, etoposide	Acute myelocytic leukemia (AML)
DCT	daunorubicin, cytarabine, thioguanine	Acute myelocytic leukemia (AML)
DHAP	dexamethasone, cytarabine, cisplatin	Non-Hodgkin lymphoma
DI	doxorubicin, ifosfamide, mesna	Sarcoma
Dox>>CMF, Sequential	doxorubicin, cyclophosphamide, methotrexate, fluorouracil	Breast
EAP	etoposide, doxorubicin, cisplatin	Gastric
EBVP	epirubicin, bleomycin, vinblastine, prednisone	Hodgkin lymphoma
EC	etoposide, carboplatin	Non-small-cell lung Small cell lung
ELF	etoposide, leucovorin, fluorouracil	Gastric
EMA 86	etoposide, mitoxantrone, cytarabine	Acute myelocytic leukemia (AML)
EP	etoposide, cisplatin	Adenocarcinoma Non-small-cell lung Small cell lung Testicular
ESHAP	etoposide, methylprednisolone, cytarabine, cisplatin	Non-Hodgkin lymphoma
EV	estramustine, vinblastine	Prostate
EVA	etoposide, vinblastine, doxorubicin	Hodgkin
FAC	fluorouracil, doxorubicin, cyclophosphamide	Breast
FAM	fluorouracil, doxorubicin, mitomycin	Adenocarcinoma Gastric
FAMTX	fluorouracil, doxorubicin, methotrexate	Gastric
FAP	fluorouracil, doxorubicin, cisplatin	Gastric
F-CL	fluorouracil, leucovorin	Colorectal
FEC	fluorouracil, epirubicin, cyclophosphamide	Breast
FED	fluorouracil, etoposide, cisplatin	Non-small-cell lung
FL	flutamide, leuprolide	Prostate
FLe	fluorouracil, levamisole	Colorectal
FNC	fluorouracil, mitoxantrone, cyclophosphamide	Breast
FOLFIRI	irinotecan, fluorouracil, leucovorin	Colorectal
FOLFOX	fluorouracil, leucovorin, oxaliplatin	Colorectal
FU/LV	fluorouracil, leucovorin	Colorectal
FZ	flutamide, goserelin	Prostate

Regimen Name	Drug Content of Regimen	Cancer Treated
HDMTX	methotrexate, leucovorin	Sarcoma (bony)
Hexa-CAF	altretamine, cyclophosphamide, methotrexate, fluorouracil	Ovarian
HI-CDAZE	daunorubicin, cytarabine, etoposide, azacitidine	Acute myelocytic leukemia (AML)
ICE	ifosfamide, carboplatin, etoposide	Small cell lung Osteosarcoma
ICE-T	ifosfamide, mesna, carboplatin, etoposide, paclitaxel	Breast, Non-small-cell sarcoma
IDMTX	methotrexate, mercaptopurine, leucovorin	Acute lymphocytic leukemia (ALL)
IDMTX/6-MP	methotrexate, leucovorin, mercaptopurine	Acute lymphocytic leukemia (ALL)
IE	ifosfamide, mesna, etoposide	Sarcoma (soft tissue)
IfoVP	ifosfamide, etoposide, mesna	Osteosarcoma
IMF	ifosfamide, methotrexate, fluorouracil	Breast
IPA	ifosfamide, cisplatin, doxorubicin	Hepatoblastoma
M-2	vincristine, carmustine, cyclophosphamide, prednisone, melphalan	Multiple myeloma
MAC-III	methotrexate, leucovorin, dactinomycin, cyclophosphamide	Gestational trophoblastic neoplasm
MACC	methotrexate, doxorubicin, cyclophosphamide, lomustine	Non-small-cell lung
MACOP-B	methotrexate, leucovorin, doxorubicin, cyclophosphamide, vincristine, prednisone, bleomycin	Non-Hodgkin lymphoma
MAID	mesna, doxorubicin, ifosfamide, dacarbazine	Sarcoma (bony and soft tissue)
m-BACOD	methotrexate, leucovorin, bleomycin, doxorubicin, cyclophosphamide, vincristine, dexamethasone	Non-Hodgkin lymphoma
MBC	methotrexate, bleomycin, cisplatin	Head/neck
MC	mitoxantrone, cytarabine	Acute myelocytic leukemia (AML)
MICE	mesna, ifosfamide, carboplatin, etoposide	Lung cancer Osteosarcoma
MINE	mesna, ifosfamide, mitoxantrone, etoposide	Non-Hodgkin lymphoma
MINE-ESHAP	mesna, ifosfamide, mitoxantrone, etoposide, methylprednisolone, cytarabine, cisplatin	Non-Hodgkin lymphoma

Appendix 3

Regimen Name	Drug Content of Regimen	Cancer Treated
mini-BEAM	carmustine, etoposide, cytarabine, melphalan	Hodgkin lymphoma
MOBP	mitomycin C, vincristine, bleomycin, cisplatin	Cervix
MOP	mechlorethamine, vincristine, procarbazine	Brain
MOPP	mechlorethamine, vincristine, procarbazine, prednisone	Hodgkin lymphoma
MOPP/ABV	mechlorethamine, vincristine, procarbazine, prednisone, doxorubicin, bleomycin, vinblastine	Hodgkin lymphoma
MOPP/ABVD	mechlorethamine, vincristine, procarbazine, prednisone, doxorubicin, bleomycin, vinblastine, dacarbazine	Hodgkin lymphoma
MP	melphalan, prednisone	Multiple myeloma
MP	mitoxantrone, prednisone	Prostate
MTX/6-MP	methotrexate, mercaptopurine	Acute lymphocytic leukemia (ALL)
MTX/6-MP/VP	methotrexate, mercaptopurine, vincristine, prednisone	Acute lymphocytic leukemia (ALL)
MTX-CDDPAdr	methotrexate, leucovorin, cisplatin, doxorubicin	Osteosarcoma
MV	mitoxantrone, etoposide	Acute myelocytic leukemia (AML)
MV	mitomycin, vinblastine	Breast
MVAC	methotrexate, vinblastine, doxorubicin, cisplatin	Bladder
MVP	mitomycin, vinblastine, cisplatin	Non-small-cell lung
MVPP	mechlorethamine, vinblastine, procarbazine, prednisone	Hodgkin lymphoma
NFL	mitoxantrone, fluorouracil, leucovorin	Breast
NOVP	mitoxantrone, vinblastine, vincristine, prednisone	Hodgkin
OPA	vincristine, prednisone, doxorubicin	Hodgkin lymphoma
OPPA	vincristine, prednisone, procarbazine, doxorubicin	Hodgkin lymphoma
PAC	cisplatin, doxorubicin, cyclophosphamide	Endometrial Ovarian
PAC-I (Indiana protocol)	cisplatin, doxorubicin, cyclophosphamide	Ovarian
PC	paclitaxel, carboplatin	Non-small-cell lung
PC	paclitaxel, cisplatin	Bladder
PCV	procarbazine, lomustine, vincristine	Brain
PE	paclitaxel, estramustine	Prostate
PFL	cisplatin, fluorouracil, leucovorin	Head/neck Gastric

Regimen Name	Drug Content of Regimen	Cancer Treated
POC	prednisone, vincristine, lomustine	Brain
ProMACE	prednisone, methotrexate, doxorubicin, cyclophosphamide, etoposide	Non-Hodgkin lymphoma
ProMACE/ CytaBOM	prednisone, methotrexate, doxorubicin, cyclophosphamide, etoposide, cytarabine, bleomycin, vincristine, leucovorin	Non-Hodgkin lymphoma
ProMACE/MOPP	prednisone, methotrexate, doxorubicin, cyclophosphamide, etoposide, mechlorethamine, vincristine, procarbazine	Non-Hodgkin lymphoma
Pt/VM	cisplatin, teniposide	Neuroblastoma
PVA	prednisone, vincristine, asparaginase	Acute lymphocytic leukemia (ALL)
PVB	cisplatin, vinblastine, bleomycin	Adenocarcinoma Testicular
PVDA	prednisone, vincristine, daunorubicin, asparaginase	Acute lymphocytic leukemia (ALL)
SMF	streptozocin, mitomycin, fluorouracil	Pancreatic
Stanford V	mechlorethamine, doxorubicin, vinblastine, vincristine, bleomycin, etoposide, prednisone	Hodgkin lymphoma
TAD	thioguanine, cytarabine, daunorubicin	Acute myelocytic leukemia (AML)
TCF	paclitaxel, cisplatin, fluorouracil	Esophageal
TIP	paclitaxel, ifosfamide, mesna, cisplatin	Esophageal Head/neck Testicular
TIT	methotrexate, cytarabine, hydrocortisone	Acute lymphocytic leukemia (ALL), to prevent spread to brain
Topo/CTX	cyclophosphamide, mesna, topotecan	Sarcoma (bony and soft tissue)
VAB-6	vinblastine, dactinomycin, bleomycin, cyclophosphamide, cisplatin	Testicular
VACAdr	vincristine, dactinomycin, cyclophosphamide, doxorubicin	Sarcoma (bony and soft tissue)
VAC Pediatric	vincristine, dactinomycin, cyclophosphamide	Bone Sarcoma
VAC Pulse	vincristine, dactinomycin, cyclophosphamide	Sarcoma
VAC Standard	vincristine, dactinomycin, cyclophosphamide	Sarcoma
VAD	vincristine, doxorubicin, dexamethasone	Multiple myeloma
VAD	vincristine, doxorubicin, dactinomycin	Wilm tumor

Regimen Name	Drug Content of Regimen	Cancer Treated
VAPEC-B	vincristine, doxorubicin, prednisone, etoposide, cyclophosphamide, bleomycin	Hodgkin lymphoma Non-Hodgkin lymphoma
VATH	vinblastine, doxorubicin, thiotepa, fluoxymesterone	Breast
VBAP	vincristine, carmustine, doxorubicin, prednisone	Multiple myeloma
VBMCP	vincristine, carmustine, cyclophosphamide, melphalan, prednisone	Multiple myeloma
VC	vinorelbine, cisplatin	Non-small-cell lung
VCAP	vincristine, cyclophosphamide, doxorubicin, prednisone	Multiple myeloma
VCMP	vincristine, cyclophosphamide, melphalan, prednisone	Multiple myeloma
VD	vinorelbine, doxorubicin	Breast
VIC	carboplatin, etoposide, ifosfamide, mesna	Non-small-cell lung
Vin/Cis	vinorelbine, cisplatin	Non-small-cell lung
VeIP	vinblastine, ifosfamide, mesna, cisplatin	Genitourinary Testicular
VIP	etoposide, ifosfamide, mesna, cisplatin	Genitourinary Lung Testicular
VM	mitomycin, vinblastine	Breast
VMCP	vincristine, melphalan, cyclophosphamide, prednisone	Multiple myeloma
VP	etoposide, cisplatin	Small cell lung
V-TAD	etoposide, thioguanine, cytarabine, daunorubicin	Acute myelocytic leukemia (AML)
5 + 2	cytarabine, daunorubicin, mitoxantrone	Acute myelocytic leukemia (AML)
7 + 3	cytarabine, daunorubicin	Acute myelocytic leukemia (AML)
7 + 3	cytarabine, mitoxantrone	Acute myelocytic leukemia (AML)
7 + 3	cytarabine, idarubicin	Acute myelocytic leukemia (AML)
8 in 1	methylprednisolone, vincristine, lomustine, procarbazine, hydroxyurea, cisplatin, cytarabine, dacarbazine	Brain

NOTE: This appendix only lists a sampling of the hundreds of Clinical Trials.

Disease Type	Trial Identifier	Trial Description
AIDS-related lymphoma	PROLOGUE-EFC4978	Phase IV randomized study of rasburicase alone versus rasburicase and allopurinol versus allopurinol alone in patients with leukemia, lymphoma, or solid tumor malignancy at risk for hyperuricemia and tumor lysis syndrome
Anal cancer	EORTC-22011	Phase II/III randomized study of radiotherapy with mitomycin and fluorouracil versus mitomycin and cisplatin in patients With locally advanced anal cancer
Anal cancer	NCRI-ACT-II	Phase III randomized study of radiotherapy and fluorouracil with either mitomycin or cisplatin and with or without maintenance therapy in patients with primary epidermoid anal cancer
Bladder cancer	EORTC-30994	Phase III randomized study of immediate versus deferred adjuvant chemotherapy after radical cystectomy in patients with stage III or IV transitional cell carcinoma of the bladder urothelium
Bladder cancer	SWOG-4B951	Phase III randomized study of methotrexate, vinblastine, doxorubicin, and cisplatin versus observation alone based on p53 gene status in patients with organ confined transitional cell carcinoma of the bladder who have undergone radical cystectomy and bilateral pelvic lymphadenectomy
Breast cancer	01062	Phase III trial comparing regimens of Adriamycin plus Cytoxan followed by either Taxotere or Taxotere plus Xeloda as adjuvant therapy for female patients with high-risk breast cancer

Disease Type	Trial Identifier	Trial Description
Breast cancer	02103	Phase II trial of 5-fluorouracil, epirubicin, cyclophosphamide (FEC100) for 4 cycles followed by docetaxel with capecitabine (wTX) with Herceptin (in HER2-positive patients only) administered as preoperative therapy for patients with locally advanced breast cancer, stages II and III (XEL377)
Breast cancer	03076	Phase III study comparing GW572016 and letrozole versus letrozole in subjects with estrogen/progesterone receptor-positive advanced or metastatic breast cancer (EGF30008)
Breast cancer	04007	Trial comparing treatment with either pegylated liposomal doxorubicin or capecitabine as first-line chemotherapy for metastatic breast cancer in women 60 years and older
Breast cancer	04028	Phase III study comparing GW572016 and capecitabine (Xeloda) versus capecitabine in women with refractory advanced or metastatic breast cancer
Breast cancer	04070	Phase II study of weekly irinotecan/carboplatin (ICb) with or without cetuximab (Erbitux) in patients with metastatic breast cancer
Breast cancer Ovarian cancer	NCI-99-C-0138	Phase I/II randomized pilot study of p53 peptide vaccine and low-dose interleukin-2 in patients with stage IV, recurrent, or progressive breast or ovarian cancer
Breast cancer	NCI-03-C-0040	Phase I/II study of vaccinia-CEA-Tricom vaccine before dose-intensive induction chemotherapy and fowlpox-CEA-Tricom vaccine after dose-intensive induction chemotherapy and immune depletion in patients with previously untreated metastatic breast cancer
Cervical cancer	AGOSG-OVAR-MO16375-MARCH	Phase IV randomized study of epoetin beta for anemia management in patients with stage IIB, III, or IVA cervical cancer treated with cisplatin and radiotherapy
Cervical cancer	EORTC-55994	Phase III randomized study of neoadjuvant cisplatin-based chemotherapy followed by radical hysterectomy versus standard therapy with concurrent radiotherapy and cisplatin-based chemotherapy in patients with stage IB2, IIA, or IIB cervical cancer

Disease Type	Trial Identifier	Trial Description
Colon cancer Prostate cancer Rectal cancer	3086	Phase II trial of ABX-EGF monotherapy in subjects with metastatic colorectal cancer following treatment with fluoropyrimidine, irinotecan, and oxaliplatin chemotherapy
Colon cancer	04062	Phase III study to investigate bevacizumab (q3w or q2w) in combination with either intermittent capecitabine plus oxaliplatin ("Xelox") (q3w) or fluorouracil/leucovorin with oxaliplatin (FOLFOX-4) versus FOLFOX-4 regimen alone as adjuvant chemotherapy in colon carcinoma (BO17920)
Colon cancer Rectal cancer	AVF3430n	Stage IV trial comparing 2 oxaliplatin/Avastin-based treatment sequences as first-line therapy for metastatic colorectal cancer; designed to compare the efficacy of these 2 treatment sequences with respect to progression-free survival (PFS) and overall survival
Gastric cancer	KYUH-UHA-GC04-03	Phase III randomized study of neoadjuvant S-1 and cisplatin in patients with potentially resectable stage III gastric cancer
Gastric cancer	QUINT-TPU-S1301	Phase III randomized study of S-1 and cisplatin versus fluorouracil and cisplatin in patients with unresectable locally advanced or metastatic gastric cancer
Gastric cancer	NYWCCC-0266	Phase I/II pilot study of oblimersen, cisplatin, and fluorouracil in patients with advanced esophageal, gastroesophageal junction, or gastric cancer
HIV	NCT00197574	Phase III study to test the hypothesis that treating HSV-2 infection in the HIV-infected partner of a heterosexual couple (meaning that one partner has HIV and the other does not) will reduce the chances that he or she will transmit the HIV virus to the uninfected partner
HIV	NCT00254046	Phase II study to research with the goal of evaluating the effect of TMC125 (a non-nucleoside reverse transcriptase inhibitor) on slowing down the growth of the HIV virus; will also investigate whether this new medication is well tolerated and to further confirm that the medication is safe to be used

Disease Type	Trial Identifier	Trial Description
Intraocular melanoma Melanoma	NCT00084656	Phase II trial studying how well giving monoclonal antibody therapy together with vaccine therapy works in treating patients with resected stage III or stage IV melanoma
Leukemia	03017	Phase III trial of fludarabine, cyclophosphamide, and rituximab versus pentostatin, cyclophosphamide, and rituximab in previously untreated or treated B-cell chronic lymphocytic leukemia
Leukemia Lymphoma	04100	Phase II study of elsamitrucin (SPI 28090) in patients with relapsed or refractory non-Hodgkin lymphoma (ELSA-2004-001)
Leukemia	5022	Phase II trial of talabostat (PT-100) and rituximab in patients with advanced chronic lymphocytic leukemia (CLL) who have failed a fludarabine regimen (PTH-203)
Lung cancer	2033	Phase III trial of cisplatin/etoposide/radiotherapy with or without consolidation docetaxel in patients with inoperable, locally advanced stage III non-small-cell lung cancer
Lung cancer	3012	Randomized trial of carboplatin/gemcitabine versus gemcitabine alone in performance status 2 (PS2) patients with advanced (stage IIIB or IV) non-small-cell lung cancer
Lung cancer	4107	Phase III study of docetaxel or pemetrexed with or without cetuximab in patients with recurrent or progressive non-small-cell lung cancer after platinum-based therapy (IMCL CP02-0452)
Lung cancer	4126	Phase I/pilot trial of Alimta in combination with cisplatin in previously untreated extensive stage small-cell lung cancer (ES-SCLC) (H3E-US-X049)
Lymphoma	02057	Phase II trial of Neulasta (pegfilgrastim) versus Neupogen (filgrastim) to treat neutropenia post autologous peripheral blood stem cell transplant for patients with non-Hodgkin lymphoma
Lymphoma	4129	Phase II study of Velcade in patients with relapsed or refractory indolent lymphoma

Disease Type	Trial Identifier	Trial Description
Lymphoma	NCI-01-C-0030	Phase II study of etoposide, vincristine, cyclophosphamide, doxorubicin, and rituximab in patients with previously untreated AIDS-related non-Hodgkin lymphoma
Melanoma	NCT00089063	Phase II trial studying vaccine therapy and sargramostim to see how well they work compared to vaccine therapy alone in treating patients who have undergone surgery for stage IIB, stage IIC, stage III, or stage IV melanoma
Melanoma	NCT00110019	Phase III trial studying carboplatin, paclitaxel, and sorafenib to see how well they work compared to carbo-platin and paclitaxel in treating patients with unresectable stage III or stage IV melanoma
Myeloma	3047	Phase II trial of Velcade (PS341, bortezomib) in Velcade-naive patients with multiple myeloma who have undergone high-dose melphalan followed by autologous peripheral blood stem cell transplantation and failed to achieve a complete response
Neuroblastoma	COG-ANBL0032	Phase III randomized study of adjuvant isotretinoin with or without monoclonal antibody Ch14.18, interleukin-2, and sargramostim (GM-CSF) in patients with neuroblastoma who have completed myeloablative therapy and autologous stem cell transplantation
Neuroblastoma	FHCRC-1697.00	Phase III randomized study of prednisone and cyclosporine or tacrolimus with versus without mycophenolate mofetil in patients with newly diagnosed chronic graft-versus-host disease
Ovarian cancer	2044	Phase III trial of induction chemotherapy with gemcitabine and carboplatin followed by paclitaxel consolidation versus paclitaxel and carboplatin followed by paclitaxel consolidation in patients with advanced primary epithelial ovarian or primary peritoneal cancer
Prostate cancer	3085	Phase III study of satraplatin plus prednisone or placebo plus prednisone in patients with hormone-refractory prostate cancer previously treated with one cytotoxic chemotherapy regimen

Disease Type	Trial Identifier	Trial Description
Soft tissue sarcoma	NCI-00-C-0092F	Phase III pilot randomized study of filgrastim-SD/01 versus filgrastim (G-CSF) with concurrent chemotherapy in patients with newly diagnosed sarcoma
Soft tissue sarcoma	COG-ARST0331	Phase III study of vincristine, dactinomycin, and cyclophosphamide with or without radiotherapy in patients with newly diagnosed low-risk rhabdomyosarcoma

Cancer Classification/Grading/Staging Systems

American Joint Commission on Cancer (AJCC) staging system
Ann Arbor lymphoma staging system
Astler-Coller colorectal cancer staging system
Bennett lymphoma classification system
Boden-Gibb testicular cancer staging system
Borrmann gastric tumor classification system
Breslow melanoma microstaging system
Butchart tumor staging system
Chang medulloblastoma staging system
Child-Pugh liver cirrhosis classification system
CIN (cervical intraepithelial neoplasia) classification system
Clark malignant melanoma microstaging system
Dukes colon cancer classification system
Dukes-Astler-Coller colon cancer classification system
Durie-Salmon multiple myeloma classification system
Eastern Cooperative Oncology Group (ECOG) performance status scale
Edmondson-Steiner hepatocellular carcinoma grading system
Enneking musculoskeletal tumor staging system
Evans neuroblastoma staging system
International Federal of Gynecology and Obstetrics (FIGO) staging system
French-American-British (FAB) hematologic malignancy classification system
Gleason prostate tumor score
AJCC host performance status scale
International Staging System (ISS) for multiple myeloma
Jewett prostate cancer classification system
Jewett-Marshall bladder cancer scale
Karnofsky performance status scale
Kiel leukemia and lymphoma classification system
Kernohan astrocytoma grading system
Lukes-Collins non-Hodgkin lymphoma classification system
Mayo-St. Ann astrocytoma grading system
M. D. Anderson cancer grading system
Rappaport lymphoma classification system
Revised European American Lymphoma (REAL) classification system
Robson renal cell carcinoma staging system
Russell soft tissue sarcoma classification system
Rye Hodgkin disease classification system
Whitmore-Jewett prostate carcinoma staging system
Wolfe breast carcinoma classification
World Health Organization (WHO) classification system
Zubrod performance status scale

TNM Staging

Tumor (T)

T	Primary tumor, size, and invasiveness
TX	Primary tumor cannot be assessed
T0	No evidence of primary tumor
Tis	Carcinoma in situ
T1-T4	Presence of tumors; higher number indicates increased size, extent, or degree of penetration

Node (N)

N	Regional lymph nodes, presence or absence
NX	Regional lymph nodes cannot be assessed
N0	No regional lymph node metastasis
N1-N3	Regional lymph node metastasis; high number indicates greater involvement

Metastasis (M)

M	Distant metastasis, presence or absence of distant metastasis, including lymph nodes that are not regional
MX	Distant metastasis cannot be assessed
M0	No distant metastasis
M1	Distant metastasis

Clinical and Pathological Staging

a	Autopsy classification or stage
c	Clinical classification or stage
p	Pathologic classification or stage
r	Recurrent classification or stage
y	Classification during or after multimodality treatment

Other Descriptors

GX, G1–G4	Histopathologic grade
LX, L0, L1	Lymphatic vessel invasion
RX, RO-R2	Residual tumor
SX, SO-S2	Scleral invasion, serum markers
VX, V0-V2	Venous invasion

Bladder Cancer
Jewett Staging

Stage A	Submucosal invasion but no involvement of muscle
Stage B	Bladder wall or muscle invasion
Stage B1	Superficial
Stage B2	Deep
Stage C	Extension through serosa into perivesical fat (around bladder)
Stage D	Lymph node and distant metastases
Stage D1	Regional nodes
Stage D2	Distant nodes and other distant metastases

Breast Cancer
TNM Staging
Tumor (T)

TX	Primary tumor cannot be assessed
T0	No evidence of primary tumor found
Tis	Carcinoma in situ: intraductal carcinoma, or lobular carcinoma in situ, or Paget disease of the nipple with no tumor (Note: Paget disease associated with a tumor is classified according to the size of the tumor.)
T1	Tumor <2 cm in greatest dimension
T1a	<0.5 cm in greatest dimension
T1b	>0.5 cm but <1 cm in greatest dimension
T1c	>1 cm but not >2 cm in greatest dimension
T2	Tumor >2 cm but not >5 cm in greatest dimension
T3	Tumor >5 cm in greatest dimension
T4	Tumor of any size with direct extension to chest wall or skin
T4a	Extension to chest wall
T4b	Edema (including peau d'orange), or ulceration of the skin of the breast, or satellite skin nodules confined to the same breast
T4c	Findings of both 4a and 4b
T4d	Inflammatory carcinoma

Node (N)

NX	Regional lymph nodes cannot be assessed
N0	No regional lymph node metastasis
N1	Metastasis to movable ipsilateral axillary node(s)
N2	Metastasis to ipsilateral axillary node(s) fixed to one another or to other structures
N3	Metastasis to ipsilateral internal mammary lymph

Cancer Classification

Metastasis (M)

MX   Presence of distant metastasis cannot be assessed
M0   No distant metastases are found
M1   Distant metastases are present

Colorectal Cancer
Dukes Staging

Stage A   Confined to mucosa
Stage B   Varies by system
Stage C   Positive lymph nodes
Stage D   Distant metastases

Gynecologic Cancer
International Federation of Gynecologists and Obstetricians (FIGO) Staging

Stage 0   Carcinoma in situ, intraepithelial carcinoma; cases of stage 0 should not be included in any therapeutic statistics for invasive carcinoma

Stage I   Carcinoma is strictly confined to the cervix

  Stage IA   Invasive cancer identified only microscopically; invasion is limited to measured stromal invasion of <5 mm deep taken from the base of the epithelium, either surface or glandular, from which it originates

    Stage IA1   Measured invasion of stroma <3 mm deep and <7 mm wide

    Stage IA2   Measured invasion of stroma >3 mm and <5 mm deep and <7 mm wide

  Stage IB   Clinical lesions confined to the cervix or preclinical lesions >IA

  Stage IB1   Clinical lesions <4 cm in size

  Stage IB2   Clinical lesions >4 cm in size

Stage II   Carcinoma extends beyond the cervix but has not extended onto pelvic wall; carcinoma involves the vagina, but not as far as the lowest third

  Stage IIA   No obvious parametrial involvement

  Stage IIB   With parametrial involvement

Stage III   Carcinoma has extended onto the pelvic wall

  Stage IIIA   No extension onto the pelvic wall, but involvement of the lowest third of the vagina

  Stage IIIB   Extension onto the pelvic wall or hydronephrosis or nonfunctioning kidney

Stage IV	Carcinoma has extended beyond the true pelvis or has clinically involved the mucosa of the bladder or rectum
Stage IVA	Spread of the growth to adjacent organs
Stage IVB	Spread to distant organs

Lymphoma, Hodgkin and Non-Hodgkin
Ann Arbor Staging

Stage I	Involvement of a single lymph node region
Stage IE	A single extralymphatic organ or site
Stage II	Involvement of 2 or more lymph node regions on same side of diaphragm
Stage II3	Number of lymph node regions involved may be indicated by a subscript
Stage IIE	Localized involvement of extralymphatic organ or site and of 1 or more lymph node regions on the same side of the diaphragm
Stage III	Involvement of lymph node regions on both sides of diaphragm
Stage IIIE	Localized involvement of extralymphatic organ or site
Stage IIIS	Involvement of spleen
Stage IIISE	Both stage IIIE and IIIS. Also written Stage III+SE
Stage IV	Diffuse or disseminated multifocal involvement of one or more extralymphatic organs or tissues with or without associated lymph node enlargement
Stage IVE	Used when extranodal lymphoid malignancies arise in tissues separate from, but near, the major lymphatic aggregates

Extralymphatic sites of involvement use letter code and plus sign (+).

N	nodes
H	liver
L	lung
M	bone marrow
S	spleen
P	pleura
O	bone
D	skin

Revised European American Lymphoma (REAL) Classification System

Excellent prognosis	Average 5-year survival rate of 70%
Good prognosis	Average 5-year survival rate of 50–70%
Fair prognosis	Average 5-year survival rate of 30–49%

A55

Poor prognosis   Average 5-year survival rate of <30%

Lung Cancer Staging

Stage 0	Carcinoma in situ
Stage IA	T1 N0 M0
Stage IB	T2 N0 M0
Stage IIA	T1 N1 M0
Stage IIB	T2 N1 M0; T3 N0 M0
Stage IIIA	T3 N1 M0; T1 N2 M0; T2 N2 M0; T3 N2 M0
Stage IIIB	T4 N0 M0; T4 N1 M0; T4 N2 M0; T1 N3 M0; T2 N3 M0; T3 N3 M0; T4 N3 M0
Stage IV	Any T Any N M1

Malignant Melanoma Staging

Stage I	Localized, without metastases to distant or regional nodes (allows localized disease <5 cm from initial tumor within primary lymphatic drainage area
Stage II	Regionalized, involvement of regional nodes
Stage III	Disseminated, visceral, or lymphatic metastases or multiple cutaneous or subsequent metastases

Melanoma Cancer Staging

Stage 0	Tis N0 M0
Stage IA	T1a N0 M0
Stage IB	T1b N0 M0; T2a N0 M0
Stage IIA	T2b N0 M0; T3a N0 M0
Stage IIB	T3b N0 M0; T4a N0 M0
Stage IIC	T4b N0 M0
Stage III	Any T N1 M0; Any T N2 M0; Any T N3 M0
Stage IV	Any T any N M1

Melanoma TNM Staging

Tumor (T)

TX	Primary tumor cannot be assessed (e.g., shave biopsy or regressed melanoma).
T0	No evidence of primary tumor

Tis	Melanoma in situ
T1	Tumor <1.0-mm thick with or without ulceration
T1a	Tumor <1.0-mm thick and Clark level II or III, no ulceration
T1b	Tumor <1.0-mm thick and Clark level IV or V or with ulceration
T2	Tumor >1.0-mm but not >2.0-mm thick, with or without ulceration
T2a	Tumor >1.0-mm but not >2.0-mm thick, no ulceration
T2b	Tumor >1.0-mm but not >2.0-mm thick, with ulceration
T3	Tumor >2.0-mm but not >4-mm thick, with or without ulceration
T3a	Tumor >2.0-mm but not >4-mm thick, no ulceration
T3b	Tumor >2.0-mm thick, but not >4 mm, with ulceration
T4	Tumor >4.0-mm thick, with or without ulceration
T4a	Tumor >4.0-mm thick, no ulceration
T4b	Tumor >4.0-mm thick, with ulceration

Node (N)

NX	Regional lymph nodes cannot be assessed
N0	No regional lymph node metastasis
N1	Metastasis to 1 lymph node
N1a	Clinically occult (microscopic) metastasis
N1b	Clinically apparent (macroscopic) metastasis
N2	Metastasis to 2 or 3 regional nodes or intralymphatic regional metastasis without nodal metastases
N2a	Clinically occult (microscopic) metastasis
N2b	Clinically apparent (macroscopic) metastasis
N2c	Satellite or in-transit metastasis without nodal metastasis
N3	Metastasis in 4 or more regional nodes, or matted lymph nodes, or in transit metastasis or satellite(s) with metastatic regional node(s)

Metastasis (M)

MX	Distant metastasis cannot be assessed
M0	No distant metastasis
M1	Distant metastasis
M1a	Metastasis to skin, subcutaneous tissues, or distant lymph nodes
M1b	Metastasis to lung
M1c	Metastasis to all other visceral sites or distant metastasis at any site associated with elevated levels of serum lactic dehydrogenase

Breslow Depth of Invasion for Melanoma

0.75 mm	Comparable with Clark level II
>0.75–1.5 mm	Comparable with Clark level III
>1.5–4.0 mm	Comparable with Clark level IV
>4.0 mm	Comparable with Clark level V

Cancer Classification

Clark Level of Invasion for Melanoma

Level I	Confined to epidermis (in situ); never metastasizes; 100% cure rate
Level II	Invasion into papillary dermis; invasion past basement membrane (localized)
Level III	Tumor filling papillary dermis (localized), and compressing the reticular dermis
Level IV	Invasion of reticular dermis (localized)
Level V	Invasion of subcutaneous tissue (regionalized by direct extension)

Prostate Cancer Staging

Stage A	Can be subdivided based on the number of cell clusters (foci) seen on microscopic examination
Stage B	Difference between Stage A and Stage B is whether nodule(s) are clinically palpable (or visibly seen) in prostate
Stage C	Dividing line between Stage B and Stage C is microscopically evident capsular invasion
Stage D	Determinant is presence of metastatic disease identified either clinically or microscopically

Appendix 6
Drug Abbreviations and Names

Drug Abbreviation	Drug Description
ABI-007	A Cremophor ELP-free, albumin-stabilized nanoparticle formulation of the natural taxane paclitaxel with antineoplastic activity. This formulation solubilizes paclitaxel without the use of Cremophor ELP and permits the administration of larger doses of this agent, which would be toxic in a Cremophor ELP-containing formulation due to Cremophor ELP's toxicity profile. Cremophor ELP is a nonionic solubilizer made by reacting castor oil with ethylene oxide in a molar ratio of 1:35, followed by a purification step. (Abraxane)
ABT-510	A synthetic peptide that mimics the anti-angiogenic activity of the endogenous protein thrombospondin-1 (TSP-1). ABT-510 inhibits the actions of several pro-angiogenic growth factors important to tumor neovascularization; these pro-angiogenic growth factors include vascular endothelial growth factor (VEGF), basic fibroblast growth factor (bFGF)), hepatocyte growth factor (HGF), and interleukin 8 (IL-8).
ABT-751	An orally bioavailable antimitotic sulfonamide. ABT-751 binds to the colchicine-binding site on beta-tubulin and inhibits the polymerization of microtubules, thereby preventing tumor cell replication. Also disrupts tumor neovascularization, reducing tumor blood flow and so inducing a cytotoxic effect.
AE-941	A multifunctional antiangiogenic agent derived from shark cartilage with potential antineoplastic activity. Competitively inhibits the binding of proangiogenic vascular endothelial growth factor (VEGF) to its cell receptor, thereby inhibiting endothelial cell proliferation. Also inhibits matrix metalloproteinases (MMPs), stimulates tissue plasminogen activator (tPA), and activates caspase-mediated apoptotic pathways in endothelial cells. (Neovastat)
AEE-788	An orally bioavailable multiple-receptor tyrosine kinase inhibitor. Inhibits phosphorylation of the tyrosine kinases of epidermal growth factor receptor (EGFR), human epidermal growth factor receptor 2 (HER2), and vascular endothelial growth factor receptor 2 (VEGF2), resulting in receptor inhibition, the inhibition of cellular proliferation, and induction of tumor cell and tumor-associated endothelial cell apoptosis.
AG-013736	An orally bioavailable tyrosine kinase inhibitor. AG-013736 inhibits the proangiogenic cytokines vascular endothelial growth factor (VEGF) and platelet-derived growth factor receptor (PDGF), thereby exerting an anti-angiogenic effect.
AG-858	A recombinant cancer vaccine made with tumor-derived heat shock protein-70 (HSP70) peptide complexes. Tumor-derived HSP70-peptide complexes used in vaccine preparations have been shown to prime tumor immunity and tumor-specific T cells in animal models. (autologous heat-shock protein-70 peptide vaccine)

Drug Abbreviations and Names

Drug Abbreviation	Drug Description
AMD-3100	A bicyclam with hematopoietic stem cell-mobilizing properties. AMD-3100 blocks the binding of stromal cell-derived factor (SDF-1alpha) to the cellular receptor CXCR4, resulting in hematopoietic stem cell (HSC) release from bone marrow and HSC movement into the peripheral circulation.
AMG-706	An orally bioavailable multiple-receptor tyrosine kinase inhibitor with potential antineoplastic activity. AMG-706 selectively targets and inhibits vascular endothelial growth factor (VEGFR), platelet-derived growth factor (PDGFR), kit, and Ret receptors, thereby inhibiting angiogenesis and cellular proliferation.
AMN-107	An orally available aminopyrimidine with antineoplastic activity. Designed to overcome imatinib resistance, AMN-107 is a tyrosine kinase inhibitor that binds to and inhibits the Bcr-Abl fusion protein, an abnormal chimeric tyrosine kinase expressed in Philadelphia chromosome-positive (Ph+) chronic myeloid leukemia (CML) cells. Also inhibits the receptor tyrosine kinases for platelet-derived growth factor (PDGF) and for c-kit, a receptor tyrosine kinase activated in gastrointestinal stromal tumor (GIST). AMN107 interrupts phosphorylation of these tyrosine kinases and their downstream signaling targets, resulting in decreased cellular proliferation and the induction of apoptosis.
AZD-2171	An indole ether quinazoline derivative with antineoplastic properties. Competing with adenosine triphosphate, AZD-2171 binds to and inhibits all 3 vascular endothelial growth factor receptor (VEGF-1,-2,-3) tyrosine kinases, thereby blocking VEGF-signaling, angiogenesis, and tumor cell growth.
BMS-214662	A nonsedating benzodiazepine derivative with antineoplastic activity. Inhibits the enzyme farnesyl protein transferase, resulting in apoptosis of tumor cells. Farnesyl protein transferase modifies several proteins posttranslationally (farnesylation), including Ras, an oncoprotein implicated in the pathogenesis of many human tumors. May also reverse the malignant phenotype of H-Ras-transformed cells. This agent has been shown to be active against tumor cells with and without Ras mutations.
BMS-275291	A sulfhydryl-based second-generation matrix metalloproteinase (MMP) inhibitor with potential antineoplastic activity. Selectively inhibits several MMPs (MMP 1, 2, 8, 9, and 14), thereby inducing extracellular matrix degradation, and inhibiting angiogenesis, tumor growth and invasion, and metastasis.
BMS-354825	An orally bioavailable synthetic small molecule-inhibitor of SRC-family protein-tyrosine kinases. Binds to and inhibits the growth-promoting activities of these kinases. Has been shown to overcome the resistance to imatinib of chronic myeloid leukemia (CML) cells harboring BCR-ABL kinase domain point mutations.
BMS-599626	An orally bioavailable pan-HER tyrosine kinase inhibitor with potential antineoplastic activity. Inhibits human epidermal growth factor receptors (HER) HER1, HER2 and HER4, thereby inhibiting the proliferation of tumor cells that overexpress these receptors.

Drug Abbreviation	Drug Description
CC-8490	A benzopyran with potential antineoplastic activity. Acts as a selective estrogen receptor modulator (SERM), inhibiting the proliferation of estrogen-sensitive breast cancer cells. Also inhibits growth and induces apoptosis of glioblastoma cells via a mechanism independent of estrogen receptor-related mechanisms.
CI-1033	An orally bioavailable quinazoline with potential antineoplastic and radiosensitizing activities. Binds to the intracellular domains of pan-erbB tyrosine kinases, irreversibly inhibiting their signal transduction functions and resulting in apoptosis and suppression of tumor cell proliferation. erbB is a member of the epidermal growth factor receptor (EGFR) family and is implicated in the malignant transformation of many solid tumors, including breast, ovarian, prostate, lung, and brain cancers. Also acts as a radiosensitizing agent and displays synergistic activity with other chemotherapeutic agents.
CP-724,714	An orally bioavailable quinazoline with potential antineoplastic activity. Selectively binds to the intracellular domain of HER2, reversibly inhibiting its tyrosine kinase activity and resulting in suppression of tumor cell growth. HER2, a member of the epidermal growth factor receptor (EGFR) family, is overexpressed in many adenocarcinomas, particularly breast cancers.
DJ-927	A semisynthetic orally available taxane derivative with potent antineoplastic properties. Binds to tubulin, promoting microtubule assembly and stabilization and preventing microtubule depolymerization, thereby inhibiting cell proliferation. This agent may be useful for treating multidrug resistant tumors. More potent than paclitaxel and docetaxel and is the first oral taxane derivative.
E7389	A synthetic analogue of halichondrin B, a substance derived from a marine sponge (Lissodendoryx species) with antineoplastic activity. Binds to the vinca domain of tubulin and inhibits the polymerization of tubulin and the assembly of microtubules, resulting in inhibition of mitotic spindle assembly, induction of cell cycle arrest at G2/M phase, and, potentially, tumor regression.
EF-5	A 2-nitroimidazole with radiosensitizing properties. Etanidazole depletes glutathione and inhibits glutathione transferase, thereby enhancing the cytotoxicity of ionizing radiation. This agent may also be useful as an imaging agent for identifying hypoxic, drug-resistant regions of primary tumors or metastases.
EGb761	A standardized ginkgo biloba extract with antioxidant and neuroprotective activities. Has been shown to inhibit the proliferation of certain tumor cells in vitro. (ginkgo biloba)
EP-2101	Proprietary cancer DNA vaccine that contains multiple natural and modified epitopes derived from the 4 tumor associated antigens, CEA, HER2/neu, p53, and MAGE 2/3. Also includes CAP1-6D, a heteroclitic CEA analog, and PADRE, a proprietary universal T-cell epitope that serves to enhance the immunogenicity of the epitopes. Agent has been shown to elicit cytotoxic T-lymphocyte responses against tumor cells expressing these multiple epitopes.

A61

Appendix 6

Drug Abbreviation	Drug Description
FR901228	A bicyclic depsipeptide antibiotic isolated from the bacterium Chromobacterium violaceum. After intracellular activation, depsipeptide binds to and inhibits histone deacetylase, thereby affecting the regulation of gene expression and inducing cell differentiation, cell cycle arrest, and apoptosis. This agent also inhibits hypoxia-induced angiogenesis and depletes several HSP90-dependent oncoproteins.
GTI-2040	A 20-mer antisense oligonucleotide complementary to a coding region in the mRNA of the R2 small subunit component of human ribonucleotide reductase. Decreases mRNA and protein levels of R2 in vitro and may inhibit tumor cell proliferation in human tumors in vivo.
GW-786034	A multifunctional antiangiogenic agent derived from shark cartilage with potential antineoplastic activity. Competitively inhibits the binding of proangiogenic vascular endothelial growth factor (VEGF) to its cell receptor, thereby inhibiting endothelial cell proliferation. Agent also inhibits matrix metalloproteinases (MMPs), stimulates tissue plasminogen activator (tPA), and activates caspase-mediated apoptotic pathways in endothelial cells. (Neovastat)
IPI-504	A small-molecule inhibitor of heat shock protein-90 (HSP90) with antiproliferative and antineoplastic activity. Binds to and inhibits the cytosolic chaperone functions of HSP90, which maintains the stability and functional shape of many oncogenic signaling proteins and may be overexpressed or overactive in tumor cells. IPI-504-mediated inhibition of HSP90 promotes the proteasomal degradation of oncogenic signaling proteins in susceptible tumor cell populations, which may result in the induction of apoptosis.
KRN-5500	A semisynthetic derivative of the nucleoside-like antineoplastic antibiotic spicamycin, originally isolated from the bacterium Streptomyces alanosinicus. Inhibits protein synthesis by interfering with endoplasmic reticulum and Golgi apparatus functions. Agent also induces cell differentiation and caspase-dependent apoptosis.
MLN-2704	An immunoconjugate that consists of a humanized monoclonal antibody (MLN-591), directed against prostate-specific membrane antigen linked to a maytansinoid (DM1). The monoclonal antibody moiety of MLN-2704 binds to tumor cells expressing prostate-specific membrane antigen; MLN-27-4 is then internalized into the tumor cell where the DM1 maytansinoid moiety binds to tubulin and inhibits tubulin polymerization and microtubule assembly, resulting in a disruption of microtubule activity and cell division, and cell death.
MLN-518	A piperazinyl quinazoline receptor tyrosine kinase inhibitor with antineoplastic activity. Inhibits the autophosphorylation of FLT3 (FMS-like tyrosine kinase-3), c-KIT and platelet-derived growth factor (PDGF) receptor tyrosine kinases, thereby inhibiting cellular proliferation and inducing apoptosis.

Drug Abbreviation	Drug Description
MS-275	A synthetic benzamide derivative. Binds to and inhibits histone deacetylase, an enzyme that regulates chromatin structure and gene transcription. Appears to exert dose-dependent effects in human leukemia cells including p21(CIP1/WAF1)-dependent growth arrest and differentiation at low drug concentrations; a marked induction of reactive oxygen species (ROS); mitochondrial damage; caspase activation; and, at higher concentrations, apoptosis. p21(CIP1/WAF1) is an inhibitor of cyclin-dependent kinases; in normal cells, its expression has been associated with cell-cycle exit and differentiation.
OGX-011	A mixed-backbone antisense oligodeoxynucleotide with chemosensitizing properties. Inhibits testosterone-repressed prostate message-2 (TRPM-2). Administration abrogates the anti-apoptotic effect of TRPM-2, thereby sensitizing cells to chemotherapy and resulting in tumor cell death. TRPM-2 is an antiapoptotic clusterin that is overexpressed by prostate cancer cells and is associated with chemoresistance.
OTI-010	Multipotent self-renewing adherent non-hematopoietic stromal cells harvested from a patient's bone marrow and grown in vitro. When injected back into the patient, autologous expanded mesenchymal stem cells may differentiate into various mesenchyme-derived cell types and, in some instances, may augment bone marrow engraftment after whole-body irradiation. (Stromagen)
PI-88	A sulfated oligosaccharide. PI-88 inhibits heparinase activity and heparin sulfate binding to fibroblast growth factor (FGF) and vascular endothelial growth factor (VEGF), resulting in decreased tumor proliferation, inhibition of angiogenesis, and inhibition of metastasis.
PKC-412	A synthetic indolocarbazole protein kinase C (PKC) inhibitor. As a nonspecific inhibitor of protein kinase C enzymes, midostaurin inhibits oncogenic PKC signal transduction pathways involved in the regulation of the cell cycle in tumor cells, thereby initiating tumor cell apoptosis.
PPI-2458	A synthetic derivative of fumagillin with antineoplastic and cytotoxic properties. Irreversibly inhibits the enzyme methion-ine aminopeptidase type 2 (MetAP2), thereby preventing abnormal cell growth and angiogenesis. Reported to have a better toxicity profile compared to other agents of its class.
PSC-833	An analogue of cyclosporin-A. Inhibits p-glycoprotein, the multidrug resistance efflux pump, thereby restoring the retention and activity of some drugs in some drug-resistant tumor cells. This agent also induces caspase-mediated apoptosis. (Amdray, Valspodar)
PV-701	An attenuated, replication-competent, oncolytic strain of New-castle disease virus. Selectively lyses tumor cells. Selectivity of this agent is related to defects in the interferon-mediated antiviral response found in tumor cells.

Drug Abbreviation	Drug Description
QS-21	A purified, natural saponin isolated from the soapbark tree with potential immunoadjuvant properties. When coadministered with vaccine peptides, it may increase total antitumoral vaccine-specific antibody responses and cytotoxic T-cell responses.
RK-0202	An oral polymer matrix–based rinse formulation that contains N-acetylcysteine, an antioxidant amino acid derivative with anti-inflammatory properties. May alleviate symptoms of radiation-induced oral mucositis.
Ro 50-3821	A pegylated form of recombinant human erythropoietin, a glycosylated protein naturally produced in the kidney that stimulates erythrocyte production in the bone marrow. Methoxypolyethylene glycol epoetin beta may reverse anemias induced by cancer therapy.
S-1	An oral fluoropyrimidine antagonist composed of tegafur combined with two modulators of 5-fluorouracil (5-FU) activity, 5-chloro-2,4-dihydroxypyridine (CDHP) and potassium oxonate, in a molar ratio of 1:0.4:1. Tegafur is a prodrug of 5-fluorouracil, an antimetabolite that inhibits thymidylate synthase, thereby inhibiting DNA synthesis and cell division, and competes with uridine triphosphate, thus inhibiting RNA and protein synthesis. CDHP is a reversible inhibitor of dihydropyrimidine dehydrogenase (DPD), the liver enzyme responsible for rapid catabolism of 5-FU into inactive metabolites. Potassium oxonate preferentially localizes in the gut and inhibits the enzyme orotate phosphoribosyltransferase (the major enzyme responsible for 5-FU activation), thereby decreasing activation of 5-FU in the gut and activated 5-FU-related gastrointestinal toxicity.
SB-715992	A synthetic small molecule with antineoplastic properties. Selectively inhibits kinesin spindle protein (KSP), resulting in inhibition of mitotic spindle assembly, induction of cell cycle arrest during the mitotic phase, and cell death in tumor cells that overexpress KSP.
SCH-58500	A genetically-engineered adenovirus that contains the gene that encodes the human tumor-suppressor protein p53. This viral vector delivers p53 into tumor cells in order to initiate p53-dependent apoptosis and p53-induced cell cycle arrest. (recombinant adenovirus-p53)
SGN-00101	A recombinant chimeric protein composed of the heat shock protein-65 (Hsp65) from Mycobacterium bovis, and the human papilloma viral (HPV) protein E7. Hsp65, similar to other members of its family of proteins, elicits a strong immune response and may be used to design vaccines against a number of different cancers. E7 protein is involved in carcinogenesis of anal and cervical tumors, and represents a tumor antigen that may be specifically targeted by lymphocytes.
SJG-136	A pyrrolobenzodiazepine dimer with potential antineoplastic activity. Binds to the minor groove of DNA and induces inter-strand cross-links between two N-2 guanine positions, thereby inhibiting DNA replication and transcription.

Drug Abbreviation	Drug Description
TAC-101	A retinobenzoic acid with potential antineoplastic activity. Inhibits retinoblastoma-gene product phosphorylation and increases the presence of 2 cyclin-dependent kinase (CDK) inhibitors, resulting in cell cycle arrest. Agent also causes a cytotoxic decline in cyclin A and thymidylate synthase expression.
TLK-286	A modified glutathione analog. Selectively activated by glutathione S-transferase P1-1 into an alkylating metabolite that forms covalent linkages with nucleophilic centers in tumor cell DNA, thereby inducing a cellular stress response and cytotoxicity, and decreasing tumor proliferation. (Telcyta)
TNP-470	A synthetic analog of fumagillin, an antibiotic isolated from the fungus Aspergillus fumigatus Fresenius with antineoplastic activity. Binds to and irreversibly inactivates methionine aminopeptidase-2 (MetAP2), resulting in endothelial cell cycle arrest late in the G1 phase and inhibition of tumor angiogenesis. Agent may also induce the p53 pathway, thereby stimulating the production of cyclin-dependent kinase inhibitor p21 and inhibiting angiogenesis.
TPI 287	A synthetic, third-generation taxane with potential antineoplastic activity. Binds to tubulin and stabilizes microtubules, resulting in inhibition of microtubule assembly/disassembly dynamics, cell cycle arrest at the G2/M phase, and apoptosis.
UCN-01	A synthetic derivative of staurosporine with antineoplastic activity. 7-hydroxystaurosporine inhibits many phosphokinases, including the serine/threonine kinase AKT, calcium-dependent protein kinase C, and cyclin-dependent kinases. This agent arrests tumor cells in the G1/S of the cell cycle and prevents nucleotide excision repair by inhibiting the G2 checkpoint kinase chk1, resulting in apoptosis.
XK469R	The racemic form of a synthetic quinoxaline phenoxypropionic acid derivative with antineoplastic properties. Selectively inhibits topoisomerase II by stabilizing the enzyme-DNA intermediates in which topoisomerase subunits are covalently linked to DNA through 5-phosphotyrosyl linkages, thereby interfering with DNA repair and replication, RNA and protein synthesis. Agent possesses unusual solid tumor selectivity and activity against multidrug-resistant cancer cells.
ZD-4054	An orally available selective antagonist of the endothelin-A (ET-A) receptor with potential antineoplastic activity. Binds selectively to the ET-A receptor, thereby inhibiting endothelin-mediated mechanisms that promote tumor cell proliferation.
ZD-6474	An orally bioavailable 4-anilinoquinazoline. ZD-6474 selectively inhibits the tyrosine kinase activity of vascular endothelial growth factor receptor 2 (VEGF2), thereby blocking VEGF-stimulated endothelial cell proliferation and migration and reducing tumor vessel permeability. Agent also blocks the tyrosine kinase activity of epidermal growth factor receptor (EGFR), a receptor tyrosine kinase that mediates tumor cell proliferation and migration and angiogenesis.

Appendix 7
Sample Reports

BREAST CANCER FINAL CLINIC VISIT

SUBJECTIVE: This 50-year-old patient was seen in the final review clinic today. The patient was diagnosed with right breast infiltrating ductal carcinoma at age 49, primary tumor being 2.3 x 2 cm, grade 3. It was a receptor-positive tumor with lymphovascular invasion and perineural channel involvement with close margins by about 1 mm at the resection site. The specimen contained ductal carcinoma in situ (DCIS) grade 3 with comedonecrosis. There were a total of 7 out of 12 right axillary nodes involved with metastasis, several with extranodal extension into the perinodal lymphatics. The patient had been assessed and was started on adjuvant AC (Adriamycin and cyclophosphamide) and Taxol systemic chemotherapy.

On examination of the right chest wall prior to chemotherapy, she was found to have a bit of skin puckering with a tiny, 3-mm size nodule in the skin. The patient subsequently completed 3 cycles of AC as well as 3 cycles of Taxol. At that time she was found to have obvious nodular disease in the chest wall without any dominant mass in the breast. In view of this she underwent a modified radical mastectomy. The mastectomy specimen, however, showed a 2-cm diameter tumor, SBR (Scarff Bloom-Richardson) grade 3 with the tumor located 2 mm from the superior, inferior, and deep margins and extending into the base of the nipple and the adjacent dermis of the skin. There was also a lymphovascular invasion noted. High-grade DCIS was found.

Subsequent to the mastectomy, she was started on radiation to the right chest wall and regional nodes. The patient completed radiation 3 months ago and had a considerable amount of moist skin desquamation that took a couple of weeks to heal with Flamazine cream application. She has done well since then and has been seen for ongoing follow up according to MA21 protocol. Since then she had a left breast mammogram and is going to have a MUGA scan done next month.

Interestingly, the patient informed me that 4 out of 11 workers in the printing place where she has been working for 25 years have developed breast cancer and 3 of them were treated by me. Apparently there is a fifth woman who has just been diagnosed with this. The Department of Health is involved with assessing this work environment. It is likely a cluster phenomenon.

As far as the patient is concerned, she is doing well and has gone back to work in an office capacity in an auto parts department. She has no systemic concerns whatsoever.

She does not have any shortness of breath, cough, or chest pain. No bony aches or pains. Her weight is steady and bowel and bladder function normally.

OBJECTIVE: She appears well on examination. The irradiated right chest wall has a moderate amount of lingering skin erythema. No skin recurrences are noted in the right chest wall. She has a patch of a papular, pimple-like appearance on the right posterior chest wall's irradiated skin. She has been known to have these lesions erupt sporadically, and they do not appear to be recurrences. Left breast is normal. She does not have swelling in the right arm. There is no hepatomegaly.

ASSESSMENT AND PLAN: As she is going to be followed by her personal physician close to her home, I have wished her well and have not given her a return appointment. The patient had been started on tamoxifen, which she is continuing without any side effects for the time being.

BREAST CANCER METASTATIC TO BRAIN CLINIC NOTE

SUBJECTIVE: This 65-year-old patient was seen in the clinic following referral with a diagnosis of previously noted breast cancer with recurrent disease in the right axilla and lungs and currently 2 small foci in the right occipital lobe of the brain, 0.5-cm nodules for assessment and treatment.

The patient appeared quite well and was accompanied by her husband. She was well aware of time and place and was cogently conversant.

The patient had been initially assessed by me in March of this year for consideration of palliative radiation to the right axillary mass. Following a lengthy discussion and the fact that she had previous high-dose radiation to this area, I did not feel that adding radiation currently would have any great significant effect in reducing the bulk of the tumor, let alone controlling the disease completely. The patient also was quite glad that this was the opinion that was offered and wanted to continue palliative analgesic management for her neurological symptoms.

The patient had been recently started on Decadron 4 mg b.i.d. to ensure she would not progress in terms of her having nausea and other side effects. The patient states that she has absolutely no symptoms of headaches, double vision, or any problems with gait. She has no cough, shortness of breath, or chest pains. She has no hemoptysis or hematemesis or any melena. She has been able to eat a normal diet and has kept her weight steady. She looks after the right axillary fungating mass with local measures. The mass drains occasional blood-tinged fluid. Apart from that, she has remained relatively stable.

OBJECTIVE: She had been investigated earlier with CT scans of her chest and was found to have no lung abnormality and normal mediastinal compartments.

The patient subsequently had chest CT scans in May when a new lesion measuring 1.3 x 0.9 cm was noted in the posterior aspect of the left upper lobe. Again, there was no measurable hilar or mediastinal adenopathy or any pleural effusion. The 3.1 x 1.1-cm right axillary mass had remained essentially unchanged. Since then the patient has had problems with nausea and some amount of vomiting and chest discomfort and moderate amount of cough but no hemoptysis. She has had no significant chest pain.

A CT scan of her chest was ordered in addition to a CT scan of her head. This scan showed slight progression of the right axillary mass increasing from 3 cm in size to 4.7 x 2.1 cm in size. In addition there was a left hilar mass that was new, measuring 2.5 x 1.2 cm, and a left posterior mid-lung lesion measuring 1.6 cm was slightly enlarged. She also had hilar adenopathy of 2.5 x 1.2 cm with a few anterior mediastinal nodes measuring up to 1.5 cm. There were no lesions noted in the pleura or any pleural effusion. At the periphery of the right hepatic lobe posteriorly there was a 7-mm hypodense lesion, but the adrenal glands were clear. This was thought to represent advancing disease in her lungs and mediastinum.

A CT scan of her head done at the same time showed a 0.5 x 0.5-cm small, enhancing lesion surrounded by edema at the left parietoccipital region, consistent with metastasis. The remaining cerebral hemispheres, ventricles, and basal cisterns were normal.

The neurological examination, including bilateral pupillary reaction, cranial nerve assessment, and strength in her arms and legs, was quite normal. She had no evidence of any lateralizing signs. Her visual acuity was excellent, both central and peripheral. She was diagnosed with glaucoma in the past and that medication has been stopped.

ASSESSMENT: The patient was a bit surprised to hear of the advancing lung disease. Her husband had to remind the patient that she was made aware of this after her last CT scan examination.

PLAN: In light of the lack of adverse changes, I did not feel that radiating the brain would offer any great benefit to her. I will discuss with my oncology colleague the possibility of getting an MRI to see if there are any other changes besides the obvious nodule noted on the CT scan in the left parietoccipital area and, if so, will consider radiation. The patient was currently more interested in getting her driver's license back, which was suspended after her intracranial disease was reported to the Department of Transportation. The patient will be contacted soon following my discussion with my oncology colleague. I have asked her to continue with Decadron 2-mg tablets in the interim before a final decision is made.

CHEMOTHERAPY TREATMENT NOTE FOR BREAST CARCINOMA

SUBJECTIVE: The patient returns for her fourth cycle of FEC100 chemotherapy for her postmenopausal, 3.8 cm, grade 2, N1 M0 breast carcinoma that is ER positive, PR negative, and HER2/neu pending.

She has quite a bit of nausea throughout the cycle. Interestingly, she lost her voice around the fifth day and then things resolved in a couple of days. Around the sixth day, she had epigastric discomfort that was quite prevalent throughout the retrosternal area. She had to use Percocet for it. The epigastric discomfort was present for 3 days but seemed to gradually wane over the last 2 days.

The patient has had this chest discomfort throughout her chemotherapy repeatedly, despite the use of ranitidine, Magic Mouthwash, and antiemetics. We are questioning whether this is some form of esophageal spasm, especially considering her underlying Crohn's disease. I am going to switch her to Pantoloc and lower the dose of her chemotherapy by 15% because she has quite considerable discomfort. She has been reviewed twice in the emergency department and has been cleared from the cardiac point of view. The history of this recurring after each cycle of chemotherapy is not in keeping with cardiac problems.

OBJECTIVE: Her blood counts today are not suitable. We are 4 days from her chemotherapy, so I am not really surprised. We will have to repeat them before the next cycle.

PLAN: She will be treated at 85% in comparison to full dose only if her ANC is 1.5 or greater. I will see her in 3 weeks for her fifth cycle.

ADDENDUM: I received a follow-up report from an outside institution regarding her breast cancer. They now state she has 2 positive lymph nodes. I need to clarify that with the pathologist there.

DISTAL PANCREATOMY AND SPLENECTOMY

PREOPERATIVE DIAGNOSIS: Pancreatic malignancy.

POSTOPERATIVE DIAGNOSIS: Pancreatic malignancy.

PROCEDURE PERFORMED: Distal pancreatomy and splenectomy.

ANESTHESIA: General.

INDICATIONS FOR PROCEDURE: This gentleman presented with a several-month history of back pain and abdominal pain. A CT scan showed a mass in the body of the pancreas with stranding around the area. An MRI suggested there was obstruction of the splenic vein and encasement of the splenic artery in the pancreas, but the superior mesenteric vessels were clear. There was no obvious evidence of metastatic disease. A fine-needle aspiration of the lesion suggested that it was probably a low-grade malignancy, although the pathologist could not be definite. Based on this and his young age, we elected to go forward with a resection.

FINDINGS: The patient did have a resectable lesion in the body of the pancreas. There was no gross evidence of any metastatic disease. There were a fair amount of soft lymph nodes around the celiac artery and a larger one in the superior pancreatic area. These were all quite soft. There were a lot of inflammatory changes around the body of the pancreas that may relate to the aspiration that was done.

DESCRIPTION OF PROCEDURE: Under satisfactory general anesthetic and in the supine position, the patient's abdomen was prepped and draped in usual fashion. He received 1 g of cefazolin and Flagyl, and a Foley catheter had been inserted.

The abdomen was opened through a chevron-type incision. The gastrocolic ligament was taken down to completely mobilize the colon off of the stomach. The left gastric epiploica was divided to completely mobilize the stomach up and off of the spleen. Findings at this time suggested that the lesion was resectable. I could follow the right colic vein back to the superior mesenteric vessels and the tumor appeared to be lateral to this. I could partially dissect up along this area fairly nicely, and the pancreas toward the head looked quite normal. The pancreas looked okay in this region. When we went above the pancreas to explore this area further, there was a large lymph node in this area. There was also some edema. This lymph node was taken and submitted separately to the pathologist. The lymphadenopathy extended all the way medially toward the celiac plexus, which would have made a complete dissection of the lymph node–bearing area impossible because of the extent of the lymphadenopathy. Certainly, the hope in this instance is that these are all benign inflammatory nodes that may relate to the aspiration, as they had not been identified on previous radiologic investigations. As I came down superiorly, I could identify the veins superior to the pancreas. At this point, the hemostasis appeared to be quite acceptable. Ligatures throughout this procedure were of 2-0 silk.

At this point, I started to dissect along the anterior border of the portal vein. Just before I was going to get through this area superiorly, we got into a branch and there was a very large amount of bleeding. I put some pressure in this area while the patient was crossmatched, and we acquired blood. Once the blood was available, I continued the dissection underlying the pancreas because this was the only way we could approach the portal vein. The pancreas was divided with electrocautery. What appeared to happen is that there was a little branch superiorly in the portal vein, probably an accessory branch because of the obstructed splenic vein. This had been avulsed, and in so doing there was a tear along the entire portal vein. Needless to say, the vein bled a fair bit from this tear. Pressure was placed above and below, and with some difficulty the tear in the superior mesenteric vein was closed with a running 4-0 Prolene suture. There was fairly significant blood loss at this point because we could only control it with pressure as we divided this.

The anesthetist was very good in keeping up with the blood loss, and there was no hypotension or even tachycardia associated with this as we replaced blood while we completed this. At this point, the area appeared to be quite dry.

The vascular surgeon came in to assess the patient intraoperatively at this time and again later, once the dissection was completed, he came in to explore the vein with us to see if there was any question of it being compromised or any problems with the vein. Once we had control, the dissection was left alone with a small amount of pressure. I went laterally and brought up the spleen. The remaining attachments to both the stomach with the short gastric arteries were ligated with 2-0 silk and the colon was taken down. The spleen and the tail of the pancreas were brought up en masse. The splenic artery and vein were brought up with the specimen as it came over more medially. As we continued along this section, the adventitial and vascular attachments down toward the duodenum were taken down to mobilize the spleen, and these were taken down as well. There appeared to be some thickening posteriorly and it was difficult to tell grossly whether or not this lesion was extending through the capsule of the pancreas. There did not appear to be any obvious large tumor posteriorly. The dissection was continued until the entire specimen was removed and submitted to the pathologist.

Further vessels in this area were oversewn with 3-0 Vicryl suture. There continued to be a bit of oozing from the portal vein and another 4-0 Prolene suture was used to close this. At this point, the vascular surgeon again reassessed the situation.

We mobilized up the splenic vein to make sure that we had not, in fact, completely obstructed the splenic vein, and there appeared to be good lumen left behind with maybe just a little bit of narrowing superiorly where this branch was entering. When we divided the splenic vein, this was in a very tiny branch as it joined into the portal vein. I suspect this was because the splenic vein was completely obstructed. My further suspicion was the reason we got into this larger vein superiorly was that it was dilated with the obstruction of the splenic vein as a tributary for blood to come back from the spleen. At this point, the hemostasis appeared to be satisfactory.

As I performed a laparotomy, I noted that the bowel was somewhat edematous. I suspected this was because we had put some pressure on the vein for some period of time as we controlled this. The superior mesenteric artery had good pulsation to it, and the bowel looked to be quite healthy, except for the edema that could be seen. I thought there was a possibility we could have a prolonged ileus, and for this reason it would be advantageous to add a gastrostomy tube.

Accordingly, two 2-0 chromic sutures were placed in the stomach and an incision was made in the stomach. A #22 Malecot tube was placed in the stomach for use as a gastrostomy. The Malecot was brought out through a separate stab incision in the left upper quadrant. It was matured in a Stamm-type fashion and sutured to the skin with 0 silk sutures. Through a separate stab incision in the right upper quadrant, a Jackson-Pratt drain was passed, looping along the pancreas into the left upper quadrant. The open end of the pancreas had the duct oversewn with a 2-0 silk suture, and the pancreas itself had some interrupted horizontal mattress sutures to compress the distal end. There appeared to be a good volume of pancreas left behind. The splenic artery itself was suture ligated with 2-0 silk. Hemostasis appeared to be acceptable at this time.

The wound was then closed in layers with #1 Vicryl, and the skin was closed with staples. Sponge, needle, and instrument counts were reported correct on all occasions. Blood loss was estimated at 2000 mL, and the patient received a 4-unit transfusion. As mentioned above, he was stable throughout the procedure and transferred to the recovery room in stable condition.

I did contact the pathologist and gave the specimen to him in a fresh fashion so there was no concern with autolysis of the pancreas that would make histologic evaluation of the pancreas less than ideal.

INVASIVE DUCTAL CARCINOMA RADIATION THERAPY CONSULTATION

REASON FOR CONSULTATION: This 65-year-old patient was seen at the request of her primary physician for assessment of adjuvant treatment for recently diagnosed left breast invasive ductal carcinoma, postmenopausal, receptor positive, T1 N1 M0. She had already seen our oncologist and was recommended to have adjuvant AC chemotherapy. She is going to start the second cycle today.

HISTORY OF PRESENT ILLNESS: Her history is that of right contralateral breast ductal carcinoma in situ (DCIS) diagnosed in 1995 when she had a lumpectomy carried out. She did not receive adjuvant systemic or radiation treatment. The patient has had regular mammograms since then, which date back to the 1980s. At one time she was found to have a cluster of microcalcifications that were apparently biopsied, but these were benign. The patient had no breast-related symptoms other than palpating a small nodule in the left breast lateral to the nipple around the 3 o'clock direction approximately a year ago. She had noticed no skin changes or any nipple eversion, bleeding, or discharge from the nipple. This was being followed and mammograms were always negative. As the nodule seemed to be getting slightly firmer, she had been assessed by her family physician and eventually had a mammogram and ultrasounds arranged. The examination confirmed the abnormality almost directly under the nipple, deep in the substance of the breast. In view of this, she had an ultrasound-guided biopsy that was consistent with invasive ductal carcinoma, SBR grade 2, with perineural invasion.

With this diagnosis, the patient had a left breast lumpectomy and sentinel lymph node mapping. Two out of the 4 sentinel lymph nodes resected were positive. The primary was 1.5 cm and SBR grade 3. The resection margins were quite close, 0.2 mm and 0.02 mm at some of the edges. The specimen also contained DCIS. The patient did well postoperatively. The question of re-excision was raised with the surgeons, but it was felt that since the primary lesion had been shaved off of the fascia and the margins had been clear, there was no necessity for re-excision.

The receptors for HER2/neu oncoprotein were obtained, and there was overexpression of the HER2/neu oncoprotein. The patient subsequently was recommended to have AC systemic chemotherapy.

PAST MEDICAL HISTORY: Her risk factors are that of menarche onset at age 14 and menopause at 49. She was on hormone replacement therapy with Estraderm patch 50 mcg for a few years, subsequently lowered to 25 mcg. She was also on progesterone tablets, which she took until 10 years ago. Apparently she had a considerable amount of bilateral breast engorgement and discomfort and eventually stopped this therapy. Her first pregnancy occurred at age 27. She is G3, P3. She breast fed her children.

MEDICATIONS: She currently takes Fosamax, calcium with vitamin D, and lorazepam.

ALLERGIES: She has an allergy to Demerol and surgical tape, but definitely not to sulfa drugs.

HABITS: She was a minimal smoker for 30 years or so, up to 7 cigarettes a day. She stopped smoking in 1985. She drinks alcohol occasionally.

FAMILY HISTORY: There is no breast or ovarian cancer in the family.

PHYSICAL EXAMINATION: On examination, she appeared well. There were no nodes palpable in the head, neck, or axillae. The previous lumpectomy scar on the right breast had healed well. No recurrences were noted in the right breast. Left axillary and breast scars have both healed well. The periareolar skin had residual blue dye from the sentinel lymph node mapping procedure. There was not much induration in the breast scar, which was around the areola and extending into the axillary tail area in the 2 o'clock direction. No abnormal nodules were felt. Lungs were clear. There was no swelling of her left arm. There was no hepatomegaly.

ASSESSMENT AND RECOMMENDATIONS: I have gone over in detail the tumor pathology as it pertains to advocating adjuvant radiation. I have reviewed the CT planning details preceding her radiation treatments. I have also reviewed the possible side effects pertaining to radiation, both acute and chronic, after 21 days of treatment, which would include breast as well as boost scar radiation. We have obtained consent from the patient. The patient will call me immediately after her last cycle to plan the radiation. She is going to be started on tamoxifen at that time and following completion of radiation will be taking Herceptin.

LEUKEMIA CLINIC NOTE

SUBJECTIVE: The patient is a pleasant, 58-year-old gentleman who likely has early B-cell chronic lymphocytic leukemia (CLL) as shown on flow cytometry. The patient is generally feeling well. He has no fever, no night sweats, and no weight loss. He has had no recent serious infections, although he does say he gets nasal infections that cause some small lymphadenopathy but resolves. He had noticed no epistaxis or other areas of bleeding.

The patient has a history of lower GI bleed in 2004. The patient has no chest pain or shortness of breath. He has no abdominal discomfort.

The patient has a daughter who had a bone marrow transplant at age 8 for myelodysplasia with some blast cells. The daughter is now 21 and doing very well in college.

OBJECTIVE: On examination the patient looks well. He has no cervical, supraclavicular, or infraclavicular adenopathy. Heart sounds are normal. Abdomen is soft and nontender with no masses and no organomegaly.

White count is 12.1, hemoglobin 14.3, and platelets 305,000.

ASSESSMENT: The patient's chronic lymphocytic leukemia remains under excellent control. We had a good discussion today. He likely has stage 0 chronic lymphocytic leukemia, although a second flow cytometry was inconclusive.

PLAN: We will continue to follow him closely. He realizes that some patients never require treatment for CLL but that others do require treatment and that CLL can become serious. Certainly, at this point the patient's CLL is under excellent control, stage 0 disease, and his lymphocytosis is under excellent control. I will arrange to see the patient again in the spring of next year.

LUNG CANCER WITH METASTATIS DEATH SUMMARY

DISCHARGE DIAGNOSIS: Carcinoma of the lung, metastatic to the liver.

HISTORY OF PRESENT ILLNESS: The patient was a 71-year-old man admitted for palliative care with a diagnosis of carcinoma of the lung. His diagnosis was preceded by several weeks of rapidly declining health with pneumonia. Since his diagnosis, his general condition had deteriorated quite rapidly, and he has been taking nasal oxygen. Recently he had been unsteady on his feet, had taken to sleeping in a La-Z-Boy, and was unable to lie flat because of shortness of breath. The 24 hours prior to his admission, it was evident to his family that he could no longer be cared for safely at home and he was admitted to our unit.

HOSPITAL COURSE: On admission the patient was virtually gasping for breath with marked chest congestion. He settled down fairly well with subcutaneous morphine and oxygen masking. The following day, however, his condition deteriorated further with acute respiratory distress. His medications were adjusted to ensure comfort, which had been requested by his family on his admission. The patient passed away peacefully with his family at his side.

MELANOMA (T2B N0) CLINIC NOTE

SUBJECTIVE: The patient and his wife were present today. The patient is seen today in follow up for T2b N0, stage IIA superficial spreading melanoma status post excision. He had a sentinel lymph node biopsy from his right and left axillae. These biopsies were negative for involvement. He has a small palpable lymph node in the left groin. On previous fine-needle aspiration, the lesion was nondiagnostic. In discussion with the patient's surgeon, an ultrasound-guided biopsy of the lesion was arranged.

OBJECTIVE: The pathology report reports the 2 biopsies showed minute fragments of fibrofatty tissue. Multiple sections showed no evidence of malignancy in this very scanty specimen.

ASSESSMENT: I have done everything possible up to this point to try and determine whether or not the lesion in the left groin is a lesion of concern. His PET scan was negative, 2 needle biopsies of the lesion have been negative, and the lesion does not appear to be changing in size. Having said that, the lesion is still palpable and there is evidence of a 1.5-cm lesion in the left groin, palpable in the upper part of the left groin.

PLAN: The patient will have to decide, in discussion with his surgeon, whether or not he wishes to pursue the route of observation or of surgery. I will leave further management of the left groin lymph node between the patient and his surgeon. I have arranged to see him in 3 months' time for on-going follow up. He will have his LFTs and LDH prior to that return visit.

It is also of note that the patient's family physician has observed that the patient has had a drop in hemoglobin recently. The etiology of this is not entirely clear, and it is currently being investigated and managed by his family physician.

The patient and his wife are happy with the care and information that they have been provided up to this point. I believe that the patient is going to contact his surgeon for an opinion with regard to further management of the left groin lymph node. I have not made a recommendation one way or another as to whether or not surgery should be performed, and I will leave this decision between the patient and his surgeon.

MELANOMA (T4B NX) CLINIC NOTE

SUBJECTIVE: The patient has returned today for follow up with regard to her high-risk melanoma. She had a T4b NX, nodular stage IIC melanoma excised from her left calf. She has had a skin graft performed. The Breslow thickness is 5.8 mm. She has osteoporosis and is being followed for this. The patient's physician is trying to arrange for her to receive Forteo.

OBJECTIVE: She had some subtle uptake on her bone scan in the left femoral neck region. I have carefully questioned the patient today as to whether or not she is having any symptoms in this region. She denies any history of any resting pain, bone pain, or any pain at night in the left hip region. She had recent liver function tests performed, and they were all in acceptable range. Her LDH was 623.

The patient appeared her stated age. She had no palpable adenopathy. Respiratory and cardiovascular exams were normal. There was no obvious hepatosplenomegaly. There was no inguinal or femoral adenopathy. Examination of her skin graft showed no significant changes compared to the last time. There were 2 small moles on the scar, about 3 to 4 mm in size, that were unchanged. They did not appear to be typical of recurrent lesions.

ASSESSMENT: The patient appears to be doing relatively well.

PLAN: I will see her again in 3 months' time. She will have a bone scan, chest x-ray, and ultrasound prior to return as well as LFTs and an LDH.

NON-HODGKIN LYMPHOMA DEATH SUMMARY

DEATH DIAGNOSIS: The patient died due to complications of her lymphoma, aspiration pneumonia, and Clostridium difficile colitis.

HISTORY OF PRESENT ILLNESS: The patient is a 73-year-old female admitted for palliative care assessment and management of chronic interstitial lung disease, non-Hodgkin lymphoma, Clostridium difficile colitis, radiation pneumonitis, and aspiration pneumonia.

HOSPITAL COURSE: It became more apparent on admission that the patient had a very poor life expectancy. She was short of breath already at the time of admission, which responded well to morphine. She also needed a Dilaudid pump due to increasing pain in both legs. We initially started the pump at 0.5 mg per hour. The pump was increased to 1.5 mg per hour with a 1.5-mg bolus every 15 minutes p.r.n.

Swallowing continued to be a concern, with failed swallowing assessment while in hospital. However, the patient did tolerate some thickened fluids and enjoyed these quite a bit. She also experienced some gastroesophageal reflux disease, which responded well to Mylanta 15 to 30 mL p.o. q.i.d. p.r.n.

Shortness of breath and leg pain became more prominent, which again responded well to her Dilaudid pump being increased as well as p.r.n. morphine. She also required Versed 1 mg subcutaneously every hour p.r.n. for increasing agitation toward the end of her life. Ventolin also was given to provide increased ventilation and decreased sensation of shortness of breath. She also developed thrush, which was treated with nystatin.

The diarrhea recurred, likely due to the fact that p.o. medications at that time were more difficult to administer, and she did not receive Flagyl that day. She developed fever, and it was presumed that the fever was either due to recurrence of aspiration pneumonia or Clostridium difficile colitis.

She died due to complications of her diagnoses. She was comfortable at the time of death.

SIGMOID COLON CARCINOMA CHEMOTHERAPY CLINIC NOTE

SUBJECTIVE: The patient is a 74-year-old woman with T1 N1 MX poorly differentiated carcinoma of the sigmoid colon. She had her original resection 6 months ago, and this is her fifth course of capecitabine.

She continues to tolerate her medication well. She has most notably had quite profound fatigue and a bit of constipation. She notices that she has a persistent nauseous feeling that starts about a week after her course of capecitabine and continues until about 3 days before her next course. Last cycle she tried Dramamine, but it gave her no relief. Nonetheless, she continues to eat normally, but she has done very little in the way of activity, and she admits this is partly because she really has nothing to do.

There has been no other change in her medications. She continues on her Celexa and Risperdal, and her depressive symptoms have been under good control.

OBJECTIVE: She has not had any leg edema. We note she has had a slowly decreasing protein and albumin level.

Her laboratory investigations today reveal a white blood count of 5400 with an absolute neutrophil count of 3700. She has a platelet count of 328,000. Hemoglobin is 10.6, which has slowly dropped down from 13.3 with a little decrement each visit. Her AST, LDH, alkaline phosphatase, gamma-GT, electrolytes, and calcium are all normal. Her unconjugated bilirubin is 22, staying just slightly above normal.

ASSESSMENT: The patient continues to tolerate her capecitabine. We did notice she looks paler today, but her hemoglobin still is not in a range that requires transfusion or augmentation.

PLAN: I have asked her to discontinue the Dramamine and have given her a prescription for metoclopramide to see if we can improve her symptoms. Because most of her sensation of nausea is in her upper chest, I wonder if there might be some merit in putting her on a proton pump inhibitor, and we will consider that next time. I have given her a prescription for capecitabine with limited use once again, and she is fine to go ahead with her fifth course of her chemotherapy.

UTERINE CARCINOMA DEATH SUMMARY

DEATH DIAGNOSIS: The patient was an 87-year-old female admitted for palliative care assessment and management of gastrointestinal bleed/vaginal bleeding with presumed uterine cancer and uncontrolled atrial fibrillation.

HISTORY OF PRESENT ILLNESS: The patient is an 87-year-old female transferred for palliative care assessment and management of uncontrolled atrial fibrillation, gastrointestinal bleeding, and vaginal bleeding with presumed diagnosis of cancer of the uterus.

HOSPITAL COURSE: The patient settled onto the floor and complained very little. She continued to experience bright red blood per vagina as well as melenic stool. I reviewed the situation of transfusions with the patient's daughter, and we agreed together to forego further transfusions, as they would only prolong suffering. As a result, she was not transfused while on our floor.

The patient complained of some right wrist pain, and subsequent x-rays were negative with regard to fracture but did reveal osteopenia.

During hospitalization oral intake was declining, and overall the patient was showing signs of nearing the end. There was some agitation noted with washing as well as increasing anxiety. As a result, she was started on Ativan 0.5 to 1 mg p.o. b.i.d. Some pain was noted as well, and as a result she was given more regular Dilaudid. It became more apparent that a pump would provide better pain relief. As a result, later during the hospitalization she was started on a pain pump with Dilaudid running at 0.5 mg/h with a 1-mg bolus p.r.n. every 15 minutes. I also left an order for Versed and scopolamine for increased secretions and agitation.

She died due to complications of her diagnosis. She was comfortable at the time of death.

Appendix 8
Common Terms by Procedure

Breast Cancer Final Clinic Visit
AC and Taxol systemic chemotherapy
Adriamycin and cyclophosphamide (AC)
axillary node
bony aches or pains
bowel and bladder function
cluster phenomenon
comedonecrosis
deep margin
ductal carcinoma in situ (DCIS)
extranodal extension
Flamazine cream
hepatomegaly
high-grade DCIS
infiltrating ductal carcinoma
irradiated skin
lymphovascular invasion
modified radical mastectomy
MUGA scan
multiple gated acquisition (MUGA)
nodular disease
papular appearance
perineural channel involvement
perinodal lymphatics
primary tumor
receptor-positive tumor
regional node
Scarff Bloom-Richardson (SBR)
skin desquamation
skin erythema
tamoxifen

Breast Cancer Metastatic to Brain Clinic Note
adverse change
axillary fungating mass
axillary mass
basal cistern
blood-tinged fluid

cerebral hemisphere
cranial nerve assessment
double vision
fungating mass
hematemesis
hemoptysis
hepatic lobe
hilar adenopathy
high-dose radiation
intracranial disease
lateralizing sign
left upper lobe
lung abnormality
mediastinal adenopathy
mediastinal compartment
mediastinal node
melena
midlung lesion
neurological symptom
palliative analgesic management
palliative radiation
parietoccipital region
pleural effusion
pupillary reaction
recurrent disease
shortness of breath

Chemotherapy Treatment Note for Breast Carcinoma
antiemetic
blood count
Crohn's disease
epigastric discomfort
ER positive
esophageal spasm
estrogen receptor (ER)
FEC100 chemotherapy
HER2/neu
Magic Mouthwash

Pantoloc
progesterone receptor (PR)
PR positive
ranitidine

Distal Pancreatomy and Splenectomy

autolysis
blood loss
cefazolin
celiac artery
celiac plexus
chevron-type incision
2-0 chromic suture
distal pancreatomy
en masse
fine-needle aspiration
Flagyl
Foley catheter
gastric epiploica
gastrocolic ligament
gastrostomy tube
general anesthetic
hemostasis
horizontal mattress suture
inflammatory change
interrupted horizontal mattress sutures
Jackson-Pratt drain
laparotomy
ligature
low-grade malignancy
lymphadenopathy
lymph node-bearing area
#22 Malecot tube
metastatic disease
pancreatic malignancy
portal vein
4-0 Prolene suture
prolonged ileus
prepped and draped
recovery room
right upper quadrant
satisfactory general anesthetic

2-0 silk suture
splenectomy
splenic artery
splenic vein
sponge, needle, and instrument counts
stable condition
Stamm-type fashion
stranding
superior mesenteric vessel
usual fashion
vascular attachment
vascular surgeon
3-0 Vicryl suture

Invasive Ductal Carcinoma Radiation Therapy Consultation

AC systemic chemotherapy
Adriamycin and cyclophosphamide (AC)
adjuvant radiation treatment
adjuvant systemic treatment
axillary tail area
breast engorgement
ductal carcinoma in situ (DCIS)
Estraderm patch
Fosamax
hepatomegaly
Herceptin
HER2/neu oncoprotein
hormone replacement therapy
induration
invasive ductal carcinoma
lorazepam
lumpectomy scar
menarche
microcalcification
nipple eversion
ovarian cancer
perineural invasion
radiation treatment
receptor positive
reexcision
SBR grade 2

Common Terms

Scarff Bloom-Richardson (SBR)
sentinel lymph node mapping procedure
systemic treatment
tamoxifen
ultrasound-guided biopsy

Leukemia Clinic Note

B-cell chronic lymphocytic leukemia
blast cell
bone marrow transplant
cervical adenopathy
chronic lymphocytic leukemia (CLL)
epistaxis
flow cytometry
gastrointestinal (GI)
GI bleed
infraclavicular adenopathy
lymphadenopathy
myelodysplasia
supraclavicular adenopathy

Lung Cancer with Metastarsis Death Summary

acute respiratory distress
carcinoma of the lung
chest congestion
metastatic
palliative care
shortness of breath

Melanoma (T2b N0) Clinic Note

axilla
fibrofatty tissue
fine-needle aspiration
lymph node
nondiagnostic
palpable lymph node
PET scan
positron emission tomography (PET)
sentinel lymph node biopsy

superficial spreading melanoma
ultrasound-guided biopsy

Melanoma (T4b NX) Clinic Note

adenopathy
bone pain
bone scan
Breslow thickness
femoral adenopathy
Forteo
inguinal adenopathy
liver function test (LFT)
nodular stage IIC melanoma
osteoporosis
palpable adenopathy
recurrent lesion
resting pain
stage IIC melanoma

Non-Hodgkin Lymphoma Death Summary

aspiration pneumonia
assessment and management
bolus
chronic interstitial lung disease
Clostridium difficile colitis
colitis
Dilaudid pump
gastroesophageal reflux disease
interstitial lung disease
lymphoma
Mylanta
non-Hodgkin lymphoma
nystatin
palliative care
radiation pneumonitis
shortness of breath
thrush
Ventolin
Versed

Sigmoid Colon Carcinoma Chemotherapy Clinic Note

absolute neutrophil count
alkaline phosphatase
capecitabine
Celexa
Dramamine
electrolytes
gamma-GT
hemoglobin
leg edema
metoclopramide
platelet count
poorly differentiated carcinoma
proton pump inhibitor
Risperdal
sigmoid colon
unconjugated bilirubin
white blood count

Uterine Carcinoma Death Summary

assessment and management
atrial fibrillation
bright red blood per vagina
Dilaudid
gastrointestinal bleeding
increased secretions
osteopenia
palliative care
scopolamine
uncontrolled atrial fibrillation
uterine cancer
vaginal bleeding
Versed

Common Terms

ABDOMINAL DISTENTION (POSTOPERATIVE)
Hormone, Posterior Pituitary
Pitressin® [US]
Pressyn® AR [Can]
Pressyn® [Can]
vasopressin

ACQUIRED IMMUNODEFICIENCY SYNDROME (AIDS)
Antiretroviral Agent, Fusion Protein
    Inhibitor
enfuvirtide
Fuzeon™ [US/Can]
Antiretroviral Agent, Non-nucleoside
    Reverse Transcriptase Inhibitor
    (NNRTI)
Kaletra™ [US/Can]
lopinavir and ritonavir
Antiretroviral Agent, Nucleoside
    Reverse Transcriptase Inhibitor
    (NRTI)
abacavir, lamivudine, and zidovudine
Trizivir® [US]
Antiretroviral Agent, Protease Inhibitor
atazanavir
fosamprenavir
Lexiva™ [US]
Reyataz® [US]
Antiretroviral Agent, Reverse
    Transcriptase Inhibitor
    (Nucleoside)
abacavir and lamivudine
emtricitabine
emtricitabine and tenofovir
Emtriva™ [US]
Epzicom™ [US]
Truvada™ [US]

Antiretroviral Agent, Reverse
    Transcriptase Inhibitor (Nucleotide)
emtricitabine and tenofovir
tenofovir
Truvada™ [US]
Viread™ [US]
Antiviral Agent
Apo-Zidovudine® [Can]
AZT™ [Can]
Combivir® [US/Can]
Crixivan® [US/Can]
delavirdine
didanosine
Epivir-HBV® [US]
Epivir® [US]
Fortovase® [US/Can]
Heptovir® [Can]
Hivid® [US/Can]
indinavir
Invirase® [US/Can]
lamivudine
nelfinavir
nevirapine
Norvir® SEC [Can]
Norvir® [US/Can]
Novo-AZT [Can]
Rescriptor® [US/Can]
Retrovir® [US/Can]
ritonavir
saquinavir
stavudine
3TC® [Can]
Videx® EC [US/Can]
Videx® [US/Can]
Viracept® [US/Can]
Viramune® [US/Can]
zalcitabine
Zerit® [US/Can]
zidovudine

zidovudine and lamivudine
Nonnucleoside Reverse Transcriptase
 Inhibitor (NNRTI)
 efavirenz
 Sustiva® [US/Can]
Nucleoside Reverse Transcriptase
 Inhibitor (NRTI)
 abacavir
 Ziagen® [US/Can]
Protease Inhibitor
 Agenerase® [US/Can]
 amprenavir

ANEMIA

Anabolic Steroid
 Anadrol® [US]
 oxymetholone
Androgen
 Deca-Durabolin® [Can]
 Durabolin® [Can]
 nandrolone
Antineoplastic Agent
 cyclophosphamide
 Cytoxan® [US/Can]
 Procytox® [Can]
Colony-Stimulating Factor
 Aranesp® [US/Can]
 darbepoetin alfa
 epoetin alfa
 Epogen® [US]
 Eprex® [Can]
 Procrit® [US]
Electrolyte Supplement, Oral
 Apo-Ferrous Gluconate® [Can]
 Apo-Ferrous Sulfate® [Can]
 Dexferrum® [US]
 Dexiron™ [Can]
 Femiron® [US-OTC]
 Feosol® [US-OTC]
 Feostat® [US-OTC]
 Feratab® [US-OTC]
 Fer-Gen-Sol [US-OTC]

Fergon® [US-OTC]
Fer-In-Sol® [US-OTC/Can]
Fer-Iron® [US-OTC]
Ferodan™ [Can]
Ferretts [US-OTC]
Ferro-Sequels® [US-OTC]
ferrous fumarate
ferrous gluconate
ferrous sulfate
Fe-Tinic™ 150 [US-OTC]
Hemocyte® [US-OTC]
Hytinic® [US-OTC]
INFeD® [US]
Infufer® [Can]
Ircon® [US-OTC]
iron dextran complex
Nephro-Fer® [US-OTC]
Niferex® 150 [US-OTC]
Niferex® [US-OTC]
Novo-Ferrogluc [Can]
Nu-Iron® 150 [US-OTC]
Palafer® [Can]
polysaccharide-iron complex
Slow FE® [US-OTC]
Growth Factor
 Aranesp® [US/Can]
 darbepoetin alfa
Immune Globulin
 BayGam® [US/Can]
 immune globulin (intramuscular)
Immunosuppressant Agent
 antithymocyte globulin (equine)
 Apo-Cyclosporine® [Can]
 Atgam® [US/Can]
 cyclosporine
 Gengraf® [US]
 Neoral® [US/Can]
 Restasis™ [US]
 Rhoxal-cyclosporine [Can]
 Sandimmune® I.V. [Can]
 Sandimmune® [US]

Iron Salt
  iron sucrose
  Venofer® [US/Can]
Recombinant Human Erythropoietin
  Aranesp® [US/Can]
  darbepoetin alfa
Vitamin
  Fero-Grad 500® [US-OTC]
  ferrous sulfate and ascorbic acid
  ferrous sulfate, ascorbic acid, and
    vitamin B-complex
  ferrous sulfate, ascorbic acid,
    vitamin B-complex, and folic acid
Vitamin, Water Soluble
  Apo-Folic® [Can]
  cyanocobalamin
  folic acid
  Nascobal® [US]
  Scheinpharm B12 [Can]
  Twelve Resin-K® [US]

ANESTHESIA (GENERAL)

Barbiturate
  Brevital® Sodium [US/Can]
  methohexital
General Anesthetic
  Amidate® [US/Can]
  desflurane
  Diprivan® [US/Can]
  enflurane
  Ethrane® [US/Can]
  etomidate
  Forane® [US]
  halothane
  isoflurane
  Ketalar® [US/Can]
  ketamine
  propofol
  sevoflurane
  Sevorane AF™ [Can]
  Suprane® [US/Can]
  Ultane® [US]

ANESTHESIA (LOCAL)

Local Anesthetic
  AK-T-Caine™ [US]
  Alcaine® [US/Can]
  Americaine® Anesthetic Lubricant [US]
  Americaine® [US-OTC]
  Ametop™ [Can]
  Anbesol® Baby [US-OTC/Can]
  Anbesol® Maximum Strength [US-OTC]
  Anbesol® [US-OTC]
  Anestacon® [US]
  Anusol® Ointment [US-OTC]
  Babee® Teething® [US-OTC]
  Band-Aid® Hurt-Free™ Antiseptic
    Wash [US-OTC]
  benzocaine
  benzocaine, butyl aminobenzoate,
    tetracaine, and benzalkonium
    chloride
  benzocaine, gelatin, pectin, and
    sodium carboxymethylcellulose
  Benzodent® [US-OTC]
  Betacaine® [Can]
  bupivacaine
  Burnamycin [US-OTC]
  Burn Jel [US-OTC]
  Burn-O-Jel [US-OTC]
  Carbocaine® [Can]
  Cepacol® [Can]
  Cepacol® Gold [US-OTC]
  Cepacol® Maximum Strength [US-OTC]
  Cepacol Viractin® [US-OTC]
  Cetacaine® [US]
  cetylpyridinium
  cetylpyridinium and benzocaine
  Chiggerex® [US-OTC]
  Chiggertox® [US-OTC]
  chloroprocaine
  Citanest® Plain [US/Can]
  cocaine
  Cylex® [US-OTC]

Detane® [US-OTC]
dibucaine
Diocaine® [Can]
dyclonine
ethyl chloride
ethyl chloride and
   dichlorotetrafluoroethane
Flucaine® [US]
Fluoracaine® [US]
Fluro-Ethyl® [US]
Foille® Medicated First Aid [US-OTC]
Foille® Plus [US-OTC]
Foille® [US-OTC]
Gebauer's Ethyl Chloride® [US]
HDA® Toothache [US-OTC]
hexylresorcinol
Hurricaine® [US]
Itch-X® [US-OTC]
Kank-A® [Can]
Lanacane® [US-OTC]
LidaMantle® [US]
lidocaine
lidocaine and epinephrine
Lidodan™ [Can]
Lidoderm® [US/Can]
LidoSite™ [US]
L-M-X™ 4 [US-OTC]
L-M-X™ 5 [US-OTC]
Marcaine® Spinal [US]
Marcaine® [US/Can]
mepivacaine
Mycinettes® [US-OTC]
Naropin® [US/Can]
Nesacaine®-CE [Can]
Nesacaine®-MPF [US]
Nesacaine® [US]
Novocain® [US/Can]
Nupercainal® [US-OTC]
Ophthetic® [US]
Opticaine® [US]
Orabase®-B [US-OTC]
Orajel® Baby Nighttime [US-OTC]
Orajel® Baby [US-OTC]
Orajel® Maximum Strength [US-OTC]

Orajel® [US-OTC]
Orasol® [US-OTC]
Polocaine® MPF [US]
Polocaine® [US/Can]
Pontocaine® [US/Can]
Pontocaine® With Dextrose [US]
pramoxine
Prax® [US-OTC]
Premjact® [US-OTC]
prilocaine
procaine
ProctoFoam® NS [US-OTC]
proparacaine
proparacaine and fluorescein
ropivacaine
Sensorcaine®-MPF [US]
Sensorcaine® [US/Can]
Solarcaine® Aloe Extra Burn Relief
   [US-OTC]
Solarcaine® [US-OTC]
Sucrets® Original [US-OTC]
Sucrets® [US-OTC]
tetracaine
tetracaine and dextrose
Topicaine® [US-OTC]
Trocaine® [US-OTC]
Tronolane® [US-OTC]
Xylocaine® MPF [US]
Xylocaine® MPF With Epinephrine [US]
Xylocaine® [US/Can]
Xylocaine® Viscous [US]
Xylocaine® With Epinephrine [Can]
Xylocard® [Can]
Zilactin® Baby [US-OTC/Can]
Zilactin®-B [US-OTC/Can]
Zilactin® [Can]
Zilactin-L® [US-OTC]
Local Anesthetic, Amide Derivative
   Chirocaine® [Can]
   levobupivacaine
Local Anesthetic, Injectable
   Chirocaine® [Can]
   levobupivacaine

ANESTHESIA (OPHTHALMIC)
Local Anesthetic
  Flucaine® [US]
  Fluoracaine® [US]
  proparacaine and fluorescein

ASPERGILLOSIS
Antifungal Agent
  Abelcet® [US/Can]
  Amphocin® [US]
  Amphotec® [US/Can]
  amphotericin B cholesteryl sulfate
    complex
  amphotericin B (conventional)
  amphotericin B lipid complex
  Ancobon® [US/Can]
  flucytosine
  Fungizone® [US/Can]
  VFEND® [US]
  voriconazole
Antifungal Agent, Systemic
  AmBisome® [US/Can]
  amphotericin B liposomal
  Cancidas® [US/Can]
  caspofungin

BLADDER IRRIGATION
Antibacterial, Topical
  acetic acid

BOWEL CLEANSING
Laxative
  castor oil
  Citro-Mag® [Can]
  Colyte® [US/Can]
  Fleet® Enema [US-OTC/Can]
  Fleet® Phospho®-Soda Accu-Prep™
    [US-OTC]
  Fleet® Phospho®-Soda Oral Laxative
    [Can]
  Fleet® Phospho®-Soda [US-OTC]

GlycoLax™ [US]
GoLYTELY® [US]
Klean-Prep® [Can]
Lyteprep™ [Can]
magnesium citrate
MiraLax™ [US]
NuLYTELY® [US]
PegLyte® [Can]
polyethylene glycol-electrolyte
  solution
Purge® [US-OTC]
sodium phosphates
TriLyte™ [US]
Visicol™ [US]
Laxative, Bowel Evacuant
  HalfLytely® and Bisacodyl [US]
  polyethylene glycol-electrolyte
    solution and bisacodyl

BOWEL STERILIZATION
Aminoglycoside (Antibiotic)
  Myciguent [US-OTC]
  Neo-Fradin™ [US]
  neomycin
  Neo-Rx [US]

CACHEXIA
Progestin
  Apo-Megestrol® [Can]
  Lin-Megestrol [Can]
  Megace® OS [US]
  Megace® [US/Can]
  megestrol acetate
  Nu-Megestrol [Can]

CANDIDIASIS
Antifungal Agent
  Abelcet® [US/Can]
  Absorbine Jr.® Antifungal [US-OTC]
  Aftate® Antifungal [US-OTC]
  Aloe Vesta® 2-n-1 Antifungal [US-
    OTC]
  Amphocin® [US]

Amphotec® [US/Can]
amphotericin B cholesteryl sulfate complex
amphotericin B (conventional)
amphotericin B lipid complex
Ancobon® [US/Can]
Apo-Fluconazole® [Can]
Apo-Ketoconazole® [Can]
Baza® Antifungal [US-OTC]
Bio-Statin® [US]
Blis-To-Sol® [US-OTC]
butoconazole
Candistatin® [Can]
Canesten® Topical [Can]
Canesten® Vaginal [Can]
Carrington Antifungal [US-OTC]
ciclopirox
Clotrimaderm [Can]
clotrimazole
Cruex® Cream [US-OTC]
1-Day™ [US-OTC]
Dermasept Antifungal [US-OTC]
Dermazole [Can]
Diflucan® [US/Can]
econazole
Ecostatin® [Can]
Exelderm® [US/Can]
Femizol-M™ [US-OTC]
Femstat® One [Can]
fluconazole
flucytosine
Fungi-Guard [US-OTC]
Fungizone® [US/Can]
Fungoid® Tincture [US-OTC]
Gen-Fluconazole [Can]
Gold Bond® Antifungal [US-OTC]
Gynazole-1® [US]
Gyne-Lotrimin® 3 [US-OTC]
itraconazole
ketoconazole
Ketoderm® [Can]
Lamisil® Topical

Loprox® [US/Can]
Lotrimin® AF Athlete's Foot Cream [US-OTC]
Lotrimin® AF Athlete's Foot Solution [US-OTC]
Lotrimin® AF Jock Itch Cream [US-OTC]
Lotrimin® AF Powder/Spray [US-OTC]
Micaderm® [US-OTC]
Micatin® [US-OTC/Can]
miconazole
Micozole [Can]
Micro-Guard® [US-OTC]
Mitrazol™ [US-OTC]
Monistat® 1 Combination Pack [US-OTC]
Monistat® 3 [US-OTC]
Monistat® 7 [US-OTC]
Monistat® [Can]
Monistat-Derm® [US]
Mycelex®-3 [US-OTC]
Mycelex®-7 [US-OTC]
Mycelex® Twin Pack [US-OTC]
Mycelex® [US]
Mycostatin® [US/Can]
naftifine
Naftin® [US]
Nilstat® [Can]
Nizoral® A-D [US-OTC]
Nizoral® [US/Can]
Novo-Fluconazole [Can]
Novo-Ketoconazole [Can]
Nyaderm [Can]
nystatin
Nystat-Rx® [US]
Nystop® [US]
oxiconazole
Oxistat® [US/Can]
Oxizole® [Can]
Pedi-Dri® [US]
Penlac™ [US/Can]
Pitrex [Can]

PMS-Nystatin [Can]
Spectazole® [US/Can]
Sporanox® [US/Can]
sulconazole
Terazol® 3 [US]
Terazol® 7 [US]
Terazol® [Can]
terbinafine (topical)
terconazole
Tinactin® Antifungal Jock Itch [US-OTC]
Tinactin® Antifungal [US-OTC]
Tinaderm [US-OTC]
Ting® [US-OTC]
tioconazole
Tip Tap Toe [US-OTC]
tolnaftate
Triple Care® Antifungal [OTC]
Trivagizole-3® [Can]
Vagistat®-1 [US-OTC]
Zeasorb®-AF [US-OTC]
Antifungal Agent, Systemic
AmBisome® [US/Can]
amphotericin B liposomal
Antifungal/Corticosteroid
nystatin and triamcinolone

CARCINOMA

Androgen
Andriol® [Can]
Androderm® [US/Can]
AndroGel® [US/Can]
Android® [US]
Andropository [Can]
bicalutamide
Casodex® [US/Can]
Deca-Durabolin® [Can]
Delatestryl® [US/Can]
Depotest® 100 [Can]
Depo®-Testosterone [US]
Durabolin® [Can]
Everone® 200 [Can]
Methitest® [US]

methyltestosterone
nandrolone
Striant™ [US]
Teslac® [US/Can]
Testim™ [US]
Testoderm® [Can]
testolactone
Testopel® [US]
testosterone
Testred® [US]
Virilon® [US]
Antiandrogen
Alti-CPA [Can]
Androcur® [Can]
Androcur® Depot [Can]
Apo-Flutamide® [Can]
cyproterone (Canada only)
Euflex® [Can]
Eulexin® [US/Can]
flutamide
Gen-Cyproterone [Can]
Novo-Flutamide [Can]
PMS-Flutamide [Can]
Antineoplastic Agent
Adriamycin® [Can]
Adriamycin PFS® [US]
Adriamycin RDF® [US]
Adrucil® [US/Can]
Alkeran® [US/Can]
altretamine
aminoglutethimide
Anandron® [Can]
anastrozole
Apo-Megestrol® [Can]
Apo-Methotrexate® [Can]
Apo-Tamox® [Can]
Arimidex® [US/Can]
BiCNU® [US/Can]
Blenoxane® [US/Can]
bleomycin
Camptosar® [US/Can]
Carac™ [US]
carboplatin

carmustine
CeeNU® [US/Can]
chlorambucil
cisplatin
Cosmegen® [US/Can]
cyclophosphamide
Cytadren® [US]
cytarabine
Cytosar® [Can]
Cytosar-U® [US]
Cytoxan® [US/Can]
dacarbazine
dactinomycin
docetaxel
doxorubicin
Droxia™ [US]
DTIC® [Can]
DTIC-Dome® [US]
Efudex® [US/Can]
Eligard® [US]
Emcyt® [US/Can]
estramustine
Etopophos® [US]
etoposide
etoposide phosphate
Fareston® [US/Can]
floxuridine
Fluoroplex® [US]
fluorouracil
FUDR® [US/Can]
gemcitabine
Gemzar® [US/Can]
Gen-Hydroxyurea [Can]
Gen-Tamoxifen [Can]
Gliadel® [US]
Herceptin®[US/Can]
Hexalen® [US/Can]
Hycamtin® [US/Can]
Hydrea® [US/Can]
hydroxyurea
Idamycin® [Can]
Idamycin PFS® [US]
idarubicin

Ifex® [US/Can]
ifosfamide
irinotecan
Leukeran® [US/Can]
leuprolide acetate
Lin-Megestrol [Can]
lomustine
Lupron Depot-Ped® [US]
Lupron Depot® [US/Can]
Lupron® [US/Can]
Lysodren® [US/Can]
mechlorethamine
Megace® OS [US]
Megace® [US/Can]
megestrol acetate
melphalan
methotrexate
mitomycin
mitotane
mitoxantrone
Mustargen® [US/Can]
Mutamycin® [US/Can]
Mylocel™ [US]
Navelbine® [US/Can]
Nilandron® [US]
nilutamide
Nolvadex®-D [Can]
Nolvadex® [US/Can]
Novantrone® [US/Can]
Novo-Tamoxifen [Can]
Nu-Megestrol [Can]
Oncovin® [Can]
Onxol™ [US]
paclitaxel
Paraplatin-AQ [Can]
Paraplatin® [US]
Photofrin® [US/Can]
Platinol®-AQ [US]
PMS-Tamoxifen [Can]
porfimer
Procytox® [Can]
raltitrexed (Canada only)
ratio-Methotrexate [Can]

Rheumatrex® [US]
Rubex® [US]
streptozocin
Tamofen® [Can]
tamoxifen
Taxol® [US/Can]
Taxotere® [US/Can]
teniposide
thiotepa
Tomudex® [Can]
Toposar® [US]
topotecan
toremifene
trastuzumab
Trexall™ [US]
Velban® [Can]
VePesid® [US/Can]
Viadur® [US/Can]
vinblastine
Vincasar® PFS® [US/Can]
vincristine
vinorelbine
Vumon® [US/Can]
Zanosar® [US/Can]
Antineoplastic Agent, Alkylating Agent
Temodal™ [Can]
Temodar® [US/Can]
temozolomide
Antineoplastic Agent, Anthracycline
Ellence® [US/Can]
epirubicin
Pharmorubicin® [Can]
valrubicin
Valstar® [Can]
Valtaxin® [Can]
Antineoplastic Agent, Antibiotic
Ellence® [US/Can]
epirubicin
Pharmorubicin® [Can]
Antineoplastic Agent, Antimetabolite
capecitabine
Xeloda® [US/Can]

Antineoplastic Agent, Estrogen
    Receptor Antagonist
Faslodex® [US]
fulvestrant
Antineoplastic Agent, Hormone
    (Antiestrogen)
Femara® [US/Can]
letrozole
Antineoplastic Agent, Miscellaneous
Aromasin® [US/Can]
denileukin diftitox
exemestane
ONTAK® [US]
Antineoplastic Agent, Monoclonal
    Antibody
Avastin™ [US]
bevacizumab
Antiviral Agent
    interferon alfa-2b and ribavirin
        combination pack
Rebetron® [US/Can]
Biological Response Modulator
    aldesleukin
    BCG vaccine
    ImmuCyst® [Can]
    interferon alfa-2b and ribavirin
        combination pack
    Oncotice™ [Can]
    Pacis™ [Can]
    Proleukin® [US/Can]
    Rebetron® [US/Can]
    TheraCys® [US]
    TICE® BCG [US]
Estrogen and Androgen Combination
    Estratest® H.S. [US]
    Estratest® [US/Can]
    estrogens (esterified) and
        methyltestosterone
Estrogen Derivative
    Alora® [US]
    C.E.S.® [Can]
    Climara® [US/Can]
    Congest [Can]

Delestrogen® [US/Can]
Depo®-Estradiol [US/Can]
Esclim® [US]
Estrace® [US/Can]
Estraderm® [US/Can]
estradiol
Estradot® [Can]
Estrasorb™ [US]
Estring® [US/Can]
EstroGel® [US/Can]
estrogens (conjugated/equine)
estrone
Femring™ [US]
Gynodiol® [US]
Menostar™ [US]
Oesclim® [Can]
Premarin® [US/Can]
Vagifem® [US/Can]
Vivelle-Dot® [US]
Vivelle® [US/Can]
Gonadotropin-Releasing Hormone
    Analog
goserelin
Zoladex® LA [Can]
Zoladex® [US/Can]
Gonadotropin Releasing Hormone
    Antagonist
abarelix
Plenaxis™ [US]
Luteinizing Hormone-Releasing
    Hormone Analog
buserelin acetate (Canada only)
Trelstar™ Depot [US/Can]
Trelstar™ LA [US]
triptorelin
Progestin
Alti-CPA [Can]
Alti-MPA [Can]
Androcur® [Can]
Androcur® Depot [Can]
Apo-Medroxy® [Can]
Crinone® [US/Can]
cyproterone (Canada only)

Depo-Provera® Contraceptive [US]
Depo-Provera® [US/Can]
Gen-Cyproterone [Can]
Gen-Medroxy [Can]
hydroxyprogesterone caproate
medroxyprogesterone acetate
Novo-Medrone [Can]
Prochieve™ [US]
Progestasert® [US]
progesterone
Prometrium® [US/Can]
Provera® [US/Can]
Somatostatin Analog
octreotide
Sandostatin LAR® [US/Can]
Sandostatin® [US/Can]
Thyroid Product
Armour® Thyroid [US]
Cytomel® [US/Can]
Eltroxin® [Can]
Levothroid® [US]
levothyroxine
Levoxyl® [US]
liothyronine
liotrix
Nature-Throid® NT [US]
Novothyrox [US]
Synthroid® [US/Can]
thyroid
Thyrolar® [US/Can]
Triostat® [US]
Unithroid® [US]
Westhroid® [US]
Vaccine, Recombinant
Avastin™ [US]
bevacizumab

CIRRHOSIS
Bile Acid Sequestrant
cholestyramine resin
Novo-Cholamine [Can]
Novo-Cholamine Light [Can]
PMS-Cholestyramine [Can]

Prevalite® [US]
Questran® Light Sugar Free [Can]
Questran® Light [US]
Questran® [US/Can]
Chelating Agent
Cuprimine® [US/Can]
Depen® [US/Can]
penicillamine
Electrolyte Supplement, Oral
Alcalak [US-OTC]
Alka-Mints® [US-OTC]
Amitone® [US-OTC]
Apo-Cal® [Can]
Calcarb 600 [US-OTC]
Calci-Chew® [US-OTC]
Calci-Mix® [US-OTC]
Calcite-500 [Can]
Cal-Citrate® 250 [US-OTC]
calcium carbonate
calcium citrate
calcium glubionate
calcium lactate
Cal-Gest [US-OTC]
Cal-Mint [US-OTC]
Caltrate® 600 [US-OTC]
Caltrate® [Can]
Chooz® [US-OTC]
Citracal® [US-OTC]
Florical® [US-OTC]
Mylanta® Children's [US-OTC]
Nephro-Calci® [US-OTC]
Os-Cal® 500 [US-OTC]
Os-Cal® [Can]
Osteocit® [Can]
Oysco 500 [US-OTC]
Oyst-Cal 500 [US-OTC]
Titralac™ Extra Strength [US-OTC]
Titralac™ [US-OTC]
Tums® 500 [US-OTC]
Tums® E-X [US-OTC]
Tums® Smooth Dissolve [US-OTC]
Tums® Ultra [US-OTC]
Tums® [US-OTC]

Immunosuppressant Agent
Alti-Azathioprine [Can]
Apo-Azathioprine® [Can]
Azasan® [US]
azathioprine
Gen-Azathioprine [Can]
Imuran® [US/Can]
Vitamin D Analog
Calciferol™ [US]
Drisdol® [US/Can]
ergocalciferol
Ostoforte® [Can]
Vitamin, Fat Soluble
AquaMEPHYTON® [Can]
Aquasol A® [US]
Konakion [Can]
Mephyton® [US/Can]
Palmitate-A® [US-OTC]
phytonadione
vitamin A

CISPLATIN TOXICITY
Antidote
sodium thiosulfate
Versiclear™ [US]

COLONIC EVACUATION
Laxative
Alophen® [US-OTC]
Apo-Bisacodyl® [Can]
Bisac-Evac™ [US-OTC]
bisacodyl
Bisacodyl Unisert® [US-OTC]
Carter's Little Pills® [Can]
Correctol® Tablets [US-OTC]
Doxidan® (reformulation) [US-OTC]
Dulcolax® [US-OTC/Can]
Femilax™ [US-OTC]
Fleet® Bisacodyl Enema [US-OTC]
Fleet® Stimulant Laxative [US-OTC]
Gentlax® [US-OTC]
Modane Tablets® [US-OTC]
Veracolate [US-OTC]

CONDYLOMA ACUMINATUM

Antiviral Agent
  interferon alfa-2b and ribavirin
    combination pack
  Rebetron® [US/Can]
Biological Response Modulator
  Alferon® N [US/Can]
  interferon alfa-2a
  interferon alfa-2b
  interferon alfa-2b and ribavirin
    combination pack
  interferon alfa-n3
  Intron® A [US/Can]
  Rebetron® [US/Can]
  Roferon-A® [US/Can]
Immune Response Modifier
  Aldara™ [US/Can]
  imiquimod
Keratolytic Agent
  Condyline™ [Can]
  Condylox® [US]
  Podocon-25™ [US]
  Podofilm® [Can]
  podofilox
  podophyllum resin
  Wartec® [Can]

CONSTIPATION

Laxative
  Acilac [Can]
  Agoral® Maximum Strength
    Laxative [US-OTC]
  Alophen® [US-OTC]
  Apo-Bisacodyl® [Can]
  Apo-Lactulose® [Can]
  Bausch & Lomb® Computer Eye
    Drops [US-OTC]
  Bisac-Evac™ [US-OTC]
  bisacodyl
  Bisacodyl Unisert® [US-OTC]
  Carter's Little Pills® [Can]
  castor oil

Cholac® [US]
Citrucel® [US-OTC]
Constilac® [US]
Constulose® [US]
Correctol® Tablets [US-OTC]
Doxidan® (reformulation) [US-OTC]
Dulcolax® Milk of Magnesia [US-OTC]
Dulcolax® [US-OTC/Can]
Enulose® [US]
Equalactin® [US-OTC]
Evac-U-Gen [US-OTC]
ex-lax® Maximum Strength [US-OTC]
ex-lax® [US-OTC]
Femilax™ [US-OTC]
Fiberall® [US]
FiberCon® [US-OTC]
FiberEase™ [US-OTC]
Fiber-Lax® [US-OTC]
FiberNorm™ [US-OTC]
Fleet® Babylax® [US-OTC]
Fleet® Bisacodyl Enema [US-OTC]
Fleet® Enema [US-OTC/Can]
Fleet® Glycerin Suppositories
  Maximum Strength [US-OTC]
Fleet® Glycerin Suppositories [US-OTC]
Fleet® Liquid Glycerin Suppositories
  [US-OTC]
Fleet® Phospho®-Soda Accu-Prep™
  [US-OTC]
Fleet® Phospho®-Soda Oral Laxative
  [Can]
Fleet® Phospho®-Soda [US-OTC]
Fleet® Stimulant Laxative [US-OTC]
Fletcher's® Castoria® [US-OTC]
Generlac® [US]
Genfiber® [US-OTC]
Gentlax® [US-OTC]
glycerin
Hydrocil® [US-OTC]
Konsyl-D® [US-OTC]
Konsyl® Easy Mix [US-OTC]

Drugs by Indication

Konsyl® Orange [US-OTC]
Konsyl® Tablets [US-OTC]
Konsyl® [US-OTC]
Kristalose™ [US]
lactulose
Laxilose [Can]
magnesium hydroxide
magnesium hydroxide and mineral
  oil emulsion
magnesium oxide
magnesium sulfate
Mag-Ox® 400 [US-OTC]
malt soup extract
Maltsupex® [US-OTC]
Metamucil® [Can]
Metamucil® Smooth Texture [US-
  OTC]
Metamucil® [US-OTC]
methylcellulose
Modane® Bulk [US-OTC]
Modane Tablets® [US-OTC]
Novo-Mucilax [Can]
Osmoglyn® [US]
Perdiem® Fiber Therapy [US-OTC]
Phillips'® Fibercaps [US-OTC]
Phillips'® Milk of Magnesia [US-
  OTC]
Phillips' M-O® [US-OTC]
PMS-Lactulose [Can]
polycarbophil
psyllium
Purge® [US-OTC]
Reguloid® [US-OTC]
Sani-Supp® [US-OTC]
Senexon® [US-OTC]
senna
Senna-Gen® [US-OTC]
Sennatural™ [US-OTC]
Senokot® Children's [US-OTC]
Senokot® [US-OTC]
SenokotXTRA® [US-OTC]
Serutan® [US-OTC]

sodium phosphates
sorbitol
Uro-Mag® [US-OTC]
Veracolate [US-OTC]
Visicol™ [US]
X-Prep® [US-OTC]
Laxative, Stimulant
  docusate and senna
  Peri-Colace®) (reformulation) [US-
    OTC]
  Senokot-S® [US-OTC]
Stool Softener
  Albert® Docusate [Can]
  Apo-Docusate-Calcium® [Can]
  Apo-Docusate-Sodium® [Can]
  Colace® [US-OTC/Can]
  Colax-C® [Can]
  Diocto® [US-OTC]
  docusate
  docusate and senna
  Docusoft-S™ [US-OTC]
  DOK™ [US-OTC]
  DOS® [US-OTC]
  D-S-S® [US-OTC]
  Dulcolax® Stool Softener [US-OTC]
  Enemeez® [US-OTC]
  Fleet® Sof-Lax® [US-OTC]
  Genasoft® [US-OTC]
  Novo-Docusate Calcium [Can]
  Novo-Docusate Sodium [Can]
  Peri-Colace®) (reformulation) [US-
    OTC]
  Phillips'® Stool Softener Laxative
    [US-OTC]
  PMS-Docusate Calcium [Can]
  PMS-Docusate Sodium [Can]
  Regulex® [Can]
  Selax® [Can]
  Senokot-S®) [US-OTC]
  Silace [US-OTC]
  Soflax™ [Can]
  Surfak® [US-OTC]

CRYPTOCOCCOSIS

Antifungal Agent
Abelcet® [US/Can]
Amphocin® [US]
Amphotec® [US/Can]
amphotericin B cholesteryl sulfate complex
amphotericin B (conventional)
amphotericin B lipid complex
Ancobon® [US/Can]
Apo-Fluconazole® [Can]
Diflucan® [US/Can]
fluconazole
flucytosine
Fungizone® [US/Can]
Gen-Fluconazole [Can]
itraconazole
Novo-Fluconazole [Can]
Sporanox® [US/Can]
Antifungal Agent, Systemic
AmBisome® [US/Can]
amphotericin B liposomal

CYTOMEGALOVIRUS

Antiviral Agent
cidofovir
Cytovene® [US/Can]
foscarnet
Foscavir® [US/Can]
ganciclovir
Vistide® [US]
Vitrasert® [US/Can]
Antiviral Agent, Ophthalmic
fomivirsen (Canada only)
Vitravene™ [Can]
Immune Globulin
Carimune™ [US]
CytoGam® [US]
cytomegalovirus immune globulin (intravenous-human)
Flebogamma® [US]
Gamimune® N [US/Can]

Gammagard® S/D [US/Can]
Gammar®-P I.V. [US]
Gamunex® [US/Can]
immune globulin (intravenous)
Iveegam EN [US]
Iveegam Immuno® [Can]
Octagam® [US]
Panglobulin® [US]
Polygam® S/D [US]
Venoglobulin®-S [US]

DERMATOMYCOSIS

Antifungal Agent
Aloe Vesta® 2-n-1 Antifungal [US-OTC]
Apo-Ketoconazole® [Can]
Baza® Antifungal [US-OTC]
Carrington Antifungal [US-OTC]
Dermazole [Can]
Femizol-M™ [US-OTC]
Fulvicin-U/F® [Can]
Fungoid® Tincture [US-OTC]
Grifulvin® V [US]
griseofulvin
Gris-PEG® [US]
ketoconazole
Ketoderm® [Can]
Lotrimin®) AF Powder/Spray [US-OTC]
Micaderm® [US-OTC]
Micatin® [US-OTC/Can]
miconazole
Micozole [Can]
Micro-Guard® [US-OTC]
Mitrazol™ [US-OTC]
Monistat® 1 Combination Pack [US-OTC]
Monistat®) 3 [US-OTC]
Monistat® 7 [US-OTC]
Monistat® [Can]
Monistat-Derm® [US]
naftifine
Naftin® [US]

Nizoral® A-D [US-OTC]
Nizoral® [US/Can]
Novo-Ketoconazole [Can]
oxiconazole
Oxistat® [US/Can]
Oxizole® [Can]
Triple Care® Antifungal [OTC]
Zeasorb®-AF [US-OTC]

ENCEPHALITIS (HERPES VIRUS)

Antiviral Agent
acyclovir
Alti-Acyclovir [Can]
Apo-Acyclovir® [Can]
Gen-Acyclovir [Can]
Nu-Acyclovir [Can]
ratio-Acyclovir [Can]
Zovirax® [US/Can]

ESSENTIAL THROMBOCYTHEMIA (ET)

Platelet Reducing Agent
Agrylin® [US/Can]
anagrelide

FACTOR IX DEFICIENCY

Antihemophilic Agent
Bebulin® VH [US]
factor IX complex (human)
Profilnine® SD [US]
Proplex® T [US]

FACTOR VIII DEFICIENCY

Blood Product Derivative
Alphanate® [US]
antihemophilic factor (human)
Hemofil® M [US/Can]
Humate-P® [US/Can]
Koate®-DVI [US]
Monarc® M [US]
Monoclate-P® [US]

Hemophilic Agent
anti-inhibitor coagulant complex
Autoplex® T [US]
Feiba VH Immuno® [Can]
Feiba VH® [US]

FEBRILE NEUTROPENIA

Colony-Stimulating Factor
Neulasta™ [US]
pegfilgrastim
Quinolone
ciprofloxacin
Cipro® [US/Can]
Cipro® XL [Can]
Cipro® XR [US]

FEVER

Antipyretic
Abenol® [Can]
Acephen® [US-OTC]
acetaminophen
Advil® Children's [US-OTC]
Advil® Infants' [US-OTC]
Advil® Junior [US-OTC]
Advil® Migraine [US-OTC]
Advil® [US-OTC/Can]
Aleve® [US-OTC]
Amigesic® [US/Can]
Anaprox® DS [US/Can]
Anaprox® [US/Can]
Apo-Acetaminophen® [Can]
Apo-Ibuprofen® [Can]
Apo-Napro-Na® [Can]
Apo-Napro-Na DS® [Can]
Apo-Naproxen® [Can]
Apo-Naproxen SR® [Can]
Asaphen [Can]
Asaphen E.C. [Can]
Ascriptin® Extra Strength [US-OTC]
Ascriptin® [US-OTC]
Aspercin Extra [US-OTC]
Aspercin [US-OTC]
Aspergum® [US-OTC]

aspirin
Aspirin Free Anacin® Maximum Strength [US-OTC]
Atasol® [Can]
Bayer® Aspirin Extra Strength [US-OTC]
Bayer® Aspirin Regimen Adult Low Strength [US-OTC]
Bayer® Aspirin Regimen Children's [US-OTC]
Bayer® Aspirin Regimen Regular Strength [US-OTC]
Bayer® Aspirin [US-OTC]
Bayer® Extra Strength Arthritis Pain Regimen [US-OTC]
Bayer® Plus Extra Strength [US-OTC]
Bayer® Women's Aspirin Plus Calcium [US-OTC]
Bufferin® Extra Strength [US-OTC]
Bufferin® [US-OTC]
Buffinol Extra [US-OTC]
Buffinol [US-OTC]
Cetafen Extra® [US-OTC]
Cetafen® [US-OTC]
Comtrex® Sore Throat Maximum Strength [US-OTC]
Easprin® [US]
EC-Naprosyn® [US]
Ecotrin® Low Strength [US-OTC]
Ecotrin® Maximum Strength [US-OTC]
Ecotrin® [US-OTC]
ElixSure™ Fever/Pain [US-OTC]
Entrophen® [Can]
FeverALL® [US-OTC]
Genapap® Children [US-OTC]
Genapap® Extra Strength [US-OTC]
Genapap® Infant [US-OTC]
Genapap® [US-OTC]
Genebs® Extra Strength [US-OTC]
Genebs® [US-OTC]
Gen-Naproxen EC [Can]
Genpril® [US-OTC]

Halfprin® [US-OTC]
Ibu-200 [US-OTC]
ibuprofen
I-Prin [US-OTC]
Mapap® Arthritis [US-OTC]
Mapap® Children's [US-OTC]
Mapap® Extra Strength [US-OTC]
Mapap® Infants [US-OTC]
Mapap® [US-OTC]
Menadol® [US-OTC]
Midol® Maximum Strength Cramp Formula [US-OTC]
Mono-Gesic® [US]
Motrin® Children's [US-OTC/Can]
Motrin® IB [US-OTC/Can]
Motrin® Infants' [US-OTC]
Motrin® Junior Strength [US-OTC]
Motrin® Migraine Pain [US-OTC]
Motrin® [US/Can]
Naprelan® [US]
Naprosyn® [US/Can]
naproxen
Naxen® [Can]
Novasen [Can]
Novo-Naproc EC [Can]
Novo-Naprox [Can]
Novo-Naprox Sodium [Can]
Novo-Naprox Sodium DS [Can]
Novo-Naprox SR [Can]
Novo-Profen® [Can]
Nu-Ibuprofen [Can]
Nu-Naprox [Can]
Pamprin® Maximum Strength All Day Relief [US-OTC]
Pediatrix [Can]
Redutemp® [US-OTC]
Riva-Naproxen [Can]
Salflex® [US/Can]
salsalate
Silapap® Children's [US-OTC]
Silapap® Infants [US-OTC]
sodium salicylate
St Joseph® Adult Aspirin [US-OTC]

Sureprin 81™ [US-OTC]
Tempra® [Can]
Tylenol® 8 Hour [US-OTC]
Tylenol® Arthritis Pain [US-OTC]
Tylenol® Children's [US-OTC]
Tylenol® Extra Strength [US-OTC]
Tylenol® Infants [US-OTC]
Tylenol® Junior Strength [US-OTC]
Tylenol® Sore Throat [US-OTC]
Tylenol® [US-OTC/Can]
Ultraprin [US-OTC]
Valorin Extra [US-OTC]
Valorin [US-OTC]
ZORprin® [US]

GENITAL HERPES

Antiviral Agent
famciclovir
Famvir® [US/Can]
valacyclovir
Valtrex® [US/Can]

GENITAL WART

Immune Response Modifier
Aldara™ [US/Can]
imiquimod

GLIOMA

Antineoplastic Agent
CeeNU® [US/Can]
lomustine
Antiviral Agent
interferon alfa-2b and ribavirin
combination pack
Rebetron® [US/Can]
Biological Response Modulator
interferon alfa-2b
interferon alfa-2b and ribavirin
combination pack
Intron® A [US/Can]
Rebetron® [US/Can]

GRAFT VERSUS HOST DISEASE

Immunosuppressant Agent
antithymocyte globulin (equine)
Apo-Cyclosporine® [Can]
Atgam® [US/Can]
CellCept® [US/Can]
cyclosporine
Gengraf® [US]
muromonab-CD3
mycophenolate
Myfortic® [US]
Neoral® [US/Can]
Orthoclone OKT® 3 [US/Can]
Prograf® [US/Can]
Protopic® [US/Can]
Restasis™ [US]
Rhoxal-cyclosporine [Can]
Sandimmune® I.V. [Can]
Sandimmune® [US]
tacrolimus

GRANULOMATOUS DISEASE, CHRONIC

Biological Response Modulator
Actimmune® [US/Can]
interferon gamma-1b

HEMATOLOGIC DISORDER

Adrenal Corticosteroid
A-HydroCort® [US]
A-methapred® [US]
Apo-Prednisone® [Can]
Aristocort® Forte Injection [US]
Aristocort® Intralesional Injection [US]
Aristocort® Tablet [US/Can]
Aristospan® Intraarticular Injection
[US/Can]
Aristospan® Intralesional Injection
[US/Can]
betamethasone (systemic)
Celestone® Soluspan® [US/Can]

Celestone® [US]
Cortef® Tablet [US/Can]
corticotropin
cortisone acetate
Cortone® [Can]
Decadron® [US/Can]
Deltasone® [US]
Depo-Medrol® [US/Can]
Dexamethasone Intensol® [US]
dexamethasone (systemic)
DexPak® TaperPak® [US]
Diodex® [Can]
H.P. Acthar® Gel [US]
hydrocortisone (systemic)
Hydrocortone® Phosphate [US]
Kenalog® Injection [US/Can]
Medrol® [US/Can]
methylprednisolone
Orapred™ [US]
Pediapred® [US/Can]
PMS-Dexamethasone [Can]
Prednicot® [US]
prednisolone (systemic)
Prednisol® TBA [US]
prednisone
Prednisone Intensol™ [US]
Prelone® [US]
Solu-Cortef® [US/Can]
Solu-Medrol® [US/Can]
Sterapred® DS [US]
Sterapred® [US]
triamcinolone (systemic)
Winpred™ [Can]

HEMOLYTIC DISEASE OF THE NEWBORN
Immune Globulin
BayRho-D® Full-Dose [US/Can]
BayRho-D® Mini-Dose [US]
MICRhoGAM® [US]
Rho^D immune globulin
RhoGAM® [US]
Rhophylac® [US]
WinRho SDF® [US]

HEMOPHILIA
Antihemophilic Agent
antihemophilic factor (porcine)
Hyate:C® [US]
Vasopressin Analog, Synthetic
Apo-Desmopressin® [Can]
DDAVP® [US/Can]
desmopressin acetate
Minirin® [Can]
Octostim® [Can]
Stimate™ [US]

HEMOPHILIA A
Antihemophilic Agent
factor VIIa (recombinant)
Niastase® [Can]
NovoSeven® [US]
Blood Product Derivative
Advate [US]
Alphanate® [US]
antihemophilic factor (human)
antihemophilic factor (recombinant)
factor VIIa (recombinant)
Helixate® FS [US/Can]
Hemofil® M [US/Can]
Humate-P® [US/Can]
Koate®-DVI [US]
Kogenate® [Can]
Kogenate® FS [US/Can]
Monarc® M [US]
Monoclate-P® [US]
Niastase® [Can]
NovoSeven® [US]
Recombinate™ [US/Can]
ReFacto® [US/Can]

HEMOPHILIA B
Antihemophilic Agent
AlphaNine® SD [US]
BeneFix® [US/Can]
factor IX
factor VIIa (recombinant)

Immunine® VH [Can]
Mononine® [US/Can]
Niastase® [Can]
NovoSeven® [US]
Blood Product Derivative
factor VIIa (recombinant)
Niastase® [Can]
NovoSeven® [US]

HEMORRHAGE

Adrenergic Agonist Agent
Adrenalin® [US/Can]
epinephrine
Antihemophilic Agent
Bebulin® VH [US]
factor IX complex (human)
Profilnine® SD [US]
Proplex® T [US]
Ergot Alkaloid and Derivative
ergonovine
Hemostatic Agent
Amicar® [US/Can]
aminocaproic acid
aprotinin
Avitene® Flour [US]
Avitene® Ultrafoam [US]
Avitene® UltraWrap™ [US]
Avitene® [US]
cellulose, oxidized regenerated
collagen hemostat
EndoAvitene® [US]
gelatin (absorbable)
Gelfilm® [US]
Gelfoam® [US]
Helistat® [US]
Instat™ MCH [US]
Surgical® Fibrillar [US]
Surgicel® NuKnit [US]
Surgicel® [US]
SyringeAvitene™ [US]
Thrombin-JMI® [US]
thrombin (topical)
Thrombogen® [US]

Thrombostat™ [Can]
Trasylol® [US/Can]
Progestin
Alti-MPA [Can]
Apo-Medroxy® [Can]
Aygestin® [US]
Camila™ [US]
Crinone® [US/Can]
Depo-Provera® Contraceptive [US]
Depo-Provera® [US/Can]
Errin™ [US]
Gen-Medroxy [Can]
hydroxyprogesterone caproate
Jolivette™ [US]
medroxyprogesterone acetate
Micronor® [US/Can]
Nora-BE™ [US]
norethindrone
Norlutate® [Can]
Nor-QD® [US]
Novo-Medrone [Can]
Prochieve™ [US]
Progestasert® [US]
progesterone
Prometrium® [US/Can]
Provera® [US/Can]
Vitamin, Fat Soluble
AquaMEPHYTON® [Can]
Konakion [Can]
Mephyton® [US/Can]
phytonadione

HEMORRHAGE (PREVENTION)
Antihemophilic Agent
Cyklokapron® [US/Can]
tranexamic acid

HEMOSIDEROSIS
Antidote
deferoxamine
Desferal® [US/Can]
PMS-Deferoxamine [Can]

HEMOSTASIS
Hemostatic Agent
  Crosseal™ [US]
  fibrin sealant kit
  Tisseel® VH [US/Can]

HEPATIC CIRRHOSIS
Diuretic, Potassium Sparing
  amiloride
  Midamor® [Can]

HEPATITIS A
Immune Globulin
  BayGam® [US/Can]
  immune globulin (intramuscular)
Vaccine, Inactivated Virus
  Avaxim® [Can]
  Avaxim®-Pediatric [Can]
  Epaxal Berna® [Can]
  Havrix® [US/Can]
  hepatitis A vaccine
  VAQTA® [US/Can]

HEPATITIS B
Antiretroviral Agent, Non-nucleoside
  Reverse Transcriptase Inhibitor
  (NNRTI)
  adefovir
  Hepsera™ [US]
Antiviral Agent
  Epivir-HBV® [US]
  Epivir® [US]
  Heptovir® [Can]
  interferon alfa-2b and ribavirin
    combination pack
  lamivudine
  Rebetron® [US/Can]
  3TC® [Can]
Biological Response Modulator
  interferon alfa-2b
  interferon alfa-2b and ribavirin
    combination pack

Intron® A [US/Can]
Rebetron® [US/Can]
Immune Globulin
  BayHep B® [US/Can]
  hepatitis B immune globulin
  Nabi-HB® [US]
Vaccine, Inactivated Virus
  Comvax® [US]
  Engerix-B® [US/Can]
  Haemophilus B conjugate and
    hepatitis B vaccine
  hepatitis B vaccine
  Recombivax HB® [US/Can]

HEPATITIS C
Antiviral Agent
  interferon alfa-2b and ribavirin
    combination pack
  Rebetron® [US/Can]
Biological Response Modulator
  interferon alfa-2b
  interferon alfa-2b and ribavirin
    combination pack
  Intron® A [US/Can]
  Rebetron® [US/Can]
Interferon
  Infergen® [US/Can]
  interferon alfacon-1
  Pegasys® [US/Can]
  peginterferon alfa-2a
  peginterferon alfa-2b
  PEG-Intron™ [US/Can]

HERPES SIMPLEX
Antiviral Agent
  acyclovir
  Alti-Acyclovir [Can]
  Apo-Acyclovir® [Can]
  Cytovene® [US/Can]
  famciclovir
  Famvir® [US/Can]
  foscarnet
  Foscavir® [US/Can]

ganciclovir
Gen-Acyclovir [Can]
Nu-Acyclovir [Can]
ratio-Acyclovir [Can]
trifluridine
Viroptic® [US/Can]
Vitrasert® [US/Can]
Zovirax® [US/Can]
Antiviral Agent, Topical
Abreva® [US-OTC]
docosanol

HERPES ZOSTER

Analgesic, Topical
capsaicin
Zostrix®-HP [US-OTC/Can]
Zostrix® [US-OTC/Can]
Antiviral Agent
acyclovir
Alti-Acyclovir [Can]
Apo-Acyclovir® [Can]
famciclovir
Famvir® [US/Can]
Gen-Acyclovir [Can]
Nu-Acyclovir [Can]
ratio-Acyclovir [Can]
valacyclovir
Valtrex® [US/Can]
Zovirax® [US/Can]

HISTOPLASMOSIS

Antifungal Agent
Amphocin® [US]
amphotericin B (conventional)
Apo-Ketoconazole® [Can]
Fungizone® [US/Can]
itraconazole
ketoconazole
Ketoderm® [Can]
Nizoral® A-D [US-OTC]
Nizoral® [US/Can]
Novo-Ketoconazole [Can]
Sporanox® [US/Can]

HODGKIN DISEASE

Antineoplastic Agent
Adriamycin® [Can]
Adriamycin PFS® [US]
Adriamycin RDF® [US]
BiCNU® [US/Can]
Blenoxane® [US/Can]
bleomycin
carmustine
CeeNU® [US/Can]
chlorambucil
cisplatin
cyclophosphamide
Cytoxan® [US/Can]
dacarbazine
doxorubicin
DTIC® [Can]
DTIC-Dome® [US]
Gliadel® [US]
Idamycin® [Can]
Idamycin PFS® [US]
idarubicin
Leukeran® [US/Can]
lomustine
Matulane® [US/Can]
mechlorethamine
Mustargen® [US/Can]
Natulan® [Can]
Oncovin® [Can]
Platinol®-AQ [US]
procarbazine
Procytox® [Can]
Rubex® [US]
streptozocin
thiotepa
Velban® [Can]
vinblastine
Vincasar® PFS® [US/Can]
vincristine
Zanosar® [US/Can]

HYPERAMMONEMIA
Ammonium Detoxicant
Acilac [Can]
Apo-Lactulose® [Can]
Cholac® [US]
Constilac® [US]
Constulose® [US]
Enulose® [US]
Generlac® [US]
Kristalose™ [US]
lactulose
Laxilose [Can]
PMS-Lactulose [Can]
sodium phenylacetate and sodium benzoate
Ucephan® [US]

HYPERCALCEMIA
Bisphosphonate Derivative
Actonel® [US/Can]
alendronate
Aredia® [US/Can]
Bonefos® [Can]
clodronate disodium (Canada only)
Didronel® [US/Can]
etidronate disodium
Fosamax® [US/Can]
Gen-Etidronate [Can]
Novo-Alendronate [Can]
Ostac® [Can]
pamidronate
risedronate
zoledronic acid
Zometa® [US/Can]
Chelating Agent
edetate disodium
Endrate® [US]
Polypeptide Hormone
Calcimar® [Can]
calcitonin
Caltine® [Can]
Miacalcin® NS [Can]

Miacalcin® [US]
Urinary Tract Product
Calcibind® [US/Can]
cellulose sodium phosphate

HYPERCHOLESTEROLEMIA
Antihyperlipidemic Agent, Miscellaneous
colesevelam
Colestid® [US/Can]
colestipol
WelChol® [US/Can]
Antilipemic Agent, 2-Azetidinone
ezetimibe
ezetimibe and simvastatin
Ezetrol® [Can]
Vytorin™ [US]
Zetia™ [US]
Antilipemic Agent, HMG-CoA Reductase Inhibitor
amlodipine and atorvastatin
Caduet® [US]
Bile Acid Sequestrant
cholestyramine resin
colesevelam
Novo-Cholamine [Can]
Novo-Cholamine Light [Can]
PMS-Cholestyramine [Can]
Prevalite® [US]
Questran® Light Sugar Free [Can]
Questran® Light [US]
Questran® [US/Can]
WelChol® [US/Can]
HMG-CoA Reductase Inhibitor
Advicor™ [US]
Altoprev™ [US]
Apo-Lovastatin® [Can]
Apo-Pravastatin® [Can]
Apo-Simvastatin® [Can]
atorvastatin
fluvastatin
Gen-Lovastatin [Can]
Gen-Simvastatin [Can]

Lescol® [US/Can]
Lescol® XL [US]
Lin-Pravastatin [Can]
Lipitor® [US/Can]
lovastatin
Mevacor® [US/Can]
niacin and lovastatin
Novo-Lovastatin [Can]
Novo-Pravastatin [Can]
Nu-Lovastatin [Can]
PMS-Lovastatin [Can]
PMS-Pravastatin [Can]
Pravachol® [US/Can]
pravastatin
ratio-Lovastatin [Can]
ratio-Pravastatin [Can]
ratio-Simvastatin [Can]
Riva-Simvastatin [Can]
simvastatin
Zocor® [US/Can]
Vitamin, Water Soluble
  Advicor™ [US]
  niacin and lovastatin

HYPERKALEMIA
Antidote
  Kayexalate® [US/Can]
  Kionex™ [US]
  PMS-Sodium Polystyrene Sulfonate [Can]
  sodium polystyrene sulfonate
  SPS® [US]
Electrolyte Supplement, Oral
  Alcalak [US-OTC]
  Alka-Mints® [US-OTC]
  Amitone® [US-OTC]
  Apo-Cal® [Can]
  Brioschi® [US-OTC]
  Calcarb 600 [US-OTC]
  Calci-Chew® [US-OTC]
  Calci-Mix® [US-OTC]
  Calcite-500 [Can]
  Cal-Citrate® 250 [US-OTC]

calcium carbonate
calcium citrate
calcium glubionate
calcium lactate
calcium phosphate (tribasic)
Cal-Gest [US-OTC]
Cal-Mint [US-OTC]
Caltrate® 600 [US-OTC]
Caltrate® [Can]
Chooz® [US-OTC]
Citracal® [US-OTC]
Florical® [US-OTC]
Mylanta® Children's [US-OTC]
Nephro-Calci® [US-OTC]
Neut® [US]
Os-Cal® 500 [US-OTC]
Os-Cal® [Can]
Osteocit® [Can]
Oysco 500 [US-OTC]
Oyst-Cal 500 [US-OTC]
Posture® [US-OTC]
sodium bicarbonate
Titralac™ Extra Strength [US-OTC]
Titralac™ [US-OTC]
Tums® 500 [US-OTC]
Tums® E-X [US-OTC]
Tums® Smooth Dissolve [US-OTC]
Tums® Ultra [US-OTC]
Tums® [US-OTC]

HYPERLIPIDEMIA
Antihyperlipidemic Agent,
  Miscellaneous
  Apo-Fenofibrate® [Can]
  Apo-Feno-Micro® [Can]
  Apo-Gemfibrozil® [Can]
  bezafibrate (Canada only)
  Bezalip® [Can]
  Colestid® [US/Can]
  colestipol
  fenofibrate
  gemfibrozil
  Gen-Fenofibrat Micro [Can]

Gen-Gemfibrozil [Can]
Lipidil Micro® [Can]
Lipidil Supra® [Can]
Lofibra™ [US]
Lopid® [US/Can]
Novo-Fenofibrate [Can]
Novo-Gemfibrozil [Can]
Nu-Fenofibrate [Can]
Nu-Gemfibrozil [Can]
PMS-Bezafibrate [Can]
PMS-Fenofibrate Micro [Can]
PMS-Gemfibrozil [Can]
TriCor® [US/Can]
Antilipemic Agent, HMG-CoA
   Reductase Inhibitor
  Crestor® [US/Can]
  rosuvastatin
Bile Acid Sequestrant
  cholestyramine resin
  Novo-Cholamine [Can]
  Novo-Cholamine Light [Can]
  PMS-Cholestyramine [Can]
  Prevalite® [US]
  Questran® Light Sugar Free [Can]
  Questran® Light [US]
  Questran® [US/Can]
HMG-CoA Reductase Inhibitor
  Advicor™ [US]
  niacin and lovastatin
Vitamin, Water Soluble
  Advicor™ [US]
  niacin
  niacin and lovastatin
  Niacor® [US]
  Niaspan® [US/Can]
  Nicotinex [US-OTC]
  Slo-Niacin® [US-OTC]

HYPERMAGNESEMIA
Diuretic, Loop
  Apo-Furosemide® [Can]
  bumetanide
  Bumex® [US/Can]

Burinex® [Can]
Demadex® [US]
Edecrin® [US/Can]
ethacrynic acid
furosemide
Lasix® Special [Can]
Lasix® [US/Can]
torsemide
Electrolyte Supplement, Oral
  calcium chloride
  calcium gluconate

HYPERPARATHYROIDISM
Calcimimetic
  cinacalcet
  Sensipar™ [US]
Vitamin D Analog
  doxercalciferol
  Hectorol® [US/Can]
  paricalcitol
  Zemplar™ [US/Can]

HYPERPHOSPHATEMIA
Antacid
  ALternaGel® [US-OTC]
  Alu-Cap® [US-OTC]
  aluminum hydroxide
  Amphojel® [Can]
  Basaljel® [Can]
Electrolyte Supplement, Oral
  Alcalak [US-OTC]
  Alka-Mints® [US-OTC]
  Amitone® [US-OTC]
  Apo-Cal® [Can]
  Calcarb 600 [US-OTC]
  Calci-Chew® [US-OTC]
  Calci-Mix® [US-OTC]
  Calcite-500 [Can]
  calcium acetate
  calcium carbonate
  Cal-Gest [US-OTC]
  Cal-Mint [US-OTC]
  Caltrate® 600 [US-OTC]

Caltrate® [Can]
Chooz® [US-OTC]
Florical® [US-OTC]
Mylanta® Children's [US-OTC]
Nephro-Calci® [US-OTC]
Os-Cal® 500 [US-OTC]
Os-Cal® [Can]
Oysco 500 [US-OTC]
Oyst-Cal 500 [US-OTC]
PhosLo® [US]
Titralac™ Extra Strength [US-OTC]
Titralac™ [US-OTC]
Tums® 500 [US-OTC]
Tums® E-X [US-OTC]
Tums® Smooth Dissolve [US-OTC]
Tums® Ultra [US-OTC]
Tums® [US-OTC]
Phosphate Binder
Renagel® [US/Can]
sevelamer

HYPERPLASIA, VULVAR SQUAMOUS

Estrogen Derivative
Alora® [US]
Cenestin® [US/Can]
C.E.S.® [Can]
Climara® [US/Can]
Congest [Can]
Delestrogen® [US/Can]
Depo®-Estradiol [US/Can]
Esclim® [US]
Estrace® [US/Can]
Estraderm® [US/Can]
estradiol
Estradot® [Can]
Estrasorb™ [US]
Estratab® [Can]
Estring® [US/Can]
EstroGel® [US/Can]
estrogens (conjugated A/synthetic)
estrogens (conjugated/equine)
estrogens (esterified)

estrone
estropipate
Femring™ [US]
Gynodiol® [US]
Menest® [US/Can]
Menostar™ [US]
Oesclim® [Can]
Ogen® [US/Can]
Ortho-Est® [US]
Premarin® [US/Can]
Vagifem® [US/Can]
Vivelle-Dot® [US]
Vivelle® [US/Can]

HYPERPROLACTINEMIA

Ergot Alkaloid and Derivative
Apo-Bromocriptine® [Can]
bromocriptine
Parlodel® [US/Can]
PMS-Bromocriptine [Can]
Ergot-like Derivative
cabergoline
Dostinex® [US/Can]

HYPERTHYROIDISM

Antithyroid Agent
Iosat™ [US-OTC]
methimazole
Pima® [US]
potassium iodide
propylthiouracil
Propyl-Thyracil® [Can]
SSKI® [US]
Tapazole® [US/Can]
Beta-Adrenergic Blocker
Apo-Propranolol® [Can]
Inderal® LA [US/Can]
Inderal® [US/Can]
InnoPran XL™ [US]
Nu-Propranolol [Can]
propranolol
Propranolol Intensol™ [US]

HYPERTRIGLYCERIDEMIA

Antihyperlipidemic Agent,
  Miscellaneous
  Apo-Gemfibrozil® [Can]
  gemfibrozil
  Gen-Gemfibrozil [Can]
  Lopid® [US/Can]
  Novo-Gemfibrozil [Can]
  Nu-Gemfibrozil [Can]
  PMS-Gemfibrozil [Can]
Antilipemic Agent, 2-Azetidinone
  ezetimibe and simvastatin
  Vytorin™ [US]
HMG-CoA Reductase Inhibitor
  Apo-Simvastatin® [Can]
  Gen-Simvastatin [Can]
  ratio-Simvastatin [Can]
  Riva-Simvastatin [Can]
  simvastatin
  Zocor® [US/Can]
Vitamin, Water Soluble
  niacin
  Niacor® [US]
  Niaspan® [US/Can]
  Nicotinex [US-OTC]
  Slo-Niacin® [US-OTC]

HYPERURICEMIA

Enzyme
  Elitek™ [US]
  rasburicase
Uricosuric Agent
  Apo-Sulfinpyrazone® [Can]
  Benuryl™ [Can]
  Nu-Sulfinpyrazone [Can]
  probenecid
  sulfinpyrazone
Xanthine Oxidase Inhibitor
  allopurinol
  Aloprim™ [US]
  Apo-Allopurinol® [Can]
  Zyloprim® [US/Can]

HYPOALDOSTERONISM

Diuretic, Potassium Sparing
  amiloride
  Midamor® [Can]

HYPOCALCEMIA

Electrolyte Supplement, Oral
  Alcalak [US-OTC]
  Alka-Mints® [US-OTC]
  Amitone® [US-OTC]
  Apo-Cal® [Can]
  Calcarb 600 [US-OTC]
  Calci-Chew® [US-OTC]
  Calci-Mix® [US-OTC]
  Calcite-500 [Can]
  Cal-Citrate® 250 [US-OTC]
  calcium carbonate
  calcium chloride
  calcium citrate
  calcium glubionate
  calcium gluconate
  calcium lactate
  calcium phosphate (tribasic)
  Cal-Gest [US-OTC]
  Cal-Mint [US-OTC]
  Caltrate® 600 [US-OTC]
  Caltrate® [Can]
  Chooz® [US-OTC]
  Citracal® [US-OTC]
  Florical® [US-OTC]
  Mylanta® Children's [US-OTC]
  Nephro-Calci® [US-OTC]
  Os-Cal® 500 [US-OTC]
  Os-Cal® [Can]
  Osteocit® [Can]
  Oysco 500 [US-OTC]
  Oyst-Cal 500 [US-OTC]
  Posture® [US-OTC]
  Titralac™ Extra Strength [US-OTC]
  Titralac™ [US-OTC]
  Tums® 500 [US-OTC]
  Tums® E-X [US-OTC]
  Tums® Smooth Dissolve [US-OTC]

Tums® Ultra [US-OTC]
Tums® [US-OTC]
Vitamin D Analog
  Calciferol™ [US]
  Calcijex® [US]
  calcitriol
  DHT™ Intensol™ [US]
  DHT™ [US]
  dihydrotachysterol
  Drisdol® [US/Can]
  ergocalciferol
  Hytakerol® [US/Can]
  Ostoforte® [Can]
  Rocaltrol® [US/Can]

HYPOCHLOREMIA
Electrolyte Supplement, Oral
  ammonium chloride

HYPOCHLORHYDRIA
Gastrointestinal Agent, Miscellaneous
  glutamic acid

HYPOGLYCEMIA
Antihypoglycemic Agent
  B-D™ Glucose [US-OTC]
  Dex4 Glucose [US-OTC]
  diazoxide
  GlucaGen® Diagnostic Kit [US]
  GlucaGen® [US]
  glucagon
  Glucagon Diagnostic Kit [US]
  Glucagon Emergency Kit [US]
  glucose (instant)
  Glutol™ [US-OTC]
  Glutose™ [US-OTC]
  Hyperstat® I.V. [Can]
  Hyperstat® [US]
  Insta-Glucose® [US-OTC]
  Proglycem® [US/Can]

HYPOGONADISM
Androgen
  Andriol® [Can]
  Androderm® [US/Can]
  AndroGel® [US/Can]
  Android® [US]
  Andropository [Can]
  Delatestryl® [US/Can]
  Depotest® 100 [Can]
  Depo®-Testosterone [US]
  Everone® 200 [Can]
  Methitest® [US]
  methyltestosterone
  Striant™ [US]
  Testim™ [US]
  Testoderm® [Can]
  Testopel® [US]
  testosterone
  Testred® [US]
  Virilon® [US]
Diagnostic Agent
  Factrel® [US]
  gonadorelin
  Lutrepulse™ [Can]
Estrogen Derivative
  Alora® [US]
  Cenestin® [US/Can]
  C.E.S.® [Can]
  Climara® [US/Can]
  Congest [Can]
  Delestrogen® [US/Can]
  Depo®-Estradiol [US/Can]
  Esclim® [US]
  Estrace® [US/Can]
  Estraderm® [US/Can]
  estradiol
  Estradot® [Can]
  Estrasorb™ [US]
  Estratab® [Can]
  Estring® [US/Can]
  EstroGel® [US/Can]
  estrogens (conjugated A/synthetic)

estrogens (conjugated/equine)
estrogens (esterified)
estrone
estropipate
ethinyl estradiol
Femring™ [US]
Gynodiol®) [US]
Menest® [US/Can]
Menostar™ [US]
Oesclim® [Can]
Ogen® [US/Can]
Ortho-Est® [US]
Premarin® [US/Can]
Vagifem® [US/Can]
Vivelle-Dot® [US]
Vivelle® [US/Can]

HYPOKALEMIA
Diuretic, Potassium Sparing
  Aldactone® [US/Can]
  amiloride
  Dyrenium® [US]
  Midamor® [Can]
  Novo-Spiroton [Can]
  spironolactone
  triamterene
Electrolyte Supplement, Oral
  Apo-K® [Can]
  Effer-K™ [US]
  Glu-K® [US-OTC]
  K+8 [US]
  K+10 [US]
  Kaon-Cl®-10 [US]
  Kaon-Cl® 20 [US]
  Kaon® [US]
  Kay Ciel® [US]
  K+ Care® ET [US]
  K+ Care® [US]
  K-Dur® 10 [US]
  K-Dur® 20 [US]
  K-Dur® [Can]
  Klor-Con® 8 [US]
  Klor-Con® 10 [US]

Klor-Con®/25 [US]
Klor-Con®/EF [US]
Klor-Con® M [US]
Klor-Con® [US]
K-Lor™ [US/Can]
Klotrix® [US]
K-Lyte/Cl® 50 [US]
K-Lyte/Cl® [US]
K-Lyte® DS [US]
K-Lyte® [US/Can]
K-Phos® MF [US]
K-Phos® Neutral [US]
K-Phos® No. 2 [US]
K-Tab® [US]
Micro-K® 10 Extencaps® [US]
Micro-K® Extencaps [US-OTC/Can]
Neutra-Phos®-K [US-OTC]
Neutra-Phos® [US-OTC]
potassium acetate
potassium acetate, potassium
   bicarbonate, and potassium citrate
potassium bicarbonate
potassium bicarbonate and
   potassium chloride, effervescent
potassium bicarbonate and
   potassium citrate, effervescent
potassium chloride
potassium gluconate
potassium phosphate
potassium phosphate and sodium
   phosphate
Roychlor® [Can]
Rum-K® [US]
Slow-K® [Can]
Tri-K® [US]
Uro-KP-Neutral® [US]

HYPOMAGNESEMIA
Electrolyte Supplement, Oral
  Almora® [US-OTC]
  Chloromag® [US]
  Dulcolax® Milk of Magnesia [US-OTC]
  Mag Delay® [US-OTC]

Mag G® [US-OTC]
magnesium chloride
magnesium gluconate
magnesium hydroxide
magnesium oxide
magnesium sulfate
Magonate® Sport [US-OTC]
Magonate® [US-OTC]
Mag-Ox® 400 [US-OTC]
Mag-SR® [US-OTC]
Magtrate®) [US-OTC]
Phillips'® Milk of Magnesia [US-OTC]
Slow-Mag® [US-OTC]
Uro-Mag® [US-OTC]

HYPONATREMIA

Electrolyte Supplement, Oral
Altamist [US-OTC]
Ayr® Baby Saline [US-OTC]
Ayr® Saline Mist [US-OTC]
Ayr® Saline [US-OTC]
Breathe Right® Saline [US-OTC]
Brioschi® [US-OTC]
Broncho Saline® [US-OTC]
Entsol® [US-OTC]
Fleet® Enema [US-OTC/Can]
Fleet® Phospho®-Soda Accu-Prep™
[US-OTC]
Fleet® Phospho®-Soda Oral Laxative
[Can]
Fleet® Phospho®-Soda [US-OTC]
Muro 128® [US-OTC]
Nasal Moist® [US-OTC]
NaSal™ [US-OTC]
Na-Zone® [US-OTC]
Neut® [US]
Ocean® [US-OTC]
Pediamist® [US-OTC]
Pretz® Irrigation [US-OTC]
SalineX® [US-OTC]
SeaMist® [US-OTC]
Simply Saline™ [US-OTC]
sodium acetate

sodium bicarbonate
sodium chloride
sodium phosphates
Visicol™ [US]
Wound Wash Saline™ [US-OTC]

HYPOPARATHYROIDISM

Diagnostic Agent
Forteo™ [US]
teriparatide
Vitamin D Analog
Calciferol™ [US]
Calcijex® [US]
calcitriol
DHT™ Intensol™ [US]
DHT™ [US]
dihydrotachysterol
Drisdol® [US/Can]
ergocalciferol
Hytakerol® [US/Can]
Ostoforte® [Can]
Rocaltrol® [US/Can]

HYPOPHOSPHATEMIA

Electrolyte Supplement, Oral
K-Phos® MF [US]
K-Phos® Neutral [US]
K-Phos® No. 2 [US]
Neutra-Phos®-K [US-OTC]
Neutra-Phos® [US-OTC]
potassium phosphate
potassium phosphate and sodium
phosphate
Uro-KP-Neutral® [US]
Vitamin D Analog
Calciferol™ [US]
Calcijex® [US]
calcitriol
DHT™ Intensol™ [US]
DHT™ [US]
dihydrotachysterol
Drisdol® [US/Can]
ergocalciferol

Hytakerol® [US/Can]
Ostoforte® [Can]
Rocaltrol® [US/Can]

HYPOPROTHROMBINEMIA
Vitamin, Fat Soluble
AquaMEPHYTON® [Can]
Konakion [Can]
Mephyton® [US/Can]
phytonadione

HYPOTHYROIDISM
Thyroid Product
Armour® Thyroid [US]
Cytomel® [US/Can]
Eltroxin® [Can]
Levothroid® [US]
levothyroxine
Levoxyl® [US]
liothyronine
liotrix
Nature-Throid® NT [US]
Novothyrox [US]
Synthroid® [US/Can]
thyroid
Thyrolar® [US/Can]
Triostat® [US]
Unithroid® [US]
Westhroid® [US]

IDIOPATHIC THROMBOCYTOPENIA PURPURA
Immune Globulin
BayGam® [US/Can]
Carimune™ [US]
Flebogamma® [US]
Gamimune® N [US/Can]
Gammagard® S/D [US/Can]
Gammar®-P I.V. [US]
Gamunex® [US/Can]
immune globulin (intramuscular)
immune globulin (intravenous)

Iveegam EN [US]
Iveegam Immuno® [Can]
Octagam® [US]
Panglobulin® [US]
Polygam® S/D [US]
Venoglobulin®-S [US]

IMMUNODEFICIENCY
Enzyme
Adagen™ [US/Can]
pegademase (bovine)
Immune Globulin
Carimune™ [US]
Flebogamma® [US]
Gamimune® N [US/Can]
Gammagard® S/D [US/Can]
Gammar®-P I.V. [US]
Gamunex® [US/Can]
immune globulin (intravenous)
Iveegam EN [US]
Iveegam Immuno® [Can]
Octagam® [US]
Panglobulin® [US]
Polygam® S/D [US]
Venoglobulin®-S [US]

IRON DEFICIENCY ANEMIA
Iron Salt
ferric gluconate
Ferrlecit® [US]

ISCHEMIA
Blood Viscosity Reducer Agent
Albert® Pentoxifylline [Can]
Apo-Pentoxifylline SR® [Can]
Nu-Pentoxifylline SR [Can]
pentoxifylline
Pentoxil® [US]
ratio-Pentoxifylline [Can]
Trental® [US/Can]
Platelet Aggregation Inhibitor
abciximab

ReoPro® [US/Can]
Vasodilator
  ethaverine
  papaverine
  Para-Time S.R.® [US]

KAPOSI SARCOMA
Antineoplastic Agent
  Caelyx® [Can]
  daunorubicin citrate (liposomal)
  DaunoXome® [US]
  Doxil® [US]
  doxorubicin (liposomal)
  Onxol™ [US]
  paclitaxel
  Taxol® [US/Can]
  Velban® [Can]
  vinblastine
Antineoplastic Agent, Miscellaneous
  alitretinoin
  Panretin® [US/Can]
Biological Response Modulator
  interferon alfa-2a
  interferon alfa-2b
  Intron® A [US/Can]
  Roferon-A® [US/Can]
Retinoic Acid Derivative
  alitretinoin
  Panretin® [US/Can]

LEUKAPHERESIS
Blood Modifiers
  Pentaspan® [US/Can]
  pentastarch

LEUKEMIA
Antineoplastic Agent
  Adriamycin® [Can]
  Adriamycin PFS® [US]
  Adriamycin RDF® [US]
  Apo-Methotrexate® [Can]
  asparaginase
  busulfan

Busulfex® [US/Can]
Cerubidine® [US/Can]
chlorambucil
cladribine
cyclophosphamide
cytarabine
Cytosar® [Can]
Cytosar-U® [US]
Cytoxan® [US/Can]
daunorubicin hydrochloride
doxorubicin
Droxia™ [US]
Elspar® [US/Can]
etoposide
fludarabine
Fludara® [US/Can]
Gen-Hydroxyurea [Can]
Hydrea® [US/Can]
hydroxyurea
Ifex® [US/Can]
ifosfamide
Kidrolase® [Can]
Lanvis® [Can]
Leukeran® [US/Can]
Leustatin™ [US/Can]
mechlorethamine
mercaptopurine
methotrexate
mitoxantrone
Mustargen® [US/Can]
Myleran® [US/Can]
Mylocel™ [US]
Nipent® [US/Can]
Novantrone® [US/Can]
Oncaspar® [US]
Oncovin® [Can]
pegaspargase
pentostatin
Procytox® [Can]
Purinethol® [US/Can]
ratio-Methotrexate [Can]
Rheumatrex® [US]
Rubex® [US]

teniposide
thioguanine
Toposar® [US]
tretinoin (oral)
Trexall™ [US]
VePesid® [US/Can]
Vesanoid® [US/Can]
Vincasar® PFS® [US/Can]
vincristine
Vumon® [US/Can]
Antineoplastic Agent, Miscellaneous
  arsenic trioxide
  Trisenox™ [US]
Antineoplastic Agent, Monoclonal
  Antibody
  alemtuzumab
  Campath® [US]
Antineoplastic Agent, Natural Source
  (Plant) Derivative
  gemtuzumab ozogamicin
  Mylotarg® [US/Can]
Antineoplastic, Tyrosine Kinase
  Inhibitor
  Gleevec® [US/Can]
  imatinib
Antiviral Agent
  interferon alfa-2b and ribavirin
    combination pack
  Rebetron® [US/Can]
Biological Response Modulator
  interferon alfa-2a
  interferon alfa-2b
  interferon alfa-2b and ribavirin
    combination pack
  Intron® A [US/Can]
  Rebetron® [US/Can]
  Roferon-A® [US/Can]
Immune Globulin
  Carimune™ [US]
  Flebogamma® [US]
  Gamimune® N [US/Can]
  Gammagard® S/D [US/Can]
  Gammar®-P I.V. [US]

  Gamunex® [US/Can]
  immune globulin (intravenous)
  Iveegam EN [US]
  Iveegam Immuno® [Can]
  Octagam® [US]
  Panglobulin® [US]
  Polygam® S/D [US]
  Venoglobulin®-S [US]

LYMPHOMA

Antineoplastic Agent
  Adriamycin® [Can]
  Adriamycin PFS® [US]
  Adriamycin RDF® [US]
  Apo-Methotrexate® [Can]
  asparaginase
  BiCNU® [US/Can]
  Blenoxane® [US/Can]
  bleomycin
  carmustine
  CeeNU® [US/Can]
  chlorambucil
  cisplatin
  cyclophosphamide
  cytarabine
  Cytosar® [Can]
  Cytosar-U® [US]
  Cytoxan® [US/Can]
  doxorubicin
  Elspar® [US/Can]
  etoposide
  Gliadel® [US]
  Idamycin® [Can]
  Idamycin PFS® [US]
  idarubicin
  Ifex® [US/Can]
  ifosfamide
  Kidrolase® [Can]
  Leukeran® [US/Can]
  lomustine
  Matulane® [US/Can]
  mechlorethamine
  methotrexate

mitoxantrone
Mustargen® [US/Can]
Natulan® [Can]
Novantrone® [US/Can]
Oncaspar® [US]
Oncovin® [Can]
pegaspargase
Platinol®-AQ [US]
procarbazine
Procytox® [Can]
ratio-Methotrexate [Can]
Rheumatrex® [US]
Rituxan® [US/Can]
rituximab
Rubex® [US]
teniposide
thiotepa
Toposar® [US]
Trexall™ [US]
Velban® [Can]
VePesid® [US/Can]
vinblastine
Vincasar® PFS® [US/Can]
vincristine
Vumon® [US/Can]
Antineoplastic Agent, Monoclonal
    Antibody
  Bexxar® [US]
  ibritumomab
  tositumomab and iodine I 131
    tositumomab
  Zevalin™ [US]
Antiviral Agent
  interferon alfa-2b and ribavirin
    combination pack
  Rebetron® [US/Can]
Biological Response Modulator
  interferon alfa-2a
  interferon alfa-2b
  interferon alfa-2b and ribavirin
    combination pack
  Intron® A [US/Can]
  Rebetron® [US/Can]

Roferon-A® [US/Can]
Colony-Stimulating Factor
  Leukine™ [US/Can]
  sargramostim
Radiopharmaceutical
  Bexxar® [US]
  ibritumomab
  tositumomab and iodine I 131
    tositumomab
  Zevalin™ [US]
Retinoic Acid Derivative
  bexarotene
  Targretin® [US/Can]
Vitamin A Derivative
  bexarotene
  Targretin® [US/Can]
Vitamin, Fat Soluble
  bexarotene
  Targretin® [US/Can]

LYMPHOMATOUS MENINGITIS

Antineoplastic Agent, Antimetabolite
    (Purine)
  cytarabine (liposomal)
  DepoCyt™ [US/Can]

MALARIA

Aminoquinoline (Antimalarial)
  Apo-Hydroxyquine® [Can]
  Aralen® [US/Can]
  chloroquine phosphate
  hydroxychloroquine
  Plaquenil® [US/Can]
  primaquine
Antimalarial Agent
  Apo-Mefloquine® [Can]
  atovaquone and proguanil
  Fansidar® [US]
  Lariam® [US/Can]
  Malarone™ [US/Can]
  mefloquine
  quinine

Quinine-Odan™ [Can]
sulfadoxine and pyrimethamine
Folic Acid Antagonist (Antimalarial)
Daraprim® [US/Can]
pyrimethamine
Sulfonamide
sulfadiazine
Tetracycline Derivative
Adoxa™ [US]
Apo-Doxy® [Can]
Apo-Doxy Tabs® [Can]
Doryx® [US]
Doxy-100® [US]
Doxycin [Can]
doxycycline
Doxytec [Can]
Monodox® [US]
Novo-Doxylin [Can]
Nu-Doxycycline [Can]
Periostat® [US]
Vibramycin® [US]
Vibra-Tabs® [US/Can]

MALIGNANT EFFUSION

Antineoplastic Agent
thiotepa

MALIGNANT PLEURAL MESOTHELIOMA

Antineoplastic Agent, Antimetabolite
Alimta® [US]
pemetrexed
Antineoplastic Agent, Antimetabolite
(Antifolate)
Alimta® [US]
pemetrexed

MALNUTRITION

Electrolyte Supplement, Oral
Anuzinc [Can]
Orazinc® [US-OTC]
Rivasol [Can]
Zincate® [US]
zinc sulfate

Nutritional Supplement
cysteine
glucose polymers
Moducal® [US-OTC]
Polycose® [US-OTC]
Trace Element
Iodopen® [US]
Molypen® [US]
M.T.E.-4® [US]
M.T.E.-5® [US]
M.T.E.-6® [US]
M.T.E.-7® [US]
Multitrace™-4 Neonatal [US]
Multitrace™-4 Pediatric [US]
Multitrace™-4 [US]
Multitrace™-5 [US]
Neotrace-4® [US]
Pedtrace-4® [US]
P.T.E.-4® [US]
P.T.E.-5® [US]
Selepen® [US]
trace metals
zinc chloride
Vitamin
ADEKs [US-OTC]
Advanced NatalCare® [US]
A-Free Prenatal [US]
Aminate Fe-90 [US]
Anemagen™ OB [US]
Cal-Nate™ [US]
CareNate™ 600 [US]
Centrum® Kids Rugrats™ Complete
[US-OTC]
Centrum® Kids Rugrats™ Extra
Calcium [US-OTC]
Centrum® Kids Rugrats™ Extra C
[US-OTC]
Centrum® Performance™ [US-OTC]
Centrum® Silver® [US-OTC]
Centrum® [US-OTC]
Chromagen® OB [US]
Citracal® Prenatal Rx [US]
Duet® DHA [US]

Duet® [US]
Flintstones® Complete [US-OTC]
Flintstones® Original [US-OTC]
Flintstones® Plus Calcium [US-OTC]
Flintstones® Plus Extra C [US-OTC]
Flintstones® Plus Iron [US-OTC]
Folbee [US]
Folgard RX 2.2® [US]
Folgard® [US-OTC]
folic acid, cyanocobalamin, and
  pyridoxine
Foltx® [US]
Geritol® Tonic [US-OTC]
Iberet®-500 [US-OTC]
Iberet-Folic-500® [US]
Iberet® [US-OTC]
Infuvite® Adult [US]
Infuvite® Pediatric [US]
KPN Prenatal [US]
M.V.I.®-12 [US]
M.V.I.-Adult® [US]
M.V.I.-Pediatric® [US]
My First Flintstones® [US-OTC]
NataChew™ [US]
NataFort® [US]
NatalCare® CFe 60 [US]
NatalCare® GlossTabs™ [US]
NatalCare® PIC Forte [US]
NatalCare® PIC [US]
NatalCare® Plus [US]
NatalCare® Rx [US]
NatalCare® Three [US]
NataTab™ CFe [US]
NataTab™ FA [US]
NataTab™ Rx [US]
Nestabs® CBF [US]
Nestabs® FA [US]
Nestabs® RX [US]
Niferex®-PN Forte [US]
Niferex®-PN [US]
NutriNate® [US]
OB-20 [US]
Obegyn™ [US]

One-A-Day® 50 Plus Formula [US-
  OTC]
One-A-Day® Active Formula [US-
  OTC]
One-A -Day® Essential Formula
  [US-OTC]
One-A-Day® Kids Bugs Bunny and
  Friends Complete [US-OTC]
One-A-Day® Kids Bugs Bunny and
  Friends Plus Extra C [US-OTC]
One-A-Day® Kids Extreme Sports
  [US-OTC]
One-A-Day® Kids Scooby-Doo!
  Complete [US-OTC]
One-A-Day® Kids Scooby Doo! Plus
  Calcium [US-OTC]
One-A-Day® Maximum Formula
  [US-OTC]
One-A-Day® Men's Formula [US-
  OTC]
One-A-Day® Today [US-OTC]
One-A-Day® Women's Formula
  [US-OTC]
Poly-Vi-Flor® [US]
Poly-Vi-Flor® With Iron [US]
Poly-Vi-Sol® [US-OTC]
Poly-Vi-Sol® with Iron [US-OTC]
PreCare®[US]
Prenatal 1-A-Day [US]
Prenatal AD [US]
Prenatal H [US]
Prenatal MR 90 Fe™ [US]
Prenatal MTR with Selenium [US]
Prenatal Plus [US]
Prenatal Rx 1 [US]
Prenatal U [US]
Prenatal Z [US]
Prenate Elite™ [US]
Prenate GT™ [US]
Soluvite-F [US]
StrongStart™ [US]
Stuartnatal® Plus 3™ [US-OTC]
Stuart Prenatal® [US-OTC]

Theragran® Heart Right™ [US-OTC]
Theragran-M® Advanced Formula
 [US-OTC]
Tricardio B [Can]
Trinate [US]
Tri-Vi-Flor® [US]
Tri-Vi-Flor® with Iron [US]
Tri-Vi-Sol® [US-OTC]
Tri-Vi-Sol® with Iron [US-OTC]
Ultra NatalCare® [US]
Vicon Forte® [US]
Vicon Plus® [US-OTC]
Vi-Daylin® ADC + Iron [US-OTC]
Vi-Daylin® ADC [US-OTC]
Vi-Daylin® Drops [US-OTC]
Vi-Daylin®/F ADC + Iron [US]
Vi-Daylin®/F ADC [US]
Vi-Daylin®/F + Iron [US]
Vi-Daylin®/F [US]
Vi-Daylin® + Iron Drops [US-OTC]
Vi-Daylin® + Iron Liquid [US-OTC]
Vi-Daylin® Liquid [US-OTC]
Vitaball® [US-OTC]
Vitacon Forte [US]
vitamins (multiple/injectable)
vitamins (multiple/oral)
vitamins (multiple/pediatric)
vitamins (multiple/prenatal)
Vitamin, Fat Soluble
 Aqua Gem E® [US-OTC]
 Aquasol A® [US]
 Aquasol E® [US-OTC]
 E-Gems® [US-OTC]
 Key-E® Kaps [US-OTC]
 Key-E® [US-OTC]
 Palmitate-A® [US-OTC]
 vitamin A
 vitamin E
Vitamin, Water Soluble
 Allbee® C-800 + Iron [US-OTC]
 Allbee® C-800 [US-OTC]
 Allbee® with C [US-OTC]
 Aminoxin® [US-OTC]

Apatate® [US-OTC]
Betaxin® [Can]
DiatxFe™ [US]
Diatx™ [US]
Gevrabon® [US-OTC]
NephPlex® Rx [US]
Nephrocaps® [US]
Nephron FA® [US]
Nephro-Vite® Rx [US]
Nephro-Vite® [US]
pyridoxine
Stresstabs® B-Complex + Iron [US-
 OTC]
Stresstabs® B-Complex [US-OTC]
Stresstabs® B-Complex + Zinc [US-
 OTC]
Surbex-T® [US-OTC]
Thiamilate® [US-OTC]
thiamine
Trinsicon® [US]
vitamin B complex combinations
Z-Bec® [US-OTC]

MASTOCYTOSIS
Histamine H2 Antagonist
 Alti-Ranitidine [Can]
 Apo-Cimetidine® [Can]
 Apo-Famotidine® [Can]
 Apo-Ranitidine® [Can]
 cimetidine
 famotidine
 Gen-Cimetidine [Can]
 Gen-Famotidine [Can]
 Gen-Ranitidine [Can]
 Novo-Cimetidine [Can]
 Novo-Famotidine [Can]
 Novo-Ranidine [Can]
 Nu-Cimet [Can]
 Nu-Famotidine [Can]
 Nu-Ranit [Can]
 Pepcid® AC [US-OTC/Can]
 Pepcid® I.V. [Can]
 Pepcid® [US/Can]

PMS-Cimetidine [Can]
PMS-Ranitidine [Can]
ranitidine hydrochloride
ratio-Famotidine [Can]
Rhoxal-famotidine [Can]
Rhoxal-ranitidine [Can]
Riva-Famotidine [Can]
Tagamet® HB 200 [US-OTC/Can]
Tagamet® [US]
Zantac® 75 [US-OTC/Can]
Zantac® [US/Can]
Mast Cell Stabilizer
cromolyn sodium
Gastrocrom® [US]

MELANOMA

Antineoplastic Agent
Blenoxane® [US/Can]
bleomycin
CeeNU® [US/Can]
cisplatin
Cosmegen® [US/Can]
dacarbazine
dactinomycin
Droxia™ [US]
DTIC® [Can]
DTIC-Dome® [US]
Gen-Hydroxyurea [Can]
Hydrea® [US/Can]
hydroxyurea
lomustine
Mylocel™ [US]
Platinol®-AQ [US]
teniposide
Vumon® [US/Can]
Antiviral Agent
interferon alfa-2b and ribavirin
combination pack
Rebetron® [US/Can]
Biological Response Modulator
interferon alfa-2a
interferon alfa-2b

interferon alfa-2b and ribavirin
combination pack
Intron® A [US/Can]
Rebetron® [US/Can]
Roferon-A® [US/Can]

METHEMOGLOBIN

Antidote
methylene blue
Vitamin, Water Soluble
ascorbic acid
C-500-GR™ [US-OTC]
Cecon® [US-OTC]
Cevi-Bid® [US-OTC]
C-Gram [US-OTC]
Dull-C® [US-OTC]
Proflavanol C™ [Can]
Revitalose C-1000® [Can]
riboflavin
Vita-C® [US-OTC]

MOUTH INFECTION

Antibacterial, Topical
dequalinium (Canada only)
Antifungal Agent, Topical
dequalinium (Canada only)

MOUTH PAIN

Pharmaceutical Aid
Cepastat® Extra Strength [US-OTC]
Cepastat® [US-OTC]
Chloraseptic®Gargle [US-OTC]
Chloraseptic® Mouth Pain Spray
[US-OTC]
Chloraseptic® Rinse [US-OTC]
Chloraseptic® Spray for Kids [US-
OTC]
Chloraseptic® Spray [US-OTC]
Pain-A-Lay® [US-OTC]
phenol

MYCOBACTERIUM AVIUM-INTRACELLULARE
Antibiotic, Aminoglycoside
  streptomycin
Antibiotic, Miscellaneous
  Mycobutin® [US/Can]
  rifabutin
  Rifadin® [US/Can]
  rifampin
  Rimactane® [US]
  Rofact™ [Can]
Antimycobacterial Agent
  ethambutol
  Etibi® [Can]
  Myambutol® [US]
Antitubercular Agent
  streptomycin
Carbapenem (Antibiotic)
  imipenem and cilastatin
  meropenem
  Merrem® I.V. [US/Can]
  Primaxin® [US/Can]
Leprostatic Agent
  clofazimine
  Lamprene® [US/Can]
Macrolide (Antibiotic)
  azithromycin
  Biaxin® [US/Can]
  Biaxin® XL [US/Can]
  clarithromycin
  ratio-Clarithromycin [Can]
  Zithromax® [US/Can]
Quinolone
  ciprofloxacin
  Cipro® [US/Can]
  Cipro® XL [Can]
  Cipro® XR [US]

MYCOSIS (FUNGOIDES)
Psoralen
  methoxsalen
  8-MOP® [US/Can]
  Oxsoralen-Ultra® [US/Can]
  Oxsoralen® [US/Can]
  Ultramop™ [Can]
  Uvadex® [US/Can]

MYELODYSPLASTIC SYNDROME (MDS)
Antineoplastic Agent, Antimetabolite
  (Pyrimidine)
  azacitidine
  Vidaza™ [US]

MYELOMA
Antineoplastic Agent
  Adriamycin® [Can]
  Adriamycin PFS® [US]
  Adriamycin RDF® [US]
  Alkeran® [US/Can]
  BiCNU® [US/Can]
  carmustine
  cisplatin
  cyclophosphamide
  Cytoxan® [US/Can]
  doxorubicin
  Gliadel® [US]
  melphalan
  Platinol®-AQ [US]
  Procytox® [Can]
  Rubex® [US]
  teniposide
  Vumon® [US/Can]
Proteasome Inhibitor
  bortezomib
  Velcade™ [US]

NEOPLASTIC DISEASE (TREATMENT ADJUNCT)

Adrenal Corticosteroid
A-HydroCort® [US]
A-methapred® [US]
Apo-Prednisone® [Can]
Aristocort® Forte Injection [US]
Aristocort® Intralesional Injection [US]
Aristocort® Tablet [US/Can]
Aristospan® Intraarticular Injection [US/Can]
Aristospan® Intralesional Injection [US/Can]
betamethasone (systemic)
Celestone® Soluspan® [US/Can]
Celestone® [US]
Cortef® Tablet [US/Can]
corticotropin
cortisone acetate
Cortone® [Can]
Decadron® [US/Can]
Deltasone® [US]
Depo-Medrol® [US/Can]
Dexamethasone Intensol® [US]
dexamethasone (systemic)
DexPak® TaperPak® [US]
Diodex® [Can]
H.P. Acthar® Gel [US]
hydrocortisone (systemic)
Hydrocortone® Phosphate [US]
Kenalog® Injection [US/Can]
Medrol® [US/Can]
methylprednisolone
Orapred™ [US]
Pediapred® [US/Can]
PMS-Dexamethasone [Can]
Prednicot® [US]
prednisolone (systemic)
Prednisol® TBA [US]
prednisone
Prednisone Intensol™ [US]
Prelone® [US]

Solu-Cortef® [US/Can]
Solu-Medrol® [US/Can]
Sterapred® DS [US]
Sterapred® [US]
triamcinolone (systemic)
Winpred™ [Can]

NEPHROTOXICITY (CISPLATIN-INDUCED)

Antidote
amifostine
Ethyol® [US/Can]

NEURALGIA

Analgesic, Topical
Antiphlogistine Rub A-535 Capsaicin [Can]
Antiphlogistine Rub A-535 No Odour [Can]
ArthriCare® for Women Extra Moisturizing [US-OTC]
ArthriCare® for Women Multi-Action [US-OTC]
ArthriCare® for Women Silky Dry [US-OTC]
ArthriCare® for Women Ultra Strength [US-OTC]
Capsagel® [US-OTC]
capsaicin
Capzasin-HP® [US-OTC]
Mobisyl® [US-OTC]
Myoflex® [US-OTC/Can]
Sportscreme® [US-OTC]
triethanolamine salicylate
Zostrix®-HP [US-OTC/Can]
Zostrix® [US-OTC/Can]
Nonsteroidal Antiinflammatory Drug (NSAID)
Asaphen [Can]
Asaphen E.C. [Can]
Ascriptin® Extra Strength [US-OTC]
Ascriptin® [US-OTC]
Aspercin Extra [US-OTC]

Aspercin [US-OTC]
aspirin
Bayer® Aspirin Extra Strength [US-OTC]
Bayer® Aspirin Regimen Adult Low Strength [US-OTC]
Bayer® Aspirin Regimen Children's [US-OTC]
Bayer® Aspirin Regimen Regular Strength [US-OTC]
Bayer® Aspirin [US-OTC]
Bayer® Extra Strength Arthritis Pain Regimen [US-OTC]
Bayer® Plus Extra Strength [US-OTC]
Bayer® Women's Aspirin Plus Calcium [US-OTC]
Bufferin® Extra Strength [US-OTC]
Bufferin® [US-OTC]
Buffinol Extra [US-OTC]
Buffinol [US-OTC]
Easprin® [US]
Ecotrin® Low Strength [US-OTC]
Ecotrin® Maximum Strength [US-OTC]
Ecotrin® [US-OTC]
Entrophen® [Can]
Halfprin® [US-OTC]
Novasen [Can]
St Joseph® Adult Aspirin [US-OTC]
Sureprin 81™ [US-OTC]
ZORprin® [US]

NEUROBLASTOMA

Antineoplastic Agent
Adriamycin® [Can]
Adriamycin PFS® [US]
Adriamycin RDF® [US]
Alkeran® [US/Can]
Cosmegen® [US/Can]
cyclophosphamide
Cytoxan® [US/Can]
dacarbazine
dactinomycin
doxorubicin

DTIC® [Can]
DTIC-Dome® [US]
melphalan
Oncovin® [Can]
Procytox® [Can]
Rubex® [US]
teniposide
Vincasar® PFS® [US/Can]
vincristine
Vumon® [US/Can]

NEUTROPENIA

Colony-Stimulating Factor
filgrastim
Neupogen® [US/Can]

ORAL LESION

Local Anesthetic
benzocaine, gelatin, pectin, and sodium carboxymethylcellulose

OSTEOSARCOMA

Antineoplastic Agent
Adriamycin® [Can]
Adriamycin PFS® [US]
Adriamycin RDF® [US]
Apo-Methotrexate® [Can]
cisplatin
doxorubicin
methotrexate
Platinol®-AQ [US]
ratio-Methotrexate [Can]
Rheumatrex® [US]
Rubex® [US]
Trexall™ [US]

OSTOMY CARE

Protectant, Topical
A and D® Ointment [US-OTC]
Baza® Clear [US-OTC]
Clocream® [US-OTC]
Sween Cream® [US-OTC]
vitamin A and vitamin D

PAIN

Analgesic, Miscellaneous
acetaminophen and tramadol
Ultracet™ [US]
Analgesic, Narcotic
acetaminophen and codeine
Actiq® [US/Can]
alfentanil
Alfenta® [US/Can]
Anexsia® [US]
Apo-Butorphanol® [Can]
aspirin and codeine
Astramorph/PF™ [US]
Avinza™ [US]
Bancap HC® [US]
belladonna and opium
B&O Supprettes® [US]
Buprenex® [US/Can]
buprenorphine
butalbital, aspirin, caffeine, and
codeine
butorphanol
Capital® and Codeine [US]
Ceta-Plus® [US]
codeine
Codeine Contin® [Can]
Co-Gesic® [US]
Coryphen® Codeine [Can]
Damason-P® [US]
Darvocet A500™ [US]
Darvocet-N® 50 [US/Can]
Darvocet-N® 100 [US/Can]
Darvon-N® [US/Can]
Darvon® [US]
Demerol® [US/Can]
DepoDur™ [US]
dihydrocodeine, aspirin, and caffeine
Dilaudid-HP-Plus® [Can]
Dilaudid-HP® [US/Can]
Dilaudid® Sterile Powder [Can]
Dilaudid® [US/Can]
Dilaudid-XP® [Can]

Dolophine® [US/Can]
Duragesic® [US/Can]
Duramorph® [US]
Endocet® [US/Can]
Endodan® [US/Can]
fentanyl
Fiorinal®-C 1/2 [Can]
Fiorinal®-C 1/4 [Can]
Fiorinal® With Codeine [US]
hycet™ [US]
hydrocodone and acetaminophen
hydrocodone and aspirin
hydrocodone and ibuprofen
Hydromorph Contin® [Can]
hydromorphone
Hydromorphone HP [Can]
Infumorph® [US]
Kadian® [US/Can]
Levo-Dromoran® [US]
levorphanol
Lorcet® 10/650 [US]
Lorcet®-HD [US]
Lorcet® Plus [US]
Lortab® [US]
Margesic® H [US]
Maxidone™ [US]
meperidine
meperidine and promethazine
Meperitab® [US]
M-Eslon® [Can]
Metadol™ [Can]
methadone
Methadone Intensol™[US]
Methadose® [US/Can]
Morphine HP® [Can]
Morphine LP® Epidural [Can]
morphine sulfate
M.O.S.-Sulfate® [Can]
MS Contin® [US/Can]
MSIR® [US/Can]
nalbuphine
Norco® [US]
Nubain® [US/Can]

Numorphan® [US/Can]
opium tincture
Oramorph SR® [US]
Oxycocet® [Can]
Oxycodan® [Can]
oxycodone
oxycodone and acetaminophen
oxycodone and aspirin
OxyContin® [US/Can]
Oxydose™ [US]
OxyFast® [US]
OxyIR® [US/Can]
oxymorphone
paregoric
pentazocine
pentazocine and acetaminophen
Percocet®-Demi [Can]
Percocet® [US/Can]
Percodan® [US/Can]
Phrenilin® With Caffeine and
  Codeine [US]
PMS-Butorphanol [Can]
PMS-Hydromorphone [Can]
PMS-Morphine Sulfate SR [Can]
PMS-Oxycodone-Acetaminophen
  [Can]
Pronap-100® [US]
propoxyphene
propoxyphene and acetaminophen
propoxyphene and aspirin
ratio-Emtec [Can]
ratio-Lenoltec [Can]
ratio-Morphine SR [Can]
remifentanil
RMS® [US]
Roxanol 100® [US]
Roxanol®-T [US]
Roxanol® [US]
Roxicet® 5/500 [US]
Roxicet™ [US]
Roxicodone™ Intensol™ [US]
Roxicodone™ [US]
Stadol NS™ [Can]

Stadol® [US]
Stagesic® [US]
Statex® [Can]
Sublimaze® [US]
Subutex® [US]
sufentanil
Sufenta® [US/Can]
Supeudol® [Can]
Synalgos®-DC [US]
642® Tablet [Can]
Talwin® NX [US]
Talwin® [US/Can]
Tecnal C 1/2 [Can]
Tecnal C 1/4 [Can]
Triatec-8 [Can]
Triatec-8-Strong [Can]
Triatec-30 [Can]
Tylenol® Elixir with Codeine [Can]
Tylenol® No. 1 [Can]
Tylenol® No. 1 Forte [Can]
Tylenol® No. 2 with Codeine [Can]
Tylenol® No. 3 with Codeine [Can]
Tylenol® No. 4 with Codeine [Can]
Tylenol® with Codeine [US/Can]
Tylox® [US]
Ultiva™ [US/Can]
Vicodin® ES [US]
Vicodin® HP [US]
Vicodin® [US]
Vicoprofen® [US/Can]
Zydone® [US]
Analgesic, Nonnarcotic
  Abenol® [Can]
  Acephen® [US-OTC]
  acetaminophen
  acetaminophen and
    diphenhydramine
  acetaminophen and
    phenyltoloxamine
  acetaminophen and tramadol
  acetaminophen, aspirin, and caffeine
  Acular LS™ [US]
  Acular® P.F. [US]

Acular® [US/Can]
Advil® Children's [US-OTC]
Advil® Infants' [US-OTC]
Advil® Junior [US-OTC]
Advil® Migraine [US-OTC]
Advil® [US-OTC/Can]
Aleve® [US-OTC]
Alti-Flurbiprofen [Can]
Amigesic® [US/Can]
Anaprox® DS [US/Can]
Anaprox® [US/Can]
Ansaid® [US/Can]
Apo-Acetaminophen® [Can]
Apo-Diclo® [Can]
Apo-Diclo Rapide® [Can]
Apo-Diclo SR® [Can]
Apo-Diflunisal® [Can]
Apo-Etodolac® [Can]
Apo-Flurbiprofen® [Can]
Apo-Ibuprofen® [Can]
Apo-Indomethacin® [Can]
Apo-Keto® [Can]
Apo-Keto-E® [Can]
Apo-Ketorolac® [Can]
Apo-Ketorolac Injectable® [Can]
Apo-Keto SR® [Can]
Apo-Mefenamic® [Can]
Apo-Nabumetone® [Can]
Apo-Napro-Na® [Can]
Apo-Napro-Na DS® [Can]
Apo-Naproxen® [Can]
Apo-Naproxen SR® [Can]
Apo-Oxaprozin® [Can]
Apo-Piroxicam® [Can]
Apo-Sulin® [Can]
Asaphen [Can]
Asaphen E.C. [Can]
Ascriptin® Extra Strength [US-OTC]
Ascriptin® [US-OTC]
Aspercin Extra [US-OTC]
Aspercin [US-OTC]
Aspergum® [US-OTC]
aspirin

Aspirin Free Anacin® Maximum
    Strength [US-OTC]
Atasol® [Can]
Bayer® Aspirin Extra Strength [US-
    OTC]
Bayer® Aspirin Regimen Adult Low
    Strength [US-OTC]
Bayer® Aspirin Regimen Children's
    [US-OTC]
Bayer® Aspirin Regimen Regular
    Strength [US-OTC]
Bayer® Aspirin [US-OTC]
Bayer® Extra Strength Arthritis Pain
    Regimen [US-OTC]
Bayer® Plus Extra Strength [US-OTC]
Bayer® Women's Aspirin Plus
    Calcium [US-OTC]
Bufferin® Extra Strength [US-OTC]
Bufferin® [US-OTC]
Buffinol Extra [US-OTC]
Buffinol [US-OTC]
Cataflam® [US/Can]
Cetafen Extra® [US-OTC]
Cetafen® [US-OTC]
choline magnesium trisalicylate
Clinoril® [US]
Comtrex® Sore Throat Maximum
    Strength [US-OTC]
Daypro® [US/Can]
diclofenac
Diclotec [Can]
diflunisal
Dolobid® [US]
Easprin® [US]
EC-Naprosyn® [US]
Ecotrin® Low Strength [US-OTC]
Ecotrin® Maximum Strength [US-OTC]
Ecotrin® [US-OTC]
ElixSure™ Fever/Pain [US-OTC]
Entrophen® [Can]
etodolac
Excedrin® Extra Strength [US-OTC]
Excedrin® Migraine [US-OTC]

Excedrin® P.M. [US-OTC]
Feldene® [US/Can]
Fem-Prin® [US-OTC]
fenoprofen
FeverALL® [US-OTC]
flurbiprofen
Froben® [Can]
Froben-SR® [Can]
Genaced™ [US-OTC]
Genapap® Children [US-OTC]
Genapap® Extra Strength [US-OTC]
Genapap® Infant [US-OTC]
Genapap® [US-OTC]
Genebs® Extra Strength [US-OTC]
Genebs® [US-OTC]
Genesec® [US-OTC]
Gen-Nabumetone [Can]
Gen-Naproxen EC [Can]
Gen-Piroxicam [Can]
Genpril® [US-OTC]
Goody's® Extra Strength Headache
   Powder [US-OTC]
Goody's® Extra Strength Pain Relief
   [US-OTC]
Goody's PM® Powder [US]
Halfprin® [US-OTC]
Ibu-200 [US-OTC]
ibuprofen
Indocid® [Can]
Indocid® P.D.A. [Can]
Indocin® I.V. [US]
Indocin® SR [US]
Indocin® [US/Can]
Indo-Lemmon [Can]
indomethacin
Indotec [Can]
I-Prin [US-OTC]
ketoprofen
ketorolac
Legatrin PM® [US-OTC]
Lodine® [US/Can]
Lodine® XL [US]
Mapap® Arthritis [US-OTC]

Mapap® Children's [US-OTC]
Mapap® Extra Strength [US-OTC]
Mapap® Infants [US-OTC]
Mapap® [US-OTC]
meclofenamate
Meclomen® [Can]
mefenamic acid
Menadol® [US-OTC]
Midol® Maximum Strength Cramp
   Formula [US-OTC]
Mono-Gesic® [US]
Motrin® Children's [US-OTC/Can]
Motrin® IB [US-OTC/Can]
Motrin® Infants' [US-OTC]
Motrin® Junior Strength [US-OTC]
Motrin® Migraine Pain [US-OTC]
Motrin® [US/Can]
nabumetone
Nalfon® [US/Can]
Naprelan® [US]
Naprosyn® [US/Can]
naproxen
Naxen® [Can]
Norgesic™ Forte [US/Can]
Norgesic™ [US/Can]
Novasen [Can]
Novo-Difenac® [Can]
Novo-Difenac-K [Can]
Novo-Difenac® SR [Can]
Novo-Diflunisal [Can]
Novo-Flurprofen [Can]
Novo-Keto [Can]
Novo-Keto-EC [Can]
Novo-Ketorolac [Can]
Novo-Methacin [Can]
Novo-Naproc EC [Can]
Novo-Naprox [Can]
Novo-Naprox Sodium [Can]
Novo-Naprox Sodium DS [Can]
Novo-Naprox SR [Can]
Novo-Pirocam® [Can]
Novo-Profen® [Can]
Novo-Sundac [Can]

Nu-Diclo [Can]
Nu-Diclo-SR [Can]
Nu-Diflunisal [Can]
Nu-Flurprofen [Can]
Nu-Ibuprofen [Can]
Nu-Indo [Can]
Nu-Ketoprofen [Can]
Nu-Ketoprofen-E [Can]
Nu-Mefenamic [Can]
Nu-Naprox [Can]
Nu-Pirox [Can]
Nu-Sundac [Can]
Ocufen® [US/Can]
orphenadrine, aspirin, and caffeine
Orphengesic Forte [US]
Orphengesic [US]
Orudis® KT [US-OTC]
Orudis® SR [Can]
Oruvail® [US/Can]
oxaprozin
Pain-Off [US-OTC]
Pamprin® Maximum Strength All
   Day Relief [US-OTC]
Pediatrix [Can]
Pennsaid® [Can]
Percogesic® Extra Strength [US-OTC]
Percogesic® [US-OTC]
Pexicam® [Can]
Phenylgesic® [US-OTC]
piroxicam
piroxicam and cyclodextrin (Canada
   only)
PMS-Diclofenac [Can]
PMS-Diclofenac SR [Can]
PMS-Mefenamic Acid [Can]
Ponstan® [Can]
Ponstel® [US/Can]
ratio-Ketorolac [Can]
Redutemp® [US-OTC]
Relafen® [US/Can]
Rhodacine® [Can]
Rhodis™ [Can]
Rhodis-EC™ [Can]

Rhodis SR™ [Can]
Rhoxal-nabumetone [Can]
Rhoxal-oxaprozin [Can]
Riva-Diclofenac [Can]
Riva-Diclofenac-K [Can]
Riva-Naproxen [Can]
Salflex® [US/Can]
salsalate
Silapap® Children's [US-OTC]
Silapap® Infants [US-OTC]
sodium salicylate
Solaraze™ [US]
St Joseph® Adult Aspirin [US-OTC]
sulindac
Sureprin 81™ [US-OTC]
Tempra® [Can]
Tolectin® DS [US]
Tolectin® [US/Can]
tolmetin
Toradol® IM [Can]
Toradol® [US/Can]
tramadol
Tylenol® 8 Hour [US-OTC]
Tylenol® Arthritis Pain [US-OTC]
Tylenol® Children's [US-OTC]
Tylenol® Extra Strength [US-OTC]
Tylenol® Infants [US-OTC]
Tylenol® Junior Strength [US-OTC]
Tylenol® PM Extra Strength [US-OTC]
Tylenol® Severe Allergy [US-OTC]
Tylenol® Sore Throat [US-OTC]
Tylenol® [US-OTC/Can]
Ultracet™ [US]
Ultram® [US/Can]
Ultraprin [US-OTC]
Utradol™ [Can]
Valorin Extra [US-OTC]
Valorin [US-OTC]
Vanquish® Extra Strength Pain
   Reliever [US-OTC]
Voltaren Ophthalmic® [US]
Voltaren Rapide® [Can]
Voltaren® [US/Can]

Voltaren®-XR [US]
Voltare Ophtha® [Can]
ZORprin® [US]
Decongestant/Analgesic
  Advil® Cold, Children's [US-OTC]
  Advil® Cold & Sinus [US-OTC/Can]
  Dristan® Sinus Tablet [US-OTC/Can]
  Motrin® Cold and Sinus [US-OTC]
  Motrin® Cold, Children's [US-OTC]
  pseudoephedrine and ibuprofen
  Sudafed® Sinus Advance [Can]
Local Anesthetic
  Alcaine® [US/Can]
  Diocaine® [Can]
  ethyl chloride
  ethyl chloride and
    dichlorotetrafluoroethane
  Fluro-Ethyl® [US]
  Gebauer's Ethyl Chloride® [US]
  Ophthetic® [US]
  proparacaine
Neuroleptic Agent
  Apo-Methoprazine® [Can]
  methotrimeprazine (Canada only)
  Novo-Meprazine [Can]
  Nozinan® [Can]
Nonsteroidal Antiinflammatory Drug
    (NSAID)
  Doan's® Extra Strength [US-OTC]
  Doan's® [US-OTC]
  magnesium salicylate
  Momentum® [US-OTC]
Nonsteroidal Antiinflammatory Drug
    (NSAID), Oral
  floctafenine (Canada only)

PAIN (ANOGENITAL)

Anesthetic/Corticosteroid
  Analpram-HC® [US]
  Enzone® [US]
  Epifoam® [US]
  Pramosone® [US]
  Pramox® HC [Can]

pramoxine and hydrocortisone
  ProctoFoam®-HC [US/Can]
  Zone-A Forte® [US]
  Zone-A® [US]
Local Anesthetic
  AK-T-Caine™ [US]
  Americaine® Anesthetic Lubricant
    [US]
  Americaine® [US-OTC]
  Ametop™ [Can]
  Anbesol® Baby [US-OTC/Can]
  Anbesol® Maximum Strength [US-
    OTC]
  Anbesol® [US-OTC]
  Anusol® Ointment [US-OTC]
  Babee® Teething® [US-OTC]
  benzocaine
  Benzodent® [US-OTC]
  Cepacol® Maximum Strength [US-
    OTC]
  Cepacol Viractin® [US-OTC]
  Chiggerex® [US-OTC]
  Chiggertox® [US-OTC]
  Cylex® [US-OTC]
  Detane® [US-OTC]
  dibucaine
  dyclonine
  Foille® Medicated First Aid [US-OTC]
  Foille® Plus [US-OTC]
  Foille® [US-OTC]
  HDA® Toothache [US-OTC]
  Hurricaine® [US]
  Itch-X® [US-OTC]
  Lanacane® [US-OTC]
  Mycinettes® [US-OTC]
  Nupercainal® [US-OTC]
  Opticaine® [US]
  Orabase®-B [US-OTC]
  Orajel® Baby Nighttime [US-OTC]
  Orajel® Baby [US-OTC]
  Orajel® Maximum Strength [US-OTC]
  Orajel® [US-OTC]
  Orasol® [US-OTC]

Pontocaine® [US/Can]
pramoxine
Prax® [US-OTC]
ProctoFoam® NS [US-OTC]
Solarcaine® [US-OTC]
Sucrets® [US-OTC]
tetracaine
Trocaine® [US-OTC]
Tronolane® [US-OTC]
Zilactin® Baby [US-OTC/Can]
Zilactin®-B [US-OTC/Can]

PAIN (BONE)
Radiopharmaceutical
Metastron® [US/Can]
strontium-89

PAIN (MUSCLE)
Analgesic, Topical
dichlorodifluoromethane and
trichloromonofluoromethane
Fluori-Methane® [US]

PARACOCCIDIOIDOMYCOSIS
Antifungal Agent
Apo-Ketoconazole® [Can]
ketoconazole
Ketoderm® [Can]
Nizoral® A-D [US-OTC]
Nizoral® [US/Can]
Novo-Ketoconazole [Can]

PHEOCHROMOCYTOMA (DIAGNOSIS)
Alpha-Adrenergic Agonist
Catapres® [US/Can]
clonidine

PERIANAL WART
Immune Response Modifier
Aldara™ [US/Can]
imiquimod

PLATELET AGGREGATION (PROPHYLAXIS)
Antiplatelet Agent
Apo-Dipyridamole FC® [Can]
Asaphen [Can]
Asaphen E.C. [Can]
Ascriptin® Extra Strength [US-OTC]
Ascriptin® [US-OTC]
Aspercin Extra [US-OTC]
Aspercin [US-OTC]
Aspergum® [US-OTC]
aspirin
Bayer® Aspirin Extra Strength [US-OTC]
Bayer® Aspirin Regimen Adult Low Strength [US-OTC]
Bayer® Aspirin Regimen Children's [US-OTC]
Bayer® Aspirin Regimen Regular Strength [US-OTC]
Bayer® Aspirin [US-OTC]
Bayer® Extra Strength Arthritis Pain Regimen [US-OTC]
Bayer® Plus Extra Strength [US-OTC]
Bayer® Women's Aspirin Plus Calcium [US-OTC]
Bufferin® Extra Strength [US-OTC]
Bufferin® [US-OTC]
Buffinol Extra [US-OTC]
Buffinol [US-OTC]
dipyridamole
Easprin® [US]
Ecotrin® Low Strength [US-OTC]
Ecotrin® Maximum Strength [US-OTC]
Ecotrin® [US-OTC]
Entrophen® [Can]
Halfprin® [US-OTC]
Novasen [Can]
Novo-Dipiradol [Can]
Persantine® [US/Can]
St Joseph® Adult Aspirin [US-OTC]

Sureprin 81™ [US-OTC]
ZORprin® [US]

PNEUMOCYSTIS CARINII

Antibiotic, Miscellaneous
  Apo-Trimethoprim® [Can]
  NeuTrexin® [US]
  Primsol® [US]
  Proloprim® [US/Can]
  trimethoprim
  trimetrexate glucuronate
Antiprotozoal
  atovaquone
  Mepron® [US/Can]
  NebuPent® [US]
  Pentacarinat® [Can]
  Pentam-300® [US]
  pentamidine
Sulfonamide
  Apo-Sulfatrim® [Can]
  Bactrim™ DS [US]
  Bactrim™ [US]
  Novo-Trimel [Can]
  Novo-Trimel D.S. [Can]
  Nu-Cotrimox® [Can]
  Septra® DS [US/Can]
  Septra® Injection [Can]
  Septra® [US/Can]
  sulfamethoxazole and trimethoprim
Sulfone
  dapsone

POLYCYTHEMIA VERA

Antineoplastic Agent
  busulfan
  Busulfex® [US/Can]
  mechlorethamine
  Mustargen® [US/Can]
  Myleran® [US/Can]

POLYMYOSITIS

Antineoplastic Agent
  Apo-Methotrexate® [Can]
  chlorambucil
  cyclophosphamide
  Cytoxan® [US/Can]
  Leukeran® [US/Can]
  methotrexate
  Procytox® [Can]
  ratio-Methotrexate [Can]
  Rheumatrex® [US]
  Trexall™ [US]
Immunosuppressant Agent
  Alti-Azathioprine [Can]
  Apo-Azathioprine® [Can]
  Azasan® [US]
  azathioprine
  Gen-Azathioprine [Can]
  Imuran® [US/Can]

PORPHYRIA

Blood Modifier
  hemin
  Panhematin® [US]
Phenothiazine Derivative
  Apo-Chlorpromazine® [Can]
  chlorpromazine
  Largactil® [Can]
  Novo-Chlorpromazine [Can]

PURPURA

Immune Globulin
  Carimune™ [US]
  Flebogamma® [US]
  Gamimune® N [US/Can]
  Gammagard® S/D [US/Can]
  Gammar®-P I.V. [US]
  Gamunex® [US/Can]
  immune globulin (intravenous)
  Iveegam EN [US]
  Iveegam Immuno® [Can]
  Octagam® [US]

Panglobulin® [US]
Polygam® S/D [US]
Venoglobulin®-S [US]
Immunosuppressant Agent
Alti-Azathioprine [Can]
Apo-Azathioprine® [Can]
Azasan® [US]
azathioprine
Gen-Azathioprine [Can]
Imuran® [US/Can]

PURPURA (THROMBOCYTOPENIC)
Antineoplastic Agent
Oncovin® [Can]
Vincasar® PFS® [US/Can]
vincristine

RETINOBLASTOMA
Antineoplastic Agent
Cosmegen® [US/Can]
cyclophosphamide
Cytoxan® [US/Can]
dactinomycin
Procytox® [Can]

RHABDOMYOSARCOMA
Antineoplastic Agent
Alkeran® [US/Can]
Cosmegen® [US/Can]
cyclophosphamide
Cytoxan® [US/Can]
dactinomycin
etoposide
melphalan
Oncovin® [Can]
Procytox® [Can]
Toposar® [US]
VePesid® [US/Can]
Vincasar® PFS® [US/Can]
vincristine

SARCOIDOSIS
Corticosteroid, Topical
Aclovate® [US]
alclometasone
amcinonide
Amcort® [Can]
ApexiCon™ E [US]
ApexiCon™ [US]
Aquacort® [Can]
Aquanil™ HC [US]
Aristocort® A Topical [US]
Aristocort® Topical [US]
Betaderm® [Can]
Betaject™ [Can]
betamethasone (topical)
Beta-Val® [US]
Betnesol® [Can]
Betnovate® [Can]
CaldeCORT® [US]
Capex™ [US/Can]
Carmol-HC® [US]
Celestoderm®-EV/2 [Can]
Celestoderm®-V [Can]
Cetacort® [US]
clobetasol
Clobevate® [US]
Clobex™ [US]
clocortolone
Cloderm® [US/Can]
Cordran® SP [US]
Cordran® [US/Can]
Cormax® [US]
Cortagel® Maximum Strength [US]
Cortaid® Intensive Therapy [US]
Cortaid® Maximum Strength [US]
Cortaid®Sensitive Skin With Aloe [US]
Corticool® [US]
Cortizone®-5 [US]
Cortizone®-10 Maximum Strength [US]
Cortizone®-10 Plus Maximum Strength [US]

Cortizone® 10 Quick Shot [US]
Cortizone® for Kids [US]
Cutivate™ [US]
Cyclocort® [US/Can]
Dermarest® Dri-Cort [US]
Derma-Smoothe/FS® [US/Can]
Dermatop® [US/Can]
Dermovate® [Can]
Dermtex® HC [US]
Desocort® [Can]
desonide
DesOwen® [US]
Desoxi® [Can]
desoximetasone
diflorasone
Diprolene® AF [US]
Diprolene® Glycol [Can]
Diprolene® [US]
Diprosone® [Can]
Ectosone [Can]
Elocom® [Can]
Elocon® [US]
Embeline™ E [US]
Embeline™ [US]
Florone® [US/Can]
fluocinolone
fluocinonide
Fluoderm [Can]
flurandrenolide
fluticasone (topical)
Gen-Clobetasol [Can]
halcinonide
halobetasol
Halog® [US/Can]
hydrocortisone (topical)
Hytone® [US]
Kenalog® in Orabase® [US/Can]
Kenalog® Topical [US/Can]
LactiCare-HC® [US]
Lidemol® [Can]
Lidex-E® [US]
Lidex® [US/Can]
Locoid® [US/Can]

LoKara™ [US]
Luxiq® [US]
Lyderm® [Can]
Lydonide [Can]
Maxivate® [US]
mometasone furoate
Nasonex® [US/Can]
Novo-Clobetasol [Can]
Nupercainal® Hydrocortisone Cream
    [US]
Nutracort® [US]
Olux® [US]
Oracort [Can]
Pandel® [US]
PMS-Desonide [Can]
Post Peel Healing Balm [US]
prednicarbate
Prevex® B [Can]
Psorcon® E™ [US]
Psorcon® [US/Can]
Sarnol®-HC [US]
Summer's Eve® SpecialCare™
    Medicated Anti-Itch Cream [US]
Synalar® [US/Can]
Taro-Desoximetasone [Can]
Taro-Sone® [Can]
Temovate E® [US]
Temovate® [US]
Texacort® [US]
Theracort® [US]
Tiamol® [Can]
Ti-U-Lac® H [Can]
Topicort®-LP [US]
Topicort® [US/Can]
Topisone® [Can]
Topsyn® [Can]
Triacet™ Topical [US]
Triaderm [Can]
triamcinolone (topical)
Triderm® [US]
Tridesilon® [US]
Ultravate® [US/Can]
urea and hydrocortisone

Uremol® HC [Can]
Valisone® Scalp Lotion [Can]
Westcort® [US/Can]

SARCOMA

Antineoplastic Agent
  Adriamycin® [Can]
  Adriamycin PFS® [US]
  Adriamycin RDF® [US]
  Apo-Methotrexate® [Can]
  Blenoxane® [US/Can]
  bleomycin
  cisplatin
  Cosmegen® [US/Can]
  dacarbazine
  dactinomycin
  doxorubicin
  DTIC® [Can]
  DTIC-Dome® [US]
  Ifex® [US/Can]
  ifosfamide
  methotrexate
  Oncovin® [Can]
  Platinol®-AQ [US]
  ratio-Methotrexate [Can]
  Rheumatrex® [US]
  Rubex® [US]
  Trexall™ [US]
  Velban® [Can]
  vinblastine
  Vincasar® PFS® [US/Can]
  vincristine

SOFT TISSUE INFECTION

Aminoglycoside (Antibiotic)
  AKTob® [US]
  Alcomicin® [Can]
  amikacin
  Amikin® [US/Can]
  Apo-Tobramycin® [Can]
  Diogent® [Can]
  Garamycin® [Can]
  gentamicin

Nebcin® [Can]
PMS-Tobramycin [Can]
SAB-Gentamicin [Can]
tobramycin
Tobrex® [US/Can]
Tomycine™ [Can]
Antibiotic, Carbacephem
  Lorabid® [US/Can]
  loracarbef
Antibiotic, Carbapenem
  ertapenem
  Invanz® [US/Can]
Antibiotic, Miscellaneous
  Alti-Clindamycin [Can]
  Apo-Clindamycin® [Can]
  Cleocin HCl® [US]
  Cleocin Pediatric® [US]
  Cleocin Phosphate® [US]
  Cleocin® [US]
  clindamycin
  Clindoxyl® [Can]
  Dalacin® C [Can]
  Dalacin® T [Can]
  Novo-Clindamycin [Can]
  Vancocin® [US/Can]
  vancomycin
Antibiotic, Penicillin
  pivampicillin (Canada only)
Antibiotic, Quinolone
  Iquix® [US]
  Levaquin® [US/Can]
  levofloxacin
  Quixin™ [US]
Antifungal Agent, Systemic
  Fucidin® [Can]
  Fucithalmic® [Can]
  fusidic acid (Canada only)
Cephalosporin (First Generation)
  Ancef® [US]
  Apo-Cefadroxil® [Can]
  Apo-Cephalex® [Can]
  Biocef® [US]
  cefadroxil

cefazolin
cephalexin
cephalothin
cephradine
Duricef® [US/Can]
Keflex® [US]
Keftab® [Can]
Novo-Cefadroxil [Can]
Novo-Lexin® [Can]
Nu-Cephalex® [Can]
Panixine DisperDose™ [US]
Velosef® [US]

Cephalosporin (Second Generation)
Apo-Cefaclor® [Can]
Apo-Cefuroxime® [Can]
Ceclor® CD [US]
Ceclor® [US/Can]
cefaclor
Cefotan® [US/Can]
cefotetan
cefoxitin
cefpodoxime
cefprozil
Ceftin® [US/Can]
cefuroxime
Cefzil® [US/Can]
Kefurox® [Can]
Mefoxin® [US/Can]
Novo-Cefaclor [Can]
Nu-Cefaclor [Can]
PMS-Cefaclor [Can]
Raniclor™ [US]
ratio-Cefuroxime [Can]
Vantin® [US/Can]
Zinacef® [US/Can]

Cephalosporin (Third Generation)
Cedax® [US]
cefixime
Cefizox® [US/Can]
cefotaxime
ceftazidime
ceftibuten
ceftizoxime

ceftriaxone
Claforan® [US/Can]
Fortaz® [US/Can]
Rocephin® [US/Can]
Suprax® [US/Can]
Tazicef® [US]

Cephalosporin (Fourth Generation)
cefepime
Maxipime® [US/Can]

Macrolide (Antibiotic)
azithromycin
dirithromycin
Dynabac® [US]
Zithromax® [US/Can]

Penicillin
Alti-Amoxi-Clav® [Can]
amoxicillin
amoxicillin and clavulanate
    potassium
Amoxil® [US/Can]
ampicillin
ampicillin and sulbactam
Apo-Amoxi® [Can]
Apo-Amoxi-Clav [Can]
Apo-Ampi® [Can]
Apo-Cloxi® [Can]
Apo-Pen VK® [Can]
Augmentin ES-600® [US]
Augmentin® [US/Can]
Augmentin XR™ [US]
Bicillin® C-R 900/300 [US]
Bicillin® C-R [US].
Bicillin® L-A [US]
carbenicillin
Clavulin® [Can]
cloxacillin
dicloxacillin
DisperMox™ [US]
Dycil® [Can]
Gen-Amoxicillin [Can]
Geocillin® [US]
Lin-Amox [Can]
Moxilin® [US]

Nadopen-V® [Can]
nafcillin
Nallpen® [Can]
Novamoxin® [Can]
Novo-Ampicillin [Can]
Novo-Cloxin [Can]
Novo-Pen-VK®[Can]
Nu-Amoxi [Can]
Nu-Ampi [Can]
Nu-Cloxi® [Can]
Nu-Pen-VK® [Can]
oxacillin
Pathocil® [Can]
penicillin G benzathine
penicillin G benzathine and
   penicillin G procaine
penicillin G (parenteral/aqueous)
penicillin G procaine
penicillin V potassium
Permapen® Isoject® [US]
Pfizerpen-AS® [Can]
Pfizerpen® [US/Can]
piperacillin
piperacillin and tazobactam sodium
PMS-Amoxicillin [Can]
Principen® [US]
PVF® K [Can]
ratio-AmoxiClav
Riva-Cloxacillin [Can]
Tazocin® [Can]
ticarcillin
ticarcillin and clavulanate potassium
Ticar® [US]
Timentin® [US/Can]
Trimox® [US]
Unasyn® [US/Can]
Unipen® [Can]
Veetids® [US]
Wycillin® [Can]
Zosyn® [US]
Quinolone
   Apo-Oflox® [Can]

ciprofloxacin
Cipro® [US/Can]
Cipro® XL [Can]
Cipro® XR [US]
Floxin® [US/Can]
lomefloxacin
Maxaquin® [US]
ofloxacin

SOFT TISSUE SARCOMA
Antineoplastic Agent
   Adriamycin® [Can]
   Adriamycin PFS® [US]
   Adriamycin RDF® [US]
   Cosmegen® [US/Can]
   dactinomycin
   doxorubicin
   Rubex® [US]

STOMATITIS
Local Anesthetic
   Cepacol® Maximum Strength [US-
      OTC]
   dyclonine
   Sucrets® [US-OTC]
Skin and Mucous Membrane Agent
   Gelclair™ [US]
   maltodextrin
   Multidex® [US-OTC]
   OraRinse™ [US-OTC]

THROMBOCYTOPENIA
Anticoagulant, Thrombin Inhibitor
   argatroban
Enzyme
   alglucerase
   Ceredase® [US]
Platelet Growth Factor
   Neumega® [US]
   oprelvekin

THROMBOCYTOPENIA (HEPARIN-INDUCED)
Anticoagulant (Other)
  lepirudin
  Refludan® [US/Can]

THROMBOCYTOSIS
Antineoplastic Agent
  Droxia™ [US]
  Gen-Hydroxyurea [Can]
  Hydrea® [US/Can]
  hydroxyurea
  Mylocel™ [US]

THROMBOLYTIC THERAPY
Anticoagulant (Other)
  anisindione
  Apo-Warfarin® [Can]
  Coumadin® [US/Can]
  dalteparin
  enoxaparin
  Fragmin® [US/Can]
  Gen-Warfarin [Can]
  Hepalean® [Can]
  Hepalean® Leo [Can]
  Hepalean®-LOK [Can]
  heparin
  Hep-Lock® [US]
  Innohep® [US/Can]
  Lovenox® HP [Can]
  Lovenox® [US/Can]
  Taro-Warfarin [Can]
  tinzaparin
  warfarin
Fibrinolytic Agent
  Abbokinase® [US]
  Activase® rt-PA [Can]
  Activase® [US]
  alteplase
  Cathflo™ Activase® [US/Can]
  Retavase® [US/Can]
  reteplase

  Streptase® [US/Can]
  streptokinase
  urokinase

TOXOPLASMOSIS
Antibiotic, Miscellaneous
  Alti-Clindamycin [Can]
  Apo-Clindamycin® [Can]
  Cleocin HCl® [US]
  Cleocin Pediatric® [US]
  Cleocin Phosphate® [US]
  Cleocin® [US]
  clindamycin
  Clindoxyl® [Can]
  Dalacin® C [Can]
  Dalacin® T [Can]
  Dalacin® Vaginal [Can]
  Novo-Clindamycin [Can]
Folic Acid Antagonist (Antimalarial)
  Daraprim® [US/Can]
  pyrimethamine
Sulfonamide
  sulfadiazine

TRANSFUSION REACTION
Antihistamine
  Alavert™ [US-OTC]
  Aler-Dryl [US-OTC]
  Aller-Chlor® [US-OTC]
  Allerdryl® [Can]
  AllerMax® [US-OTC]
  Allernix [Can]
  Apo-Hydroxyzine® [Can]
  Apo-Loratadine® [Can]
  Atarax® [US/Can]
  azatadine
  Banophen® [US-OTC]
  Benadryl® Allergy [US-OTC/Can]
  Benadryl® Dye-Free Allergy [US-OTC]
  Benadryl® Gel Extra Strength [US-OTC]
  Benadryl® Gel [US-OTC]

Benadryl® Injection [US]
brompheniramine
chlorpheniramine
Chlorphen [US-OTC]
Chlor-Trimeton® [US-OTC]
Chlor-Tripolon® [Can]
Claritin® Hives Relief [US-OTC]
Claritin® Kids [Can]
Claritin® [US-OTC/Can]
clemastine
cyproheptadine
Dayhist® Allergy [US-OTC]
dexchlorpheniramine
Diabetic Tussin® Allergy Relief [US-OTC]
Dimetapp® Children's ND [US-OTC]
Diphen® AF [US-OTC]
Diphenhist [US-OTC]
diphenhydramine
Diphen® [US-OTC]
Genahist® [US-OTC]
Hydramine® [US-OTC]
hydroxyzine
Hyrexin-50® [US]
loratadine
Nolahist® [US-OTC/Can]
Novo-Hydroxyzin [Can]
Novo-Pheniram® [Can]
Periactin® [Can]
phenindamine
PMS-Diphenhydramine [Can]
PMS-Hydroxyzine [Can]
Siladryl® Allergy [US-OTC]
Silphen® [US-OTC]
Tavist® Allergy [US-OTC]
Tavist® ND [US-OTC]
Vistaril® [US/Can]
Phenothiazine Derivative
Phenadoz™ [US]
Phenergan® [US/Can]
promethazine

TUMOR (BRAIN)
Antineoplastic Agent
BiCNU® [US/Can]
carboplatin
carmustine
CeeNU® [US/Can]
Gliadel® [US]
lomustine
Matulane® [US/Can]
mechlorethamine
Mustargen® [US/Can]
Natulan® [Can]
Paraplatin-AQ [Can]
Paraplatin® [US]
procarbazine
Biological Response Modulator
interferon alfa-2b
Intron® A [US/Can]

VENEREAL WART
Biological Response Modulator
Alferon® N [US/Can]
interferon alfa-n3

VITAMIN B5 DEFICIENCY
Vitamin, Water Soluble
pantothenic acid

VITAMIN B6 DEFICIENCY
Vitamin, Water Soluble
Aminoxin® [US-OTC]
pyridoxine

VITAMIN B12 DEFICIENCY
Vitamin, Water Soluble
cyanocobalamin
Nascobal® [US]
Scheinpharm B12 [Can]
Twelve Resin-K® [US]

VITAMIN B DEFICIENCY
Vitamin, Water Soluble
  vitamin B complex with vitamin C
  vitamin B complex with vitamin C
    and folic acid

VITAMIN C DEFICIENCY
Vitamin, Water Soluble
  ascorbic acid
  C-500-GR™ [US-OTC]
  Cecon® [US-OTC]
  Cevi-Bid® [US-OTC]
  C-Gram [US-OTC]
  Dull-C® [US-OTC]
  Proflavanol C™ [Can]
  Revitalose C-1000® [Can]
  sodium ascorbate
  Vita-C® [US-OTC]
  vitamin B complex with vitamin C
  vitamin B complex with vitamin C
    and folic acid

VITAMIN D DEFICIENCY
Vitamin D Analog
  Calciferol™ [US]
  cholecalciferol
  Delta-D® [US]
  Drisdol® [US/Can]
  D-Vi-Sol® [Can]
  ergocalciferol
  Ostoforte® [Can]

VITAMIN K DEFICIENCY
Vitamin, Fat Soluble
  AquaMEPHYTON® [Can]
  Konakion [Can]
  Mephyton® [US/Can]
  phytonadione

VOMITING, CHEMOTHERAPY-RELATED
Selective 5-HT3 Receptor Antagonist
  Anzemet® [US/Can]
  dolasetron
  granisetron
  Kytril® [US/Can]
  ondansetron
  Zofran® ODT [US/Can]
  Zofran® [US/Can]

National Cancer Institute (NCI) Comprehensive Cancer Centers

ALABAMA

UAB Comprehensive Cancer Center
University of Alabama
1824 Sixth Avenue South, Room 237
Birmingham, Alabama 35293-3300
(205) 934-5077
www.ccc.uab.edu

ARIZONA

Arizona Cancer Center
University of Arizona
1501 North Campbell Avenue
Tucson, Arizona 85724
(520) 626-7925
www.azcc.arizona.edu

CALIFORNIA

Beckman Research Institute, City of Hope
1500 East Duarte Road
Duarte, California 91010-3000
(626) 256-4673
www.cityofhope.org

Salk Institute
10010 North Torrey Pines Road
La Jolla, California 92037
(858) 453-4100, extension 1386
www.salk.edu

The Burnham Institute
10901 North Torrey Pines Road
La Jolla, California 92037-1099
(858) 646-3100
www.burnhaminstitute.org

UCSD Cancer Center, Rebecca and John Moores
University of California at San Diego
9500 Gilman Drive
La Jolla, California 92093-0658
(858) 822-1222
cancer.ucsd.edu

Jonsson Comprehensive Cancer Center
University of California at Los Angeles
Factor Building, Room 8-684
10833 Le Conte Avenue
Los Angeles, California 90095-1781
(310) 825-5268
www.cancer.mednet.ucla.edu

USC/Norris Comprehensive Cancer Center
University of Southern California
1441 Eastlake Avenue, NOR 8302L
Los Angeles, California 90089-9181
(323) 865-0816
ccnt.hsc.usc.edu

Chao Family Comprehensive Cancer Center
University of California at Irvine
101 The City Drive
Building 23, Rt. 81, Room 406
Orange, California 92868
(714) 456-6310
www.ucihs.uci.edu/cancer

UC Davis Cancer Center
4501 X Street, Suite 3003
Sacramento, California 95817
(916) 734-5800
cancer.ucdmc.ucdavis.edu

UCSF Comprehensive Cancer Center & Cancer Research Institute
University of California at San Francisco
2340 Sutter Street, Box 0128
San Francisco, California 94115-0128
(415) 502-1710
cc.ucsf.edu

COLORADO
University of Colorado Cancer Center
University of Colorado Health Sciences Center
RC1-South Tower
Mail Stop 8111, P.O. Box 6511
Aurora, Colorado 80045-0511
(303) 724-3155
www.uccc.info

CONNECTICUT
Yale Cancer Center
Yale University School of Medicine
333 Cedar Street, Box 208028
New Haven, Connecticut 06520-8028
(203) 785-4371
www.info.med.yale.edu/ycc

DISTRICT OF COLUMBIA
Lombardi Cancer Research Center
Georgetown University Medical Center
3800 Reservoir Road, N.W.
Washington, DC 20057
(202) 687-2110
lombardi.georgetown.edu

FLORIDA
H. Lee Moffitt Cancer Center & Research Institute
University of South Florida
12902 Magnolia Drive
Tampa, Florida 33612-9497
(813) 615-4261
www.moffitt.usf.edu

HAWAII
Cancer Research Center of Hawaii
University of Hawaii at Manoa
1236 Lauhala Street
Honolulu, Hawaii 96813
(808) 586-3013
www.crch.org

ILLINOIS
University of Chicago Cancer Research Center
5841 South Maryland Avenue, MC 2115
Chicago, Illinois 60637-1470
Tel: (773) 702-6180
www-uccrc.uchicago.edu

Robert H. Lurie Comprehensive Cancer Center
Northwestern University
676 North Saint Clair Street, Suite 1200
Chicago, Illinois 60611
(312) 908-5250
www.cancer.northwestern.edu

INDIANA
Indiana University Cancer Center
Indiana Cancer Pavilion
535 Barnhill Drive, Room 455
Indianapolis, Indiana 46202-5289
(317) 278-0070
www.iucc.iu.edu

Purdue University Cancer Center
Hansen Life Sciences Research Building
South University Street
West Lafayette, Indiana 47907-1524
(765) 494-9129
www.pharmacy.purdue.edu/~ccenter

IOWA

Holden Comprehensive Cancer Center
5970 "Z" JPP
200 Hawkins Drive
Iowa City, Iowa 52242
(319) 353-8620
www.cancer.vh.org

MAINE

The Jackson Laboratory
600 Main Street
Bar Harbor, Maine 04609-0800
(207) 288-6041
www.jax.org

MARYLAND

The Sidney Kimmel Comprehensive Cancer Center
Johns Hopkins Hospital
401 North Broadway
The Weinberg Building, Suite 1100
Baltimore, Maryland 21231
(410) 955-8822
www.hopkinskimmelcancercenter.org/index.cfm

MASSACHUSETTS

Dana-Farber/Harvard Cancer Center
Dana-Farber Cancer Institute
44 Binney Street, Room 1628
Boston, Massachusetts 02115
(617) 632-4266
www.dfhcc.harvard.edu

Center for Cancer Research
Massachusetts Institute of Technology
77 Massachusetts Avenue, Room E17-110
Cambridge, Massachusetts 02139-4307
(617) 253-8511
web.mit.edu/ccr/index.html

MICHIGAN

Comprehensive Cancer Center
University of Michigan
6302 CGC/0942
1500 East Medical Center Drive
Ann Arbor, Michigan 48109-0942
(734) 936-1831
www.cancer.med.umich.edu

Barbara Ann Karmanos Cancer Institute
Wayne State University School of Medicine
4100 John R
Detroit, Michigan 48201
(313) 576-8660
www.karmanos.org

MINNESOTA

University of Minnesota Cancer Center
MMC 806, 420 Delaware Street, S.E.
Minneapolis, Minnesota 55455
(612) 624-8484
www.cancer.umn.edu

Mayo Clinic Cancer Center
Mayo Clinic Rochester
200 First Street, S.W.
Rochester, Minnesota 55905
(507) 284-3753
www.mayoclinic.org/cancercenter-rst

MISSOURI

Siteman Cancer Center
Washington University School of Medicine
660 South Euclid Avenue, Campus Box 8109
St. Louis, Missouri 63110
(314) 362-8020
www.siteman.wustl.edu

NEBRASKA
University of Nebraska Medical Center/Eppley Cancer Center
600 South 42nd Street
Omaha, Nebraska 68198-6805
(402) 559-4238
www.unmc.edu/cancercenter

NEW HAMPSHIRE
Norris Cotton Cancer Center
Dartmouth-Hitchcock Medical Center
One Medical Center Drive, Hinman
Box 7920
Lebanon, New Hampshire 03756-0001
(603) 653-9000
www.dartmouth.edu/dms/nccc/index.htm

NEW JERSEY
The Cancer Institute of New Jersey
Robert Wood Johnson University
Hospital
Robert Wood Johnson Medical School
195 Little Albany Street, Room 2002B
New Brunswick, New Jersey 08903
(732) 235-8064
www-cinj.umdnj.edu

NEW MEXICO
UNM Cancer Research & Treatment Center
MSC 08 4630
1 University of New Mexico
2325 Camino de Salud, NE
Albuquerque, NM 87131
(505) 272-5622
cancer.unm.edu

NEW YORK
Cancer Research Center
Albert Einstein College of Medicine
Chanin Building, Room 209
1300 Morris Park Avenue
Bronx, New York 10461
(718) 430-2302
www.aecom.yu.edu/cancer

Roswell Park Cancer Institute
Elm & Carlton Streets
Buffalo, New York 14263-0001
(716) 845-5772
www.roswellpark.org

Cold Spring Harbor Laboratory
P.O. Box 100
Cold Spring Harbor, New York 11724
(516) 367-8383
www.cshl.org

NYU Cancer Institute
New York University Medical Center
550 First Avenue
New York, New York 10016
(212) 263-8950
www.nyucancerinstitute.org

Memorial Sloan-Kettering Cancer Center
1275 York Avenue
New York, New York 10021
(212) 639-2000
www.mskcc.org

Herbert Irving Comprehensive Cancer Center
College of Physicians & Surgeons
Columbia University
161 Fort Washington Avenue
11th Floor, Room 1153
New York, New York 10032
(212) 305-5201
www.ccc.columbia.edu

NORTH CAROLINA

UNC Lineberger Comprehensive Cancer Center
University of North Carolina at Chapel Hill
School of Medicine, CB-7295
102 West Drive
Chapel Hill, North Carolina 27599-7295
(919) 966-3036
www.cancer.med.unc.edu

Duke Comprehensive Cancer Center
Duke University Medical Center
Box 3843
Durham, North Carolina 27710
(919) 684-5613
www.cancer.duke.edu

Comprehensive Cancer Center
Wake Forest University
Bowman Gray School of Medicine
Medical Center Boulevard
Winston-Salem, North Carolina 27157-1082
(336) 716-7971
www.bgsm.edu/cancer

OHIO

Case Comprehensive Cancer Center
Case Western Reserve University
11100 Euclid Avenue, Wearn 151
Cleveland, Ohio 44106-5065
(216) 844-8562
www.cancer.case.edu

Comprehensive Cancer Center, Arthur G. James Cancer Hospital and Richard J. Solove Research Institute
Ohio State University
A458 Starling Loving Hall
320 West 10th Avenue
Columbus, Ohio 43210
(614) 293-7521
www.jamesline.com

OREGON

OHSU Cancer Institute
Oregon Health & Science University
3181 S.W. Sam Jackson Park Road, CR145
Portland, Oregon 97201-3098
(503) 494-1617
www.ohsu.edu/oci

PENNSYLVANIA

Fox Chase Cancer Center
7701 Burholme Avenue
Philadelphia, Pennsylvania 19111
(215) 728-2781
www.fccc.edu

Kimmel Cancer Center
Thomas Jefferson University
233 South 10th Street
BLSB, Room 1050
Philadelphia, Pennsylvania 19107-5799
(888) 955-1212
www.kcc.tju.edu

The Wistar Institute
3601 Spruce Street
Philadelphia, Pennsylvania 19104-4268
(215) 898-3926
www.wistar.upenn.edu

University of Pittsburgh Cancer Institute
UPMC Cancer Pavilion
5150 Centre Avenue, Suite 500
Pittsburgh, Pennsylvania 15232
(412) 623-3205
www.upci.upmc.edu

TENNESSEE

St. Jude Children's Research Hospital
332 North Lauderdale
Memphis, Tennessee 38105-2794
(901) 495-3982
www.stjude.org

Vanderbilt-Ingram Cancer Center
Vanderbilt University
691 Preston Research Building
Nashville, Tennessee 37232-6838
(615) 936-1782
www.vicc.org

TEXAS

M.D. Anderson Cancer Center
University of Texas
1515 Holcombe Boulevard, Box 91
Houston, Texas 77030
(713) 792-2121
www.mdanderson.org

San Antonio Cancer Institute
University of Texas Health Science
Center at San Antonio
7703 Floyd Curl Drive, MSC 7772
San Antonio, Texas 78229-3900
(210) 567-2710
www.saci.uthscsa.edu

UTAH

Huntsman Cancer Institute
University of Utah
2000 Circle of Hope
Salt Lake City, Utah 84112-5550
(801) 585-3281
www.hci.utah.edu

VERMONT

Vermont Cancer Center
University of Vermont
149 Beaumont Ave., HRSF326
Burlington, Vermont 05405
(802) 656-4414
www.vermontcancer.org/

VIRGINIA

Cancer Center
University of Virginia,
Health Sciences Center
Jefferson Park Ave., Room 617E
Charlottesville, Virginia 22908
(434) 243-9926
www.healthsystem.virginia.edu/internet
/cancer

Massey Cancer Center
Virginia Commonwealth University
P.O. Box 980037
Richmond, Virginia 23298-0037
(804) 828-0450
www.vcu.edu/mcc

WASHINGTON

Fred Hutchinson Cancer Research Center
P.O. Box 19024, D1-060
Seattle, Washington 98109-1024
(206) 667-4305
www.fhcrc.org

WISCONSIN

Comprehensive Cancer Center
University of Wisconsin
600 Highland Avenue, Room K4/610
Madison, Wisconsin 53792-0001
(608) 263-8610
www.cancer.wisc.edu